Ambulatory Medicine Case Book

Ambulatory Medicine Case Book

Joyce P. Doyle, M.D.
Associate Professor of Medicine
Program Director, Internal Medicine Residency
Department of Medicine
Division of General Medicine
Emory University School of Medicine
Atlanta, Georgia

Laura J. Martin, M.D.
Assistant Professor in Medicine
Coordinator of Ambulatory Medicine Conferences
Department of Medicine
Division of General Medicine
Emory University School of Medicine
Atlanta, Georgia

LIPPINCOTT WILLIAMS & WILKINS
A **Wolters Kluwer** Company
Philadelphia · Baltimore · New York · London
Buenos Aires · Hong Kong · Sydney · Tokyo

Acquisitions Editor: Richard Winters
Developmental Editor: Stacy L. Baze
Supervising Editor: Steven P. Martin
Production Editor: Janet Domingo
Manufacturing Manager: Colin J. Warnock
Cover Designer: Christine Jenny
Compositor: Compset, Inc.
Printer: RR Donnelley Willard

© 2002 by LIPPINCOTT WILLIAMS & WILKINS
530 Walnut Street
Philadelphia, PA 19106-3780 USA
LWW.com

Printed in the USA

Library of Congress Cataloging-in-Publication Data

Ambulatory medicine case book/ [edited by] Joyce P. Doyle, Laura J. Martin.
    p. ; cm.
  Includes bibliographical references and index.
  ISBN 0-7817-3064-3
  1. Ambulatory medical care—Case studies. I. Doyle, Joyce P. II. Martin, Laura J.
  [DNLM: 1. Ambulatory Care—Case Report. WB 101 A4975 2001]
  RC66 .A434 2001
  616'.09—dc21   2001038874

Care has been taken to confirm the accuracy of the information presented and to describe generally accepted practices. However, the authors, editors, and publisher are not responsible for errors or omissions or for any consequences from application of the information in this book and make no warranty, expressed or implied, with respect to the currency, completeness, or accuracy of the contents of the publication. Application of this information in a particular situation remains the professional responsibility of the practitioner.

The authors, editors, and publisher have exerted every effort to ensure that drug selection and dosage set forth in this text are in accordance with current recommendations and practice at the time of publication. However, in view of ongoing research, changes in government regulations, and the constant flow of information relating to drug therapy and drug reactions, the reader is urged to check the package insert for each drug for any change in indications and dosage and for added warnings and precautions. This is particularly important when the recommended agent is a new or infrequently employed drug.

Some drugs and medical devices presented in this publication have Food and Drug Administration (FDA) clearance for limited use in restricted research settings. It is the responsibility of the health care providers to ascertain the FDA status of each drug or device planned for use in their clinical practice.

10 9 8 7 6 5 4 3 2 1

Contents

Contributing Authors

Holly Avey, M.P.H.
Doctoral Student
Department of Health Promotion and Behavior
University of Georgia
Health Educator,
Office of Health Promotion
Grady Health System
80 Butler Street SE
Atlanta, Georgia 30303

Rebecca Babcock Bair, M.D.
Hospitalist
Monte Sol Medical Group
Santa Fe, New Mexico 87505

Henry Baffoe-Bonnie, M.D.
Instructor in Medicine
Division of General Medicine
Emory University School of Medicine
69 Butler Street
Atlanta, Georgia 30303

Michael Benjamin, M.D.
Hematology-Oncology Fellow
Winship Cancer Institute
Emory University School of Medicine
1639 Pierce Drive
Atlanta, Georgia 30322

Lisa B. Bernstein, M.D.
Assistant Professor in Medicine
Division of General Medicine
Emory University School of Medicine
69 Butler Street
Atlanta, Georgia 30303

Susan Borys, M.D.
Associate, Department of Internal Medicine
Geisinger Medical Group
Northumberland, Pennsylvania 17857

Donald Brady, M.D.
Assistant Professor in Medicine
Division of General Medicine
Emory University School of Medicine
69 Butler Street
Atlanta, Georgia 30303

Yvonne J. Braver, M.D.
Associate Staff
Department of General Internal Medicine
The Cleveland Clinic Foundation
9500 Euclid Avenue
Cleveland, Ohio 44195

Timothy A. Briscoe, Pharm.D., C.D.E
Clinical Pharmacist Specialist
Primary Care Clinics
Grady Health System
69 Butler Street
Atlanta, Georgia 30303

Erica Brownfield, M.D.
Assistant Professor in Medicine
Associate Director, Medical Clerkship
Division of General Medicine
Emory University School of Medicine
69 Butler Street
Atlanta, Georgia 30303

Jada Bussey-Jones, M.D.
Assistant Professor in Medicine
Division of General Medicine
Emory University School of Medicine
69 Butler Street
Atlanta, Georgia 30303

Murtaza Cassoobhoy, M.D.
Assistant Professor in Medicine
Division of General Medicine
Emory University School of Medicine
69 Butler Street
Atlanta, Georgia 30303

Sanjukta Rinku Chatterjee, M.D.
Assistant Professor in Medicine
Emory University School of Medicine
Veterans Affairs Medical Center
Atlanta, Georgia 30322

Michael T. Compton, M.D.
Postdoctoral Fellow in Community Psychiatry/
    Public Health
Department of Psychiatry and Behavioral
Sciences
Resident in Preventive Medicine
Department of Family and Preventive Medicine
Emory University School of Medicine
80 Butler Street
Atlanta, Georgia 30303

Doyt Conn, M.D.
Professor of Medicine
Director, Division of Rheumatology
Emory University School of Medicine
69 Butler Street
Atlanta, Georgia 30303

George Deriso, M.D.
Hospitalist
Crawford Long Hospital
Emory Healthcare
69 Butler Street
Atlanta, Georgia 30303

Gregory Diamonti, M.D.
Fellow
Division of Digestive Diseases
Emory University School of Medicine
69 Butler Street
Atlanta, Georgia 30303

Lorenzo Di Francesco, M.D.
Assistant Professor in Medicine
Division of General Medicine
Emory University School of Medicine
69 Butler Street
Atlanta, Georgia 30303

Joyce P. Doyle, M.D.
Associate Professor of Medicine
Director
Internal Medicine Residency
Division of General Medicine
Emory University School of Medicine
69 Butler Street
Atlanta, Georgia 30303

Daniel D. Dressler, M.D.
Instructor in Medicine
Division of General Medicine
Emory University School of Medicine
69 Butler Street
Atlanta, Georgia 30303

Byard F. Edwards, M.D.
Assistant Professor in Medicine
Division of Nephrology
Emory University School of Medicine
69 Butler Street
Atlanta, Georgia 30303

John Evans, M.D.
Instructor in Internal Medicine
Harvard Medical School
Massachusetts General Hospital
55 Fruit Street
Boston, Massachusetts 02114

Janice G. Farrehi, M.D.
Clinical Assistant Professor in Medicine
Michigan State University College of
    Osteopathic Medicine
4255 Beecher Road
Flint, Michigan, 48532

Jonathan M. Flacker, M.D.
Assistant Professor in Medicine
    and Geriatrics
Division of General Medicine
Emory University School of Medicine
Director, Grady Geriatrics Center
69 Butler Street
Atlanta, Georgia 30303

Andrew C. Furman, M.D.
Assistant Professor in Psychiatry
Department of Psychiatry
Emory University School of Medicine
Assistant Chief of Service
Department of Psychiatry
Grady Memorial Hospital
69 Butler Street
Atlanta, Georgia 30303

Nina S. Garas, M.D.
Assistant Professor in Medicine
Division of General Medicine
Emory University School of Medicine
69 Butler Street
Atlanta, Georgia 30303

Inginia Genao, M.D.
Assistant Professor in Medicine
Division of General Medicine
Emory University School of Medicine
69 Butler Street
Atlanta, Georgia 30303

Yacob Ghebremeskel, M.D.
Instructor in Medicine
Division of General Medicine
Emory University School of Medicine
69 Butler Street
Atlanta, Georgia 30303

Charles R. Harper, M.D.
Assistant Professor in Medicine
Division of General Medicine
Emory University School of Medicine
Director
Urgent Care Center
Grady Memorial Hospital
69 Butler Street
Atlanta, Georgia 30303

Stacy M. Higgins, M.D.
Instructor in Medicine
Division of General Medicine
Emory University School of Medicine
69 Butler Street
Atlanta, Georgia 30303

Nurcan Ilksoy, M.D.
Assistant Professor in Medicine
Division of General Medicine
Emory University School of Medicine
69 Butler Street
Atlanta, Georgia 30303

Terry A. Jacobson, M.D.
Director
Office of Health Promotion and Disease
* Prevention*
Associate Professor of Medicine
Emory University School of Medicine
69 Butler Street
Atlanta, Georgia, 30303

Jennifer Kleinbart, M.D.
Assistant Professor in Medicine
Division of General Medicine
Emory University School of Medicine
Atlanta, Georgia 30303

Michael D. Koplon, M.D.
Internal Medicine Private Practice
6005 Park Avenue
Memphis, Tennessee, 38119

Sunil Kripalani, M.D., M.Sc.
Instructor in Medicine
Division of General Medicine
Emory University School of Medicine
69 Butler Street
Atlanta, Georgia 30303

S. Sam Lim, M.D.
Fellow
Division of Rheumatology
Emory University School of Medicine
69 Butler Street
Atlanta, Georgia 30303

Atul V. Marathe, M.D.
Fellow
Division of Digestive Diseases
Emory University School of Medicine
1639 Pierce Drive
Atlanta, Georgia 30322

Ira C. Marathe, M.D.
Primary Care Service
Veterans Affairs Medical Center
Emory University School of Medicine
1670 Clairmont Road
Decatur, Georgia 30033

Laura J. Martin, M.D.
Assistant Professor in Medicine
Division of General Medicine
Emory University School of Medicine
69 Butler Street
Atlanta, Georgia, 30303

Calvin O. McCall, M.D.
Assistant Professor in Dermatology
Department of Dermatology
Emory University School of Medicine
69 Butler Street
Atlanta, Georgia 30303

Lesley S. Miller, M.D.
Instructor in Medicine
Division of General Medicine
Emory University School of Medicine
69 Butler Street
Atlanta, Georgia 30303

Naveen V. Narahari, M.D.
Instructor in Medicine
Division of General Medicine
Emory University School of Medicine
69 Butler Street
Atlanta, Georgia 30303

Anuradha Paranjape, M.D., M.P.H.
Instructor in Medicine
Division of General Medicine
Emory University School of Medicine
69 Butler Street
Atlanta, Georgia 30303

Foreword

Physicians-in-training traditionally have learned their craft by studying cases. The *Ambulatory Medical Case Book,* edited by Joyce P. Doyle, M.D., and Laura J. Martin, M.D., M.P.H., captures this long tradition and breaks new ground by focusing on the ambulatory setting. The book grew from a comprehensive series of teaching conferences under the direction of Drs. Doyle and Martin presented by the faculty in the Division of General Medicine to the residents in the General Medicine Clinic at Grady Memorial Hospital. The clinical topics chosen for presentation were those encountered in outpatients seen in the clinic. Each case in the book illustrates key clinical points followed by a concise discussion of the issues faced by the clinician caring for such a patient. The book provides up-to-date references to establish an evidence-based approach. The cases developed by the editors and their colleagues have been enormously successful teaching tools.

Today, physicians are faced with the need to see patients in a highly efficient manner while making no compromise in terms of quality of care. We now expect quality to be better than ever in terms of following the most recently developed guidelines, avoiding medical errors, and being cost efficient. Although intensely challenging for physicians, much of this is to the good for both patients and doctors. The *Ambulatory Medical Case Book* is a response to the modern practice of outpatient medicine. The authors of each case provide succinct, useful clinical guides to the care of the majority of clinical problems encountered in an ambulatory practice. Their recommendations are evidence-based and cost efficient. Their approach reflects the clinical experience of practitioners in a large urban hospital teaching clinic that provides more than 50,000 patient-visits per year, and trains more than 150 residents per year. In this fast-paced setting, the approach offered by the editors and their colleagues works to enhance the quality of care by providing a practical and concise approach to clinical problems.

Our residents and medical students found the curriculum of cases invaluable. I believe it will be equally invaluable for residents, students, teachers, and practicing physicians who work in outpatient settings across the country. This book should find a home in the clinic, the conference room, and the medical library, where physicians and physicians-in-training seek answers to the immediate problems of the patients they see. The *Ambulatory Medicine Case Book* meets the demands of today's practice. It provides a perfect compliment to the physician's knowledge and skill that can be applied immediately to enhance quality in modern ambulatory care.

William T. Branch, Jr., M.D.
Carter Smith, Sr. Professor of Medicine
Vice Chairman for Primary Care
Director, Division of General Medicine
Emory University School of Medicine

Preface

In recent years ambulatory medicine has become increasingly emphasized as an integral component of internal medicine and primary care residency training programs in the United States. Indeed, primary care practitioners are expected to be on the forefront in diagnosing and treating a wide range of medical conditions on an outpatient basis. In our effort to teach ambulatory medicine to our residents at Emory University School of Medicine, we have developed a three-year curriculum of ambulatory medicine conferences. These conferences, which are interactive case-based discussions led by faculty members from the Division of General Medicine, have formed the foundation of the *Ambulatory Medicine Case Book.*

The case-based method of teaching and learning has proven to be very popular and highly effective among our colleagues and housestaff. In the *Ambulatory Medicine Case Book,* we have included case-based topics that we believe are at the core of ambulatory internal medicine and primary care. These case discussions are evidence-based and clinically oriented. We hope that you will find these discussions to be both interesting and didactic.

The majority of authors contributing to the *Ambulatory Medicine Case Book* are currently, or were previously, on the staff of Emory University School of Medicine. We thank each author for his or her illustriousness and enthusiasm. We also thank the following people: Dr. William T. Branch, our Division Director, who has provided much vision and support leading to the development of the Ambulatory Medicine Case Book; Mr. Richard Winters, Executive Editor, and Ms. Stacey Baze, Developmental Editor at Lippincott, Williams & Wilkins for their insight and assistance; Dr. Michael Lubin, for his advice and support; Mr. Daryl Todd, Clinical Manager, General Medical Clinics, Grady Memorial Hospital, for his support; and Ms. Joanne Boykin, Ms. Jacci Hurd, Ms. Lavonda Miles, and Ms. Betty Webb for their administrative assistance. Finally, we thank our families for all of their support and love.

Joyce P. Doyle
Laura J. Martin

I
Asthma and Allergy

1
Asthma

Laura J. Martin

1. What are some of the inflammatory mediators involved in asthma?
2. How is asthma diagnosed?
3. How is the severity of asthma classified?
4. What pharmacologic treatments are available to treat adult asthma in the ambulatory setting?
5. What does the Expert Panel recommend on treating adult asthma with pharmacologic therapy?

Discussion

What Are Some of the Inflammatory Mediators Involved in Asthma?

Asthma is an inflammatory condition of the airways characterized by airway hyper-responsiveness and edema, acute bronchoconstriction, and mucous plug formation. As a result of these processes, reversible airway obstruction occurs. The inflammatory response involved in an asthma exacerbation includes mast cells and macrophages, along with eosinophils, T-lymphocytes, neutrophils, basophils, and platelets. These cells produce inflammatory mediators, such as histamine, bradykinin, platelet-activating factor, prostaglandins, and leukotrienes (LTC4, LTD4, and LTE4), that lead to bronchoconstriction.

How Is Asthma Diagnosed?

In 1997, The National Asthma Education and Prevention Program of the National Heart, Lung, and Blood Institute (NHLBI) published the national guidelines "Expert Panel Report 2: Guidelines for the Diagnosis and Management of Asthma." According to these guidelines, the practitioner should diagnose asthma by establishing the following:

1. A history of recurrent symptoms of airway inflammation. Classic symptoms include wheezing, shortness of breath, chest tightness, and/or cough. The symptoms are usually most pronounced at night and in the early morning hours. The absence of symptoms at the time of the visit does not exclude an asthma diagnosis.
2. Reversible airflow obstruction using spirometry. Airflow obstruction is established by a forced expiratory volume in 1 second (FEV_1) of less than 80% pre-

dicted and a FEV_1/ forced vital capacity (FVC) of less than 65% or below the lower limits of normal. Reversibility of obstruction can be shown when the FEV_1 increases by greater than or equal to 12% and by at least 200 mL after using a short-term β agonist such as albuterol. If spirometry does not show significant obstruction and asthma is highly suspected, then additional tests may be considered, including monitoring peak expiratory flow rate (PEFR) twice daily over a 1- to 2-week period to assess diurnal variation and/or bronchoprovocation with methacholine, histamine, or exercise. If these additional tests are negative, then the patient is less likely to have asthma.

3. Exclusion of alternative diagnoses. Chronic obstructive pulmonary disease (COPD), heart disease, and foreign bodies can cause airway obstruction.

How Is the Severity of Asthma Classified?

According to the Expert Panel, asthma severity can be classified based on clinical features before treatment. The four levels or severity, starting with the least severe, are mild intermittent, mild persistent, moderate persistent, and severe persistent (Table 1.1).

What Pharmacologic Therapy Is Available to Treat Adult Asthma in the Ambulatory Setting?

Beta2 agonists are potent bronchodilators that can be administered in a short-acting form such as albuterol or in a long-acting form such as salmeterol. Beta2 agonists

Table 1.1. Classification of Asthma Severity

	Symptoms[a]	Nighttime Symptoms	Lung Function
Step 4. Severe persistent	Continual symptoms Limited physical activity Frequent exacerbations	Frequent	FEV_1 or PEF ≤60% predicted PEF variability >30%
Step 3. Moderate persistent	Daily symptoms Daily use of inhaled short-acting β2 agonist Exacerbations affect activity Exacerbations at least twice a week	More than once a week	FEV_1 or PEF >60%–<80% predicted PEF variability >30%
Step 2. Mild persistent	Symptoms more than twice a week but less than once a day Exacerbations may affect activity	More than twice a month	FEV_1 or PEF ≥80% predicted PEF variability 20% to 30%
Step 1. Mild intermittent	Symptoms no more than twice a week Asymptomatic and normal PEF between exacerbations Exacerbations brief	No more than twice a month	FEV_1 or PEF ≥80% predicted PEF variability <20%

FEV_1, forced expiratory volume in 1 second; PEF, peak expiratory flow.
[a]Only one of the features of severity is needed to place the patient into that category.
Adapted from National Asthma Education and Prevention Program. Expert Panel Report 2: guidelines for diagnosis and management of asthma. Bethesda: National Heart, Lung and Blood Institute, 1997. National Institutes of Health Publication No. 97-4051; with permission.

have been shown to relax bronchial smooth muscle. Short-acting beta2 agonists are used on an as needed basis in patients with all degrees of asthma severity to treat acute symptoms. Long-acting β2 agonists, such as salmeterol, are recommended for use in patients with moderate to severe persistent asthma along with an antiinflammatory medication such as an inhaled steroid.

Inhaled corticosteroids are potent antiinflammatory medications indicated for use in patients with persistent asthma. It is recommended that patients use inhaled steroids with spacers to optimize absorption and prevent oral thrush. Rinsing the mouth with water after use also has been shown to reduce the incidence of oral thrush. High-dose inhaled steroids including fluticasone and budesonide are available for use in patients with moderate to severe persistent asthma. High-dose inhaled steroids have been shown to have significant systemic absorption in some patients, leading to adrenal suppression, cataracts, and bone loss.

Cromolyn and nedocromil inhibit inflammatory cell activation and mediator release. These agents may be used as an initial therapy for long-term control in children. They are also used as prophylactic treatment before exercise and unavoidable exposure to known allergens.

Leukotriene modifiers, including the leukotriene receptor antagonists and 5-lipoxygenase inhibitors, have been shown to decrease symptoms and increase PEFR in some patients with mild persistent asthma. In patients who gain benefit, the dose of inhaled steroids can sometimes be reduced.

Theophylline SR is sometimes used as a second-line agent in patients with persistent asthma. Theophylline is a methylxanthine bronchodilator that has been shown to increase contractility of respiratory muscles in some patients. Theophylline levels should be monitored to prevent toxicity. Numerous medications can affect the clearance of theophylline.

Oral steroids are sometimes needed on a long-term basis to treat patients with severe persistent asthma. In patients with any severity level, sometimes a short-term oral steroid course can be useful in moderate to severe acute exacerbations to reduce airway inflammation.

What Does the Expert Panel Report 2 Recommend on how to Initiate Pharmacologic Therapy?

According to the Expert Panel, a step approach is recommended. The practitioner uses clinical judgment to determine the amount and frequency of medication needed to suppress airway inflammation as indicated by asthma severity (Table 1.2). The preferred approach is to initiate therapy at a higher level at the onset to obtain quick control and then step down therapy to the minimal amount needed to maintain control. Regular follow-up visits at 1- to 6-month intervals are recommended. Education of the patient is essential for achieving optimal asthma control. Patients should be counseled on avoiding precipitating factors that can cause asthma exacerbations. Step-down therapy should be considered once control of symptoms is sustained.

Consider stepping up therapy if control of symptoms is not maintained. Before stepping up therapy, remember to review the patient's compliance, avoidance of precipitating factors, and technique of using inhalers.

Table 1.2. Step Approach for Treating Adult Asthma in the Ambulatory Setting

	Daily Medications
Step 4. Severe persistent	Inhaled steroid (high dose)
	Long-acting inhaled β2 agonist or theophylline SR, or long-acting β2-agonist tablets
Step 3. Moderate persistent	Either inhaled steroid (medium dose) or inhaled steroid (low to medium dose) plus long-acting β2 agonist, or theophylline SR, or long-acting β2-agonist tablets
	If necessary inhaled steroid (medium to high dose) plus long-acting β2 agonist, or theophylline SR, or long-acting β2-agonist tablets
	Short-acting inhaled β2 agonist as needed for acute symptoms
Step 2. Mild persistent	Inhaled steroid (low dose) or cromolyn or nedocromil
	Theophylline SR is an alternative, but not preferred
	Leukotriene modifier may be considered
	Short-acting inhaled β2 agonist as needed for acute symptoms
Step 1. Mild intermittent	No daily medication needed: short-acting inhaled β2 agonist as needed for acute symptoms

Adapted from National Asthma Education and Prevention Program. Expert Panel Report 2: guidelines for the diagnosis and management of asthma. Bethesda: National Heart, Lung and Blood Institute, 1997. National Institutes of Health Publication No. 97-4051; with permission.

Case

A 51-year-old woman presents to your office to evaluate symptoms of wheezing. In recent months, she has experienced three to four episodes per week of wheezing, shortness of breath, and chest tightness. In the past month, she has awakened at night approximately three times with symptoms of wheezing and cough. She feels that her symptoms may be related to ragweed season. There are no symptoms of recent viral illnesses. There is no previous history of respiratory or cardiac disease. Her past medical history is pertinent for allergic rhinitis. She currently smokes about five cigarettes per day. Her medications include fexofenadine and a beclomethasone nasal inhaler.

Physical examination reveals a blood pressure of 124/70 mm Hg; pulse is 76 beats/min; respiratory rate is 16 breaths/min. HEENT (head, eyes, ear, nose, throat) examination is remarkable for edematous nasal mucosa. Lung examination reveals mild diffuse expiratory wheezing. The remainder of the examination is unremarkable.

1. Which findings help substantiate a diagnosis of asthma in this patient?
2. Are there any precipitating factors that may trigger her symptoms?
3. What pharmacologic therapy should be initiated?
4. What type of patient education would be helpful in treating this patient?

Case Discussion

Which Findings Help Substantiate a Diagnosis of Asthma in This Patient?

This patient has classic symptoms of asthma, including episodic wheezing, chest tightness, shortness of breath, and cough. Her history of allergic rhinitis as well as the physical findings of wheezing on lung examination increase the likelihood that she has asthma. To confirm the diagnosis, spirometry is performed, which reveals an initial FEV_1 equal to 74% of predicted, FEV_1/FVC of 60%, and a post-inhaled β2-agonist FEV_1 equal to 95% of predicted. These results are consistent with the presence of reversible airflow obstruction. Chest radiography performed to rule out alternative lung disease is unremarkable.

Are There Any Precipitating Factors that May Trigger Her Symptoms?

She has a history of allergic rhinitis and sensitivity to ragweed, indicating that she may have allergic asthma. Patients with allergic-type asthma have formation of antigen-specific immunoglobulin E antibody to specific aeroallergens. This type of allergic reaction can be divided into an early response, with degranulation of mast cells causing bronchoconstriction within minutes, and a late response several hours later when inflammatory cells and newly produced mediators cause further bronchospasm. Allergen skin testing and/or blood radioallergosorbent tests (RASTs) can be performed in some patients with allergic asthma to detect the presence of IgE antibody to specific antigens. Common aeroallergens include dust mites, pollen, molds, and animal dander. Counseling should be provided to susceptible patients on environmental avoidance of airborne triggers. Besides aeroallergens, other precipitating factors that can sometimes trigger asthma symptoms include viral upper respiratory tract infections, exercise, gastroesophageal reflux, aspirin or nonsteroidal antiinflammatory drugs, sulfiting agents, chemical irritants, and psychosocial factors.

What Pharmacologic Therapy Should Be Initiated?

Her asthma severity can be classified as mild persistent in that she has asthma symptoms greater than two times per week but less than one time per day, with nocturnal symptoms greater than two times per month. In this patient, initial treatment may comprise a medium-dose inhaled steroid with a short-acting β2 agonist as needed for symptoms. If control of symptoms is not obtained, therapy should be stepped up until control is maintained. After symptoms have shown sustained improvement, step down to the minimal therapy needed to maintain control should be initiated.

What Type of Patient Education Would Be Helpful in Treating This Patient?

Patient education is an essential component of asthma care. In accordance with the Expert Panel guidelines, members of the health-care team should discuss with her at each visit the basic facts about asthma, roles of medications, proper use of inhalers, spacers, and self-monitory skills such as the use of a peak flow meter. Counseling on tobacco cessation and avoidance of second-hand smoke is important in all patients with asthma. Yearly influenza vaccination is recommended. A written daily management plan as well as a written action plan for exacerbations enables patients to take an active role in the treatment of asthma.

Suggested Reading

Global Initiative for Asthma Management and Prevention. Bethesda: NHLBI/WHO Workshop Report, U.S. Department of Health and Human Services, 1995 (revised 1998). Publication No. 95-3659.

Lemanske R F, Busse W W. Asthma. *JAMA* 1997;278:1855–1873.

National Asthma Education and Prevention Program. Expert Panel Report 2: guidelines for the diagnosis and management of asthma. Bethesda: National Heart, Lung and Blood Institute. 1997. National Institutes of Health Publication No. 97-4051.

Practice parameters for the diagnosis and treatment of asthma. *J. Allergy Clin Immunol* 1995;96(5 Pt 2): 707–870.

2

Allergic Rhinitis

Sanjukta Rinku Chatterjee

1. What are the causes and clinical presentations of allergic rhinitis?
2. What are the underlying pathophysiologic processes that result in allergic rhinitis?
3. What is the initial workup of allergic rhinitis?
4. What are the mainstay treatments of allergic rhinitis?

Discussion

What Are the Etiologies and Clinical Presentations of Allergic Rhinitis?

Allergic rhinitis has been estimated to affect 20 to 40 million people in the United States. Estimated cost for medications, office visits, and lost productivity at work is $5.6 billion annually. Many studies have shown that allergic rhinitis can have significant effects on quality of life issues such as missed days or poorer performance at work or school, fatigue, cognitive impairment, and headaches. Treatment of allergic rhinitis has been shown in several studies to have beneficial effects on common coexisting medical conditions such as asthma, sinusitis, and otitis media.

Allergic rhinitis can be divided into three main subtypes: seasonal, perennial, and episodic. The most common allergens causing seasonal allergic rhinitis include pollen from trees and grasses, as well as molds and ragweed. The location and timing of pollen dispersion vary widely, but in general it appears that tree pollens are more common in early to mid-spring, grasses in late spring and early summer, and weeds from late summer until early fall. Perennial allergic rhinitis occurring throughout the year is typically triggered by allergens that may exist more chronically, such as dust mites and molds. Episodic allergic rhinitis is usually triggered by specific inciting factors, such as certain animal exposures, which may be intermittent. There also may be in the same individual various combinations of all three subtypes.

The clinical presentation of allergic rhinitis typically includes symptoms such as nasal congestion, rhinorrhea, sneezing, nasal pruritus, and postnasal drip. Ocular pruritus may be experienced as well.

Typical physical examination findings relate to inflammation of the nasal mucosa, including pale, boggy, and swollen nasal mucosa with pale pink or bluish gray discoloration and clear rhinorrhea. Nasal polyps may be seen, as may scleral injection and clear discharge. Dark discolorations beneath the eyes, known as "allergic shiners," may exist, as may a transverse crease across the nasal bridge caused by repetitive upward rubbing of the irritated nose (the "allergic salute").

What Are the Underlying Pathophysiologic Processes that Result in Allergic Rhinitis?

The underlying pathophysiology of allergic rhinitis begins after initial exposure to an allergen leads to the production of allergen-specific IgE-producing lymphocytes. The IgE produced binds to receptors on the surface of mast cells and basophils, causing sensitization of the nasal mucosa.

Reexposure to the allergen causes crosslinking of the receptors and bound IgE on the cells' surfaces, which leads to degranulation of the cells with release of inflammatory mediators such as histamine, prostaglandins, and leukotrienes. Histamine affects multiple end-organ targets on the nasal mucosa, such as sensory nerve endings, glandular tissue, and blood vessels, leading to the classic signs and symptoms of allergic rhinitis.

There is an early or immediate phase reaction associated with mainly mast cells and subsequent mediator release, particularly involving histamine. Symptoms that predominate include pruritus and sneezing, for which antihistamines are quite effective. This reaction occurs within minutes of allergen exposure. The late phase reaction, occurring typically within 4 to 8 hours of allergen exposure, is associated mainly with basophils, eosinophils, and lymphocytes, with subsequent mediator release. Nasal congestion is prominent, for which steroid sprays can be very useful.

What Is the Initial Workup of Allergic Rhinitis?

Initial workup begins with a thorough history and physical examination. The history should focus on determining the specific allergens involved. Information should be gathered as to the pattern of symptoms such as seasonal versus year-round, daily versus episodic, and whether symptoms are worse indoors versus outdoors. Specific triggers may be identified sometimes, such as certain animals. Duration and frequency of symptoms, as well as a thorough environmental history, are important factors in the initial workup of allergic rhinitis. Response to any treatments and allergen avoidance, if tried, should be documented as well.

Once suspected allergens are identified, skin testing is the next appropriate step. Initially, skin-prick testing is performed; if needed, intradermal testing can be performed as well. Skin-prick testing is the most commonly used test to target specific allergens responsible for the symptoms of allergic rhinitis. In certain patients, such as those with extensive dermatitis or dermatographism, *in vitro* testing can be conducted using a test known as the RAST (or radioallergosorbent) test. The testing of total immunoglobulin E (IgE) levels, peripheral eosinophilia, and nasal smears have not proven to be useful and are not routinely indicated. Positive reactions to specific allergens on skin-prick testing must be correlated with the patient's history and symptoms to determine their clinical significance.

What Are the Mainstay Treatments of Allergic Rhinitis?

Treatment of allergic rhinitis begins first and foremost with allergen avoidance. Reducing exposure to pollen, for instance, may involve staying indoors as much as possible and keeping doors and windows closed. The use of specific types of air filters may offer some relief as well. Decreasing exposure to dust mites involves measures such as avoiding carpeting and encasing bedding, such as mattresses, box springs, and pillows, in allergen-proof covers. Avoiding animals that are known triggers is recommended.

Oral antihistamines block the histamine-mediated effects on the nasal mucosa. They effectively improve symptoms of rhinorrhea, sneezing, and pruritus, but are less effective in treating nasal congestion. Typical first-generation oral antihistamines, such as chlorpheniramine and diphenhydramine, have been very effective, but can cause sedation leading to possible performance impairment.

Newer, second-generation antihistamines have now become preferable due to fewer side effects associated with sedation. Second-generation antihistamines include medications such as cetirizine, fexofenadine, and loratadine. Two second-generation antihistamines, terfenadine and astemizole, were withdrawn from the U.S. market when they were found to cause prolongation of the QT interval, which could lead to ventricular arrhythmias such as torsades de pointes. This risk was highest when they were used in combination with medications such as macrolide antibiotics and azole antifungal agents.

Intranasal antihistamines, such as azelastine, may help reduce rhinorrhea, sneezing, and pruritus.

Oral decongestants, such as pseudoephedrine can reduce nasal congestion. However, they can be associated with side effects such as insomnia and nervousness. Topical nasal preparations, such as oxymetazoline and phenylephrine, can be used as well. Prolonged use of these nasal sprays for more than 3 to 5 days can be associated with rebound nasal congestion, known as rhinitis medicamentosa, and the duration of use should be limited.

Many combination antihistamine–decongestant preparations are available that can help relieve nasal congestion in addition to pruritus, rhinorrhea, and sneezing.

It is now felt by many that perhaps the most effective medications for the treatment of allergic rhinitis are the nasal corticosteroids. They possess antiinflammatory activity through several mechanisms, one of which is believed to be the inhibition of cytokine production and secretion. They are effective against all the major symptoms of allergic rhinitis, including sneezing, pruritus, rhinorrhea, and congestion. Nasal corticosteroids available include beclomethasone, budesonide, flunisolide, fluticasone, mometasone, and triamcinolone.

There are no significant systemic side effects of steroid nasal sprays in adults, and local side effects are usually minimal, including nasal irritation, burning, and slight bleeding, with rare cases of septal perforation. Patients should be warned that for some preparations, it might take several days to see the full benefit of treatment.

Cromolyn sodium nasal spray inhibits degranulation of mast cells and thus prevents the release of mediators responsible for the allergic reaction. It has no antihistaminic effects, so it is most useful for pretreatment of the allergic reaction and should be taken prior to known exposures.

Anticholinergic nasal sprays, such as ipratropium bromide, are most effective in reduction of rhinorrhea, with very little effect on the other symptoms of allergic rhinitis.

The newest class of treatment is leukotriene receptor antagonists, which are thought to afford mainly antiinflammatory effects. There are a limited number of studies addressing the effectiveness of this class of medication, and the evidence is conflicting. There are some data to indicate a potential benefit, especially when used in combination with an antihistamine, but further studies are needed. Currently available oral leukotriene receptor antagonists include zafirlukast and montelukast.

Finally, studies have shown that allergen immunotherapy can be an effective treatment modality for many patients. Allergen immunotherapy is generally considered in situations such as when the patient has failed multiple medical therapies, or there have been significant side effects of medications so that the patient is not able to tolerate them. Immunotherapy is given by a series of injections of gradually increasing amounts of diluted, specific allergens over a period of years, with the goal of reducing clinical symptoms. There are several theories about the mechanism by which immunotherapy works, but the one most commonly cited involves the production of IgG blocking antibodies, which block IgE binding. Benefits of immunotherapy may be seen within a few months of initiation of treatment. Treatment is usually continued for 3 to 5 years (and should be discontinued if there are no improvements in 1 year). The effects of immunotherapy in patients who have a good response may last anywhere from a few years to indefinitely.

Risks of immunotherapy vary from minor local irritation at the injection site, to mild systemic reactions, and rarely anaphylaxis.

In the majority of patients, a combination of medical therapies, such as an antihistamine and nasal steroid spray, can be quite effective, and certainly treatment should be tailored for each individual patient.

Case

A 25-year-old woman comes to your office complaining of persistent nasal congestion and rhinorrhea for the past few months. She notes that in the past 1 to 2 weeks her symptoms seem to have worsened, especially with regard to pruritus and sneezing. On further questioning, she says she moved from New York to Atlanta over 1 year ago to enjoy the warm weather. She is an avid biker and has been spending more time outdoors recently, as spring has started. She does say that during last spring season, which began just after she arrived here, she did not experience these symptoms. Since she moved, she has bought an old house, which she is currently renovating. She lives with her pet cat, her long-time companion.

She says she has tried over-the-counter medications and nasal sprays, but they do not seem to help. On examination, she appears to have some mild rhinorrhea and scleral injection. There is a slightly dark discoloration under her eyes. On nasal examination, the mucosa appears to be pale, boggy, and swollen with clear mucous strands. No polyps are clearly visualized. Her tympanic membranes are normal, with no bulging and with good light reflex. There is no sinus tenderness and no lymphadenopathy, and her lungs are clear.

1. What key elements in her history lead to the diagnosis?
2. What workup should be initiated?
3. What is an optimal treatment strategy?

Case Discussion

What Key Elements in Her History Lead to the Diagnosis?

The first significant part of her history involves her move from one part of the country to another, where she is exposed to new allergens. Note that she did not develop symptoms until after her move, when they manifested themselves during the second spring season. Thus, there was time to be sensitized to these new allergens, so that on reexposure, an allergic reaction developed. The exacerbation of her symptoms during the spring season, when she spent time outdoors, points to seasonal allergic rhinitis with triggers such as various grass and tree pollens.

In addition, moving into an old house, a new environment for her, could have caused sensitization and subsequent allergic reactions to allergens such as dust mites and mold spores. This would lead to symptoms more consistent with perennial rhinitis. Animals also can be common triggers of allergic rhinitis, but by history, she has been exposed to this cat for years without problems, and so this is not likely to be a factor. Given the persistent pattern of symptoms as well as the history of exacerbation of her symptoms in spring and with outdoor activities, it appears she has perennial rhinitis, coexisting with seasonal rhinitis. Possible allergens contributing to her symptoms include tree and grass pollens, as well as dust mites and molds.

What Workup Should Be Initiated?

Once a thorough history and physical examination are complete, the next step is to try to identify specific allergens responsible for her symptoms. The most common and cost effective way to do this is skin testing using standardized extracts of suspected allergens. Any positive test she may have must be correlated with her history to determine the clinical significance of that particular allergen. Consider testing for grass and tree pollens, as well as house dust mites and molds.

What Is an Optimal Treatment Strategy?

The first and foremost step in her treatment plan is to practice allergen avoidance as much as possible. This includes staying indoors when possible during pollen season. Measures to minimize exposure to house dust mites include using special allergen-proof encasing for bedding, washing bed linens in hot water, and changing to hardwood floors in the house instead of carpeting. In some instances, specialized air filters may offer some relief.

She has already tried over-the-counter medications, which probably consisted of decongestants and perhaps first-generation antihistamines. Further questioning about over-the-counter medications tried should include the possible use of decongestant nasal sprays. If these were used for prolonged periods, she may have developed a component of rebound nasal congestion, also known as rhinitis medicamentosa.

If it appears that both over-the-counter antihistamines and decongestants were tried and failed, the next step is to try a second-generation, nonsedating antihistamine. If this is not effective alone, a combination antihistamine and decongestant might be tried. If symptoms persist, a nasal steroid spray should be tried either alone or in combination with the antihistamine. Nasal steroid sprays alone can be quite effective in many people and in many cases this is tried as first line therapy. She should be instructed that it may take a few days for the spray to be fully effective and that it should be taken on a regular basis.

Should she complain of excessive rhinorrhea, an anticholinergic nasal spray may be tried. Cromolyn sodium nasal spray may be used prophylactically to prevent symptom exacerbation before going outdoors, when known exposure to pollen will occur.

If multiple medications and their combinations have been tried unsuccessfully, or if she is unable to tolerate their side effects, immunotherapy can be considered as a possible treatment for her allergic rhinitis.

Suggested Reading

Busse W, Togias A, et al. Advances in allergic diseases: an update for the new millennium. *J Allergy Clin Immunol* 2000;105(part 2; suppl):593–627.

Dykewicz MS, Fineman S, et al., eds. Diagnosis and management of rhinitis: parameter documents of the joint task force on practice parameters in allergy, asthma, and immunology. *Annal Allergy Asthma Immunol* 1998;81:463–518.

Gentile D A, Friday G A, Skoner D. Management of allergic rhinitis: antihistamines and decongestants. *Immunol Allergy Clin North Am* 2000;20:355–368.

Spector S, White M, et al. Pathophysiology and pharmacotherapy of allergic rhinitis. *J Allergy Clin Immunol* 1999:103(part 2; suppl):377–404.

Van Cauwenberge P, Bachert C, et al. Consensus statement on the treatment of allergic rhinitis. European Academy of Allergy and Clinical Immunology. *Allergy* 2000;55:116–134.

Virant F. Allergic rhinitis. *Immunol Allergy Clin North Am* 2000;20:265–282.

II

Cardiovascular

3

Evaluation and Management of Atrial Fibrillation

Sunil Kripalani

1. How common is atrial fibrillation (AF)?
2. What conditions and medications are associated with AF?
3. What are the physiologic effects of AF on the cardiovascular system?
4. What issues should you address in patients who have AF?
5. Which diagnostic tests are appropriate?

Discussion

How Common Is Atrial Fibrillation (AF)?

Atrial fibrillation affects approximately 2.2 million people in the United States. Its prevalence increases with age, with a median age of 75 years at the time of diagnosis. Chronic AF rarely affects persons under 60 years of age, while it is found in approximately 9% of those 80 to 89 years of age. In outpatient geriatric clinics, the prevalence of AF reaches nearly 10%. Chronic AF should be distinguished from acute or paroxysmal AF, which is less common and is usually associated with a reversible condition.

Nearly half of patients with AF are asymptomatic at presentation. Another 32% experience palpitations, 10% have congestive heart failure, 2% have syncope, and 2% have a cerebrovascular event. After controlling for other factors, persons with AF appear to have 1.5 times the mortality of those without AF. Patients under age 60 with no structural heart disease (lone atrial fibrillation) have a much better prognosis.

What Conditions and Medications Are Associated with Atrial Fibrillation?

In developed countries, hypertensive heart disease is the most common illness associated with chronic AF. In underdeveloped areas, many cases of AF result from rheumatic heart disease, particularly in the presence of mitral stenosis or regurgitation. Other structural findings, which may lead to AF, are increased left atrial size, left ventricular hypertrophy, atrial septal defect, hypertrophic cardiomyopathy, and dilated cardiomyopathy. Congestive heart failure (CHF), chronic obstructive pulmonary disease (COPD), and diabetes are also associated with AF, but interestingly, coronary heart disease is not.

Acute AF may occur after binge drinking (the so-called holiday heart) or during alcohol withdrawal. Acute AF is also associated with severe infection, thyrotoxicosis, pulmonary embolism, pericarditis, myocarditis, myocardial infarction, preexcitation syndromes, pheochromocytoma, severe anemia, hypoxemia, and the postoperative period (especially following cardiac surgery). Finally, drugs and toxins which increase the sympathetic tone or decrease vagal tone may lead to AF. The most common culprits are alcohol, theophylline, aminophylline, β agonists, caffeine, and levothyroxine.

What Are the Physiologic Effects of Atrial Fibrillation on the Cardiovascular System?

Because atrial contraction is responsible for approximately 25% of ventricular filling, patients with AF may experience a significant reduction in their ventricular end-diastolic volume (Fig. 3.1). In an otherwise healthy heart, compensatory mechanisms help preserve cardiac output. However, when coexisting cardiac disease affects ventricular or valvular mechanics, the process of filling and emptying the left ventricle may become even less efficient, decreasing stroke volume and cardiac output by 20% to 25%. In other patients, bradycardia results in poor cardiac output. (Recall that stroke volume = left ventricular end-diastolic volume − end-systolic volume, and that cardiac output = forward stroke volume × heart rate.)

Ventricular filling may be significantly impaired when AF occurs with either mitral stenosis, or diastolic dysfunction. Filling also decreases with tachycardia, which shortens the amount of time spent in diastole. On the other hand, ventricular emptying is diminished by the presence of systolic dysfunction or aortic stenosis. Severe mitral regurgitation is another factor that reduces forward stroke volume, because a substantial amount of blood returns to the left atrium rather than exiting through the aortic outflow.

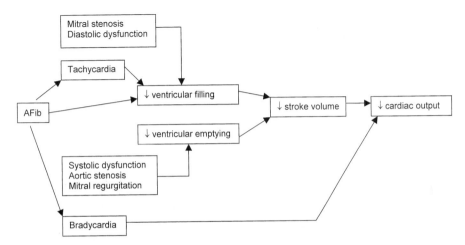

Figure 3.1. Hemodynamic effects of atrial fibrillation and associated conditions.

Occasionally, patients with AF experience low cardiac output as a result of profound bradycardia. This may result from excessive use of rate-controlling medications, or from tachycardia–bradycardia syndromes, which are more common in the elderly.

What Issues Should You Address in Patients Who Have Atrial Fibrillation?

When you see a patient with AF, you should first determine if he or she is hemodynamically stable. Other key questions are the heart rate and duration of AF. The management of AF focuses on restoration of sinus rhythm (when appropriate), maintenance of sinus rhythm, rate control, and anticoagulation (the latter is discussed in detail in another chapter).

Cardioversion is performed emergently to restore sinus rhythm when patients are hemodynamically unstable, or urgently when they are otherwise unable to tolerate AF. Conversion to sinus rhythm is most likely to succeed when the duration of AF is less than 1 year, left atrial size is less than 45 mm, and precipitating causes have been corrected. On the other hand, it is often unsuccessful when the patient has moderate or severe cardiomegaly, mitral valve disease, CHF, COPD, recurrent AF, or an inability to tolerate antiarrhythmic drugs. Even when patients with chronic AF are successfully cardioverted and placed on antiarrhythmic maintenance therapy, 35% to 60% experience a recurrence within 1 to 2 years.

The goal of rate control is to reduce the resting pulse to less than 90 beats/min and allow the active patient to perform mild or moderate exercise with no significant symptoms. Although digoxin is more commonly prescribed, the American Heart Association recommends that β blockers and nondihydropyridine calcium channel blockers (diltiazem or verapamil) be used first line. In choosing between these medications, consider the patient's activity level, blood pressure, ejection fraction, and other illnesses (Table 3.1). In hypertensive patients with AF, β blockers and nondihydropyridine calcium channel blockers can treat both the heart rate

Table 3.1. Advantages and Disadvantages of Rate-Controlling Agents

Medication	Advantages	Disadvantages
Digoxin	Good rate control at rest Indicated for CHF with low EF Does not affect blood pressure	Potential for toxicity Takes 3 h to reduce heart rate in acute setting Less effective in paroxysmal AF Ineffective during exercise
β blocker	Good rate control during exercise Antihypertensive Antianginal Helps prevent other arrhythmias Improves outcome post-MI Metoprolol and carvedilol improve outcome in stable CHF	Bronchospasm Rebound hypertension and tachycardia when abruptly discontinued Potential for hypotension
Diltiazem, verapamil	Good rate control during exercise and at rest Antihypertensive Antianginal	Peripheral edema Potential for hypotension

CHF, congestive heart failure; EF, ejection fraction; AF, atrial fibrillation; MI, myocardial infarction.

and blood pressure. Conversely, in patients with a low left ventricular ejection fraction, these agents should be used very cautiously, and digoxin becomes the therapy of choice. Patients with severe COPD or asthma may also have difficulty tolerating β blockers. In general, β blockers are more effective during exercise than at rest, and the opposite is true of digoxin. Nondihydropyridine calcium channel blockers are useful in both situations. Although β blockers and calcium channel blockers generally should not be used together, either one can be combined with digoxin for added efficacy. None of these medications help convert AF to sinus rhythm.

Which Diagnostic Tests Are Appropriate?

When a patient presents with an irregular pulse, it is appropriate to order an electrocardiogram (ECG) with rhythm strip. Be aware that AF is often confused with artifact, sinus arrhythmia, wandering atrial pacemaker, multifocal atrial tachycardia, and sinus tachycardia with frequent premature atrial depolarizations. Once the diagnosis of AF is made, an echocardiogram will provide valuable information about chamber size, ejection fraction, and valvular function.

In the patient with new-onset AF, many physicians obtain posteroanterior (PA) and lateral radiographs, looking for evidence of chronic pulmonary disease or occult pneumonia in the elderly. Because hypoxia of any etiology can cause AF, pulse oximetry is also appropriate. The level of thyroid-stimulating hormone (TSH) should be measured, whether or not the patient shows other overt manifestations of thyrotoxicosis. Even subclinical hyperthyroidism (TSH <0.5 mU/L with normal thyroid hormone levels) significantly increases the risk of AF. Finally, it is unnecessary to check cardiac enzymes in patients with new-onset AF who show no other signs of an ischemic event.

Case

Mr. K is a 67-year-old retiree who presents with palpitations that began 8 hours ago. He has noticed the problem periodically for years, usually when playing golf, but did not seek medical care because it never bothered him much. This time, however, the palpitations began at rest and have continued for the past 8 hours. There is no associated shortness of breath or chest pain. He plays golf two or three times a week, and enjoys walking the course for exercise, rather than riding a cart. He takes no medications and is unaware of any significant illnesses. He appears comfortable. Blood pressure is 155/90 mm Hg, heart rate is 104 beats/min (irregular), and respiratory rate is 12 breaths/min. Careful examination of the jugular pulsations reveals only v waves. The apical impulse is hyperdynamic but not displaced. S_1 and S_2 are present, with no murmurs or gallops. The radial pulse is weak, but the brachial pulsation is clearly irregular, with varying amplitude. Lungs are clear to auscultation. The rest of the examination is unremarkable. An ECG with rhythm strip confirms atrial fibrillation, with a heart rate of 110 beats/min.

1. What are some physical findings in AF? Because Mr. K likely has hypertensive heart disease, should we expect to find an S_4 gallop?
2. Does Mr. K need to be admitted to the hospital?
3. How should we treat his AF?

Case Discussion

What Are Some Physical Findings in AF? Since Mr. K Likely Has Hypertensive Heart Disease, Should We Expect to Find an S₄ Gallop?

Loss of the atrial contraction eliminates the *a* wave, which signifies atrial contraction, from jugular venous pulsations. It also excludes the possibility of an S_4 gallop, a sound that represents atrial contraction against a stiff ventricle. The irregular heart rate of AF produces corresponding variability in the peripheral pulse rate. Interestingly, though, because there is beat-to-beat variability in length of diastole and the amount of ventricular filling, the stroke volume varies continually. This results in varying pulse amplitudes and generally weak peripheral pulses.

Does Mr. K Need to Be Admitted to the Hospital?

No. Atrial fibrillation leads to approximately 300,000 hospitalizations annually. Although patients with new-onset AF are frequently admitted to rule out myocardial infarction, this practice is unnecessary because AF is rarely a manifestation of an otherwise asymptomatic ischemic event. Hospitalization should generally be reserved for those with cardiovascular decompensation (such as hypotension or congestive heart failure), significant underlying heart disease with a risk for impending complications, ECG evidence of ischemia or other associated arrhythmia, very rapid heart rate, or an acute neurologic event. Hospitalization also may be necessary for the treatment of another illness that precipitated AF, such as severe infection, pulmonary embolism, or thyroid storm. Also consider hospitalizing the elderly and other patients who are unable to tolerate outpatient therapy.

How Should We Treat His Atrial Fibrillation?

It is unknown how long Mr. K has had AF. His palpitations on the golf course may represent paroxysms of AF, or he may have chronic asymptomatic AF with episodes of rapid ventricular response during exercise. In either case, cardioversion alone is unlikely to maintain sinus rhythm. Because Mr. K is able to tolerate his condition quite well, apart from occasional palpitations, the decision is made not to attempt cardioversion at this time. Instead, he is given a Holter monitor to record the heart rate and rhythm over 24 hours. If the diagnosis of chronic AF is made, a trial of cardioversion and antiarrhythmic therapy would be reasonable, but there is no consensus regarding whether or not this is beneficial in stable patients with chronic AF.

At present, a β blocker is the drug of choice for management of his AF and hypertension. It will help reduce his heart rate at rest and is highly effective at preventing inappropriate tachycardia during mild or moderate exercise. He is started on atenolol 25 mg/day, with advancement to 100 mg.

Further evaluation includes a TSH and blood count, which are normal. An echocardiogram shows evidence of left ventricular hypertrophy, but no valvular disease or chamber enlargement. His risk for embolic stroke is elevated due to hypertension, and he is started on warfarin 5 mg daily, with a target international normalized ratio (INR) of 2 to 3.

Suggested Reading

Golzari H, Cebul R D, Bahler R C. Atrial fibrillation: restoration and maintenance of sinus rhythm and indications for anticoagulant therapy. *Ann Intern Med* 1996;125:311–323.

Jung F, DiMarco J P. Treatment strategies for atrial fibrillation. *Am J Med* 1998;104:272–286.

Prystowsky E N, Benson W Jr, Fuster V, et al. Management of patients with atrial fibrillation. A statement for healthcare professionals from the subcommittee on electrocardiography and electrophysiology, American Heart Association. *Circulation* 1996;93:1262–1277.

Segal J B, McNamara R L, Miller M R, et al. The evidence regarding the drugs used for ventricular rate control. *J Fam Practice* 2000;49:47–59.

4

Stroke Prevention in Chronic Atrial Fibrillation

Jennifer Kleinbart

1. What are the risk factors for thromboembolism in patients with chronic atrial fibrillation?
2. What is the benefit of anticoagulation with warfarin versus aspirin for prevention of thromboembolism in patients with nonvalvular atrial fibrillation?
3. What is the optimal target international normalized ratio?

Discussion

What Are the Risk Factors for Thromboembolism in Patients with Chronic Atrial Fibrillation?

The most important risk factor for thromboembolism is valvular or rheumatic atrial fibrillation (AF), which carries a yearly risk of thromboembolism of over 5%. These patients should routinely receive anticoagulation with warfarin. The risk of thromboembolism also increases with increasing age (Table 4.1).

The Stroke Prevention in Atrial Fibrillation study compared warfarin versus aspirin versus placebo for the prevention of thromboembolism in patients with chronic nonvalvular AF. Data from the trial's 568 patients who received placebo identified the following clinical features as risk factors for thromboembolism: (a) congestive heart failure within the preceding 3 months (relative risk of 2.6), (b) history of hypertension (relative risk of 2.2), and (c) previous thromboembolism (relative risk of 2.1). The annual rate of thromboembolism increases with the number of these risk factors as well as the presence of diabetes mellitus and increasing age (Table 4.2).

Echocardiographic findings that independently predict thromboembolism are moderate to severe left ventricular dysfunction and left atrial enlargement (>2.5 cm/m^2). The rate of thromboembolism in patients with both of these abnormalities is approximately 20% per year. Therefore, echocardiography adds important information for accurate assessment of thromboembolic risk, especially in those classified as low risk by clinical variables. Patients with neither clinical nor echocardiographic risks have a yearly rate of thromboembolism of only 1%.

Table 4.1.

Age	Yearly Risk of Thromboembolism
50–59	1.3%
60–69	2.2%
70–79	4.2%
80–89	5%–10%

What Are the Benefits and Risks of Anticoagulation with Warfarin or Aspirin for Prevention of Thromboembolism in Nonvalvular Atrial Fibrillation?

Primary prevention refers to prevention of thromboembolism in patients with no prior thromboembolic events, whereas secondary prevention refers to prevention of recurrent events in those who have a history of thromboembolism. Because patients who have experienced a thromboembolic event are at higher risk for recurrent events, the benefit of treatment is greater in these patients.

Warfarin

Patients with nonvalvular atrial fibrillation (NVAF) treated with warfarin have a significant reduction in thromboembolism of approximately 60%, as well as reduced mortality. Thirty-seven patients with NVAF and no history of thromboembolism need to be treated with warfarin for 1 year to prevent one stroke (primary prevention). For patients with a history of thromboembolism, a 68% reduction in stroke is seen among patients receiving warfarin and only 12 patients need to be treated with warfarin for 1 year to prevent one stroke. The risk of intracranial hemorrhage in patients receiving warfarin is approximately 0.3% per year compared with 0.1% per year with placebo.

Aspirin

Patients with NVAF treated with aspirin at doses of 50 to 1,300 mg/day have approximately 22% fewer strokes compared with those receiving placebo. Again, more benefit results from treatment of patients with a history of stroke: 67 patients need to be treated with aspirin for 1 year for primary prevention of one stroke and

Table 4.2.

No. of Clinical Risk Factors	Yearly Rate of Thromboembolism
0 and <60 years old	0–0.5%
0 and nondiabetic	1.4%
0	2.5%
1	7.2%
2–3	17.6%

40 for secondary stroke prevention. Patients receiving aspirin do not have lower mortality rates than those who take warfarin.

Warfarin Compared with Aspirin

A meta-analysis of trials comparing warfarin [international normalized ratio (INR) 2.0–4.0] to aspirin (75–325 mg/day) shows a 40% to 50% reduction in ischemic stroke in patients treated with warfarin. For primary prevention, 167 patients need to be treated with warfarin instead of aspirin for 1 year to prevent one stroke, whereas for secondary prevention of stroke, only 14 patients need to be treated for 1 year to prevent one stroke. Both hemorrhagic strokes and major extracranial hemorrhage occur twice as often with warfarin than aspirin, but with an absolute risk increase of only 0.2%, meaning that one extra bleed per year occurs for every 500 patients treated. Treatment of 1,000 patients with NVAF for 1 year with warfarin instead of aspirin would prevent 6 to 36 strokes, depending on the patient's risk for stroke, and cause two major extracranial bleeds.

The combination of fixed low-dose warfarin and aspirin is not as effective as adjusted-dose warfarin alone in prevention of thromboembolism and does not reduce major hemorrhage.

What Is the Optimal Target International Normalized Ratio?

The INR should be between 2.0 and 3.5. The risk of thromboembolism increases below an INR of 2.0, whereas the risk of bleeding increases over an INR of 4.0 to 5.0. Patients at higher risk for thromboembolism, especially those with prior thromboembolism, should be maintained at the higher end of this range. However, in elderly patients, a target INR of 2.0 to 2.5 may be safer because these patients are at higher risk for major bleeding events.

Case

A 60-year-old man with a history of AF diagnosed 3 years ago presents for a routine clinic visit. He has no dyspnea or other complaints and has had no complications related to AF. His only medication is aspirin 325 mg/day. When initially diagnosed with AF 3 years ago, his evaluation included an echocardiogram that showed normal valves and normal left ventricular function, normal electrolytes, and normal thyroid function testing. On examination today, his blood pressure is 160/95 mm Hg and his pulse 85 beats/min and irregular. Past blood pressures ranged from 142/88 mm Hg to 152/90 mm Hg. Cardiac examination shows an irregularly irregular rhythm, but is otherwise unremarkable.

1. What is your patient's risk for thromboembolism?
2. Given his risk for thromboembolism, how has the optimal management for stroke prevention in this patient changed?
3. How should treatment be initiated?

Case Discussion

What Is Your Patient's Risk for Thromboembolism?

Based on age (<60 years) and absence of clinical and echocardiographic risk factors, this patient's risk for thromboembolism at his last visit was <0.5% per year. Based on age alone, his risk for thromboembolism at age 60 would be approximately 2% per year. Upon reviewing the patient's record, he meets the diagnostic criteria for hypertension. Considering clinical risk factors, the diagnosis of hypertension increases his yearly rate of thromboembolism to 7%.

Given His Risk for Thromboembolism, How Has the Optimal Management for Stroke Prevention in This Patient Changed?

Previously, with this patient's low risk for thromboembolism, treatment with aspirin was appropriate. If at age 60 he did not have hypertension or other risks for thromboembolism, continued treatment with aspirin would still be reasonable. However, now with his increased risk for thromboembolism, warfarin will provide more effective stroke prevention than aspirin. With aspirin, his risk for thromboembolism would be lowered to approximately 5.6% per year, whereas warfarin would lower his risk to approximately 2.8% per year. Risks of bleeding from warfarin should be addressed prior to initiating treatment, including recent gastrointestinal bleeding, alcohol use, risk of falling, and seizure disorder.

How Should Treatment Be Initiated?

Warfarin treatment may be initiated on an outpatient basis. A loading dose of 5 mg for the first 2 days, followed by dose titration based on the INR, is associated with a lower likelihood of both excess anticoagulation and development of a hypercoagulable state. The target INR should be 2.0 to 3.5; when steady state has been reached, monitoring may be performed every 2 to 4 weeks. Patients should be educated about diet and drug interactions.

Suggested Reading

Atrial Fibrillation Investigators. Echocardiographic predictors of stroke in patients with atrial fibrillation. *Arch Intern Med* 1998;158:1316–1320.

Eskowitz M D, Levine J A. Preventing stroke in patients with atrial fibrillation. *JAMA* 1999;281:1830–1835.

Hart R G, Benavente O, McBride R, et al. Antithrombotic therapy to prevent stroke in patients with atrial fibrillation: a meta-analysis. *Ann Intern Med* 1999;131:492–501.

The Stroke Prevention in Atrial Fibrillation Investigators. Predictors of thromboembolism in atrial fibrillation: I. Clinical features of patients at risk. *Ann Intern Med* 1992;116:1–5.

The Stroke Prevention in Atrial Fibrillation Investigators. Stroke prevention in atrial fibrillation study. Final results. *Circulation* 1991;84:527–539.

5
Congestive Heart Failure

Nurcan Ilksoy

1. What are the most common causes of left ventricular systolic dysfunction?
2. How do you evaluate a patient with suspected heart failure? What diagnostic studies would you obtain to establish the diagnosis of heart failure?
3. In the patient with systolic dysfunction, what are precipitating factors for heart failure?
4. What is your risk reduction strategy to prevent the progression of heart failure?
5. What nonpharmacologic measures should be recommended to heart failure patients?
6. How do you initiate drug therapy for systolic dysfunction? Describe the treatment goals.

Discussion

What Are the Most Common Causes of Left Ventricular Systolic Dysfunction?

Congestive heart failure (CHF) is a complex syndrome, which may result from a variety of conditions affecting the myocardium, pericardium, great vessels, and valves.

The syndrome of heart failure may be predominantly left sided, right sided, or biventricular. The majority of patients with heart failure present with signs and symptoms of systolic dysfunction (left ventricular ejection fraction <40%). The most common causes of systolic dysfunction are coronary artery disease and hypertension. Coronary artery disease accounts for about two thirds of patients with systolic heart failure. Nonischemic causes, such as thyroid abnormalities, toxins (alcohol, cocaine), myocarditis, and valvular disorders, also can result in left ventricular systolic dysfunction.

How Do You Evaluate a Patient with Suspected Heart Failure? What Diagnostic Studies Would You Obtain to Establish the Diagnosis of Heart Failure?

Every patient who presents with signs or symptoms of heart failure should undergo a thorough evaluation to determine the underlying etiology of cardiac abnormality and to identify precipitating factors. The initial workup should start with a complete history and physical examination. Dyspnea on exertion, paroxysmal nocturnal dyspnea, and orthopnea are the most specific symptoms of heart failure, but it is important to remember that some patients can present with nonspecific symptoms such as fatigue, decreased appetite, and edema. A third heart sound, a displaced apical impulse, and a mitral regurgitation murmur are the most specific physical findings of left ventricular systolic dysfunction. Even though the history and physical examination provide important clues to possible etiologies of cardiac dysfunction, echocardiography or radionuclide ventriculography should be part of the evaluation. Echocardiography is the most useful diagnostic test in differentiating systolic dysfunction from diastolic dysfunction. In addition, echocardiography allows the clinician to evaluate ventricular chamber size, valvular function, and regional wall motion.

Recently, B-type natriuretic peptide (BNP) levels in plasma are being evaluated in the diagnosis of CHF in an urgent-care setting. BNP is a neurohormone released from cardiac ventricles in response to pressure and volume overload. Even though measurement of this peptide might be useful in differentiating heart failure from other causes of dyspnea, echocardiography is essential for further evaluation of heart failure.

The recommended tests for the evaluation of patients with new-onset heart failure are listed in Table 5.1. These tests are particularly helpful in identifying conditions that might mimic or precipitate the heart failure, including arrhythmias, myocardial ischemia, thyroid abnormalities, renal failure, and anemia. The decision whether to proceed with a workup for myocardial ischemia using noninvasive stress

Table 5.1. Recommended Tests for Patients with Suspected Heart Failure

Test	Finding	Suggested Diagnosis
ECG	ST-T wave changes, Q waves, atrial fibrillation, other arrhythmias	Ischemia, previous MI; Thyroid disease or heart failure aggravated by arrhythmias
Chest radiography	Pulmonary edema	Volume overload due to heart failure
CBC	Anemia	Heart failure due to or aggravated by decreased oxygen-carrying capacity
Urinalysis	Proteinuria	Nephrotic syndrome
Serum creatinine	Elevated	Volume overload due to renal failure
Serum albumin	Decreased	Increased extravascular volume due to hypoalbuminemia
TSH (obtain only if atrial fibrillation, evidence of thyroid disease, or patient >65 yr)	Abnormal	Heart failure due to or aggravated by hypo/hyperthyroidism
Ferritin (obtain only if hemochromatosis is suspected)	Increased	Hemochromatosis

ECG, electrocardiography; MI, myocardial infarction; TSH, thyroid-stimulating hormone; CBC, complete blood count.

Modified from Clinical Practice Guideline No. 11. Heart failure: management of patients with left-ventricular systolic dysfunction. U.S. Department of Health and Human Services. Agency for Health Care Policy and Research, 1994; with permission.

testing or coronary arteriography should be individualized. A decreased left ventricular ejection fraction is not a contraindication for revascularization. If there is evidence of viable myocardium on imaging studies, revascularization can improve left ventricular function. Therefore, one should perform an ischemia evaluation in patients with angina and CHF.

In the Patient with Systolic Dysfunction, What Are Precipitating Factors for Heart Failure?

Management of heart failure should start with removal of any precipitating causes such as ischemia, arrhythmias, uncontrolled hypertension, worsening valvular abnormalities, infections, substance use, and nonadherence with diet or medications. If aggravating factors cannot be identified, pharmacologic therapy should be optimized.

What Is Your Risk Reduction Strategy to Prevent the Progression of Heart Failure?

The most important goal in managing heart failure is to prevent progression by decreasing further cardiac injury. Risk reduction strategies to control coronary artery disease include smoking cessation, tight control of blood pressure, lipids, and diabetes, discontinuing cardiotoxic substances, and initiating aspirin and β blocker therapy.

What Nonpharmacologic Measures Should Be Recommended to Patients with Heart Failure?

Each patient should be encouraged to restrict sodium intake to less than 3 grams daily, monitor daily weights to facilitate diuretic dosage adjustments, and assess overall fluid balance. Moderate exercise is encouraged in the stable patient to prevent or reverse the physical deconditioning. Patients and their families should receive counseling to increase their understanding of heart failure and medication-related side effects. Close outpatient follow-up by the primary care provider serves to encourage the patient and helps to detect early signs or symptoms of volume overload or clinical deterioration. Follow-up visits should involve a complete history and physical examination and basic chemistries to monitor for possible medication side effects.

How Do You Initiate Drug Therapy for Systolic Dysfunction? Describe the Treatment Goals.

Angiotensin-Converting Enzyme Inhibitors

Goals of therapy for the patient with heart failure are not only to relieve the symptoms but also to prevent progression of left ventricular dysfunction. Consensus guidelines suggest use of angiotensin-converting enzyme (ACE) inhibitors for heart failure treatment in all patients with systolic dysfunction regardless of their symptoms (e.g., even if they are asymptomatic) unless specific contraindications or intolerance to use of these drugs exist. Clinical trials have found ACE inhibitors to have a favorable effect on the progression of left ventricular dysfunction. They have been shown to decrease mortality, reduce hospitalizations, and improve clinical status. ACE inhibitors should be initiated at a very low dose when the patient is relatively euvolemic and titrated upward until the target dose is reached. It is important to monitor renal function and serum potassium within 1 to 2 weeks of initiating therapy and periodically thereafter. If hypotension or renal insufficiency occurs, one should consider decreasing diuretics and retrying ACE inhibitors. ACE inhibitors can be used in chronic renal insufficiency as long as renal function is monitored closely and remains stable.

β Blockers

Several clinical trials have indicated that β blockers decrease morbidity and mortality and improve the clinical status of patients with chronic heart failure. They require careful administration and a low initial dose. Even low-dose treatment may cause early clinical deterioration. Avoid using in acutely ill patients.

Diuretics

Diuretics are indicated for patients with heart failure who have evidence of or a tendency toward fluid retention. Overdiuresis should be avoided because it can cause prerenal azotemia and hypotension and often leads to the inaccurate diagnosis of intolerance to ACE inhibitors. Diuretics should be used in conjunction with an ACE inhibitor and a β blocker.

Digoxin

In patients with symptomatic heart failure due to systolic dysfunction, recent data have demonstrated that digoxin improves clinical status and reduces hospitalization rates. In addition, patients with heart failure who are stable on digoxin have a significant risk of clinical deterioration when the drug is discontinued. Because digoxin has not been shown to significantly impact survival, it is recommended in patients whose symptoms persist after treatment with ACE inhibitors, β blockers, and diuretics.

Digoxin doses should be monitored and adjusted carefully in geriatric patients and those with renal insufficiency.

Other Vasodilators

In patients who are intolerant to ACE inhibitors, one should consider using the combination of hydralazine and isosorbide dinitrate or an angiotensin receptor blocker. Hydralazine and isosorbide dinitrate in combination have been shown to exercise capacity and left ventricular function but have an unclear impact on mortality. Angiotensin receptor blockers are currently under investigation for treatment of heart failure. As with ACE inhibitors, hyperkalemia, renal insufficiency, and hypotension can all occur, but angiotensin receptor blockers do not produce cough.

Aldosterone Antagonists

The Randomized Aldactone Evaluation Study in patients with severe (class IV) heart failure found that spironolactone, when added to standard therapy, had a favorable effect on mortality. When using spironolactone, potassium must be closely monitored. More studies are needed to evaluate the efficacy of aldosterone antagonists in patients with mild to moderate heart failure.

Calcium Channel Blockers

Due to negative inotropic effects, first-generation calcium channel blockers (e.g., verapamil, diltiazem) should not be used in patients with systolic dysfunction.

Second-generation agents (e.g., amlodipine) may be safer and even efficacious due to vasodilating properties. Currently, amlodipine is recommended in patients who are intolerant to ACE inhibitors or the hydralazine/isosorbide combination.

Case

A 68-year-old woman presents with progressive worsening of dyspnea on exertion over the past 2 months and increased swelling of both lower extremities. She denies concurrent chest pain or cough. She reports three-pillow orthopnea and paroxysmal nocturnal dyspnea. Her past medical history is significant for hypertension and diabetes. She takes glipizide and hydrochlorothiazide daily. On physical examination, her blood pressure is 160/90 mm Hg, pulse is 86 beats/min, and respiratory rate is 24 breaths/min. Pulse oximetry indicates 89% saturation on room air. Her lung examination reveals bibasilar crackles. The cardiac examination is remarkable for distended jugular veins, a laterally displaced apical impulse, and a third heart sound. She has 2+ pitting edema of the lower extremities bilaterally.

1. Which diagnostic tests will you obtain and why?
2. Would you admit this patient to the hospital and why?
3. Describe your medical treatment strategy.
4. What is the most appropriate next step?

Case Discussion

Which Diagnostic Tests Will You Obtain and Why?

An echocardiogram is needed to evaluate left ventricular function, chest radiography to evaluate for cardiomegaly and pulmonary congestion, and an electrocardiogram to look for evidence of ischemia and arrhythmias. A complete blood count and chemistries could uncover precipitating factors, and the baseline assessment of renal function and electrolytes are needed to direct ACE inhibitor and diuretic use.

Would You Admit This Patient to the Hospital and Why?

This patient with new-onset congestive heart failure should be admitted to the hospital for further evaluation and treatment and, in particular, to look for evidence of underlying ischemia. Management of her severe volume overloaded state and hypoxemia will require intravenous diuresis.

Upon admission to the hospital, her electrocardiogram, cardiac enzymes, and laboratory studies are all within the normal range. Chest radiography reveals cardiomegaly with pulmonary congestion, and an echocardiogram showed a left ventricular ejection fraction of 20% with severe biventricular dilatation and generalized hypokinesis. A dipyridamole thallium test is negative for evidence of ischemia.

Describe Your Medical Treatment Strategy.

After successful intravenous diuresis with furosemide, the addition and titration of a short-acting ACE inhibitor, and a daily aspirin, the patient is medically stable and ready for discharge home. Patient education for the patient and the family (which occurred throughout the hospital stay) is reinforced with discharge instructions. Discharge medications include captopril 25 mg three times daily, furosemide 40 mg daily, and aspirin 325 mg daily. She is informed of her discharge weight and instructed on performance of daily weights, sodium restriction, and participation in cardiac rehabilitation.

Two weeks later she reports substantial clinical improvement but mild dyspnea on exertion. Her blood pressure is 130/85 mm Hg, pulse 86 beats/min, and respiratory rate 18 breaths/min. She has normal jugular venous pressure and no third heart sound, but a few rales at the lung bases and trace ankle edema. Her renal function and electrolytes are within normal limit.

What Is the Most Appropriate Next Step?

You should change captopril to a long-acting ACE inhibitor, gradually increasing the ACE inhibitor to the maximum dose. As soon as she becomes stable on the ACE inhibitor and diuretic, you should initiate β blocker therapy.

Suggested Reading

ACC/AHA Task Force on Guidelines for the Evaluation and Management of the Heart Failure. *J Am Coll Cardiol* 1995;26;1376–1399.

Clinical Practice Guideline No. 11. Heart failure: management of patients with left-ventricular systolic dysfunction. U.S. Department of Health and Human Services. Agency for Health Care Policy and Research, 1994.

Consensus recommendation for the management of chronic heart failure. *Am J Cardiology* 1999;83;2A.

The Digitalis Investigation Group. The effect of digoxin on mortality and morbidity in patients with heart failure. *N Engl J Med* 1997;336:525–532.

Packer M, Gheorghiade M, et al. RAIDANCE Study. Withdrawal from digoxin from patients with chronic heart failure treated with ACEI. *N Engl J Med* 1993;329:1–7.

RALES Investigators. The effects of spironolactone on morbidity and mortality in patients with severe heart failure. *N Engl J Med* 1999;2:341:709–717.

The SAVE Investigators. Effect of captopril on mortality and morbidity in patients with LV dysfunction after MI. *N Engl J Med* 1992:327:669–677.

The SOLVD Investigators. Effect of enalapril on survival in patients with reduced LV ejection fraction and heart failure. *N Engl J Med* 1992;327:685–691.

6

Beta-Blocker Use in Patients with Heart Failure

Ben Trichon

- Discussion   *32*
- Case   *35*
- Case Discussion   *36*

1. What is the rationale for the use of β-blockers in patients with heart failure?
2. What are the demonstrated clinical benefits of β-blocker therapy in patients with heart failure?
3. Which patients with heart failure are candidates for therapy with β-blockers?
4. What are the risks of treatment with β-blockers in patients with heart failure?

Discussion

What Is the Rationale for the Use of β-Blockers in Patients with Heart Failure?

Heart failure is a major public health problem, with over 500,000 new cases annually. It is a progressive disorder and rarely resolves spontaneously. This disease progression occurs even in the absence of discrete events, such as myocardial infarction, and is associated with a high mortality rate.

Over the past decade, the treatment of heart failure has changed dramatically; instead of focusing on short-term improvements in hemodynamics, the focus now is on a more long-term strategy to favorably affect mechanisms leading to progressive ventricular failure.

The sympathetic nervous system (SNS) is activated early in the course of left ventricular (LV) systolic dysfunction. Initially, the activation of the SNS helps maintain cardiac performance by increasing contractility and heart rate, and redistributing blood flow to the central organs. Cardiac output and blood pressure are increased. Over time, however, the increased sympathetic tone is detrimental to the heart, leading to progressive myocardial injury. There are multiple mechanisms by which chronic SNS activation injures the myocardium. Elevation of cardiac output increases myocardial oxygen demand (promoting ischemia and oxidative stress), peripheral arterial vasoconstriction leads to increased afterload, and norepinephrine leads to myocyte hypertrophy and programmed cell death. Increased SNS activity also may predispose patients with heart failure to ventricular arrhythmias. Over time, these changes lead to cardiac "remodeling", in which there are changes in ventricular geometry and thickness resulting in decreased cardiac performance.

Thus, sustained activation of the SNS is a primary mechanism for progressive LV failure (reaffirmed by the linear correlation between plasma levels of norepinephrine and mortality). Reduction of the effects of the SNS on the heart via blockade of β adrenoreceptors can reduce the detrimental effects of these aforementioned processes.

What Are the Demonstrated Clinical Benefits of β-Blocker Therapy in Patients with Heart Failure?

Beta-blockers have now been evaluated in over 10,000 patients with heart failure who have participated in over 20 randomized, placebo-controlled trials. The trials have included mild to severely [New York Heart Association (NYHA) class II–IV] symptomatic patients with left ventricular ejection fractions (LVEF) of less than 45% who were already receiving treatment with angiotensin-converting enzyme (ACE) inhibitors and diuretics. Many were also receiving digitalis glycosides. A considerable number of women and patients over 65 years of age were included in these trials, with multiple etiologies for their LV systolic dysfunction. Most trials excluded patients with bradycardia (<65 beats/min) and low systolic blood pressure (<90 mm Hg). Few patients in the trials had predominantly diastolic heart failure (LVEF >45% with clinical symptoms of heart failure).

In the Cardiac Insufficiency Bisoprolol Study II, 2,647 patients with clinical heart failure were randomized to bisoprolol or placebo. Patients enrolled had moderate to severe heart failure (83% NYHA class III, and 17% NYHA class IV). Mean duration of follow-up was 16 months. The use of bisoprolol was associated with a 34% reduction in all causes of mortality (p < 0.0001), a 20% decrease in hospitalization for any reason (p < 0.0006), and a 32% reduction in risk of hospitalization for heart failure (p < 0.0001). The study was terminated early due to the dramatic mortality reduction with bisoprolol.

The Metoprolol CR/XL Randomized Intervention Trial in Congestive Heart Failure randomized 3,991 patients with moderate to severe (NYHA class II–IV) heart failure to long-acting metoprolol or placebo. Mean duration of follow-up was 12 months. Metoprolol use was associated with a 34% reduction in all-cause mortality (p < 0.00009), 38% reduction in cardiovascular deaths, 41% reduction in sudden death (p < 0.0002), and 49% reduction in death from worsening heart failure (p = 0.0023). More recently published results from the same trial demonstrated that long-acting metoprolol significantly reduced hospitalizations due to worsening heart failure, improved NYHA functional class as assessed by physicians, and patient's improved feeling of well-being.

The U.S. Carvedilol Heart Failure Trials Program (US-CHFTP) enrolled patients with heart failure in four component trials based on their symptom severity and performance on a 6-minute walk test. A total of 1,094 patients with moderate heart failure (97% NYHA class II–III) were randomized to carvedilol or placebo for a median of 7 months. The overall pooled mortality analysis demonstrated a 65% reduction in mortality among patients receiving carvedilol (p = 0.001). Sudden deaths and deaths due to progressive pump failure were reduced to the same degree. Hospitalization for cardiac causes also was reduced.

The Carvedilol Prospective Randomized Cumulative Survival (COPERNICUS) Trial results were recently presented at the European Society of Cardiology meetings. This trial included 2,200 patients with cardiomyopathies of various etiologies with symptoms at rest or with minimal exertion (NYHA class IV). All had ejection fractions estimated at <25% despite optimal therapy. The patients were randomized to carvedilol or placebo, with the dose titrated to 25 mg twice daily. Almost 80% of randomized patients were able to reach the target dose, and rates of study drug withdrawal due to intolerance were equal in both active drug and placebo groups. The use of carvedilol was associated with a 35% reduction in all causes of mortality. Benefit was seen even in patients with severe fluid retention requiring the use of intravenous diuretics. At the time of this writing, this trial has yet to be published in its final form.

The collective experience indicates that, like ACE inhibitors, long-term (>3 months) treatment with β-blockers can improve symptoms and clinical status in patients with heart failure. These agents, when added to ACE inhibitors and diuretics, increase LVEF, improve symptoms, reduce hospitalizations, and decrease all-cause mortality.

Despite this robust evidence from these and other randomized, controlled trials, there continues to be dramatic underutilization of β-blockers in appropriate patients, with estimates suggesting that only 5% to 15% of eligible patients are being treated with these agents.

Which Patients with Heart Failure Are Candidates for Therapy with β-Blockers?

All patients with stable NYHA class II through IV heart failure due to LV systolic dysfunction should receive therapy with β-blockers unless they are unable to tolerate treatment or have an accepted contraindication to their use. Treatment should not be delayed until the patient is "resistant" to other heart failure drugs; the mortality benefit is independent of symptom status, and deaths may be prevented by initiating this therapy early in the course of heart failure. These agents should be considered the standard of care in the appropriate patients.

The following patients should not be started on β-blockers:

1. Hospitalized or clinically decompensated patients requiring intravenous diuretics
2. Patients requiring intravenous inotropic therapy (i.e., dobutamine)
3. Patients with symptomatic bradycardia
4. Patients with refractory hypotension (systolic blood pressure <90 mm Hg)
5. Patients with complete heart block (in absence of implanted pacemaker)

What Are the Risks of Treatment with β-Blockers in Patients with Heart Failure?

There are several potential adverse effects of β-blocker therapy: hypotension, fluid retention and worsening of heart failure, and severe bradycardia. Hypotension can be more pronounced with those agents that concomitantly block α receptors (e.g., carvedilol). Treatment-induced vasodilation is often asymptomatic, but may produce symptoms of lightheadedness, dizziness, or syncope. Hypotension is usually seen within 24 to 48 hours of initiation of therapy and often subsides with repeated administration without any dose changes. Administering the β-blocker and vasodilator (ACE inhibitor) at different times of the day can minimize the occurrence of this side effect. If hypotension does occur, the dose of vasodilator or diuretic may be reduced temporarily and restored within several weeks.

Fluid retention and worsening heart failure symptoms can occur with initiation of β-blocker therapy. Body weight increases may begin 3 to 5 days after initiation, and if left untreated, clinical symptoms may develop within 2 weeks. It is for this reason that initiation and titration of β-blocker therapy must be implemented under close supervision. Patients must weigh themselves daily, and manage weight increases with supplemental diuretic doses until weight is restored to pretreatment levels. The chance of developing or increasing fluid retention may be minimized if diuretic dosing and volume status is optimized prior to the initiation of β-blocker therapy.

Bradycardia is usually asymptomatic, but may be severe enough to lead to hypotension or syncope. The occurrence of bradycardia is dose related. In general, if the heart rate decreases to less than 50 beats/min or second- or third-degree heart block develops, the doses of β-blockers should be decreased.

Despite the possibility of these side effects, it should be noted that over 90% of patients enrolled in the clinical trials to date have tolerated therapy with β-blockers.

Case

A 65-year-old woman presents for her routine office visit. She has had a history of heart failure for several years. Five years prior, she suffered an acute, anterior myocardial infarction, and underwent bypass grafting of three vessels. She now has an estimated LVEF of 35%. Additional medical history is notable for hypertension, type II diabetes mellitus, and hyperlipidemia. The former has been difficult to control, and her systolic dysfunction is thought to be secondary to her ischemic event and hypertension.

She has been under your care for approximately 1 year. Her exercise tolerance is reasonable; she shops, cooks, and walks 1 to 2 miles several times weekly with her husband. She occasionally becomes dyspneic walking on inclined streets or up several flights of stairs. She has no paroxysms of nocturnal dyspnea, sleeps on one pillow, and has no angina. She was last hospitalized 3 months ago with decompensated congestive heart failure thought to be secondary to excessive salt intake from a holiday dinner. She had no inducible ischemia evident at that time. Once daily medications include lisinopril 40 mg, digoxin 0.25 mg, furosemide 40 mg, aspirin 325 mg, simvastatin 40 mg, and glyburide XL 10 mg.

Physical examination findings include a blood pressure of 140/78 mm Hg and pulse of 70 beats/min (regular). The jugular venous pressure was estimated at 7 cm of water, the chest was clear to auscultation, and the cardiac examination revealed a laterally displaced apical impulse and a soft third heart sound. There was no hepatomegaly or lower extremity edema. Electrocardiography revealed normal sinus rhythm at a rate of 72 beats/minute and old Q waves in leads V1 to V3.

1. Is this patient a candidate for treatment with a β-blocker?
2. Is one β-blocker superior to another?
3. How do you initiate and titrate therapy? What is the target dose?

4. How do you manage her β-blockers if she is subsequently admitted to the hospital for congestive symptoms?

Case Discussion

Is This Patient a Candidate for Treatment with a β-Blocker?

This patient is an excellent candidate for β-blocker therapy. She has LV systolic dysfunction (LVEF of 35%) and falls into NYHA class I to II, with relatively few clinical symptoms. She has no known contraindications to therapy.

Is One β-Blocker Superior to Another?

At this time, there is no substantial evidence that one β-blocker is superior to others in the treatment of heart failure. Each of the major agents differs slightly in its pharmacologic properties. Bisoprolol and metoprolol are predominantly β1-receptor selective, whereas carvedilol is a combination β1-, β2-, and α-receptor antagonist. The latter agent also has been reported to have antioxidant properties. It is the only agent approved by the U.S. Food and Drug Administration for use in patients with heart failure. However, the major randomized, clinical trials have demonstrated significant clinical benefits with all of the above agents. It is generally accepted that the benefits in heart failure are a class effect and not restricted to one agent. There is currently a prospective trial underway randomizing patients to carvedilol or metoprolol to investigate any potential differences in magnitude of clinical benefit. Of note, no trial of β-blockers in patients with heart failure has used atenolol.

How Do You Initiate and Titrate Therapy? What Is the Target Dose?

Patients should be as close to euvolemia as possible prior to initiation of β-blocker therapy. Excess fluid retention or depletion will predispose to worsening congestion and hypotension, respectively. If patients develop worsening fluid retention during the initiation of therapy, doses of diuretics should be increased and the β-blocker continued, if possible. These transient episodes of fluid retention usually resolve with this approach. Patients should be strongly encouraged to weigh themselves daily during titration to detect early evidence of fluid retention so they may temporarily increase diuretic doses as needed.

Treatment with β-blockers should be initiated at low doses; subsequent dose escalations should be titrated gradually. Example starting doses include the following:

carvedilol	3.125 mg twice daily
bisoprolol	2.25 mg daily
metoprolol CR/XL	12.5 to 25 mg daily
metoprolol	12.5 to 25 mg twice daily

The dose may be doubled every 2 to 4 weeks if the patient has tolerated each preceding dose. Patients should be closely monitored, and signs of fluid retention, symptomatic hypotension, and/or bradycardia should be sought.

The doses of β-blockers in the major clinical trials were not determined by patients' therapeutic responses; doses were increased until a prespecified target dose was reached. Lower doses were maintained if target doses were not tolerated, but target doses were achieved in the majority of patients. Most trials did not specifically address the comparative effectiveness of different β-blocker doses. In one of the component trials of the US-CHFTP, higher doses of carvedilol (25 mg twice daily) appeared to be more effective than lower doses (6.25 mg twice daily). However, the lower doses were also associated with a substantial decrease in the risk of death and hospitalization for worsening heart failure. In practice, these agents should probably be titrated to the doses achieved in the clinical trials demonstrating clinical benefit, but low doses may be maintained if higher doses are not tolerated.

Most patients can be maintained on long-term therapy without difficulty. Clinical responses to β-blockers are not immediate; they may not become apparent until several months have passed. Even if symptoms do not improve, long-term treatment should be continued, because these agents decrease the frequency of major clinical events and death independent of their effect on symptoms.

How Do You Manage Her β-Blockers if She Is Subsequently Admitted to the Hospital for Congestive Symptoms?

Long-term treatment with β-blockers decreases the risk of hospitalization due to worsening heart failure. Withdrawal of these agents during or after an episode of congestion will not decrease the likelihood of subsequent decompensation. In fact, subsequent risk may actually increase. For this reason, if patients experience a mild degree of symptom worsening on therapy, it is reasonable to continue the β-blocker and work to achieve clinical stability by adjusting the dose of vasodilator or diuretic.

If patients require hospitalization or the use of intravenous diuretics, it is probably prudent to reduce the dose of the β-blocker briefly, but all attempts to continue their use should be made. These agents may need to be discontinued briefly during periods of severe decompensation.

Suggested Reading

Abraham W T. Beta-blockers, the new standard of therapy for mild heart failure. *Arch Intern Med* 2000; 160:1237–1247.

Bristow M R. Beta-adrenergic blockade in chronic heart failure. *Circulation* 2000;101:558–569.

Califf R M, O'Connor C M. Beta-blocker therapy for heart failure, the evidence is in, now the work begins. *JAMA* 2000;283:1335–1336.

CIBIS Investigators and Committees. A randomized trial of beta-blockade in heart failure—the cardiac insufficiency bisoprolol study (CIBIS). *Circulation* 1994;90:1765–1773.

CIBIS-II Investigators and Committees. The cardiac insufficiency bisoprolol study II (CIBIS II): a randomized controlled trial. *Lancet* 1999;353:9–13.

Eichorn E J, Bristow M R. Practical guidelines for initiation of beta-adrenergic blockade in patients with chronic heart failure. *Am J Cardiol* 1997;79:794–798.

Frishman W H. Carvedilol. *N Engl J Med* 1998;339:1759–1765.

Heidenreich P A, et al. Effect of beta-blockade on mortality in patients with heart failure: a meta-analysis of randomized clinical trials. *J Am Coll Cardiol* 1997;30:27–34.

MERIT-HF Study Group. Effect of metoprolol CR/XL in chronic heart failure: metoprolol CR/XL randomized intervention trial in congestive heart failure (MERIT-HF). *Lancet* 1999;353:2001–2007.

Packer M, et al. The effect of carvedilol on morbidity and mortality in patients with chronic heart failure. *N Engl J Med* 1996;334:1349–1355.

Packer M, Cohn J, et al. Consensus recommendations for the management of chronic heart failure. *Am J Cardiol* 1999;83:1A–79A.

7

Coronary Artery Disease Evaluation

George Deriso

1. Define unstable angina.
2. What key clinical features determine a patient's pretest probability for coronary heart disease?
3. What are contraindications to exercise stress testing?
4. When is an exercise stress test (without imaging) a reasonable choice?
5. What is the mechanism of action of dipyridamole, adenosine, and dobutamine in pharmacologic stress testing?
6. What are the advantages and disadvantages of echocardiography and radionuclide imaging?

Discussion

Define Unstable Angina.

Unstable angina is defined as angina at rest, new-onset angina within the previous 2 months, or an accelerated anginal pattern (angina at decreased workload). Patients with unstable angina require admission to the hospital for close monitoring and treatment.

What Key Clinical Features Determine a Patient's Pretest Probability for Coronary Heart Disease?

The Coronary Artery Surgery Study, involving 1,465 men and 580 women being evaluated for chest pain, identified increased age, male gender, and chest pain as major predictors of significant coronary heart disease (CHD; ≥70% luminal narrowing of at least one major artery). A subsequent study from Duke University found that in addition to age, gender, and chest pain characteristics, the probability of CHD was further increased in the presence of diabetes, a total cholesterol level of greater than 250 mg/dL, a smoking history (half a pack per day or more within the preceding 5 years or 25 pack years or greater), and Q waves or ST-T wave changes on the electrocardiography (ECG). Of these risk factors, diabetes is the strongest predictor of CHD.

What Are Contraindications to Exercise Stress Testing?

Patients undergoing exercise stress testing must have no contraindications to such testing (acute myocardial infarction in the past 2 days, unstable angina, uncontrolled arrhythmias, severe aortic stenosis, uncontrolled heart failure, pulmonary embolism, acute pericarditis, or aortic dissection).

When Is an Exercise Stress Test (Without Imaging) a Reasonable Choice?

An exercise stress test without imaging is a reasonable choice in patients who (a) are capable of exercise; (b) are not taking digoxin; and (c) have a normal resting ECG. Because criteria for diagnosing ischemia include ST segment depression or elevation provoked by exercise, the patient's resting ECG should not have ST depressions of ≥ 1 mm, a left bundle branch block, or paced rhythm.

What Is the Role and Mechanism of Action of Dipyridamole and Dobutamine Stress Testing?

In cases where a patient is unable to exercise adequately, pharmacologic stress testing may be substituted. A normal physiologic response to exercise involves increasing heart rate and inotropy, and increasing myocardial perfusion through dilatation of coronary arteries. The most commonly used drugs—adenosine, dipyridamole (Persantine), and dobutamine—have different mechanisms of action. Adenosine is a direct vasodilator that results in coronary vasodilatation. Dipyridamole results in coronary vasodilatation through inhibiting the reuptake of adenosine. Both drugs mimic the physiologic effects of exercise. During exercise, normal arteries maximally vasodilate to increase coronary perfusion during the time of increased myocardial oxygen demand. Arteries with atherosclerotic plaques cannot vasodilate during exercise and remain relatively fixed in diameter. This results in a "coronary steal phenomenon," or shunting of blood flow toward areas of the myocardium fed by normal arteries and away from areas fed by diseased arteries. The radionuclide, injected following administration of adenosine or dipyridamole, concentrates in areas with better blood flow, leaving a relative "defect" in the territory fed by the diseased artery. In the case of ischemia, the defect will be "reversible" or reperfused once the stress is removed. If an infarct or scar is present, the defect will remain constant or "fixed" regardless of stress. Dobutamine, a $\beta 1$ agonist, induces myocardial stress by increasing cardiac demand.

What Are the Advantages and Disadvantages of Echocardiography and Radionuclide Imaging?

Stress testing with cardiac imaging, although more costly, has several advantages over the standard stress test. The addition of imaging increases the sensitivity of stress testing for detecting CHD and has the capability of localizing ischemia. Imaging should be considered in patients with abnormal resting ECGs, particularly

ST segment depressions, left bundle branch block, or preexcitation syndromes such as Wolff-Parkinson-White syndrome.

The radionuclides thallium 201 and technetium 99 sestamibi are most commonly used for assessment of myocardial perfusion. Their use increases the sensitivity of exercise testing from 65% to 70%, to 80% to 85%, but has the disadvantage of being time consuming and expensive. Thallium 201 behaves like potassium; thus, energy-dependent (Na/K ATPase) cellular uptake of thallium declines with ischemia and is absent in the areas of scarring. Pulmonary uptake of thallium poststress is indicative of an elevated pulmonary capillary wedge pressure and is a negative prognostic indicator. Technetium 99 sestamibi, when given as a bolus injection, can be imaged as it passes through the heart, allowing calculation of the left ventricular ejection fraction. In addition, technetium 99 sestamibi produces superior imaging quality in obese patients due to less attenuation by soft tissue. Stress testing with radionuclide imaging has been shown to predict left main disease or triple vessel disease with a high level of accuracy and offers prognostic information.

Stress echocardiography involves the comparison of cardiac wall motion at rest and immediately after exercise or pharmacologic stress. During exercise or stress, a normal ventricle demonstrates increased contractility. Ischemia is suggested if the ventricle fails to increase contractility or develops regional wall motion abnormalities with stress. The sensitivity for detecting significant CHD is comparable with radionuclide imaging. Advantages over radionuclide imaging include lower cost and ready availability, and it can be done more quickly. The disadvantages include its limitation in patients with baseline abnormalities in ventricular function and technical difficulties due to body habitus (e.g., obesity). Of note, severe obesity also can decrease the sensitivity and specificity of radionuclide imaging.

Case

A 48-year-old man with a 5-year history of hypertension reports "indigestion" on and off for the past month. He describes an uncomfortable sensation in the chest following large spicy meals and occasionally while climbing stairs. It is not associated with shortness of breath and resolves with antacids and rest. The last episode occurred 3 days ago following a spaghetti dinner and lasted 5 to 10 minutes. He does not get this discomfort while walking several blocks on flat ground and it has not interfered with his daily activities. He denies smoking and does not have diabetes, but had a total cholesterol of 240 mg/dL last year. His father died of a "heart attack" at age 78. His only medication is lisinopril 5 mg daily. He does not drink alcohol.

The physical examination reveals an older man in no apparent distress. His blood pressure is 152/92 mm Hg, the heart rate is 90 beats/min, and body mass index is 31. Results of the cardiopulmonary examination are normal except for the presence of an S_4. An ECG performed in your office shows evidence of left ventricular hypertrophy with repolarization changes and is unchanged from a previous ECG.

Due to his age, gender, and cardiac risk factors, you are concerned about possible CHD. The chest symptoms appear to occur during times of increased cardiac demand. You estimate that the patient's pretest probability of significant CHD is about 50% and wish to order an outpatient cardiac stress test.

1. Would you choose an exercise stress test or pharmacologic stress test, and why?
2. Would you choose a stress test with or without imaging, and why?
3. Would you change his medical regimen or order further tests?

Case Discussion

Would You Choose an Exercise Stress Test or Pharmacologic Stress Test, and Why?

Because the patient is able to walk, an exercise stress test is preferable to a pharmacologic stress test and will give you information on his functional status. If he is unable to complete the exercise test protocol, you may then choose pharmacologic stress testing.

Would You Choose a Stress Test with or Without Imaging, and Why?

Use of an exercise stress test with imaging is preferable in this setting. Left ventricular hypertrophy, particularly when associated with repolarization abnormalities as in this patient (e.g., ST segment depressions of >1 mm) will decrease the specificity of the exercise stress test and increase your false-positive rate.

Would You Change His Medical Regimen or Order Further Tests?

The patient's blood pressure regimen should be modified because his blood pressure remains elevated. One option is to increase the dose of his angiotensin-converting enzyme inhibitor to 10 mg daily. With his relatively high resting heart rate, another option is to add a β1-selective β blocker. The patient should begin taking one aspirin daily for its platelet inhibitory effect. In addition, ordering a fasting lipid profile and fasting glucose for diabetes screening are appropriate, as is thyroid testing with thyroid-stimulating hormone.

Suggested Reading

ACC/AHA Guidelines for Exercise Testing. *J Am Coll Cardiol* 1997;30:260–315.

Diamond G A, Forrester J S. Analysis of probability as an aid in the clinical diagnosis of coronary artery disease. *N Engl J Med* 1979;300:1350.

Garber A M, Solomon N A. Cost effectiveness of alternative test strategies for diagnosis of coronary artery disease. *Ann Intern Med* 1999;130:719.

Mayo Clinic Cardiovascular Working Group on Stress Testing. Cardiovascular stress testing: a description of the various types of stress tests and indications for their use. *Mayo Clin Proc* 1996;71:43–52.

Pryor D B, Shaw L, McCants C B, et al. Value of the history and physical in identifying patients at increased risk for coronary artery disease. *Ann Intern Med* 1993;118:81.

8

Interpretation of Noninvasive Cardiac Testing

Charles D. Searles

1. What are the diagnostic characteristics of noninvasive tests?
2. What constitutes a positive exercise stress test result?
3. What constitutes a positive stress imaging study result?
4. What factors affect the accuracy of noninvasive testing?
5. What prognostic information is gained from noninvasive testing?
6. What is the role of electron beam (ultrafast) computed tomography and positron emission tomography scanning in the diagnosis of coronary artery disease?

Discussion

What Are the Diagnostic Characteristics of Noninvasive Tests?

When assessing the accuracy of a test, one must understand terms such as sensitivity, specificity, and predictive value of positive and negative tests. The sensitivity of noninvasive cardiac tests measures the probability that a patient with obstructive coronary artery disease (CAD) will have a positive test result, whereas the specificity measures the probability that a patient without obstructive CAD will have a negative test result. However, sensitivity and specificity by themselves do not provide all the information needed to interpret the results of noninvasive testing. Essential to test interpretation is the predictive value of the test, which can be deduced from the sensitivity and specificity, along with the pretest probability that the patient has obstructive CAD. Bayesian principles state that the predictive accuracy of a test depends on the prevalence of disease in the population under study, that is, the pretest disease prevalence influences the posttest likelihood of significant CAD:

$$\text{Sensitivity} = \frac{\text{True positive}}{\text{True positive} + \text{False negative}}$$

$$\text{Specificity} = \frac{\text{True negative}}{\text{True negative} + \text{False positive}}$$

Bayes theorem:

Probability of disease presence with a positive test =

$$\frac{\text{sensitivity} \times \text{prevalence}}{(\text{sensitivity} \times \text{prevalence}) + [(1 - \text{specificity}) \times (1 - \text{prevalence})]}$$

Probability of disease presence with a negative test =

$$\frac{(1 - \text{sensitivity}) \times \text{prevalence}}{[(1 - \text{sensitivity}) \times \text{prevalence}] + [\text{specificity} \times (1 - \text{prevalence})]}$$

These equations should not be committed to memory, but rather they are shown to emphasize the importance of knowing a patient's pretest probability of obstructive CAD, a value that the clinician has estimated from a thorough history and physical examination, with emphasis on cardiac risk factors. Application of bayesian principles to the interpretation of noninvasive testing implies that diagnostic testing may be of limited value to patients who have a very high (>80%) or very low (<20%) pretest probability of CAD. Therefore, diagnostic testing is most valuable when the pretest probability of obstructive CAD is intermediate: for example, a 50-year-old man with atypical angina whose pretest probability of CAD is felt to be 50%. In this situation, the test result has the largest effect on the posttest probability of disease and thus on clinical decisions.

When the pretest probability of obstructive CAD is high, a positive result only confirms the high probability of disease, and a negative test result may not decrease the probability of disease enough to make a clinical difference. When the pretest probability of obstructive CAD is low, a negative result only confirms the low probability of disease, and a positive result may not increase the probability of disease enough to make a difference in clinical decisions. Test ordering becomes more cost effective if the physician who is considering ordering the test estimates the pretest probability of disease (using information from a thoughtful clinical assessment), then orders the appropriate test, and, finally, properly integrates the test results with the available clinical information. It should be remembered that a test is helpful only to the extent that it provides nonredundant information—information above and beyond what was previously available from an astute clinical assessment.

What Constitutes an Abnormal Exercise Stress Test Result?

The diagnostic interpretation of the exercise test centers on the ECG ST segment response, although interpretation also should include symptomatic response, exercise capacity, and hemodynamic response. The occurrence of ischemic chest pain consistent with angina is important, particularly if it forces termination of the test. Important positive findings on stress testing include abnormalities in exercise capacity, decreased systolic blood pressure in response to exercise (>10 mm Hg decrease), and inability to achieve a heart rate in excess of 120 beats/min. However, the most commonly used definition for a positive exercise test result is greater than or equal to 1 mm of horizontal or downward sloping ST-segment depression or elevation for at least 60 to 80 msec after the end of the QRS complex, during or after exercise.

The sensitivity of exercise stress testing is about 50%, and the specificity is approximately 90%. The diagnostic value of the exercise ECG test lies in its relatively high specificity. However, the accuracy of the test appears to be improved when other clinical factors are considered in response to exercise. If typical chest discomfort occurs during exercise with ST horizontal or downward sloping depression of 1 mm or more, the predictive value for the detection of CAD is 90%. ST-segment depression of 2 mm or more accompanied by typical chest discomfort is virtually diagnostic of significant CAD. In the absence of typical angina pectoris, downward sloping or horizontal ST-segment depression of 1 mm or more has a predictive value of 70% in the detection of significant coronary stenosis, but this increases to 90% with ST-segment depression of 2 mm or more. The early onset of ST-segment depression during exercise, its long persistence following discontinuation of exercise, and ST-segment depression with low work capacity or exercise duration are all strongly associated with multivessel coronary disease. Exercise-induced QRS prolongation also appears to be a function of exercise-induced ischemia and is related to the extent of exercise-induced segmental contraction abnormalities.

What Constitutes a Positive Stress Imaging Study Result?

The two most commonly used isotopes for radionuclide myocardial perfusion imaging are thallium 201 and technetium 99m (sestamibi). Both thallium 201 and technetium 99m are most commonly imaged using single-photon emission computed tomography (SPECT). Exercise or pharmacologic techniques can be used to induce stress. When the patient can exercise to develop an appropriate level of cardiovascular stress (6–12 minutes, achieving ≥85% of predicted maximum heart rate), exercise stress testing is preferable to pharmacologic stress testing. However, if the patient cannot exercise, then pharmacologic stress testing may be preferred. Three drugs commonly used for pharmacologic stress testing are dipyridamole, adenosine, and dobutamine. Dipyridamole (which causes vasodilatation by blocking the cellular uptake of adenosine) and adenosine are the more commonly used agents for radionuclide myocardial perfusion imaging, whereas dobutamine, a positive inotrope and chronotrope, is more commonly used with echocardiography.

Radionuclide imaging is performed at rest and during stress to produce images of myocardial regional uptake that reflect relative regional blood flow. During maximal exercise or vasodilator stress, myocardial blood flow is usually increased three- to fivefold compared with rest. In the presence of significant coronary stenosis, myocardial perfusion will not increase appropriately in the territory supplied by the artery with the stenosis, creating heterogeneous uptake. Images of the heterogeneous uptake during stress are obtained and compared with baseline resting images, and areas of myocardial ischemia can then be identified, quantified, and correlated to obstruction in particular coronary arteries. Areas of myocardium that are hypoperfused during stress but demonstrate improved perfusion on resting images are interpreted as being ischemic, whereas areas of myocardium that are hypoperfused on both stress and resting images are considered as scarred, infarcted myocardium.

The largest accumulated experience in myocardial perfusion imaging has been with the tracer thallium 201, but available evidence suggests that newer technetium 99m tracers such as sestamibi have similar diagnostic accuracy. The reported sensitivity for SPECT perfusion imaging has generally ranged from 70% to 90%, and the reported specificity ranges from 60% to 90%. As is the case for exercise stress testing, stress perfusion imaging generally has a higher sensitivity for the detection of multivessel disease compared with the sensitivity for the detection of single-vessel disease.

Exercise thallium testing, simultaneous with electrocardiography, is superior to exercise electrocardiography alone in the detection of CAD, identification of multivessel disease, localization of diseased vessels, and detection of myocardial viability in regions of abnormal wall motion. This is true for patients with and without normal resting ECGs. From the published results of 4,000 exercise redistribution images with angiographic documentation, the sensitivity of exercise ECG/thallium testing averaged 82% and the specificity averaged 88%. In the same patients, conventional ECG exercise stress testing had a sensitivity ranging from 50% to 80%.

Stress echocardiography involves imaging the left ventricular (LV) walls during stress and comparing segmental motion and thickening with images obtained at rest. Echocardiographic findings suggestive of myocardial ischemia include a decrease in wall motion in one or more segments with stress, a decrease in wall thickening in one or more LV segments with stress, and compensatory hyperkinesis in complementary or nonischemic wall segments. For patients in which pharmacologic stress testing is preferred, dobutamine is the agent of choice. Dobutamine increases heart rate, systolic blood pressure, and myocardial contractility, all of which will increase myocardial oxygen demand and secondarily increase myocardial blood flow and provoke ischemia. Stress echocardiography, either with exercise or dobutamine, has been reported to have sensitivity and specificity for detecting CAD in the range for stress radionuclide myocardial perfusion imaging. As expected, the reported sensitivity of stress echocardiography for multivessel disease is higher than for single-vessel disease.

What Factors Affect the Accuracy of Noninvasive Testing?

There are important subsets of patients in whom various factors adversely affect the sensitivity and specificity of exercise ECG testing, and stress perfusion imaging or stress echocardiography may be the preferred initial diagnostic test. Dipyridamole or adenosine stress perfusion imaging is preferred in patients with baseline ECG abnormalities such as complete left bundle branch block or electronically paced ventricular rhythm. Stress perfusion imaging or stress echocardiography is preferred in patients with >1 mm ST depression at rest, preexcitation, or patients with prior revascularization. In addition, exercise ECG testing may be less specific in patients on digoxin with <1 mm ST depression, and patients with left ventricular hypertrophy (LVH) and <1 mm ST depression. Exercise ECG testing will be less sensitive in patients on β blockers, and it is generally recommended that β blockers be withheld about 48 hours before exercise stress testing for the diagnosis and initial risk stratification of patients with suspected CAD.

Exercise testing in women presents some difficulties that are not seen in men, and, at least in part, these difficulties reflect the differences in prevalence of CAD between men and women as well as differences in sensitivity and specificity. Exercise testing is less sensitive in women than in men, and it may be less specific.

There are several proposed reasons for this difference, but they are unproven. Women generally have a lower pretest likelihood of CAD than men.

Exercise testing in the elderly is more difficult to perform and interpret, and the follow-up risks of coronary angiography and revascularization are greater. The greater severity of CAD in this group increases the sensitivity of exercise testing, but it decreases the specificity.

As is the case for exercise ECG testing alone, the sensitivity of an exercise imaging study for the diagnosis of CAD appears to be lower in patients on β blockers. It is recommended that β blockers be withheld prior to exercise imaging studies for the diagnosis and initial risk stratification of patients with suspected CAD. Patients with left bundle branch block tend to have an increased prevalence of myocardial perfusion defects during exercise imaging, defects that may be reversible or fixed, and often involve the interventricular septum. These defects are frequently not borne out on coronary angiography, and are often absent during pharmacologic stress testing. Multiple studies have found that perfusion imaging with pharmacologic vasodilatation is more accurate for identifying CAD in patients with left bundle-branch block.

The sensitivity of radionuclide perfusion scans may be lower in women than in men. Artifacts due to breast or diaphragmatic attenuation of the radioactive tracer usually manifest as perfusion defects in the anterior and inferior walls, respectively. These artifacts may be improved with the use of gated technetium 99m sestamibi SPECT imaging because this technique uses an isotope with a higher energy (technetium 99m has a higher energy than thallium 201), and it allows comparison of perfusion defects with regional wall motion of the left ventricle. Exercise or pharmacologic stress echocardiography may help avoid artifacts specifically due to breast attenuation. However, echocardiographic imaging in obese persons tends to be more difficult and produces images of poorer quality.

What Prognostic Information Is Gained from Noninvasive Testing?

Noninvasive cardiac stress testing can not only provide valuable information that is needed to establish the diagnosis of CAD, but it can also estimate the prognosis in patients with chronic stable angina. In the case of exercise ECG stress testing, prognostic information may be derived from maximum exercise capacity, the amount of ST depression, and the degree of angina during exercise. The Duke treadmill score combines this information and provides a way to calculate risk. Among outpatients with suspected CAD, the two thirds of patients with scores indicating a low risk had a 4-year survival rate of 99%, and the 4% who had scores indicating high risk had a 4-year survival rate of 79% (average annual mortality rate of 5%).

A normal stress perfusion study is associated with a subsequent rate of cardiac death and myocardial infarction of less than 1% per year, even in patients with known CAD. A possible exception to this statement would be patients with exercise treadmill results that suggest high risk but who have normal perfusion scans. In contrast, several different abnormal findings on stress SPECT perfusion imaging have been associated with severe CAD and subsequent cardiac events. Large stress-induced perfusion defects and defects in multiple coronary artery territories are poor prognostic signs. Lung uptake of thallium 201 on poststress images, and/or the presence of poststress ischemic (LV) dilatation are indicators of stress-induced global dysfunction and are associated with an adverse prognosis, independent of clinical, ECG, and cardiac catheterization data. The results of SPECT perfusion imaging can be used to identify a high-risk patient subset with a greater than 3% annual mortality rate. These patients should be considered for early coronary angiography because their prognosis may be improved by revascularization.

A negative stress echocardiographic test predicts a low risk for future cardiovascular events. The prognosis is not benign in patients with a positive stress echocardiographic study, with morbid or fatal cardiovascular events more likely in patients with wall motion abnormalities after stress. However, the reported actual event rates for positive stress echocardiographic studies are variable and not as well established as for nuclear perfusion imaging. Patients with a positive ECG response to treadmill stress testing but no inducible wall motion abnormality on echocardiography have a very low rate of adverse cardiovascular events during follow-up.

What Is the Role of Electron Beam (Ultrafast) Computed Tomography and Positron Emission Tomography Scanning in the Diagnosis of Coronary Artery Disease?

Electron beam computed tomography (EBCT) permits detection and quantification of coronary artery calcium with very rapid scanning times. The calcium is quantified and reported as a calcium score. In several studies, calcium of the coronary arteries detected by EBCT was an important indicator of angiographic coronary stenosis. Although the sensitivity of EBCT is felt to be relatively high, the specificity is relatively low, and the test has an overall predictive accuracy of about 70% in typical CAD patient populations. Some studies have shown that the presence and amount of calcium detected in the coronary arteries by EBCT correlate with presence and amount of atherosclerotic plaque, whereas others have shown marked variability in repeated measures of coronary calcium in the same patient. Given the high rate of false-positive studies of EBCT (calcium does not concentrate exclusively at sites of severe coronary artery stenosis) relative to other, more established imaging modalities, the proper role of EBCT is controversial.

Positron emission tomography (PET) involves quantitative imaging of myocardial uptake of high-energy positron-emitting tracers. For the detection of CAD, the relative distribution of myocardial blood flow is examined using the tracers rubidium 82 or nitrogen 13 ammonia, initially at rest, then again during pharmacologic vasodilatation. PET offers several advantages over SPECT for the detection of CAD, including better overall diagnostic accuracy. However, one significant limitation of PET is its increased cost.

Positron emission tomography is considered to be the standard of reference for noninvasive detection of myocardial viability with nuclear techniques. The most common technique for determining viability uses nitrogen 13 ammonia as a perfusion tracer and fluoride-18-fluorodeoxyglucose (FDG) as a metabolic marker for glucose metabolism. A myocardial region that may appear to be nonfunctional can be determined to have preserved viability when there is a mismatch between the perfusion tracer and FDG uptake. This region would show little or no perfusion tracer uptake, but would demonstrate the uptake of FDG.

Case

A 56-year-old postmenopausal woman presents for the first time to your clinic. She is moderately obese, and she states that over the past month she has been experiencing periodic episodes of "sticking" in her chest lasting several minutes. The chest discomfort does not radiate to her neck or arms; it sometimes appears to be precipitated by exertion or emotional duress, but occurs other times while she is sitting quietly. Sublingual nitroglycerin mostly relieves her symptoms. The chest discomfort symptoms have led to a modest reduction in her daily activities, but the patient acknowledges that the worst part of the pain is the anxiety that it provokes. She has a history of hypertension, and she has high cholesterol. She denies smoking, a history of diabetes, and significant family history of CAD. She takes amlodipine and hydrochlorothiazide for blood pressure control and simvastatin for elevated cholesterol. Her resting ECG shows increased voltage suggesting LVH, but the ST-segment and T-wave morphology are normal.

She has brought with her the results of a recent exercise stress test with dual isotope SPECT radionuclide perfusion imaging that had been ordered by her previous health-care provider. The results indicate that she had exercised 5 minutes on the treadmill, achieving 85% of her predicted maximum heart rate. Her blood pressure and pulse response were appropriate and she had no chest discomfort. The test was discontinued because of fatigue. In the last minute of exercise, she had approximately 1 mm of horizontal ST depression in the inferior and lateral leads lasting 2 minutes of recovery.

The resting images obtained following injection of thallium 201 show small anterior and inferior defects in 5% and 7% of the LV myocardium, respectively. Stress images were obtained following injection of sestamibi at peak exercise, and these show a 7% defect inferiorly and a 25% defect anteriorly. On gated images of LV wall motion, there is no wall motion abnormality inferiorly, but there was a mild wall motion abnormality anteriorly.

1. Was the study that was obtained for this patient ordered appropriately?
2. How would you interpret the test results?
3. What would be the next step in this patient's management?

Case Discussion

Was the Study that Was Obtained for This Patient Ordered Appropriately?

Yes. Diagnostic testing is most valuable when the pretest probability of obstructive CAD is intermediate. The estimation of pretest probability in this patient would be based on the nature of her symptoms and her cardiac risk factors. This patient has several risk factors (hypertension, hyperlipidemia, postmenopause), but her symptoms are somewhat atypical for angina pectoris—stabbing pain, not predictably brought on by exertion, modest relief with nitroglycerin. Based on this information and based on comparison of this patient with similar patients who were part of large CAD data bases, this patient's pretest probability of obstructive CAD is probably 40% to 50%, which is in the intermediate range.

Exercise ECG testing in women can be problematic. The test in women may be less sensitive and less specific. In addition, the LVH on her resting ECG tends to increase the number of false-positive exercise ECG test results. Given these potential complicating conditions, it would be appropriate to use an exercise stress imaging test.

How Would You Interpret the Test Results?

In this example of an exercise stress imaging test, it is important to interpret both the exercise ECG results together with the myocardial perfusion imaging results. Both tests independently can provide important diagnostic and prognostic information, and, in patients with an intermediate pretest probability of disease, these tests together better predict the likelihood of obstructive CAD.

This patient achieved a heart rate that was adequate for interpretation of the exercise ECG (at least 85% of predicted maximum heart rate). She had 1 mm of horizontal ST depression, and this represents a positive result for ischemia. Given this positive result, the patient's probability of having obstructive CAD increases from 45% to 75%. A negative test (e.g., no ECG changes or symptoms) would decrease her probability of disease to 25%, not low enough that you would be comfortable without further testing such as coronary arteriography.

The radionuclide perfusion images showed a fixed inferior defect, which is likely diaphragmatic attenuation artifact. There appeared to be at least a 20% anterior wall reversible defect (5% defect at rest, 25% after stress), some of which may be breast attenuation artifact. However, the large size of the defect suggests that there is significant stress-induced myocardial ischemia. Positive results from myocardial perfusion imaging and exercise ECG increase the probability of obstructive CAD from a pretest probability of 45% to a posttest probability of 95%. If the patient had negative results from exercise ECG and the imaging study, the probability of disease would have decreased from 45% to 8%. This may be an acceptable level to reassure the patient that her chest discomfort is most likely not related to obstructive CAD and that the only further therapy concerning her heart would be aggressive risk factor modification.

What Would Be the Next Step in This Patient's Management?

The results of exercise stress testing and SPECT perfusion imaging can be used to identify patients at high, intermediate, or low risk for cardiac event or mortality. The patients identified as high risk by stress perfusion imaging have an annual mortality rate of 3%, and they should receive coronary arteriography because their prognosis may be improved by revascularization. Patients identified as low risk have a cardiac event rate of less than 1% annually, and coronary arteriography is not warranted.

This patient may be considered to have an intermediate risk for cardiac event. Despite the 1 mm of ST depression, which indicated that the exercise test result was positive, the fact that she is able to exercise 5 minutes without angina makes her risk of death is 1.25% per year. The results of the SPECT perfusion imaging also predict an intermediate risk for this patient. The reversible defect was moderately large, but it was associated with obstructive CAD in only one coronary artery territory. In addition, there were none of the other features of high-risk perfusion studies; there was no reported increased lung uptake of radiotracer or poststress ischemic LV dilatation, and the wall motion abnormality was mild.

In patients identified as intermediate risk by stress perfusion imaging, the decision to proceed with coronary angiography should be based on symptoms, the response to medical therapy, and the physician's and patient's thresholds for absolutely knowing the extent of CAD. For a sedentary patient with several other comorbid illnesses (e.g., cancer, severe lung disease, renal failure, etc.), the threshold for proceeding with coronary angiography would be higher than for an otherwise healthy airline pilot. In the case described above, the patient seems to be fairly healthy, but she is anxious and somewhat limited in her activities. In addition, the obstructive lesion appears to be in the territory of the left anterior descending artery with a potentially large amount of myocardium at risk. The most prudent decision would be to refer the patient for coronary angiography to define the coronary anatomy and extent of CAD.

Suggested Reading

Beller G A, Zaret B L. Contributions of nuclear cardiology to diagnosis and prognosis of patients with coronary artery disease. *Circulation* 2000;101:1465–1478.

Gibbons R J. Myocardial perfusion imaging. *Heart* 2000;83:355–360.

Gibbons R J, et al. ACC/AHA/ACP-ASIM guidelines for the management of patients with chronic stable angina. *J Am Coll Cardiol* 1999;33:2092–2197.

Patterson R E, Horowitz S F, Eisner R L. Comparison of modalities to diagnose coronary artery disease. *Semin Nucl Med* 1994;24:286–310.

9

Hypercholesterolemia in Primary Prevention

Terry A. Jacobson
Charles R. Harper

1. What are the risk factors for coronary artery disease according to the recent National Cholesterol Education Program Adult Treatment Panel III guidelines?
2. What are the most common causes of secondary "hypercholesterolemia"?
3. At what levels of low-density lipoprotein cholesterol should dietary and drug therapy be initiated in primary prevention and secondary prevention (i.e., coronary artery disease, angina, and myocardial infarction)?
4. What is the available evidence that treatment with the 3-hydroxy-3-methylglutaryl coenzyme A (HMG-CoA) reductase inhibitors (statins) reduces coronary artery disease morbidity and mortality?
5. What are the dietary recommendations for elevated cholesterol levels?
6. What are the different drugs used to treat hypercholesterolemia, and what are their side effects that require therapeutic monitoring?
7. What other evidence-based primary prevention modalities have been shown to reduce the risk for coronary artery disease?

Discussion

What Are the Risk Factors for Coronary Artery Disease According to the Recent National Cholesterol Education Program Adult Treatment Panel III Guidelines?

Matching Intensity of Therapy to Coronary Artery Disease Risk

The goal of the National Cholesterol Education Program (NCEP) is to match the coronary artery disease (CAD) risk status of an individual patient to the intensity of therapy. Those at higher risk for CAD should be treated more aggressively than patients at low risk. The guidelines essentially divide all patients into one of the following risk factor categories from the highest risk to the lowest risk: (a) patients with CAD or CAD risk equivalents; (b) patients with multiple risk factors and ele-

Table 9.1. NCEP Risk Factors*

Positive risk factors
    Age
        Male (≥45 years)
        Female (≥55 years or premature menopause without ERT)
    Family history of premature CAD (male <55 years, female <65 years)
    Current cigarette smoking
    Hypertension (≥140/90 mm Hg or on antihypertensive medication)
    Low HDL-cholesterol (<40 mg/dL)
Negative risk factor
    High HDL-cholesterol (≥60 mg/dL)

NCEP, National Cholesterol Education Program; ERT, estrogen replacement therapy; CAD, coronary artery disease; HDL, high-density lipoprotein.
*Diabetes is considered a CAD risk equivalent.

vated low-density lipoprotein (LDL) cholesterol; and (c) patients with zero to one CAD risk factors and an elevated LDL cholesterol. CAD patients include those with any documented atherosclerotic disease, such as previous myocardial infarction (MI), angina pectoris, history of percutaneous transluminal coronary angioplasty or coronary artery bypass grafting, positive coronary catheterization, or other positive diagnostic test for CAD. Those with diabetes or noncoronary forms of atherosclerosis are also considered to be at high risk for future coronary events, and are considered "CAD risk equivalents." These include patients with peripheral artery disease, abdominal aortic aneurysm, and symptomatic carotid disease (including transient ischemic attacks and carotid stroke).

The multiple risk factor patient includes patients with elevated LDL cholesterol and two of the following risk factors: age over 45 years if male, age over 55 years if female (or if prematurely menopausal, not on estrogen replacement therapy), premature family history of CAD (<55 years of age in father or first-degree male relative or <65 years of age in mother or first-degree female relative), current cigarette smoking, hypertension [≥140/90 mm Hg or currently taking antihypertensive medication] and high-density lipoprotein (HDL) cholesterol low (<40 mg/dL) (Table 9.1). A high

Age Years	Pts
20–34	−9
35–39	−4
40–44	0
45–49	3
50–54	6
55–59	8
60–64	10
65–69	11
70–74	12
75–79	13

Systolic Blood Pressure	Untreated	Treated
<120	0	0
120–129	0	1
130–139	1	2
140–159	1	2
≥160	2	3

HDL-C (mg/dL)	Pts
>60	−1
50–59	0
40–49	1
<40	2

Pts	10-Yr CHD Risk
<0	<1%
0	1%
1	1%
2	1%
3	1%
4	1%
5	2%
6	2%
7	3%
8	4%
9	5%
10	6%
11	8%
12	10%
13	12%
14	16%
15	20%
16	25%
≥17	≥30%

Total Cholesterol (mg/dL)	20–39	40–49	50–59	60–69	70–79
<160	0	0	0	0	0
160–169	4	3	2	1	0
200–239	7	5	3	1	0
240–279	9	6	4	2	1
>280	11	8	5	3	1
Cigarette Smoking					
Nonsmoker	0	0	0	0	0
Smoker	8	5	3	1	1

Figure 9.1. Assessing CHD Risk in Men

HDL level (>60 mg/dL) is considered a negative risk factor and generally reduces the risk of a patient by one risk factor.

In patients with multiple risk factors, a 10-year risk assessment is then carried out using the Framingham risk prediction tool (see Fig. 9.1). This scoring system allows clinicians to more precisely determine an individual's risk for CHD over the next 10 years. After assigning points for the different CHD risk factors, a summation score is then determined and patients are then divided into the following three risk categories: 10 year CHD risk score >20%, 10–20%, and <10%. Those patients with scores >20% are considered to be "CHD risk equivalents" and should be targeted as aggressively as patients with CHD with a goal LDL below 100mg/dl. For those patients whose risk is 10–20%, the initiation of drug therapy is considered for those with LDL levels above 130mg/dl; while those with <10% CHD risk, drug therapy is considered when LDL-C levels remain above 160mg/dl. For patients with 0–1 risk factors, it is not necessary to perform a CHD risk assessment with the Framingham score, and the level to consider drug initiation is 190mg/dl.

The patient with an elevated LDL cholesterol but with no (or only one) CAD risk factor is generally considered at lower cardiovascular risk. These patients often are younger, such as men less than 35 years of age or premenopausal women.

Counting of Risk Factors, Low-Density Lipoprotein Cholesterol Determination, and Non-HDL Cholesterol

To accurately determine a patient's risk for CAD, a full lipoprotein panel is generally required, including total cholesterol, LDL cholesterol, HDL cholesterol, and triglycerides. LDL cholesterol is generally not measured directly but is calculated using the following formula: LDL cholesterol = total cholesterol − HDL cholesterol − (triglycerides/5).

The formula breaks down when triglyceride levels are greater than 400 mg/dL, and thus a fasting level is generally required for those with high triglycerides or diabetes mellitus at baseline. Although it is recommended that all patients receive a fasting lipid level, some clinicians will do "opportunistic" screening when the patients are available in the office. This approach is generally valid unless the patient is later found to have high triglycerides or a metabolic abnormality known to affect lipids such as diabetes mellitus.

The main lipoprotein for screening, targeting, and monitoring is LDL cholesterol. The LDL cholesterol level and the patient's CHD risk status determines the goal of lipid lowering therapy and at what level to initiate diet and drug therapy. It is generally recommended that the baseline LDL value be a determination of two measurements taken 1 to 8 weeks apart because therapy is often lifetime and there can be significant intraindividual variation of up to 20 to 30 mg/dL per day. The cut-off points for the initiation of diet and drug therapy are outlined in Table 9.2.

A secondary target of drug therapy besides LDL-C, is Non-HDL Cholesterol (Non-HDL-C). This is the Total Cholesterol minus the HDL Cholesterol (TC–HDL=Non-HDL-C). Non-HDL represents the measurement of other atherogenic lipoproteins besides LDL-C, and includes very low-density lipoproteins (VLDL) and intermediate density lipoproteins (IDL). In patients with high triglycerides (>200mg/dl), the goal non-HDL-C is set at 30mg/dl higher than that for LDL-C. For example, if the goal LDL-C is less than 130, the goal Non-HDL-C is less than 160mg/dl.

Table 9.2. NCEP Guidelines: Emphasis on Low-Density Lipoprotein (LDL) Cholesterol and Risk Stratification for Treatment Goals

Risk Category	LDL Goal	LDL Level at Which to Consider Drug Therapy
CHD or CHD Risk Equivalents (10-year risk >20%)	<100 mg/dL	≥130 mg/dL (100–129 mg/dL; drug optional)
2+ Risk Factors (10-year risk ≤20%)	<130 mg/dL	10-year risk 10–20%; ≥130 mg/dL 10-year risk <10%; ≥160 mg/dL
0–1 Risk Factor	<160 mg/dL	≥190 mg/dL (160–189 mg/dL; LDL-lowering drug optional)

NCEP, National Cholesterol Education Program; CHD, coronary heart disease.

What Are the Most Common Causes of Secondary "Hypercholesterolemia"?

Before initiating therapy for hyperlipidemia, secondary causes need to be ruled out. The most common secondary causes include diabetes mellitus, hypothyroidism, nephrotic syndrome, chronic renal insufficiency, and obstructive liver disease. Generally, a fasting blood glucose level, liver function tests, thyroid-stimulating hormone (TSH), and a creatinine level should be assessed to rule out these possibilities. Treatment of secondary hyperlipidemia is aimed first at treating the underlying causes such as diabetes mellitus, hypothyroidism, or renal insufficiency before deciding upon lifetime drug therapy. Diabetes mellitus is generally associated with elevated triglycerides and low HDL cholesterol, in addition to borderline or high LDL levels. The dyslipidemia of chronic renal failure is generally characterized by hypertriglyceridemia. In addition to secondary metabolic causes, certain drug therapies may cause multiple lipid abnormalities. The most common drugs that induce lipid changes include estrogen and alcohol, which increase both triglycerides and HDL cholesterol, whereas β blockers and progesterone may lower HDL cholesterol.

At What Levels of Low-Density Lipoprotein Cholesterol Should Dietary and Drug Therapy Be Initiated in Primary Prevention and Secondary Prevention (i.e., Coronary Artery Disease, Angina, and Myocardial Infarction)?

Although the goal of lipid-lowering therapy is to reduce LDL cholesterol and improve the overall lipid profile, the ultimate goal of therapy is to reduce CAD risk and future CAD events. Diet is still the cornerstone of all hyperlipidemia therapy, and all physicians must be familiar with administering at least an NCEP step 1 "low fat, low cholesterol" diet to patients. The target goals of lipid lowering are different for secondary and primary prevention, reflecting the concept of more aggressive targeting for those at greater risk. The goal LDL levels for patients with CAD or a CAD risk equivalent is an LDL cholesterol of less than 100 mg/dL. The goal for patients without CAD and with two or greater risk factors, is LDL cholesterol less than 130 mg/dL, whereas the goal for patients without CAD and fewer than two risk factors is LDL cholesterol less than 160 mg/dL (Table 9.2). For patients with multiple risk factors whose Framingham scores exceed 20%, they are considered a CAD risk equivalent, with LDL-C goal <100 mg/dL.

Recent data suggest that patients with diabetes mellitus are at increased vascular risk and have comparable risk to nondiabetic patients with a history of MI. Thus, recent guidelines suggest that diabetes should be considered a "CAD risk equivalent" and that the target LDL goal for diabetic treatment should be similar to that for CAD patients.

What Is the Available Evidence that Treatment with the HGM-CoA Reductase Inhibitors (Statins) Reduces CAD Morbidity and Mortality?

Although the NCEP guidelines were published before the results of the clinical trials with the HMG-CoA reductase inhibitors (statins), the studies have revealed a uniform consistency in reducing CAD risk in both secondary and primary prevention. The secondary prevention trials with statins in patients with severe and moderate hypercholesterolemia (4S, CARE, LIPID) demonstrated in aggregate not only a risk reduction in nonfatal MI and CAD deaths of approximately 30%, but also a reduction in total mortality (30%), need for revascularization procedures (35%), and reduction in stroke (29%). The primary prevention trials with statins in patients with severe and moderate hyperlipidemia (WOSCOPS, AFCAPS/TexCAPS) also demonstrated comparable reductions in nonfatal MI and CAD deaths, but did not show reductions in total mortality or stroke.

In addition to studies in patients with elevated LDL cholesterol, two studies with patients with low HDL levels, also demonstrated clinical CAD risk reduction. The Veterans' Affairs High Density Lipoprotein Cholesterol Intervention Trial (VA HIT) showed that in men with CAD and isolated low HDL cholesterol, the drug gemfibrozil reduced CAD events by about 21%. In the AFCAPS/TexCAPS primary prevention trial, patients with moderate LDL elevations and borderline low HDL levels had their risk of CAD reduced by lovastatin by 37%.

What Are the Dietary Recommendations for Elevated Cholesterol Levels?

The NCEP guidelines recommend a step 1 diet for the general public, but a more restrictive step 2 diet for those with elevated LDL-C levels. The goal of the NCEP step 1 diet is to reduce total fat consumption to less than 30% of total calories, saturated fat (and trans-saturated fats) to less than 10% of all calories, and cholesterol content of food to less than 300 mg/day, and to maintain ideal body weight through proper nutrition and physical activity. The main emphasis of a step 1 diet is to reduce total and saturated fat by reducing the intake of fatty meats (e.g., hamburger, steak, bacon, hot dogs, sausage, etc), reduce or eliminate frying or baking with lard, vegetable oils, or shortening, reduce margarine and butter using nonstick sprays, and reduce dairy products rich in fat, including whole milk, ice cream, and cheese. Patients also should be told to learn to read food labels, maintain ideal body weight, exercise, and limit caloric consumption. Positive suggestions for improved eating include more meatless or vegetarian meals, leaner cuts of meat, limiting portion size, switching to monounsaturated (olive oil, peanut oil) or polyunsaturated oils (canola oil) for cooking and baking, and eating more fruits and vegetables. A step 2 NCEP diet is generally more restrictive in saturated fat intake, allowing less than 7% of calories from saturated fat. This requires greater changes in life-style, and it is generally recommended that a dietitian assist when these changes are required.

What Are the Different Drugs Used to Treat Hypercholesterolemia and What Are Their Potential Side Effects that Require Therapeutic Monitoring?

If dietary therapy fails, drug therapy should be instituted. The drugs with the greatest efficacy, safety, and evidence-based outcomes include the HMG-CoA reductase inhibitors or statins. At baseline before initiating therapy, a liver function test (LFT) should be obtained and repeated at 6 and 12 weeks after therapy because the incidence of elevated LFTs (transaminitis) is about 1.5%. If the dosage is titrated upward, a repeat LFT level also should be obtained. It is generally recommended that if LFTs increase to three times greater than the upper limit of normal (ULN) that they be discontinued or the dosage reduced. Patients can be titrated gradually, with the doubling in statin dose generally resulting in an additional 6% LDL reduction. The statins can reduce LDL by 20% to 50% depending on the statin and the dose. The two statins that induce the greatest LDL reduction (i.e., 30%–50%) include simvastatin, atorvastatin, and rosuvastatin whereas those with more modest LDL reductions (i.e., 20%–35%) include fluvastatin, pravastatin, and lovastatin. The statins should be used very carefully in certain subgroups of patients on other medications. One of the rare side effects of statin therapy, particularly in combination with certain other medications, is the increased incidence of myopathy leading to rhabdomyolysis. Although myositis is rare, occurring in 1/1,000 patients, creatine phosphokinase (CPK) elevations of more than 10 times the ULN with muscle weakness, muscle pain, or tenderness are the hallmarks of myopathy and should result in drug discontinuation. The drugs that have been shown to increase the risk of rhabdomyolysis with a statin include erythromycin or azithromax, gemfibrozil, niacin, cyclosporine, and azole antifungals.

Other safe drugs that can be used to lower LDL levels include the bile acid sequestrants (cholestyramine, colestipol) and niacin. These drugs require more patient education because they require slow dose titration schedules and have annoying but predictable side effects such as constipation or bloating with the bile acids, or flushing with niacin. The fibrate drugs (gemfibrozil, fenofibrate) and niacin, are the drugs of first choice for patients with isolated hypertriglyceridemia. Like the statins, they are also effective in mixed hyperlipidemia, or those patients with moderate elevations in LDL cholesterol and triglycerides. These drugs should be used cautiously with statins due to the risks of rhabdomyolysis and myopathy. This combination should only be used if it is determined that the benefits of therapy clearly outweigh the risks.

What Other Evidence-Based Primary Prevention Modalities Have Been Shown to Reduce the Risk for Coronary Artery Disease?

In addition to statin therapy in primary prevention, other therapies have been shown to reduce the risk of cardiovascular disease. There is excellent clinical trial data in primary prevention that low-dose aspirin, antihypertensive therapy, and possibly angiotensin-converting enzyme (ACE) inhibitors in diabetics (HOPE trial), may reduce cardiovascular risk. Although no randomized trials exist, there are strong epidemiologic data that smoking cessation and exercise also reduce risk. There are currently no data in primary prevention that suggest that estrogen, vitamin E, or folate reduces the risk of CAD, but clinical trials are ongoing.

Case

A 52-year-old man, working as a bus driver, presents to you after being told that he had "a cholesterol problem" after a routine insurance physical about 6 months ago. He has a history of well-controlled hypertension for the past 20 years and is on atenolol 50 mg and low dose hydrochlorathiazide (12.5 mg). Although he does not smoke, he is 30% above his ideal body weight at 250 pounds, but says he is very adherent to a low-salt diet. He is sedentary, but occasionally lifts weights at home twice per week. Although he states that he is in excellent physical condition, his father had a "heart attack" at the age of 45 years and a fatal stroke at 52 years. He is concerned about his family history and has recently gone on a "low-cholesterol" diet.

Physical examination shows a blood pressure of 165/100 mm Hg with a normal cuff and 145/95 mm Hg with a large cuff; pulse is 58 beats/min and regular. The patient is a slightly obese anxious male. HEENT (head, eyes, ear, nose, throat) examination shows bilateral corneal arcus and hypertensive retinopathy. The skin shows no tendon xanthomas. Heart examination shows a normal S_1/S_2 without murmur, rub, or gallop. Extremities have excellent pulses that are 2+ throughout.

Laboratory results are as follows: total cholesterol 232 mg/dL, LDL cholesterol 175 mg/dL, HDL cholesterol 33 mg/dL, triglycerides 120 mg/dL, glucose 200 mg/dL nonfasting and 112 mg/dL fasting, creatinine 1.2 mg/dL, TSH 1.5 μIU/mL, alanine aminotransferase 30 U/L, and aspartate aminotransferase 25 U/L.

1. Determine the patient's risk factors for coronary artery disease and his Framingham 10 year CAD risk score.
2. What secondary causes of hypercholesterolemia need to be ruled out before initiating therapy?
3. What is the goal low-density lipoprotein cholesterol level if dietary therapy is ineffective after 3 to 6 months on an NCEP step 2 diet? What is the goal of therapy if the patient later develops coronary artery disease or diabetes mellitus?
4. You decide to initiate statin therapy in this patient. What baseline laboratory studies are required and when should you repeat a lipid determination or other laboratory evaluation? What should be considered if a patient develops muscle pain or muscle tenderness after initiating a statin?
5. The patient is concerned about developing CAD given his family history of premature heart disease. Are there other evidence-based interventions in primary prevention that have been proven to reduce CAD risk?

Case Discussion

Determine the Patient's Risk Factors for Coronary Artery Disease and His Framingham 10 Year CAD Risk Score

In addition to an elevated LDL cholesterol of 175 mg/dL, the patient has the following risk factors: male age over 45 years, premature family history of CAD in a male relative, hypertension requiring drug treatment, and a low HDL cholesterol of 33 mg/dL. On examination he demonstrates inadequately controlled blood pressure, hypertensive retinopathy, normal peripheral pulses, and obesity. Although obesity and a sedentary life-style are CAD risk factors, they are not counted as NCEP risk factor because they mediate their effects through blood pressure and lipid changes. In counting risk factors, a high HDL level of over 60 mg/dL counts as a negative risk factor because it partially offsets some of the CAD risk. Although an elevated LDL cholesterol of over 160 mg/dL is a positive CAD risk factor, it is not counted as an NCEP risk factor because it is used in determining the threshold for dietary and drug treatment.

Using the Framingham scoring system (Fig. 9.1), the patient gets the following points: 6 for age 52, 2 for treated hypertension and a systolic blood pressure of 145, 3 for total cholesterol of 232 at age 52, 2 for a low HDL-C of 33, and 0 for being a nonsmoker. The total point score adds to 13 and represents a 10-year risk of CHD of 12%.

What Secondary Causes of Hypercholesterolemia Need to Be Ruled Out Before Initiating Therapy?

The most common secondary causes include diabetes, hypothyroidism, nephrotic syndrome, chronic renal failure, and obstructive liver disease. Normal LFT results and normal TSH, creatinine, and fasting glucose levels rule out these secondary causes. Although the patient does not meet the new American Diabetes Association criteria for diabetes (fasting glucose > .126 mg/dL confirmed in two separate blood specimens), he probably has impaired glucose tolerance and is at risk for developing diabetes. In addition he may have the beginning of the cardiovascular risk syndrome called the metabolic syndrome, characterized by insulin resistance (glucose >110 mg/dL), hypertension (≥130/85 mm), low HDL cholesterol (<40 mg/dL), elevated triglycerides (≥150 mg/dL), and obesity (waist ≥40 inches). Any patient with 3 of 5 of these risk factors may have the metabolic syndrome and may be at increased risk of developing CAD and diabetes.

What Is the Goal LDL-C Level if Dietary Therapy Is Ineffective? What Is the Goal of Therapy if the Patient Later Develops Coronary Artery Disease or Diabetes Mellitus?

The goal of therapy for a primary prevention patient with LDL levels of greater than 160 mg/dL, two or more CAD risk factors and a 10 year CAD risk score of <20% is a LDL cholesterol less than 130 mg/dL. If he develops CAD or diabetes mellitus, the goal of therapy is LDL cholesterol less than 100 mg/dL. New guidelines suggest treating diabetics as having a CAD risk equivalent because their risk for future CAD events is comparable with that of nondiabetic patients with CAD. Thus, the LDL cholesterol target for diabetic patients is the same as for those with CAD, less than 100 mg/dL.

You decide to initiate statin therapy in this patient. What baseline laboratory studies are required and when should you repeat a lipid determination or other laboratory evaluation? What should be considered if a patient develops muscle pain or muscle tenderness after initiating a statin?

Generally, a baseline LFT is required before initiating statin therapy because the risk of transaminitis is 1.5%. It is generally recommended that you repeat the LFT measurement at 6 and 12 weeks after initiating therapy, or after titrating the dose upward. Most transaminitis occurs early in the first 6 months of therapy, unless an additional hepatic metabolized drug is added. Changes in lipid levels on drug therapy can be seen within 4 to 6 weeks of therapy. CPK levels are not generally recommended at baseline. Patients should be told that if muscle pain, muscle tenderness, or muscle weakness occur after statin therapy, then they need to be evaluated and a CPK measurement determined. The following statin drug combinations increase the risk of rhabdomyolysis: erythromycin (or azithromax), cyclosporine, gemfibrozil, niacin, and azole antifungals.

The patient is concerned about developing CAD given his family history of premature heart disease. Are there other evidence-based interventions in primary prevention that have been proven to reduce CAD risk?

Several studies have indicated that besides lipid-lowering therapy with the statins, low-dose aspirin, hypertension control, and ACE inhibitors in diabetics may reduce the risk of cardiovascular disease in primary prevention. Although never studied in randomized trials, smoking cessation and increased physical activity probably also reduce the risk of CAD. No data yet exist that demonstrate that vitamin E, β-carotene, estrogen, or folate reduces the risk of CAD.

Suggested Reading

Downs J R, Clearfield M, Weis S, et al. for the AFCAPS/TexCAPS Research Group. Primary prevention of acute coronary events with lovastatin in men and women with average cholesterol levels: results of AFCAPS/TexCAPS. *JAMA* 1998;279:1615–1622.

Expert Panel. Executive summary of the third report of the National Cholesterol Education Program (NCEP) Expert Panel on Detection, Evaluation, and Treatment of High Blood Cholesterol in Adults (Adult Treatment Panel III). *JAMA* 2001;285:2486–2497.

Expert Panel. Summary of the second report of the National Cholesterol Education Program (NCEP) Expert Panel on Detection, Evaluation, and Treatment of High Blood Cholesterol in Adults (Adult Treatment Panel II). *JAMA* 1993;269:3015–3023.

Jacobson T A, Schein J R, Williamson A, et al. Maximizing the cost-effectiveness of lipid-lowering therapy. *Arch Intern Med* 1998;158:1977–1989.

Knopp R H. Drug treatment of lipid disorders. *N Engl J Med* 1999;341;498–511.

Shepherd J, Cobbe S M, Ford I, et al. for the West of Scotland Coronary Prevention Study Group. Prevention of coronary heart disease with pravastatin in men with hypercholesterolemia. *N Engl J Med* 1995;333:1301–1307.

10

Diet in the Prevention and Treatment of Coronary Artery Disease

Charles R. Harper
Terry A. Jacobson

1. When should the National Cholesterol Education Program (NCEP) step 1 or step 2 diet be started? What are the goals of therapy and how often should lipids be monitored?
2. Be familiar with the makeup of the NCEP step 1 and step 2 diets.
3. Know and understand how changes in dietary components affect low-density lipoprotein and high-density lipoprotein cholesterols and triglycerides.
4. Certain dietary supplements have been popularized in the lay press. What is the evidence supporting or refuting the use of some common dietary supplements?

Discussion

When Should the NCEP Step 1 or Step 2 Diet Be Started? What Are the Goals of Therapy and How Often Should Lipids Be Monitored?

Although specific recommendations concerning diet and the prevention of coronary artery disease (CAD) have been made for the public at large, the decision to begin the NCEP step 1 diet is based on low-density lipoprotein (LDL) cholesterol levels and the presence of cardiac risk factors. For patients without CAD and less than two cardiac risk factors, dietary therapy is recommended at LDL cholesterol levels of 160 mg/dL or higher. The goal of therapy is to reduce LDL cholesterol below 160 mg/dL. Usually a patient is started first on the step 1 diet. Lipids are checked at 6 weeks (for patient motivation) and 3 months. If after 3 months of adherence to the step 1 diet LDL cholesterol levels are not below 160 mg/dL, then a step 2 diet is initiated. Most patients require help from a registered dietitian to adhere to a step 2 diet. After initiating a step 2 diet, lipids are again monitored at 6 weeks and 3 months. If at this point the LDL cholesterol is greater than 190 mg/dL, drug treatment should be considered. Clinical discretion is advised for those patients with

Table 10.1. NCEP Dietary Guidelines

	LDL-cholesterol Initiation Level	LDL-cholesterol Goal of Therapy
Without CAD and fewer than two risk factors	>160 mg/dL	<160 mg/dL
Without CAD and two or more risk factors	>130 mg/dL	<130 mg/dL
With CAD or diabetes	>100 mg/dL	<100 mg/dL

NCEP, National Cholesterol Education Program; LDL, low-density lipoprotein; CAD, coronary artery disease.

fewer than two CAD risk factors whose LDL cholesterol remains in the 160 to 190 mg/dL range despite 6 months of dietary therapy. A lipid-lowering drug may be considered in these patients. Even after a lipid-lowering drug is started, the patient should be encouraged to continue the NCEP diet.

In patients without CAD and two or more cardiac risk factors, dietary therapy is usually recommended when LDL cholesterol levels are 130 mg/dL or higher. The goal of therapy is to reduce LDL cholesterol below 130 mg/dL. The patient is then started on a step 1 diet, and the same time line as described above is followed. If LDL cholesterol levels remain greater than 160 mg/dL after adherence to 6 months of dietary therapy, including 3 months on a step 2 diet, then drug therapy should be considered. Patients with LDL cholesterol levels that remain in the 130 to 160 mg/dL range require the clinician's judgment on the need for starting drug therapy.

Dietary therapy is recommended for CAD patients and diabetics with LDL cholesterol above 100 mg/dL. The goal is to reduce LDL cholesterol to 100 mg/dL or below. CAD patients and diabetics should start with the step 2 diet. If the goal of therapy is not reached in 6 to 12 weeks, drug therapy should be considered (Table 10.1).

Be Familiar with the Makeup of the NCEP Step 1 and Step 2 Diets.

Table 10.2 lists the major components of the NCEP diet. Both diets require that total fat not exceed 30% of total calories.

Table 10.2. Components of the NCEP Diets

Nutrient	Step 1 Diet	Step 2 Diet
Total fat	30% or less of total calories	30% or less of total calories
Saturated fatty acids	8–10% of total calories	Less than 7% of total calories
Polyunsaturated fatty acids	Up to 10% of total calories	Up to 10% of total calories
Monounsaturated fatty acids	Up to 15% of total calories	Up to 15% of total calories
Carbohydrates	55% or more of total calories	55% or more of total calories
Protein	15% of total calories	15% of total calories
Cholesterol	Less than 300 mg/day	Less than 200 mg/day
Total calories	Adequate to achieve and maintain desirable weight	Adequate to achieve and maintain desirable weight

What Are the Effects of Various Dietary Components on Lipoprotein Levels? What Are Common Sources of These Nutrients?

Dietary cholesterol was once thought to increase LDL cholesterol levels by inhibiting the synthesis of LDL receptors, thereby increasing plasma LDL cholesterol levels. Sources of dietary cholesterol include meat, egg yolk, shellfish, and organ meats. More recent evidence shows that the effects of dietary cholesterol in humans tends to be highly variable, with both hyper- and hyporesponders observed. Changes in dietary cholesterol generally have a small impact on blood lipid levels.

Saturated fatty acids raise serum LDL cholesterol levels. The mechanism is thought to involve the downregulation of the expression of the hepatic LDL receptor. Sources of saturated fats include meats, high-fat dairy products, and certain oils such as coconut and palm kernel oil. In the landmark Seven-Country Study, the incidence of CAD was independently associated with the intake of saturated fat.

Trans fatty acids (TFAs) increase LDL cholesterol and decrease high-density lipoprotein (HDL) cholesterol levels. TFAs are formed when vegetable oils are hydrogenated, changing them from the cis to the trans configuration. TFAs are widely used in the food/agriculture industry because they have a higher melting point and stay solid at room temperature. Common sources of TFA include stick margarine, shortening, commercially processed baked goods, snack foods, and fried foods. The Nurses Health Study, a prospective case control study of 80,000 women, suggested that replacing TFAs with unhydrogenated monounsaturated and polyunsaturated fatty acids may significantly reduce risk of CAD.

The polyunsaturated fatty acids (PUFAs) can be divided into omega-6 (n-6) and omega-3 (n-3) fatty acids. These groups of fatty acids are named according to the location of the first double bond in the fatty acid molecule.

The n-6 PUFAs are fats derived from seed oils such as corn, safflower, and sunflower seeds. When substituted for saturated fat, the n-6 PUFA's lower LDL cholesterol levels. Excessive amounts of n-6 oils can result in lower HDL cholesterol levels and increased obesity (9 kcal/g of oil). Therefore, it is not recommended that they make up more than 10% of the total daily caloric intake.

The n-3 fatty acids have been shown to lower triglycerides with minimal effect on LDL and HDL cholesterol levels. They have a cardioprotective effect, as documented in several randomized control–led secondary prevention trials. The n-3 fatty acids have been shown to reduce the risk of cardiac death and nonfatal myocardial infarction (MI) in patients with CAD. This was recently demonstrated in the GISSI-Prevenzione trial of 11,000 CAD patients, where the n-3 fatty acids demonstrated a relative risk reduction of 24% [number needed to treat (NNT) = 43]. This cardioprotective effect is thought to be due to their ability to prevent cardiac arrhythmias, although they also have been shown to have a beneficial effect on thrombosis and platelet reactivity. Sources of n-3 fatty acids include marine sources such as mackerel, salmon, and sardines, along with plant sources such as walnuts and to a lesser extent some vegetables. Although the n-3 fatty acids are considered an essential nutrient, there are no U.S. guidelines on recommended consumption. Current European guidelines range from 2% to 5% of total caloric intake.

Monounsaturated fatty acids (MUFAs) have received much attention in the medical and lay literature because of the large role they play in the Mediterranean diet.

When substituted for saturated fat, MUFAs lower LDL cholesterol without changing HDL cholesterol levels. MUFAs are also thought to make LDL cholesterol less susceptible to oxidation, which is an important step in the formation of atherosclerotic lesions. MUFAs are found in olive oil, canola oil, peanut oil, avocados, and almonds.

Vegetable protein in the form of soy protein has been shown to reduce LDL cholesterol levels without changing HDL cholesterol when substituted for animal fat and protein. Although not clearly delineated, it is thought that the phytoestrogens in soy play a role in its lipid-lowering effect and may increase HDL cholesterol.

Dietary fiber can be divided into two groups: insoluble fiber (wheat bran), which aids in bowel function, and soluble fiber, which may have a small cholesterol-lowering effect.

Good sources of soluble fiber are oat bran, psyllium (metamucil), and pectins from fruits and vegetables. Epidemiologic data suggest that fiber may reduce CAD.

Alcohol consumption has been associated with a decreased risk of CAD in several epidemiologic studies. Alcohol has been shown to increase HDL cholesterol. Other contributors to alcohol's cardioprotective effect include inhibition of platelet aggregation and decrease in fibrinogen levels. The negative effects of chronic heavy alcohol use include exacerbation of hypertension, cardiomyopathy, liver disease, accidents, and suicide. Thus, a public health recommendation for alcohol usage to reduce CAD risk is not appropriate (Table 10.3).

A significant challenge to most clinicians is how to provide understandable and useful dietary advice during a brief office visit. The MEDICS questionnaire can be used as a quick preliminary tool to isolate sources of fat in a patient's diet. Ideally, this could be followed up by a visit to a registered dietitian (Table 10.4).

Certain dietary supplements have been popularized in the lay press. What is the evidence supporting or refuting the use of some common dietary supplements (omega-3 fatty acid supplements, garlic capsules, vitamin E and folate) in the prevention of CAD?

In the past, the evidence for increasing the intake of n-3 fatty acids was mostly epidemiologic. More recent clinical trial evidence now exists to suggest a cardio-

Table 10.3. Effects of Various Dietary Components on Lipoprotein Levels

Name	Common Source	LDL	HDL	Triglyceride
Saturated fat	Beef, coconut oil, palm oil	↑↑	↑	↔
Monounsaturated fat	Olive oil, canola oil, avocado	↓	↔	↓ If substituted for carbohydrate
Trans fatty acids (hydrogenated oils)	Snack foods, crackers, muffins, cookies, hydrogenated oils	↑	↓	↔
Polyunsaturated omega-6	Corn oil, sunflower oil, safflower oil	↓	↓	↓ If substituted for carbohydrate
Polyunsaturated omega-3	Fish, fish oil, flax seed, meats, egg	Variable	↑	↓
Dietary cholesterol	Meats, egg	Variable	Variable	↔
Fiber	Oats, oat bran	↓	↔	↔
Soy protein	Tofu	↓	↔	↔
Alcohol		↔	↑	↑
Weight loss		↓	↑	↓

Table 10.4. MEDICS Questionnaire

Category	Ask Regarding	Skills to Learn
Meat	Beef, pork, lamb, or veal?	Learn to order leaner cuts of meat
	Portion size?	Restrict to lean portions of 4 oz or less (size of deck of cards)
	Liver or organ meats?	Avoid organ meats?
	Fowl or fish meats?	Use skinless poultry; avoid fried items
	Hot dogs or sausage?	Eat sparingly
Egg yolks	How many per week? (four for step 1, two for step 2)	Use egg whites for omelets and recipes; consider egg substitutes
Dairy products	Whole milk products?	Use skim milk or 1% milk
	Cheeses?	Use low-fat cheeses like mozzarella
	Ice cream?	Use no- or low-fat yogurt
	Cream cheese?	Use no-fat cream cheese
Invisible fats		
Baking goods	Doughnuts, cakes, pies, muffins, cookies?	Read labels and use no or low-fat items; watch muffins which can be high fat; bake with low fat recipes
Fried foods	French-fries?	Substitute fruit or pretzels for snacks
Cooking fats	Oils and spreads?	Use nonstick sprays; liquid instead of stick or tub margarine
Snacks	Ice cream, candy bars, cake, cookies, chips	Use more fruit and vegetables as snacks
Spirits	How many drinks of alcohol per week? A unit of alcohol is 1 oz of liquor, one glass of wine, one can of beer.	Limit alcohol to one to two drinks per day. Restrict further if triglycerides are high.

protective benefit from increasing n-3 consumption in patients with established CAD. Primary prevention trials do not exist at this time. The various trials are summarized in Table 10.5.

An early meta-analysis suggested that garlic oil capsules or garlic cloves may have some cholesterol lowering effect; however, the trials included in this review

Table 10.5. Trials Involving Common Dietary Supplements

Study	Design	Intervention	End points	Intervention Event Rate	Control Event Rate	NNT
GISSI-Prevenzione Trial	Randomized control, 11,324 post-MI patients, followed 42 mo	Fish oil (EPA) 850 mg daily	CAD death and nonfatal MI	6.9%	9.2%	43
DART	Randomized control, 2,033 men post-MI, followed 24 mo	Fish meal twice a week or fish oil 1,500 mg daily	Total mortality	9.3%	12.8%	28
Lyon Diet Heart Study	Randomized control, 605 post-MI patients followed 27 mo	Margarine type spread supplemented with n-3 fatty acid	CAD death and nonfatal MI	1.32%	5.5%	23
The Indian Experiment of infarct survival	Randomized control, 360 patients post MI followed 12 months	Fish oil (EPA) 1 gm/day	CAD death and nonfatal MI	24.5%	34.7%	9.8%

NNT, number needed to treat to prevent an event; EPA, eicosapentaenoic acid.

were small, and the methodology of some trials was not sound. Recently, larger, well-designed randomized placebo-controlled trials have not demonstrated a significant cholesterol-lowering effect. There is no evidence available concerning garlic and hard end points such as cardiac death or nonfatal MI.

Because of the key role the oxidation of LDL cholesterol is thought to have in the atherosclerotic process, antioxidants such as vitamin E have received increased attention. The evidence from two large randomized placebo-controlled trials does not support a role for vitamin E in the prevention of CAD. In the Heart Outcomes Prevention Evaluation Study, 9,541 patients with established CAD or multiple risk factors were evaluated. Treatment with vitamin E 400 IU daily had no apparent effect on cardiovascular outcomes. In a second larger trial, the GISSI-Prevenzione Trial, 11,324 patients less than 3 months post-MI were evaluated. Vitamin E did not have a statistically significant effect on death, nonfatal MI, or stroke. The current available evidence does not support recommending a vitamin E supplement to patients for the prevention of CAD.

Case

A 52-year-old man comes to your office 3 months after being discharged from the hospital. During his hospitalization he underwent four-vessel coronary artery bypass graft surgery. His postoperative course was uncomplicated, and he has not had any complaints since discharge. His past medical history is significant only for hypertension diagnosed 10 years ago. His medications include atenolol 100 mg daily and aspirin 325 mg daily. He has a history of smoking 45 packs of cigarettes per year (but he has not smoked for 1 month) and no alcohol use. Family history is positive for a brother with an MI at 48 years of age. On physical examination he is a slender African-American man. Blood pressure is 132/80 mm Hg, pulse is 60 beats/min, and body mass index is 24 kg/m^2. The remainder of his examination is unremarkable. His lipid profile is total cholesterol 205 mg/dL, LDL cholesterol 112 mg/dL, HDL cholesterol 40 mg/dL, and triglycerides 265 mg/dL. The patient states that he has recently been to a health and nutrition store, where it was suggested that he start taking garlic capsules, folic acid, vitamin E, and fish oil capsules daily. The patient states that he no longer eats red meat and has given up his typical breakfast consisting of a sausage biscuit, replacing it with a whole grain muffin. He wants to know what else he can do to improve his diet. On further questioning you discover he still eats cheese several times a week. He states he usually does not have much time for lunch and gets a snack out of a vending machine at work.

1. What diet should be recommended for this patient? When should this patient's lipid profile be checked again? What is the goal of therapy? How long should dietary therapy be continued before considering a lipid-lowering drug?
2. What types of food would you tell this patient to avoid because of their high saturated fat content? What tips could you give this patient in avoiding trans fatty acids?
3. This patient wants your opinion on the utility of the nutritional supplements he has purchased. How would you advise him?

Case Discussion

What Diet Should Be Recommended for This Patient? When Should This Patient's Lipid Profile Be Checked Again? What Is the Goal of Therapy? How Long Should Dietary Therapy Be Continued Before Considering a Lipid-Lowering Drug?

This patient has documented CAD and therefore should be started on the NCEP step 2 diet. The LDL cholesterol goal for this patient is less than 100 mg/dL. In an adherent patient, it is reasonable to expect a 3% to 14% decrease in serum cholesterol levels. In this patient, diet modification may be all that is required to meet NCEP LDL goals. The next lipid profile should be checked at 6 weeks, but because this is a higher risk patient due to his CAD, the usual 3- to 6-month trial of diet may not be appropriate. If NCEP LDL goals are not met in 6 to 12 weeks, then a lipid-lowering drug should be strongly considered.

What Types of Foods Would You Tell This Patient to Avoid Because of Their High Saturated Fat Content? What Tips Could You Give This Patient in Avoiding Trans Fatty Acids?

Saturated fat is found in meat but also in high-fat dairy products. This patient should be asked about his consumption of dairy products. High-fat cheeses, ice cream, and whole and 2% milk also should be avoided. Although the patient has made the correct choice to stop eating sausage, commercially baked products such as crackers, muffins, and cakes can be a source of hidden fat. These foods are likely to contain TFAs. Fried foods are also a source of TFAs, and specific questions should be asked about ingestion of fried foods. The patient could be instructed to read labels and avoid snacks using hydrogenated oils, as these are higher in TFAs. Because of the time constraints most clinicians face, referral to a dietitian is required for a step 2 diet because more complete dietary instruction concerning fat restriction is required.

This Patient Wants Your Opinion on the Utility of the Nutritional Supplements He Has Purchased. How Would You Advise Him?

There are no trials available with garlic on the prevention of MI or cardiac death. The studies with garlic that have focused on lipids as an end point have shown mixed results, with the largest trials showing a minor to nonsignificant effect. It is also difficult to recommend vitamin E at this time because two recent secondary prevention trials have not shown a mortality benefit from treatment with vitamin E.

Elevated homocysteine is now thought to be a cardiac risk factor. Folic acid has been shown to reduce homocysteine levels; however, there are no randomized control trials demonstrating a reduction in end points such as myocardial infarction (MI) or cardiac death. Recent clinical trials have supported the consumption of fish or fish oil capsules in the prevention of nonfatal MI and cardiac death. Because of the added expense involved in purchasing these supplements you might suggest to your patient that he simply eat fish twice a week.

Suggested Reading

Grundy S M. What is the desirable ratio of saturated, polyunsaturated, and monounsaturated fatty acids in the diet. *Am J Clin Nutr* 1997;66(suppl):988–990.

Katan M B, Grundy S M, Willett W C. Should a low-fat, high-carbohydrate diet be recommended for everyone. *N Engl J Med* 1997:562–567.

Krauss R M, Deckelbaum R J, Ernst R D, et al. Dietary guidelines for healthy American adults: a statement for health professionals from the Nutrition Committee, American Heart Association. *Circulation* 1996;94:1795–1800.

Kris-Etherton P M. Monounsaturated fatty acids and risk of cardiovascular disease. *Circulation* 1999;100:1253–1258.

11

Peripheral Vascular Disease

Joyce P. Doyle

1. How is intermittent claudication defined? How sensitive is the classic history of claudication and the physical examination of distal pulses in detecting peripheral vascular disease?
2. What is the significance of the ankle-brachial index and how is it measured?
3. What other noninvasive tests are available in the diagnosis and assessment of peripheral vascular disease?
4. What is the prognosis for patients with peripheral vascular disease?
5. What are the indications for urgent referral to a vascular surgeon?
6. What are the noninvasive treatments used for patients with peripheral vascular disease?

Discussion

How Is Intermittent Claudication Defined? How Sensitive Is the Classic History of Claudication and the Physical Examination of Distal Pulses in Detecting Peripheral Vascular Disease?

A thorough history and physical examination is important in the initial assessment of a patient with suspected peripheral vascular disease (PVD). However, both are relatively insensitive. For the history, intermittent claudication has been defined by the Rose criteria as having all of the following characteristics:

1. Exertional leg symptoms that include the calf
2. Symptoms that are provoked by hurrying or walking uphill
3. Symptoms that did not begin at rest
4. Symptoms that cause patients to stop or slow their pace
5. Symptoms that did not disappear with continued walking
6. Symptoms that resolved within 10 minutes of rest

If claudication symptoms are present, they are highly specific for PVD (99%). However, as demonstrated in one study, these classic symptoms are highly insensitive and are present in only 9% of patients with abnormal noninvasive lower extremity blood flow testing (using arterial waveforms, blood flow velocities, and lower extremity pressures).

Abnormal distal pulses (dorsalis pedis or posterior tibia) measured in the same study also had limited predictive value. An abnormal dorsalis pedis pulse had 50% sensitivity and 73% specificity, and abnormal posterior tibial pulse had a sensitivity of 71% and specificity of 91% in detecting PVD when compared with normals.

What Is the Significance of the Ankle-Brachial Index and How Is It Measured?

Epidemiologic studies that patients with a low ankle-brachial index (ABI) even without symptoms of intermittent claudication have increased mortality, increased cardiovascular event rate, and impairment of lower extremity function. Measuring the ABI in patients with claudication or other cardiovascular risk factors can be easily accomplished in the primary care office and is both noninvasive and accurate. The presence of PVDs is suggested by an ABI of less than 0.90 at rest.

Equipment needed to measure the ABI includes appropriate sized blood pressure cuffs and a hand-held pulse Doppler probe. The ABI is measured with the patient supine after resting for 5 minutes. Upper extremity systolic blood pressures are measured for the left and right arms in the standard fashion at the brachial arteries using a blood pressure cuff and a Doppler probe. Systolic pressures are defined as the pressure at which the pulse is audible by Doppler upon cuff deflation. Ankle blood pressures are measured by placing the blood pressure cuff above the ankle malleoli and measuring the systolic blood pressures by Doppler for both the dorsalis pedis and posterior tibial arteries.

The ABI is calculated for each lower extremity as the highest systolic blood pressure measured at the ankle (either the dorsalis pedis or posterior tibial arteries) divided by the highest upper extremity systolic blood pressure (right or left) measured at the brachial arteries. Of note, the false-negative rate of ABI for PVD can be higher in patients with diabetes mellitus or in elderly patients with stiff blood vessels. Therefore, other testing modalities should be considered where clinically indicated in patients with normal ABIs.

$$ABI = \frac{\text{ankle systolic blood pressure}}{\text{brachial artery systolic blood pressure}}$$

What Other Noninvasive Tests Are Available in the Diagnosis and Assessment of Peripheral Vascular Disease?

Patients with abnormal ABIs in whom determination of the extent and location of the vascular occlusion will impact the treatment plan may benefit from further testing. Which of these tests to use is generally a decision made by the vascular surgeon. Pulse volume recordings, offered by many vascular laboratories, are a noninvasive modality for measuring blood pressures and arterial waveforms at five sites on each lower extremity: proximal thigh, distal thigh, proximal calf, ankle, and foot. Duplex scanning is being used increasingly to noninvasively assess blood flow at the aortoiliac level and below and appears to have good test characteristics.

When invasive treatment is being considered, either arteriography or magnetic resonance angiography is generally necessary to delineate the extent of the disease.

These tests should not be used for initial diagnosis and are generally ordered by the consulting vascular surgeon.

What Is the Prognosis for Patients with Peripheral Vascular Disease?

Among patients with claudication, the prognosis for the involved limb is relatively good, with rare progression to limb-threatening ischemia. In one prospective study, without definitive treatment, the distance patients could walk without having claudication improved in about one fourth of patients, remained the same in about half, and worsened in the remaining one fourth. Over a 5-year period, 4% to 8% of patients required peripheral vascular surgery and 2% to 4% required amputation.

Peripheral vascular disease is an important clinical predictor of widespread atherosclerotic disease and increased cardiovascular mortality. Regarding cardiovascular risk, the Framingham data indicated a twofold increase in 10-year mortality rates in males and a fourfold increase in females with claudication in comparison with those without claudication. In patients who have undergone lower extremity bypass surgery, the 5-year risk of nonfatal cardiovascular events is as high as 50%. In the Bypass Angioplasty Revascularization Investigation Trial (BARI), the 5-year survival rate among those with PVD was 77% versus 90% for those with isolated coronary disease.

What Are the Indications for Urgent Referral to a Vascular Surgeon?

Indications for urgent referral to a vascular specialist include a sudden decrease in the distance at which claudication occurs, disabling claudication, rest pain, or evidence of ulcerations or tissue necrosis on examination.

What Are the Noninvasive Treatments Used for Patients with PVD?

Noninvasive treatments used for PVD include exercise, smoking cessation, other forms of cardiovascular risk reduction, and pharmacotherapy directed toward improving blood flow. To help assess progress among patients with symptoms of intermittent claudication, it is important to initially quantify and subsequently record the initial claudication distance (the distance at which pain first begins) and absolute claudication distance (the distance at which the patient can no longer ambulate).

Exercise in the form of walking has been shown in multiple studies to significantly improve claudication distance by increasing collateral blood supply. Due to the high rate of concomitant atherosclerotic heart disease, the need for a cardiac stress test should be carefully considered prior to beginning an intensive exercise program. The following features are predictive of a successful exercise program:

- Sessions three or more times weekly for a minimum of 30 minutes
- Exercise to near maximal claudication prior to resting

- At least 6 months of exercise
- Supervised programs (appear to have some advantage over home-based programs)

Smoking cessation appears to slow disease progression and improve postoperative graft patency rates in patients with intermittent claudication.

Except for exercise and smoking cessation, there are no large clinical outcomes trials looking at aggressive cardiovascular risk factor reduction in patients with PVD. However, because these patients are at high risk for cardiovascular events, they should be treated as aggressively as patients with known coronary artery disease. Thus, smoking cessation, hypertension control, lipid reduction, diabetes control, weight reduction, and exercise should be emphasized.

Three antiplatelet agents [aspirin, ticlopidine (Ticlid), and clopidogrel (Plavix)] and two other drugs [pentoxifylline (Trental) and cilostazol (Pletal)] have been studied to varying degrees in patients with PVD. Few data exist regarding aspirin use specifically in patients with PVD. Primary prevention data for PVD obtained from the Physicians' Health Study demonstrated a lower relative risk (0.54 times) of needing peripheral vascular surgery among male patients randomized to receive aspirin 325 mg every other day when compared with those receiving placebo. Due to a low event rate in this low-risk group of patients, the absolute risk reduction was very low. A collaborative overview of randomized trials of antiplatelet therapy (primarily aspirin, dipyridamole, or sulfinpyrazone) and prevention of death, myocardial infarction, and stroke, compiled by the Antiplatelet Trialist Collaboration (1994) demonstrated a nonsignificant trend toward cardiovascular risk reduction in patients with known PVD (defined by intermittent claudication, peripheral grafts, or peripheral angioplasty). Lack of significance may have been due to the small number of patients studied. Due to the high rate of coexisting cardiovascular and cerebrovascular disease among patients with PVD, aspirin (typically 325 mg daily) should be considered for use.

If a patient is intolerant to aspirin, ticlopidine (Ticlid), a platelet aggregation inhibitor, can be considered. The Swedish Ticlopidine Multicenter Study (STIMS), a randomized, double blinded, placebo-controlled trial involving 687 women and men, was designed to determine whether ticlopidine 250 mg twice daily reduces the incidence of myocardial infarction, cerebrovascular accidents, and transient ischemic attacks in patients with intermittent claudication. There was no statistical difference between groups for the end points listed, but there was a 29% mortality reduction in the ticlopidine arm, primarily due to a reduction in ischemic heart disease. Of note, the incidence of side effects with ticlopidine was very high; 22% of patients taking ticlopidine experienced diarrhea and 2% developed hematologic complications.

Clopidogrel (Plavix) blocks adenosine diphosphate–dependent activation of the glycoprotein IIb–IIIa complex, thereby inhibiting platelet aggregation. Clopidogrel was recently compared with aspirin for prevention of ischemic stroke, myocardial infarction, and vascular death in patients considered at high risk for ischemic events (CAPRIE Trial). Among the subgroup of patients with PVD, clopidogrel 75 mg daily was superior to aspirin 325 mg daily in reducing the combined end points with a relative risk reduction of 23.8% (4.86% events in the aspirin group vs. 3.71% in the clopidogrel group). The overall safety profile of clopidogrel in this trial was at least as good as aspirin.

Pentoxifylline (Trental) is approved by the U.S. Food and Drug Administration for the treatment of intermittent claudication. It is thought to decrease blood viscosity and platelet activity by increasing red blood cell flexibility. A recent meta-analysis suggested that in comparison with placebo, pentoxifylline can be effective in improving the walking capacity of patients with moderate intermittent claudication. The average increase in walking distance was 30 m on a treadmill (equivalent to 90 m on flat ground).

Cilostazol (Pletal) is a new type III phosphodiesterase inhibitor that suppresses platelet aggregation and acts as a direct arterial vasodilator. Two recent randomized, placebo-controlled trials using cilostazol 100 mg twice daily for 12 weeks or 16 weeks demonstrated significant improvement in walking distances among patients with intermittent claudication.

Case

A 52-year-old man with a 15-year history of hypertension comes to your office complaining of buttock and thigh cramping for the past several weeks. The symptoms begin after two blocks of walking, become intolerable at three blocks, and resolve after 5 minutes of rest. He has not had pain at rest. There is no associated chest pain or shortness of breath, and no history of back pain or injury. The patient has no history of diabetes mellitus. His family history is nonsignificant. He has a history of smoking 60 packs of cigarettes per year and continues to smoke 2 packs daily. He does not drink alcohol. He has been taking atenolol 50 mg daily for years.

On physical examination, his blood pressure is 162/94 mm Hg and pulse rate is 60 beats/min. He has no carotid bruits or elevated jugular venous pressure, and has a normal cardiac and pulmonary examination, and no abdominal tenderness, bruits, or appreciable aortic enlargement. His peripheral pulses are difficult to palpate but present on Doppler, and a right femoral bruit is present. There are no lower extremity or foot ulcerations.

Laboratory studies show a glucose of 82, and a total cholesterol of 260 mg/dL with LDL of 170 mg/dL, HDL of 35 mg/dL, and triglycerides of 275 mg/dL. The ABI was 0.7 on the left and 0.75 on the right.

1. Based on the patient's clinical history, at what level do you expect peripheral arterial occlusion?
2. What is the likelihood that the patient's β blocker is contributing to his symptoms?
3. Does the ankle-brachial index play a role in predicting cardiovascular risk?
4. What treatment would you initiate?

Case Discussion

Based on the Patient's Clinical History, at What Level Do You Expect Peripheral Arterial Occlusion?

The level of arterial occlusion is typically above the level of symptoms. Bilateral buttock claudication suggests more proximal aortoiliac disease.

What Is the Likelihood that the Patient's β Blocker Is Contributing to His Symptoms?

Historically, β blockers have been avoided in PVD. Beta 2 receptors present in the periphery cause vasodilatation in normal blood vessels. Thus, β blockers could increase peripheral vasoconstriction by blocking vasodilating β2 receptors, leading to unopposed α constriction. There is no evidence to support these theoretical concerns, however, and a recent meta-analysis of nine randomized controlled trials demonstrated no significant difference in degree of claudication between patients receiving β blockers versus placebo. It is unlikely that the β blocker is contributing to this man's claudication symptoms.

Does the Ankle-Brachial Index Play a Role in Predicting Cardiovascular Risk?

The ABI is a significant predictor of cardiovascular events. In one study, the 5-year cardiovascular morbidity was 12% among patients with an ABI greater than 0.70, and 60% among those with an ABI less than 0.50. An additional 2-year follow-up study in 110 patients with intermittent claudication showed a nonfatal cardiovascular event rate of 12% in patients with ABIs of greater than 0.7, 33% for ABIs of 0.5 to 0.7, and 60% for ABIs less than 0.5.

What Treatment Would You Initiate?

The recent onset and severity of this patient's symptoms as well as his low ABI warrants a referral to a vascular specialist for possible further testing and intervention. With multiple cardiovascular risk factors (e.g., hypertension, tobacco use, family history), this patient is at high risk for a future cardiovascular event. He would likely benefit from a multilevel approach to cardiovascular risk reduction, including smoking cessation, better hypertension control, lipid reduction with a statin, and aspirin therapy. It would be prudent to evaluate this patient with a cardiac stress test prior to prescribing an exercise regimen. The patient's initial claudication distance of two blocks and absolute claudication distance of three blocks should be noted and reassessed at each follow-up visit. He should be educated on symptom recognition for cardiac chest pain, stroke, and serious limb ischemia.

Suggested Reading

CAPRIE Steering Committee. A randomized, blinded trial of clopidogrel versus aspirin in patients at risk of ischemic events (CAPRIE). *Lancet* 1996;348:1329–1339.

Criqui M H, Langer R D, Fronek A, et al. Mortality over a period of 10 years in patients with peripheral arterial disease. *N Engl J Med* 1992;326:381–386.

Dawson D L, Cutler B S, Meissner M H, et al. Cilostazol has beneficial effects in treatment of intermittent claudication: results from a multicenter, randomized, prospective, double-blind trial. *Circulation* 1998;98:678–686.

Hood S C, Moher D, Barber G G. Management of intermittent claudication with pentoxifylline: meta-analysis of randomized controlled trials. *Can Med Assoc J* 1996;155:1053–1059.

Janzon L, Bergqvist D, Boberg J, et al. Prevention of myocardial infarction and stroke in patients with intermittent claudication: effects of ticlopidine. Results from STIMS, the Swedish Ticlopidine Multi-centre Study. *J Intern Med* 1990;227:301–308.

Sutton-Tyrrell K, Rihal C, Sellers M A, et al. Long-term prognostic value of clinically evident noncoronary vascular disease in patients undergoing coronary revascularization in the bypass angioplasty revascularization investigation (BARI). *Am J Cardiol* 1998;81:375–381.

12
Palpitations

Erica Brownfield

1. What are the key historical elements in evaluating patients with palpitations?
2. What are the "red flags" associated with palpitations that require urgent cardiology referral or hospitalization?
3. What are important findings from physical examination, laboratory studies, and diagnostic tests?
4. When do patients with palpitations require further diagnostic tests?

Discussion

What Are the Key Historical Elements in Evaluating Patients with Palpitations?

Palpitations, or the unpleasant awareness of the heartbeat, is a common outpatient complaint. Palpitations can result from alterations in the heart rate, rhythm, or force of contraction. There is a large variation of patient symptoms and threshold of heartbeat awareness. Palpitations are usually benign, but can be a manifestation of a potentially life-threatening condition. There are several important questions to ask patients who present with palpitations, which can help determine the cause and risk of dangerous arrhythmias.

How Would You Describe the Palpitations?

There are some descriptions of palpitations that are useful for differential diagnosis. It can be useful to have the patient tap out the palpitations to get a sense of the rate and regularity. Premature atrial or ventricular contractions usually cause "flip-flopping" of the heart or the sensation of "skipped beats." Typically, there is a pause followed by a forceful systole after the premature contraction creating these sensations. "Rapid fluttering" or "chaotic, rapid heart beats" may be secondary to atrial fibrillation or atrial flutter. A "pounding in the neck" or "beating in the throat" may be secondary to paroxysms of rapid dysrhythmias, especially reentrant supraventricular tachycardia. Slow palpitations can be secondary to sinus bradycardia or different degrees of atrioventricular (AV) nodal block.

What Is the Manner of Onset and Termination of the Palpitations?

Palpitations that begin and end abruptly or can be terminated by vagal maneuvers are characteristic of paroxysmal supraventricular tachycardias. Those that are fleeting and repetitive are typical of premature contractions. Sinus tachycardia usually resolves slowly, following the cure of the underlying cause.

Under What Circumstances Do the Palpitations Occur?

Are the palpitations associated with anxiety or panic attacks? This is often tricky, because some patients find it difficult to determine which came first. Even so, one should not attribute palpitations to a psychiatric cause until arrhythmia is ruled out. Palpitations associated with position may be caused by AV nodal tachycardia. Often the palpitations appear with standing or bending over and end with lying down. Palpitations during periods of catecholamine excess are common and can be secondary to sinus tachycardia and supraventricular and ventricular tachycardias. One recently recognized rare disorder that manifests as palpitations during minimal exertion or with emotional stress is inappropriate sinus tachycardia. There is an inappropriate increase in sinus rate secondary to hypersensitivity to β-adrenergic stimulation. Palpitations associated with near syncope, syncope, or angina should prompt a search for ventricular tachycardia.

Is There Associated Increased Cardiovascular Risk?

When evaluating palpitations, it is important to know the patient's past medical history. A history of myocardial infarction, underlying heart disease, prior arrhythmias, or thyroid disease can be useful to narrow the differential diagnosis. Likewise, cardiac risk factors, medication use, symptoms of congestive heart failure, or a family history of sudden death is important to determine cause and assess risk. The age of the patient can sometimes be helpful, with supraventricular tachycardias beginning at younger ages and atrial fibrillation typically in older age groups.

What Are the "Red Flags" Associated with Palpitations that Require Urgent Cardiology Referral or Hospitalization?

Most patients with underlying organic heart disease or any myocardial abnormality that can lead to serious arrhythmias (e.g., scar, cardiomyopathies, valvular heart disease) should be admitted for evaluation. Likewise, patients with palpitations associated with near syncope, syncope, congestive heart failure, or angina, and those with a family history of syncope or sudden death from cardiac causes also should be evaluated in a monitored environment. Patients with palpitations associated with accessory conduction pathways (i.e., Wolf-Parkinson-White syndrome) should be referred to a cardiologist who specializes in electrophysiology for consideration of radioablative therapy.

What Are Important Findings from Physical Examination, Laboratory Studies, and Diagnostic Tests?

The physical examination is sometimes helpful in determining the cause of palpitations or assessing cardiac risk. First, one should pay close attention to vital signs, especially the rate and regularity of the pulse and if the blood pressure is compromised. Usually when a patient is in the office, the palpitations are not present. Therefore, abnormalities of the pulse may be uncommon. One should examine the patient for any evidence of thyroid disease, congestive heart failure, or valvular heart disease. It also may be helpful to have the patient take a brisk walk to try to elicit any palpitations.

Laboratory tests should be limited and focused. For example, if thyroid disease is considered, the thyroid-stimulating hormone level should be determined. A complete blood count is indicated if blood loss is suspected.

A 12-lead electrocardiogram (ECG) should be ordered on all patients with palpitations. Even though the yield is low, the test is easy, harmless, and cheap and can occasionally give clues as to the origin of palpitations or help with assessing cardiac risk. In a few cases, the actual arrhythmia is detected. A short PR interval and delta waves suggest ventricular preexcitation and the substrate for supraventricular tachycardia (Wolff-Parkinson-White syndrome). Prolongation of the QT interval may suggest long QT syndrome and the risk of polymorphic ventricular tachycardia. Q waves or other evidence of prior myocardial infarction should prompt an investigation into ventricular tachycardia originating from a cardiac scar. Complete heart block can be associated with premature ventricular depolarizations and polymorphic ventricular tachycardia.

When Do Patients with Palpitations Require Further Diagnostic Tests?

In most patients with palpitations, the history, physical examination and 12-lead ECG provide enough information to narrow the differential diagnosis and assess cardiac risk. Further diagnostic testing is indicated in the following groups of patients:

1. Those in whom the initial evaluation suggests an arrhythmic cause
2. Those who are at high risk for an arrhythmia (patients with organic heart disease or any myocardial abnormality that can lead to serious arrhythmias, family history of sudden death)
3. Those who need to have an explanation of their symptoms

Ambulatory monitoring devices (Holter, continuous loop event recorders) should be used in low-risk patients whose initial history or 12-lead ECG is suggestive of a well-tolerated unsustained arrhythmia and in those who are anxious to have an explanation of their symptoms. If the palpitations are sustained or poorly tolerated, an electrophysiology study, with or without prior ambulatory monitoring, is indicated.

Case

A 55-year-old man with a history of hypertension and gout presents to your office complaining of recurrent "fluttering" in his chest over the past few weeks. He states the sensations begin when he exerts himself and last for approximately 5 to 10 minutes. He denies any associated chest pain, but feels "short-winded" and light-headed during some of the events. One time, he "almost passed out." He thought the sensations were secondary to increased tobacco use during a stressful time in his life, but even with cutting back, the symptoms persist. He is currently taking atenolol and allopurinol. He has not taken any new medicines or any over-the-counter preparations. He denies alcohol or illicit drug use. There is no family history of sudden death. On examination, his blood pressure is 130/80 mm Hg; pulse is 65 beats/min and regular; respirations are 12 breaths/min. He is in no acute distress, but appears anxious. The rest of his examination is unremarkable.

1. Are there any worrisome elements in this patient's history?
2. What will you be looking for on a 12-lead electrocardiogram?
3. What would be the next step in the evaluation of this man's palpitations?

Case Discussion

Are There Any Worrisome Elements in This Patient's History?

The history indicates the patient has palpitations that are poorly tolerated. The fact that he becomes dyspneic and has presyncope associated with the palpitations should make you concerned that he is having an arrhythmia with hemodynamic compromise. Furthermore, the patient has cardiovascular risk factors, including hypertension and tobacco use. This information can become helpful when determining the substrate for an arrhythmia.

What Will You Be Looking For on a 12-lead Electrocardiogram?

Because of his cardiac risk factors, it is important to look for ECG evidence of prior myocardial infarction (Q waves, poor R-wave progression). One should also look at the P wave for evidence of left atrial abnormality (P mitrale), left ventricular hypertrophy, and atrial premature depolarizations suggesting a substrate for atrial fibrillation. His ECG revealed normal sinus rhythm at a rate of 65 beats/min and a left bundle branch block.

What Would Be the Next Step in the Evaluation of This Man's Palpitations?

This patient should be admitted for further workup and monitoring. Because he has at least three cardiac risk factors (male, tobacco use, hypertension), an abnormal resting ECG suggesting a myocardial abnormality, and poorly tolerated palpitations, a serious arrhythmia needs to be ruled out. Once hospitalized, if cardiac monitoring does not reveal an arrhythmia, this patient should be evaluated for possible ischemia and may be a candidate for further electrophysiologic studies.

Suggested Reading

Barsky, A J et al. The clinical course of palpitations in medical outpatients. *Arch Intern Med* 1995;155: 1782–1788.
Brugada P, et al. Investigation of palpitations. *Lancet* 1993;341:1254–1258.
Zimetbaum P, Josephson M. Evaluation of patients with palpitations. *N Engl J Med* 1998;338: 1369–1373.

III
Dermatology

13
Acne

Alexia M. Torke
Calvin O. McCall

1. What is the pathogenesis of acne?
2. What diagnostic evaluation is appropriate?
3. What medications are available for acne treatment?
4. How do I choose the right medication?

Discussion

What Is the Pathogenesis of Acne?

Acne is a common disorder that affects 85% or more of adolescents and 8% of adults 25 to 34 years of age. An understanding of the pathogenesis of acne can help guide treatment.

Acne is a disorder of the pilosebaceous unit. There are four factors involved: (a) obstruction of follicles; (b) increased sebum production; (c) the organism *Propionibacterium acnes;* and (d) inflammation.

In persons with acne, increased proliferation and decreased desquamation of keratinocytes lead to obstructed follicles called microcomedos. The cause of this abnormal keratinization has not been identified, but may be due to abnormal epithelial cell differentiation, possibly induced by abnormal sebum.

In adolescence, increased production of the hormone dehydroepiandrosterone sulfate (DHEA-S) leads to increased sebum production. Although there is some evidence that DHEA-S levels are higher in girls with acne than in girls without acne, most people with acne have normal DHEA-S levels. It may be that the follicles of acne-prone individuals are more sensitive to hormonal stimulation.

Propionibacterium acnes is a gram-positive diphtheroid bacterium normally found on the skin. Sebum acts as a growth medium, so a high sebum level leads to increased *P. acnes* proliferation. *P. acnes* leads to inflammation through two mechanisms. First, the bacteria hydrolyze triglycerides to free fatty acids. Second, the bacteria attract neutrophils that release mediators of inflammation.

The characteristic lesions of acne include comedomes, inflammatory lesions (e.g., pustules, papules, and nodules) and healing inflammatory lesions, which may cause scars, or cysts. Comedones develop from plugged follicles. If there is only a microscopic opening onto the skin, the comedo appears white (closed comedo or whitehead). If the opening is dilated, it appears black (open comedo or blackhead). It is uncertain what causes the black discoloration.

What Diagnostic Evaluation Is Appropriate?

The history should include an assessment of skin care, cosmetic use, and exposure to potential irritants. Washing the face may remove sebum, but too much washing can irritate the skin. A person with acne should wash gently with a mild soap twice daily. Cosmetics and moisturizers may worsen acne, as may greases used to style hair. Water-based cosmetics and moisturizers are less comedogenic than oil-based products. Acne also can be worsened by mechanical trauma from clothing and sports equipment, as well as from picking or squeezing the skin.

Hormonal factors should be assessed in women. Are there premenstrual acne flare-ups? These may occur due to the androgenic effects of progesterone. Acne is commonly found in women with polycystic ovarian syndrome (PCOS), which is characterized by mildly elevated testosterone levels. Symptoms and signs include menstrual irregularities, obesity, hirsutism, and infertility. However, the sudden onset of virilization is a worrisome finding that requires further evaluation by an endocrinologist because it may be caused by an adrenal or ovarian tumor.

Although previously thought to be a factor, diet is not an important causative agent in acne.

What Medications Are Available for Acne Treatment?

There are many topical and systemic agents available to treat acne. Because it takes about 8 weeks for a comedo to mature, any acne medicine should be continued for that length of time to assess its effectiveness.

Topical Therapies

Topical therapies have several effects on acne. They function to resolve comedones (comedolytic agents), decrease inflammation, normalize keratinization, and inhibit *P. acnes* (Table 13.1). Topical therapies should be applied to all acne-prone areas. They are not intended for "spot treatment" of lesions.

Retinoids normalize the process of follicular keratinization, leading to fewer obstructive lesions. They also have comedolytic effects. Tretinoin is a retinoid available in many formulations. Because this medication can be irritating to the skin, a low dose should initially be used, titrating upward. The order of potency is 0.025% cream, 0.05% cream, 0.01% gel, 0.025% gel, 0.1% cream, and 0.05% solution. The final decision about which vehicle to use depends on the patient's skin type. Creams are moisturizing, whereas gels and solutions are drying.

To reduce irritation, patients should wait at least 20 to 30 minutes after washing the face to apply tretinoin. There is a microencapsulated form of tretinoin that may be less irritating to skin.

Cutaneous side effects of tretinoin include redness, drying, hypopigmentation in persons with dark skin, and photosensitivity. There have not been any reported cases of teratogenicity with tretinoin, but due to the severe birth defects caused by

Table 13.1. Effects of Topical Agents for Acne

Comedolytics
  Salicylic acid
  Adapalene
  Tretinoin
  Tazarotene
  Benzoyl peroxide
Antiinflammatory medications
  Azelaic acid
  Adapalene
Medications that alter keratinization
  Tretinoin
  Adapalene
  Azelaic acid
Propionibacterium acne inhibitors
  Benzoyl peroxide
  Antibiotics
  Azelaic acid

systemic retinoids, topical retinoids are generally avoided in women who are pregnant. Tretinoin is a pregnancy class C drug.

Adapalene is another retinoid-like agent that has both comedolytic and antiinflammatory properties. It appears to be as effective but less irritating than tretinoin. Tazarotene is a retinoid used in the treatment of both psoriasis and acne. Tazarotene is a pregnancy class X drug.

Salicylic acid, a comedolytic agent, may have antiinflammatory effects. It is less effective than tretinoin but is also less irritating.

Azelaic acid has antiinflammatory effects and may alter keratinization. It can cause pruritis, burning, and erythema. It may occasionally produce hypopigmentation in persons with dark skin.

Topical antibiotics have direct effects against *P. acnes*. Suppressing *P. acnes* leads to a decrease in inflammatory lesions. Resistance to the topical agents can occur and is prevented by combination therapy with benzoyl peroxide (BP). The most commonly prescribed topical antibiotics, clindamycin and erythromycin, are about equally effective.

Benzoyl peroxide decreases bacterial colonization and also has comedolytic effects. BP can cause stinging, redness, and drying, and occasionally causes contact dermatitis. A small test spot can be applied and watched for 48 to 72 hours before BP is applied to the face. BP is a pregnancy class C drug.

Systemic Therapy

Antibiotics and retinoids are the mainstays of systemic therapy for acne. Hormonal therapies have a role in treatment for some women.

Systemic antibiotics are more effective in decreasing *P. acnes* than topical agents. Some antibiotics, such as tetracycline, also may directly suppress inflammation. Side effects of systemic antibiotics include vaginal candidiasis and gastrointestinal symptoms. Oral antibiotics also may decrease the effectiveness of oral contraceptives. It is extremely important to discuss this possibility with a female patient before the antibiotic is started.

Tetracycline is commonly used due to its effectiveness and low cost. It is usually given at a dose of 500 mg twice daily, although 250 mg twice daily also may be effective. Tetracycline cannot be used in pregnant women or children under 12, and should be taken on an empty stomach. Erythromycin is also commonly used in doses of 250 to 500 mg twice daily. Its use is often limited by gastrointestinal side effects. Doxycycline can be taken at doses of 100 mg twice daily. Like tetracycline, doxycycline may be photosensitizing in some patients. Minocycline is thought to be more effective than other systemic antibiotics, although this has not been proven in clinical trials. This drug has some potentially serious side effects, including autoimmune hepatitis, tooth discoloration, and hypersensitivity reactions. It also may cause a bothersome blue-gray discoloration of the skin, especially in acne scars.

Isotretinoin, a systemic retinoid, is extremely effective for severe refractory acne. It alters sebum production for up to a year after discontinuation, and has antiinflammatory properties as well. Because of its extensive side effect profile, it is reserved for acne that is especially severe or that fails to respond to other therapies. A dermatologist should generally prescribe it. The most feared complications in women are teratogenicity and spontaneous abortions. For this reason, isotretinoin should be started on day 2 or 3 of the menstrual cycle after a negative pregnancy test. Women who are sexually active should use two forms of birth control. Other side effects include cheilitis, skin peeling, increased triglycerides, elevated hepatic transaminases, and depression.

Hormonal therapy is an adjunctive treatment of acne for patients with endocrine abnormalities such as PCOS. Oral contraceptives containing a progesterone with low androgenic effects, such as norethindrone, ethynodiol diacetate, or norgestimate should be selected. The estrogen component of oral contraceptives also may improve acne by increasing sex hormone–binding globulin, which reduces active free testosterone levels, and by decreasing gonadotropin secretion, which lowers ovarian androgen secretion. Oral antiandrogens such as spironolactone are also effective in women with PCOS. An oral contraceptive containing norgestimate and ethinylestradiol was recently shown to be effective in women without hormonal abnormalities.

How Do I Choose the Right Medication?

Choice of therapy should be guided by the type and severity of acne. Acne can be classified into three types: comedonal, inflammatory, and nodulocystic. Comedolytics are first-line agents for mild comedonal acne. Moderate to severe cases of comedonal acne respond well to topical retinoids, which prevent the formation of comedones.

Inflammatory acne involves papules and pustules in addition to comedones, and is usually treated with topical agents such as benzoyl peroxide, plus a topical or systemic antibiotic.

Nodulocystic acne involves the above features plus cysts or abscesses. Topical agents are not initially effective for this type of acne. Initial treatment should consist of systemic antibiotics such as tetracycline, doxycycline, or erythromycin. If these are not effective after 8 weeks, the patient should be referred for consideration of minocycline or isotretinoin.

There is evidence that combination regimens may be more effective than single agents. For example, the combination of BP plus erythromycin is more effective than either drug alone. Because some topical medications can inactivate others, one agent should be applied in the morning and the other at night.

Oral contraceptives are effective for acne in women with PCOS. There is also some evidence that women with normal hormone levels may benefit from norgestimate/ethinylestradiol pills.

Case

A 25-year-old white woman comes to your office complaining of acne. She states that she has had it since she was 12 years of age and is frustrated because she thought it would go away by now. She uses over-the-counter BP and washes her face three to four times a day. Her past medical history is unremarkable. She notes that her menses are irregular, occurring once every 3 to 4 months. On physical examination, she is mildly overweight (body mass index of 26) and has numerous open and closed comedones on her face with some papules. Her skin is dry and slightly reddened.

1. What type of acne does this patient have?
2. What should you tell this patient about her condition?
3. What medications are most appropriate?

Case Discussion

What Type of Acne Does This Patient Have?

She has mixed comedonal acne and inflammatory acne. Although many young adults with normal hormone levels continue to suffer from acne, her irregular menses and high body weight are clues that she may have PCOS. A laboratory evaluation for PCOS is appropriate.

What Should You Tell This Patient About Her Condition?

It is important to tell her that frequent scrubbing will not cure acne. In fact, it may irritate the skin further. Because her skin is irritated, she should wash only twice a day with mild soap and water. Pinching or popping pimples will often cause them to resolve more slowly and may cause scarring. She should avoid oil-based makeup, moisturizers, and hair products. Water-based or noncomedogenic products will be less likely to worsen her acne.

What Medications Are Most Appropriate?

Because she is not responding to the BP alone, addition of a topical retinoid may help, as long as she does not plan to become pregnant. She should use the two medicines at different times of day so the BP will not inactivate the retinoid. If this therapy is not successful after 8 weeks, a combination of a topical retinoid and an oral antibiotic would be a reasonable choice. If she has evidence of PCOS, an oral contraceptive containing a progesterone with low androgenic potential or spironolactone may be helpful. OCPs may improve her acne even if her hormone levels are normal.

Suggested Reading

Cunliffe W J, Caputo R, Dreno B, et al. Clinical efficacy and safety comparison of adapalene gel and tretinoin gel in the treatment of acne vulgaris: Europe and US multicenter trials. *J Am Acad Dermatol* 1997:36(suppl);126–134.

Johnson B A, Nunley J R. Topical therapy for acne vulgaris: How do you choose the best drug for each patient? *Postgrad Med* 2000:107;69–80.

Krowchuk D P. Treating acne: A practical guide. *Med Clin North Am* 2000:84;811–828.

Packman A M, Brown R H, Dunlap F E, et al. Treatment of acne vulgaris: combination of 3% erythromycin and 5% benzoyl peroxide in a gel compared to clindamycin phosphate lotion. *Int J Dermatol* 1996:35;209–211.

Redmond G P, Olson W H, Lippman J S, et al. Norgestimate and ethinyl estradiol in the treatment of acne vulgaris: a randomized, placebo-controlled trial. *Obstet Gynecol* 1997:89;615–622.

Weiss, J S. Current options for the topical treatment of acne vulgaris. *Pediatr Dermatol* 1997:14;480–488.

Wirth F. Approach to acne vulgaris. *Up to Date* 1999:7.

14
Common Skin Rashes

Lesley S. Miller
Calvin O. McCall

1. What are the basic categories of skin rashes?
2. What key history and physical examination findings are important in diagnosing four rashes commonly seen in the ambulatory setting: urticaria, candidiasis, folliculitis, and allergic contact dermatitis?
3. How are these rashes treated?
4. When is referral to a dermatologist appropriate?

Discussion

What Are the Basic Categories of Skin Rashes?

The majority of rashes can be divided into two basic categories: infectious and inflammatory. Rashes with an infectious etiology include candidiasis, tinea, bacterial folliculitis, herpes simplex virus, impetigo, and herpes zoster virus. Common inflammatory rashes include acne, atopic dermatitis, psoriasis, rosacea, and urticaria.

What Key History and Physical Examination Findings Are Important in Diagnosing Four Rashes Commonly Seen in the Ambulatory Setting: Urticaria, Candidiasis, Folliculitis, and Allergic Contact Dermatitis?

Urticaria is a common rash with no identifiable cause in up to 80% of cases. Heredity may play a role in a small number of patients. Urticaria develops from a type I immunoglobulin E (IgE)-mediated hypersensitivity reaction. IgE causes histamine release from mast cells, resulting in transudation of fluid from cutaneous blood vessels into the dermis and the characteristic urticarial wheal. There are several types of urticaria. Acute urticaria, the most common form, has an abrupt onset and clears within 1 to 6 weeks. Chronic urticaria lasts from months to decades and may be associated with autoantibodies to the mast cell IgE receptor. Adrenergic urticaria, a rare form of the disease, is associated with the formation of lesions during times of stress and may be treated with beta blockade. Physical urticaria occurs secondary to skin trauma, and may be further subdivided into heat, cold, and solar urticaria, depending on the particular stimulus that causes the lesions. Finally, angioedema, which can be life threatening, may occur with or without urticaria, and is often caused by the same stimuli.

Taking a history is the key to evaluating any patient who presents with urticaria. Important information to elicit from the patient includes a description of the onset of the lesions, their location, and any history of prior episodes. A history of recent infections and medication use is crucial. Urticaria caused by medications may persist after the discontinuation of the offending agent, so even a remote history of medication use is important. A food history is helpful, as is a history of exposure to contactants. Allergens that may contribute to this cascade of events include infections, foods, contactants, insect bites, and medications. Common medications implicated in causing urticaria are morphine, codeine, penicillin, meperidine, quinine, aspirin, nonsteroidal antiinflammatory drugs (NSAIDs), and contrast dye. Foods that trigger urticaria include eggs, fish, shellfish, milk, chocolate, cheese, yeast, spices, pork, strawberries, nuts, and tomatoes.

Physical examination in a patient with active urticaria reveals few to thousands of pruritic, short-lived wheals that may appear as erythematous papules or plaques. They are usually round to oval in shape with peripheral blanching. Individual lesions range from a few millimeters to several centimeters in size, last from 1 to 24 hours, and may be associated with secondary changes, including excoriation and purpura.

Candidiasis is a common infectious rash occurring in all age groups and in a variety of locations throughout the body. The three most common sites for candidal infection are oral, genital, and cutaneous. The evaluation of a patient with suspected candidal infection includes a scrape of the involved skin and preparation of the specimen with 10% to 20% potassium hydroxide (KOH). A positive specimen examined under light microscopy reveals budding spores and pseudohyphae. The several risk factors for candidal infection can be divided into local factors and systemic diseases. Local factors include heat, moisture, occlusion, friction, and loss of epithelium and barrier function. Systemic illnesses or conditions that predispose patients to candidiasis include diabetes mellitus, thyroid disease, and immunosuppression (e.g., acquired immunodeficiency syndrome, malignancy, and use of immunosuppressive medications). In addition, use of antibiotics may increase the burden of yeast and cause candidal infection through removal of competing bacterial organisms.

There are several distinct types of oral candidal infections. Thrush can occur in diabetic and immunocompromised patients, as well as in those using antibiotics. The characteristic white, cheesy plaques that occur on the buccal mucosa, palate, and tongue easily scrape off. Acute atrophic candidiasis is seen with use of meterdose inhalers for asthma and chronic obstructive lung disease, as well as with use of systemic antibiotics. It is characterized by painful atrophic erythematous plaques located on the dorsum of the tongue and on the gums. Dental stomatitis occurs commonly in patients with poorly fitting dentures. Finally, angular cheilitis may be a primary phenomenon or may be seen secondary to thrush or dental stomatitis. It is most common in edentulous patients and is characterized by erythema, dryness, and cracking in the corners of the mouth.

Vulvovaginitis is a form of genital candidiasis in which white plaques on a beefy red base are found on the vaginal mucosa. There are often associated satellite pustules or scaling plaques, as well as perineal involvement. A thick white vaginal discharge may be present, and is seen more commonly with pregnancy, oral contraceptive use, and immunosuppressed states. The patient often complains of genital burning, pain, and pruritis, so it is crucial to distinguish candidal vulvovaginitis from sexually transmitted diseases that may present with similar complaints. Balanitis occurs more commonly in uncircumcised men and in those with diabetes. It is usually seen on the glans penis, either as small papules and pustules, or as vesicles that eventually rupture.

Finally, cutaneous candidal infections present most often with intertrigenal involvement, including inguinal, perineal, inframammary, and finger web areas. These are areas affected by heat, moisture, and occlusion. Intertrigo appears as macerated, erythematous plaques with sharp borders, peripheral scale, and sometimes satellite pustules and ulcerations. Diabetes is an important risk factor for cutaneous candidal infection, as is obesity and antibiotic use. Paronychia caused by *Candida* species presents with erythematous, edematous nail folds with purulent discharge. This infection is seen in patients with prolonged immersion of their fingers in water, and secondary infection of the involved areas is common.

Folliculitis, an infection of the hair follicles, is most commonly caused by staphylococcal species, but may also be caused by gram-negative organisms such as *Pseudomonas aeruginosa*. Folliculitis secondary to gram-negative organisms is usually found in patients who are taking antibiotics, whereas *Pseudomonas* folliculitis (hot tub folliculitis) is caused by bathing in whirlpools and hot tubs that have not been properly disinfected. Chronic carriers of *Staphylococcus* are at highest risk for folliculitis.

The rash of staphylococcal folliculitis appears as painless, erythematous papules or pustules centered around the hair follicle. The lesions occur most often on the scalp, buttocks, and extremities. They appear in crops and heal without scarring in 7 to 10 days. The rash is usually asymptomatic but may be pruritic. With gram-negative folliculitis, patients present with multiple pustules on the face, or less commonly with deep nodular cysts. Folliculitis caused by *Pseudomonas* occurs 1 to 3 days after water exposure and presents as multiple painful, pruritic papules and pustules. The lesions resolve spontaneously in 1 to 2 weeks.

Allergic contact dermatitis is a form of eczematous dermatitis precipitated by chemical exposure. It is caused by a cell-mediated hypersensitivity reaction, and the intensity of the reaction depends on the degree of sensitivity to the allergen. The reaction is delayed on the first exposure, with an incubation period of 5 to 21 days after initial antigen contact. For subsequent exposures, the incubation period decreases to 12 to 48 hours. Common allergens that initiate this reaction include plants such as poison oak, ivy, and sumac, chemicals and metals such as nickel, rubber compounds, benzocaine, formaldehyde, and various cosmetics, including perfumes. Sensitivity to these agents is quite common, with 25% to 60% of North Americans sensitive to poison oak, ivy, and sumac, and 10% of women allergic to nickel.

Allergic contact dermatitis can be characterized as acute, subacute, and chronic. In acute allergic contact dermatitis, the rash is characterized by acute inflammatory changes: erythema, blistering, crust, and necrosis. The lesions are intensely pruritic. In the subacute stage, one finds erythema, scale, fissuring, and a scalded appearance to the skin. Finally, in the chronic stage, the skin becomes thickened and lichenified, and there may be evidence of excoriation. The key to diagnosing allergic contact dermatitis lies first in recognizing the eczematous changes, and then identifying the pattern, distribution, shape, and locations of the lesions. Plant dermatoses characteristically have a linear shape from dragging the allergen over the skin. On the other hand, a reaction from nickel in jewelry will be localized to the skin underlying the offending agent.

How Are These Rashes Treated?

The first step in treatment of *urticaria* is to identify and remove any precipitating or exacerbating factors. Topical therapy may be instituted with calamine, menthol camphor, or doxepin hydrochloride. The mainstays of treatment, however, are antihistamines. The most commonly used long-acting antihistamines are loratidine, cetirizine, and fexofenadine. Loratidine and cetirizine are efficacious, cause little sedation, and have few drug–drug interactions. The short-acting antihistamines hydroxyzine, diphenhydramine, and doxepin are still considered most effective in treating urticaria, but their use is limited by sedation. Hydroxyzine has anxiolytic effects and may be used for the particularly distressed and anxious patient, especially at bedtime. Doxepin may be the most potent agent with the longest duration of action, but it has prominent anticholinergic effects and should be used with caution in the elderly and in patients with cardiac arrhythmias.

Treatment of candidal infection begins with removing any promoting factors and optimally treating underlying predisposing diseases, such as diabetes. Drying agents may be used, including acetic acid, zinc oxide paste, and Burow solution. Topical therapy for mucosal and cutaneous infection includes polyene and azole preparations, such as ketoconazole, clotrimazole, miconazole, and econazole, applied twice daily for 14 days. Hydrocortisone topical preparations may be used with topical antifungals if the infection is associated with severe inflammation. For vulvovaginitis, miconazole may be given intravaginally at bedtime for 3 to 7 days. For recurrent or resistant infections, systemic therapy should be instituted in addition to topical therapy. Fluconazole is used to treat oral thrush and vulvovaginitis, either with a one-time dose of 150 mg or 100 mg daily for 7 days. For cutaneous infection, treatment should continue for 1 to 2 weeks.

Staphylococcal *folliculitis,* when localized, can be treated with topical clindamycin or erythromycin applied twice daily, or mupirocin 2% ointment applied three times daily. Antibacterial soaps are also helpful to decrease the bacterial burden on the skin. For more extensive infections, oral antibiotics, including dicloxacillin, cephalexin, erythromycin, or amoxicillin clavulanate, may be necessary. Eradication of the staphylococcal carrier state with systemic antibiotic therapy should be considered in cases of recurrent or recalcitrant staphylococcal folliculitis. For gram-negative folliculitis, the first step of treatment is discontinuation of antibiotics for acne. Therapy with ampicillin, trimethoprim-sulfamethoxazole, or amoxicillin clavulanate may then be instituted. For pseudomonal folliculitis, no specific therapy is necessary because the infection is self-limited and will resolve spontaneously.

Treatment for *contact dermatitis* first and foremost involves identifying and avoiding the causative allergen. For reactions involving only a small area of skin, the mainstay of treatment is with topical corticosteroids. High-potency agents may be used for up to 2 weeks, and ointments are preferred to creams. It is important to avoid these agents on the face or in intertrigenous areas and use medium potency topical steroids instead. Nonsedating antihistamines such as cetirizine and loratidine are useful for pruritis. Cold compresses with Burow solution, or acetic acid or oatmeal colloidal baths are also useful adjunctive therapies. For dermatitis involving greater than 20% of body surface area, treatment with systemic steroids is warranted. This consists of prednisone starting at a dose of 1 mg/kg given as a 2-week taper. Intramuscular triamcinolone is sometimes used as well.

When Is Referral to a Dermatologist Appropriate?

Patients with urticaria should be referred to a subspecialist if an anaphylactic reaction is associated with urticaria, or in the presence of associated collagen vascular disease. Poor control with antihistamines, a suspected contact allergic component, and association with other dermatologic conditions are additional indications for referral. In the case of candidal infections, patients with chronic mucocutaneous candidiasis, other chronic candidal infections, or inadequate response to initial treatment should be referred to a dermatologist. A dermatology referral is also appropriate for patients with folliculitis that fails to show a rapid therapeutic response to standard treatment, or allergic contact dermatitis that is either resistant to treatment or recurs frequently.

Case 1

A 63-year-old woman with diabetes mellitus presents to your office complaining of a rash under her breasts. She states that she has had a similar rash in the past, and it usually occurs in the summer. She complains of localized pruritis and intense reddening of the skin. She has had no relief with the use of an over-the-counter corticosteroid cream. Her medications include oral glipizide 5 mg daily. A physical examination reveals an obese female with macerated inframammary plaques, which are bright red-orange in color. The borders of the plaques are well demarcated. Laboratory studies reveal a glycosylated hemoglobin level of 11%.

1. What is the most likely causative agent of this rash?
2. What are this patient's risk factors for acquiring the rash, and how might they be modified?
3. How should the patient be treated?

Case Discussion

What Is the Most Likely Causative Agent of This Rash?

This patient presents with a history and physical examination that is highly suggestive of intertrigo caused by a cutaneous candidal infection.

What Are This Patient's Risk Factors for Acquiring the Rash, and How Might They Be Modified?

Uncontrolled diabetes mellitus is this patient's most significant risk factor for candidal infection. The fact that she frequently develops the rash during the summer months suggests that local factors, such as heat and moisture, play a role as well. Risk factor modification includes addressing local factors by wearing loose, breathable clothing, and keeping the area dry. Optimizing control of the patient's diabetes is crucial in reducing her risk for candidal infection, and weight loss would also reduce her risk of infection.

How Should the Rash Be Treated?

The diagnosis should be confirmed with a scrape of the rash and KOH preparation. The patient should be instructed to wear loose-fitting cotton clothing. A drying agent, like Burow solution may be used, along with air drying the affected skin several times a day. Topical preparations such as ketoconazole, clotrimazole, miconazole, or econazole should be applied to the affected area twice daily for 14 days.

Case 2

A 20-year-old college student presents to your office complaining of an intensely pruritic rash on his lower legs. He has just returned from a hiking trip. The patient states that he cannot sleep because the itching is so severe. Physical examination of the lower extremities reveals two 5-cm linear erythematous patches with overlying vesicles, some of which are draining.

1. What is the most likely diagnosis in this patient?
2. How should the rash be treated?

Case Discussion
What Is This Patient's Diagnosis?

This patient's history and physical examination are most consistent with contact dermatitis, likely from exposure to a plant of the *Rhus* genus: poison oak, ivy, or sumac.

How Should the Rash Be Treated?

The patient should first be treated with an antihistamine given the intensity of his pruritis. Because the area of skin involved in the dermatitis is minimal, high-potency topical corticosteroid creams, such as halobetasol propionate, clobetasol propionate, betamethasone, or diflorasone may be used. Use should be limited to 2 weeks, and the patient should be warned not to use these agents on the face or groin area. The patient should be advised to wear tightly woven fabrics that cover exposed skin when there is a high likelihood of encountering irritant plants.

Suggested Reading

Arndt K A, Wintroub B U, Robinson J K, et al., eds. *Primary care dermatology.* Philadelphia: WB Saunders Company, 1997.

Feldman S R, Fleischer A B Jr, McConnell C R. Most common dermatologic problems identified by internists, 1990–1994. *Arch Intern Med* 1998;158:726–730.

Fleischer A B, Feldman S R, Katz A S, et al., eds. *20 Common problems in dermatology.* New York: McGraw-Hill, 2000.

Fleischer A B Jr, Feldman S R, McConnell R C. The most common skin problems seen by family practitioners, 1990–1994. *Family Med* 1997;29:648–652.

Friedman S J. Approach to the patient with dermatitis: atopic and contact dermatitis. In: Goroll, ed. *Primary care medicine,* 3rd ed. Philadelphia: Lippincott-Raven, 1995:907–910.

Hooper B J, Goldman M P. *Primary dermatologic care.* St. Louis: CV Mosby, 1999.

Shellow W V R. Management of intertrigo and intertrigenous dermatoses. In: Goroll, ed. *Primary care medicine,* 3rd ed. Philadelphia: Lippincott-Raven, 1995:920–922.

IV

Endocrinology and Diabetes

15

Care of the Patient with Well-Controlled Type 2 Diabetes

Judith R. Rudnick

1. How is the diagnosis of type 2 diabetes made?
2. Which components of the history and physical examination are recommended at every visit for patients with type 2 diabetes?
3. Which laboratory tests are routinely monitored in patients with diabetes and at what frequency?
4. What other interventions are recommended for patients with diabetes?

Discussion

How Is the Diagnosis of Type 2 Diabetes Made?

The diagnostic criteria for diabetes have been revised recently. There are currently three ways to diagnose diabetes: a fasting glucose of at least 126 mg/dL, a random plasma glucose of at least 200 mg/dL in association with symptoms of diabetes, or a 2-hour postprandial glucose level of at least 200 mg/dL during an oral glucose tolerance test. The classic symptoms of diabetes are polyuria, polydipsia, and weight loss. The current definitions are based on population studies showing an association between plasma glucose levels and microvascular complications of diabetes. Note that assessment of glycosylated hemoglobin (HbAlc) is not currently used to diagnose diabetes.

Which Components of the History and Physical Examination Are Recommended at Every Visit for Patients with Type 2 Diabetes?

Diabetes is a chronic illness; patients with diabetes require continuing medical care to prevent acute complications of the disease (e.g., diabetic ketoacidosis, hyperosmolar coma, and hypoglycemia) and to reduce the risk of long-term macrovascular (e.g., coronary atherosclerosis, stroke, and peripheral vascular disease) and microvascular (e.g., nephropathy, neuropathy, and retinopathy) complications. Comprehensive care of the patient with diabetes includes maximizing glycemic control.

The American Diabetes Association currently recommends that patients with diabetes be seen at least quarterly until glycemic control is achieved. Patients whose therapy is being modified may need to be seen even more frequently. At every visit the following components of the history should be reviewed:

- Frequency and causes of hyper-/hypoglycemia
- Results of self-monitored glucose measurements
- Any changes in medication or diet
- Any problems with adherence to medical or dietary regimen
- Symptoms suggesting complications of diabetes (e.g., visual changes, numbness/tingling of extremities, etc.)
- Current medications
- Tobacco and alcohol use

Routine follow-up physical examination should include the following:

- Weight
- Blood pressure
- Funduscopy
- Foot examination

Check blood pressure at every visit, because hypertension is common in diabetic patients and is often present at the time of diagnosis.

All patients with type 2 diabetes are at risk for retinopathy. As many as 21% of newly diagnosed patients with type 2 diabetes have some degree of retinopathy at the time of diagnosis. Patients with type 1 diabetes generally do not develop retinopathy in the first 5 years of the disease. An annual dilated funduscopic examination performed by an ophthalmologist is recommended.

At each visit, all patients with diabetes should have a foot examination with shoes and socks removed. Patients with a "high-risk foot" are those with peripheral neuropathy, peripheral vascular disease, callous formation, limited joint mobility, or a history of amputation or ulcer.

Which Laboratory Tests Are Routinely Monitored in Diabetic Patients and at What Frequency?

An HbAlc measurement documents the degree of glycemic control at the initial assessment and as part of continuing care. Because HbAlc reflects average glycemia over 2 to 3 months, measurement about every 3 months will determine whether metabolic control has been achieved. There are no well-controlled studies that suggest a definite testing protocol. Current standards include testing twice a year for patients with stable glycemic control and every 3 months for patients whose therapy has changed or whose glucose is not well controlled. A target HbAlc measurement is a value of less than 7.0%.

Fasting lipids should be measured annually, including low-density lipoprotein (LDL) cholesterol, high density lipoprotein (HDL) cholesterol, and triglycerides. The National Cholesterol Education program recommends that patients with diabetes be classified the same as patients with known coronary disease. The target

LDL level is less than 100 mg/dL, HDL is greater than 45 mg/dL, and triglycerides less than 200 mg/dL. Lipid-lowering agents should be considered for LDL values greater than 130 mg/dL, HDL values less than 35 mg/dL, or triglycerides greater than 400 mg/dL.

A urinary albumin:creatinine ratio should be measured annually to look for evidence of microalbuminuria. If the initial test result is abnormal (>30 mg/g), a repeat test is performed for confirmation; if the second test result is negative, then a third test is recommended. A patient should have two positive test results before a diagnosis of microalbuminuria is made. For patients with documented microalbuminuria, tight blood pressure control is of paramount importance, and treatment with an angiotensin-converting enzyme (ACE) inhibitor should be strongly considered because ACE inhibitors have been shown to decrease the rate of progression of renal disease. Once a patient with microalbuminuria is already taking full doses of an ACE inhibitor, the role of continued measurement of urine albumin:creatinine ratios is less clear but may help assess response to therapy and progression of disease. A positive urinary dipstick test result for protein suggests macroalbuminuria is present (≥300 mg/24 h). A 24-hour urinary collection for protein and creatinine is warranted in these cases.

What Other Interventions Are Recommended for Patients with Diabetes?

It is recommended that patients with diabetes receive influenza vaccination annually (in the fall), because they are at higher risk for complications from influenza. Patients with diabetes also should be encouraged to receive the pneumovax if they have not previously done so.

Case

A 58-year-old woman comes to your office for a scheduled follow up visit. She has had diabetes for 8 years; she takes glipizide XL 10 mg daily as her only medication. She checks fasting sugars weekly, and they have ranged from 80 to 130 mg/dL over the past 2 months. She had a brother who died of a myocardial infarction at age 42. She has no complaints of polyuria, polydipsia, or changes in her vision. Physical examination shows a blood pressure of 140/88 mm Hg, and weight of 201 pounds. A funduscopic examination shows flat optic discs, and no hemorrhages or proliferative retinopathy. Her lungs are clear, the cardiopulmonary examination is normal, and her feet show no skin lesions, but toenails are yellowed and cracked. The most recent laboratory studies were performed prior to her last visit 3 months ago. HbAlc is 6.9%, urine albumin:creatinine ratio is 3.0 mg/g, LDL cholesterol is 118 mg/dL, HDL cholesterol is 45 mg/dL, and triglycerides are 233 mg/dL.

1. What additional information should you obtain from this patient at this visit?
2. Is this patient meeting glycemic controls?
3. Does this patient require referral to any specialist providers?
4. Does this patient require any changes or additions to her current therapy?

Case Discussion

What Additional Information Should You Obtain from This Patient at This Visit?

Most of the recommended components are recorded above. However, a tobacco and alcohol history should also be obtained. Smoking is an independent risk factor in the development of cardiovascular disease. Patients should be encouraged to quit smoking at every visit. Alcohol use can make sugars more difficult to control and is associated with blood pressure elevation.

Is This Patient Meeting Glycemic Controls?

Yes she is. The goal range of fasting blood sugar in type 2 diabetes is 80-120 mg/dL and nighttime glucose of 100-140 mg/dL (normal is less than 100 mg/dL); a change in therapy should be considered if values are greater than 140 mg/dL or less than 80 mg/dL. The target HbAlc value is less than 7%.

The patient has a home glucose monitor and checks her fasting blood sugar weekly. This patient's home values are mostly within this range. The optimal frequency of glucose monitoring for patients with type 2 diabetes is not known. The current recommendations are only that frequency be sufficient to reach glucose goals. For patients taking insulin and sulfonylureas, home glucose monitoring helps detect asymptomatic hypoglycemia. In addition, her last HbAlc value of 6.9% meets her goal. Since her last value was determined 3 months ago, she should have this repeated 3 months from now to ensure her average glycemic control remains adequate. The natural history of diabetes is for sugars to increase over time; it is routine for changes in therapy to be required as the duration of disease increases.

Does This Patient Require Referral to Any Specialist Providers?

This patient should be referred to an ophthalmologist and podiatrist. In addition to funduscopy at every visit, patients with diabetes should be checked annually with a dilated retinal examination by an ophthalmologist. Studies have shown that primary care providers do not detect early stages of retinopathy at the frequency at which it occurs. Examination by an ophthalmologist is recommended to detect diabetic retinopathy at an early stage. Laser surgery for proliferative retinopathy significantly reduces the incidence of visual loss in patients with diabetes. Untreated proliferative retinopathy leads to visual loss and complete blindness. Up to 21% of patients with type 2 diabetes will develop retinopathy and almost half of them will become blind because of it. To prevent blindness, know when your patient's last dilated retinal examination was performed. Refer patients with new funduscopic findings to the ophthalmologist promptly.

This patient also should be referred to a podiatrist to assess her cracked toenails. They should be trimmed by a podiatrist. These findings are suggestive of fungal infection, and consideration should be given to treating the underlying infection with systemic antifungal medications. Formal testing for peripheral neuropathy should be done annually (e.g., using a monofilament).

Does This Patient Require Any Changes or Additions to Her Current Therapy?

Yes, her blood pressure of 140/88 mm Hg and her lipid values are above her goal. Target blood pressure for patients with diabetes is systolic blood pressure below 130 mm Hg and diastolic blood pressure below 80 mm Hg. Once the diagnosis of hypertension is made, life-style modifications should be used in conjunction with pharmacologic therapy to reduce blood pressure. These modifications include a low-salt diet, weight loss, exercise, and limiting alcohol consumption. If her blood pressure remains elevated at subsequent visits, antihypertensive agents should be instituted until blood pressure goals are achieved.

This patient's lipids are above goal values, yet they are below the values at which therapy is recommended. Dyslipidemia in patients with diabetes is treated in order to reduce the risk of developing coronary heart disease. In lipid management, life-style modification should be the first line of therapy. If lipids remain above goal on subsequent measurements, therapy is based on the patients' other risk factors for coronary heart disease (e.g., smoking, obesity, and hypertension) as well as the individual's specific situation. The fact that this patient had a brother who died of a myocardial infarction at a young age also increases her risk for coronary heart disease, but her diabetes puts her at the highest risk of coronary heart disease even without the family history.

The addition of a daily aspirin should be considered. Large studies and meta-analysis show that people with diabetes receive the same cardiovascular protection from aspirin as nondiabetic patients.

Suggested Reading

American Diabetes Association. Diabetic retinopathy. *Diabetes Care* 2000;23(suppl):73–76.

American Diabetes Association. Report of the Expert Committee on the Diagnosis and Classification of Diabetes Mellitus. *Diabetes Care* 2000;23(suppl):4–19.

American Diabetes Association. Standards of medical care for patients with diabetes mellitus. *Diabetes Care* 2000;23(suppl):32–42.

UK Prospective Diabetes Study (UKPDS) Group. Intensive blood-glucose control with sulphonylureas or insulin compared with conventional treatment and risk of complications in patients with type 2 diabetes. *Lancet* 1998;352:837–853.

Vijan S, et al. Screening, prevention, counseling, and treatment for the complications of type II diabetes mellitus. *J Gen Intern Med* 1997;12:567–580.

16

Care of the Patient with Uncontrolled Type 2 Diabetes Mellitus

Judith R. Rudnick

1. Recognize poorly controlled diabetes. Understand how to differentiate poor compliance from disease progression. Explore resources available (e.g., pharmacy teaching and nutrition) to help patients with compliance.
2. Know the evidence showing the benefits of tight glucose control in most diabetic patients.
3. Know when tight glucose control might not be appropriate.
4. Know the classes of oral agents available to treat diabetes.

Discussion

Recognize Poorly Controlled Diabetes. Understand How to Differentiate Poor Compliance from Disease Progression. Explore the Clinical Resources Available (e.g., Pharmacy Teaching and Nutrition) to Help Patients with Compliance.

Diabetes is a chronic progressive disease. It is typical for a patient who initially requires only diet to control blood sugars to require one or more oral agents and eventually insulin. The American Diabetes Association (ADA) recommends that all patients be asked about medication and dietary compliance at every visit. If a patient is not complying with the medical regimen, one should determine the reason (e.g., side effects or cost) so that appropriate adjustments can be made.

Clinical pharmacists can help educate patients on the proper ways to take their medications. Registered dietitians also can counsel patients on an appropriate diet. Ongoing medical nutrition therapy can be effective for achieving better glycemic control.

A patient who, despite taking medication as directed, has consistently elevated blood glucose values most likely has disease progression. Depending on the patient's current regimen, higher doses, additional oral agents, or insulin may be added to achieve metabolic targets.

Know the Evidence Showing the Benefits of Tight Glucose Control in Most Diabetic Patients.

The evidence that glucose control can prevent complications of diabetes comes from two relatively recent landmark studies: the Diabetes Control and Complications Trial (DCCT) and the United Kingdom Prospective Diabetes Study (UKPDS). The DCCT, published in 1995, studied patients with type 1 diabetes. Patients enrolled in the study were randomized to standard therapy (goal: clinical well-being) or intensive treatment (goal: normalization of blood glucose). Over the study period of 7 years, the intensive treatment group had a 60% risk reduction in the occurrence of retinopathy, nephropathy, and neuropathy. Intensive therapy resulted in both a delay in the onset and a slowing of the progression of these complications. The benefits of intensive therapy were seen in patients regardless of age, sex, or duration of diabetes. These results were obtained despite the fact that the intensive treatment group did not achieve the goal of normalization of blood glucose (mean values remained 40% above normal). The intensive treatment group did have statistically significantly lower values for both mean serum glucose and glycosylated hemoglobin (HbAlc) when compared with the standard therapy group. This study was limited by the fact that only patients with type 1 diabetes were studied, whereas about 90% of patients with diabetes have the type 2 form of the disease.

The largest and longest study of patients with type 2 diabetes is the UKPDS, which enrolled over 5,000 patients with newly diagnosed type 2 diabetes. The results of the UKPDS are not as simple to interpret as the DCCT, because there were multiple study groups comparing sulfonylurea drugs both with metformin and with insulin. In addition, hypertensive patients were randomized for "tight" or "less tight" blood pressure control. The results clearly demonstrated that patients in the intensive therapy arms (regardless of which specific therapy they were given) were able to lower their HbAlc values to a median of 7% as compared with 7.9% in the standard therapy groups. Analyses of the data show that for every percentage point decrease in HbAlc (e.g., 9%–8%), there was a 35% further reduction in the risk of complications.

There are two major similarities of these study findings. First, both studies found no "threshold" for glycemic control. In other words the relationship of complications to serum glucose remained linear all the way down to normal values. Second, neither of these studies was able to demonstrate a statistically significant decrease in cardiovascular events (e.g., myocardial infarction) in the intensive treatment groups, although a trend was seen in that direction. The UKPDS did however find a decrease in microvascular complications and vision loss in hypertensive patients in the "tight" blood pressure control group.

Know When Tight Glucose Control Might Not Be Appropriate.

The ADA suggests that patients who have had diabetes for more than 20 years after puberty with minimal complications of their disease may not require tight control.

Several factors may limit the benefits of tight control:

- Comorbidities, especially those that limit life expectancy (e.g., end-stage cancer)
- Presence of advanced diabetic complications (e.g., renal failure)
- Patient inability to carry out the treatment regimen (e.g., financial constraints)

Other factors may increase the risk of hypoglycemia from tight control:

- History of severe hypoglycemia (requiring emergency treatment)
- Inability to recognize symptoms of hypoglycemia
- Advanced congestive heart failure or cerebrovascular disease
- Autonomic neuropathy
- Medications that impair detection of hypoglycemia

The above factors should be considered when discussing target glucose for any given patient. Target glucose values are individually determined based on the risk-benefit ratio of tight control.

Know the Classes of Oral Agents Available to Treat Diabetes.

There are four major classes of oral agents available to treat patients with type 2 diabetes. The choice of medications can be made based on availability, ease of administration, patient comorbidities, and preference.

Sulfonylureas have traditionally been the first-line agents when diet alone failed. They act by increasing pancreatic insulin secretion, but also may increase insulin receptor sensitivity. Doses may be increased weekly until the maximum dose is obtained. The most common side effect is hypoglycemia. Other serious side effects are hematologic (aplastic anemia, thrombocytopenia, and agranulocytosis).

Metformin is the only currently available medication of the biguanide class. It may be used alone or in combination with other oral agents or insulin. Its mechanism of action is to increase peripheral insulin sensitivity and decrease hepatic glucose production. This drug cannot be used in patients with renal, hepatic, or cardiac failure mainly because of risk of lactic acidosis. Gastrointestinal side effects (nausea, vomiting, diarrhea, and abdominal pain) are all common. Beginning with low doses (500 mg/day) and increasing the dose by 500 mg each week can reduce the incidence of gastrointestinal upset. Metformin should be given with meals. When used as monotherapy it does not generally cause hypoglycemia.

Acarbose is the currently available α-glucosidase inhibitor. It slows the digestion of carbohydrates, delays glucose absorption into the blood stream, and decreases postprandial blood glucose. The initial dose is 25 mg three times a day. Acarbose should be taken with the first bite of each meal. The gastrointestinal side effects of pain, flatulence, and diarrhea are common and are related to the action of the medication. They usually subside over 4 to 8 weeks, but many patients discontinue the drug because of these effects. It does not cause hypoglycemia, but is only effective when taken with food.

Within the thiazolidinedione class, troglitazone was the first drug approved in the United States. Due to the increased risk of hepatic failure associated with its use, it was recently withdrawn from the market. Other drugs in this class such as rosiglitazone and pioglitazone appear to have less toxicity. This class of drugs lowers glucose by improving sensitivity to insulin in muscle and adipose tissue and by inhibiting hepatic glucose production. The initial indication for this class of drug was to reduce the dose of insulin in patients who could not achieve glycemic control despite large doses (>100 units) of insulin.

Case

A 44-year-old man with type 2 diabetes returns for follow-up and a medication refill. He reports that he missed his last appointment in the diabetes clinic 2 weeks ago. He has no complaints of polyuria, polydipsia, or blurred vision; overall he feels well. He does not currently check his sugars at home because he ran out of test strips. Because he is not feeling tired or weak the way he did when he was first diagnosed with diabetes last year, he does not see the need to "stick himself." His current medication is glipizide 10 mg twice daily; he last filled his prescription at the pharmacy 6 weeks ago. On physical examination, his blood pressure is 126/78 mm Hg, and pulse is 72 beats/min. A retinal examination shows cotton-wool spots and small hemorrhages in the right eye. Lung and cardiovascular examination results are unremarkable. Extremities reveal no ulcers or calluses on the feet. His blood sugar level as measured in the clinic is 398 mg/dL. His HbA1c was 12.8% 1 month ago. He has had no other blood work the past 12 months.

1. What is the most likely reason that this patient is not meeting glycemic controls?
2. What if anything can be done for this patient while he is in clinic? How should his regimen be changed?
3. When should a second oral agent be started?

Case Discussion

What Is the Most Likely Reason that This Patient Is Not Meeting Glycemic Controls?

We know that this patient's diabetes is poorly controlled because his random sugar is 398 mg/dL; in addition, his HbA1c of 12.8% is well above the goal of 7%. The major possibilities for poor control are noncompliance with therapy, disease progression, or a combination of both. Noting that he has missed a scheduled appointment and has not refilled his medications for 6 weeks arouses suspicion of noncompliance with his medical regimen. The ADA recommends that all diabetic patients be asked about their compliance with medications at every visit. This patient, when asked, admits he takes his diabetes medication only sporadically. He explains that it is easy to forget his medication because he has not been having any problems.

What if Anything Can Be Done for This Patient while He Is in Clinic? How Should His Regimen Be Changed?

For patients with very high glucose values (>400 mg/dL), consideration should be given to obtaining laboratory tests urgently. Urine dipstick tests for ketones and serum chemistries can be performed to check for anion gap; they might be used to determine if the patient is in diabetic ketoacidosis or a hyperosmolar state. These should be performed if the patient is having symptoms such as polyuria, polydipsia, or weight loss. For this patient, if he has no ketones in his urine and is not orthostatic, further stat tests might not be warranted. In clinic it is important to make a plan with the patient that will increase his compliance.

On examination the patient has findings consistent with diabetic retinopathy; he should be asked about his last visit to the ophthalmologist. If these eye findings are new or it has been more than a year since his last visit, he should be referred for a comprehensive eye examination and possible surgical intervention. The significance of these findings should be discussed with the patient. Additionally, one should determine the urine albumin:creatinine ratio, the serum creatinine level, and the fasting lipid profile according to ADA recommendations.

Because the patient's elevated glucose in the clinic is at least partly due to medical noncompliance, it would be reasonable to have the patient resume his previous regimen. The addition of home glucose monitoring should be considered. If the patient is willing to undertake home monitoring, he will need chem strips, lancets, and a working accucheck machine. The patient should be referred to a diabetic nutritionist for counseling on appropriate diet. He begins glipizide 10 mg twice daily and is scheduled for follow-up within the month. With his degree of glucose elevation, however, it is unlikely that this will be enough to achieve control. To maintain hydration, he should be encouraged to drink water.

When Should a Second Oral Agent Be Started?

One month later, the same patient returns to clinic. He is now taking his medication regularly, he is more compliant with the diabetic diet, and is even checking his sugars at home. He continues to feel well. His fasting blood sugar level is 150 to 203 mg/dL. One week before coming to the clinic his HbA1c was 9.9%. His random blood glucose in the clinic is 187 mg/dL. His creatinine is 1.1 mg/dL, urine albumin:creatinine ratio 0.3, LDL 142 mg/dL, and HDL 46 mg/dL.

The patient has made an improvement in his glycemic control, as evidenced by a decrease in both random glucose and HbA1c. It is important to congratulate the patient on this achievement. Unfortunately his sugars are still not at goal (80–120 mg/dL). This patient is relatively young; he was diagnosed with diabetes only 2 years ago, but already has microvascular complications. He is a patient for whom tight control might not only slow the progression of his retinopathy; it might delay the onset of other complications such as nephropathy. The data are not conclusive as to whether it will decrease his risk of coronary events. Reducing his cholesterol will decrease that risk. At this time it would be reasonable to add a second oral agent, the most common choice would be metformin 500 mg daily with meals with advancement to full doses as needed and tolerated. Assuming normal liver function, one could also begin a cholesterol-lowering agent at this visit.

Suggested Reading

American Diabetes Association. Implications of the Diabetes Control and Complications Trial. *Diabetes Care* 2000;23(suppl 1):24–26.

American Diabetes Association. Implications of the United Kingdom Prospective Diabetes Study. *Diabetes Care* 2000;23(suppl 1):27–31.

American Diabetes Association. Standards of medical care for patients with diabetes mellitus. *Diabetes Care* 2000;23(suppl 1):32–42.

The Diabetes Control and Complications Trial Research Group. The effect of intensive treatment of diabetes on the development and progression of long-term complications in insulin-dependent diabetes mellitus. *N Engl J Med* 1993;329:977–986.

UK Prospective Diabetes Study (UKPDS) Group. Intensive blood-glucose control with sulphonylureas or insulin compared with conventional treatment and risk of complications inpatients with type 2 diabetes. Lancet 1998;352:837–853.

Vijan S, et al. Screening, prevention, counseling, and treatment for the complications of type II diabetes mellitus. *J Gen Intern Med* 1997;12:567–580.

17

Obesity

Laura J. Martin

- Discussion *107*
- Case *110*
- Case Discussion *110*

1. How are overweight and obesity generally defined?
2. What common medical illnesses are associated with obesity?
3. According to the National Heart, Lung, and Blood Institute guidelines, how should overweight and obese patients initially be evaluated and treated?
4. When is pharmacotherapy a consideration in the treatment of overweight and obese patients?
5. When is surgical treatment a consideration?

Discussion

How Are Overweight and Obesity Generally Defined?

Approximately 97 million American adults are classified as being overweight or obese. This represents 54.9% of adults over the age of 20 years. Obesity is a multi-factorial chronic disease with many influences, including genetic, metabolic, and social factors, among others. Numerous common medical illnesses are associated with obesity, and there is an increase in overall mortality in patients who are obese. Successful treatment of obesity should be a goal of all primary care practitioners. In 1995, the National Heart, Lung, and Blood Institute (NHLBI) and the National Institute of Diabetes and Digestive and Kidney Diseases convened the Expert Panel on the Identification, Evaluation, and Treatment of Overweight and Obesity in Adults. According to the NHLBI guidelines, clinicians should screen all patients for obesity every 2 years by calculating body mass index (BMI). Standard equations to calculate BMI are as follows:

$$BMI = weight\ (kg)/height\ (m^2)$$

$$BMI\ in\ pounds\ and\ inches = weight\ (lbs)/height\ (in^2) \times 703$$

Patients with a BMI of 25.0 to 29.9 kg/m^2 are classified as overweight, while those with a BMI of 30 kg/m^2 or greater are classified as obese (Table 17.1).

What Common Medical Illnesses Are Associated with Obesity?

In obese adults, the prevalence of type II diabetes mellitus is 2.9 times higher than in adults with normal weight. Approximately 60% of obese patients have hyperten-

Table 17.1. Classification of Overweight and Obesity

	Obesity Class	Body Mass Index (kg/m^2)
Underweight		<18.5
Normal		18.5–24.9
Overweight		25.0–29.9
Obesity	I	30.0–34.9
	II	35.0–39.9
Extreme obesity	III	≥40.0

Adapted from *Clinical guidelines on the identification, evaluation and treatment of overweight and obesity in adults.* Bethesda: National Heart, Lung, and Blood Institute/National Institute of Diabetes and Digestive and Kidney Diseases, 1998. National Institutes of Health Publication No. 98-4083, with permission.

sion. Obesity is associated with an increased risk of cardiovascular disease, hypertension, stroke, left ventricular hypertrophy, arrhythmias, congestive heart failure, myocardial infarction, angina, and peripheral vascular disease. Mortality from cardiovascular disease is nearly 50% higher in obese patients as compared with nonobese patients.

Obese women have increased mortality from gallbladder, endometrial, cervical, and ovarian cancers. Postmenopausal obese women have increased mortality from breast cancer. Obese men have a higher mortality from rectal and prostate cancers.

Other comorbid conditions associated with obesity include osteoarthritis, obstructive sleep apnea, gastroesophageal reflux disease, stress incontinence, venous stasis, hepatic steatosis, and pseudotumor cerebri.

Secondary causes of obesity are infrequently encountered. Evaluation for hypothyroidism, Cushing disease, or Prader-Willi syndrome should be performed in cases where there is sufficient clinical suspicion.

According to NHLBI Guidelines, How Should Overweight and Obese Patients Initially Be Evaluated and Treated?

As discussed above, BMI should be calculated every 2 years to diagnose obesity at an early stage. Waist circumference should be measured in patients with a BMI of 25 to 34.9 kg/m^2 to determine if there is high risk of comorbid conditions. (Patients with a BMI of greater than 35 kg/m^2 are considered to have a high risk of comorbidity independent of waist circumference measurements).

Waist circumference correlates with the amount of abdominal visceral fat. Patients with a large waist circumference and thus a large amount of abdominal fat have an increased risk of cardiovascular disease, hypertension, and type II diabetes mellitus. A waist circumference of greater than or equal to 40 inches (102 cm) in men or greater than or equal to 35 inches (88 cm) in women denotes a high risk of comorbidity.

Along with BMI and waist circumference measurements, assessment of standard risk factors for cardiovascular disease should be performed. Overweight and obese patients with significant risks should lose weight.

In general, there are three scenarios where weight loss is recommended. The first is in any obese patient with a BMI greater than or equal to 30 kg/m^2. The second is in an overweight patient with a BMI of 25 to 29.0 kg/m^2 with a large waist circumference and therefore high risk for comorbidity. The third is in an overweight patient with a BMI of 25 to 29.9 kg/m^2 with at least two risk factors for comorbid conditions.

The clinician should participate in motivating patients to lose weight. Personalized counseling on each patient's risk factors may improve motivation.

The recommended initial weight loss goal in obese patients is 10% of baseline weight at a rate of 1 to 2 pounds per week. This can be accomplished by placing the patient on a low-calorie diet resulting in an energy deficit of 500 to 1,000 kcal per day. The low-calorie diet should be consistent with the National Cholesterol Education Program (NCEP) step 1 or 2 diet with total fat intake less than 30% of total calories. In general, 1,000 to 1,200 kcal per day for women and 1,200 to 1,500 kcal per day for men can be recommended. In overweight patients, an energy deficit of 300 to 500 kcal per day can be recommended resulting in loss of about half a pound per week. Dietary measures should be continued for a period of 6 months.

Physical activity is helpful in maintaining weight loss. The initial activity goal recommended for most patients is 30 to 40 minutes of exercise 3 to 5 days per week. A long-term activity goal is 30 minutes of moderately intense exercise on a daily basis. Besides exercise, other strategies that may help patients to lose weight include food diaries, physical activity logs, behavioral modification, stress management, and social support. A reevaluation of weight loss therapy should be performed after 6 months.

Among patients who lose greater than 10% of body weight after 6 months, up to 80% will regain it over the long term. Studies have shown that patients who maintain regular continued contact with their clinician for continuing support and monitoring are less likely to regain weight. Among patients who do not lose 10% of body weight after 6 months to 1 year, the clinician should evaluate if the patient has sufficient motivation to continue weight loss efforts.

When Is Pharmacotherapy a Consideration in the Treatment of Overweight or Obesity?

If dietary and life-style measures alone do not result in substantial weight loss after six months, pharmacotherapy can be added in selected patients. These patients include those with a BMI greater than 30 kg/m^2 or a BMI greater than 27 kg/m^2 with two or more comorbid conditions (such as hypertension, hyperlipidemia, coronary artery disease, type II diabetes mellitus, or obstructive sleep apnea). Currently sibutramine and orlistat are two widely prescribed weight loss medications that are approved by the U.S. Food and Drug Administration.

Sibutramine is a serotonin-norepinephrine reuptake inhibitor that is metabolized in the liver. It induces a decrease in appetite leading to a decrease in oral intake and subsequent weight loss. Side effects include an increase in blood pressure and heart rate, dry mouth, anorexia, headache, insomnia, and constipation. Sibutramine should be used with caution or not at all in patients with hypertension and cardiovascular disease. It should not be used with selective serotonin reuptake inhibitors (SSRIs) or monoamine oxidase (MAO) inhibitors. Recommended initial dosage is 10 mg per day. After 4 weeks, the dose can be titrated up to 15 mg per day if needed. After 4 weeks of the maximal dose, if adequate weight loss is not achieved, then an alternative weight loss therapy should be considered.

Orlistat prevents absorption of approximately 30% of dietary fat by inhibiting lipase. Side effects include flatus, bloating, oily fecal spotting, and increased urinary oxalate. Patients should be advised to strictly adhere to a low-fat diet while taking this medication because the severity of gastrointestinal side effects tend to correlate with the amount of fat ingested. Orlistat should not be prescribed in patients with chronic malabsorption or cholestasis. It should be used with caution in patients with a history of hyperoxaluria or calcium oxalate nephrolithiasis. Recommended dosing is 120 mg orally three times daily with meals.

When Is Surgical Treatment a Consideration?

Surgical therapy sometimes plays a role in treating selected obese patients who have a very high risk for comorbid conditions and have not met their weight loss goals with trials of life-style modification and pharmacotherapy. According to the American College of Endocrinology, surgical therapy can be considered in patients with a BMI greater than or equal to 40 kg/m^2 or a BMI of 35 to 39.9 kg/m^2 with comorbid conditions, who have been obese for at least 5 years and have no history of alcohol abuse or major psychiatric disorders. Surgical consideration should be limited to those patients 18 to 65 years of age. Surgical methods include gastric stapling (vertical banded gastroplasty) and gastric bypass. Gastric bypass has been shown to produce significantly more weight loss on a long-term basis than gastroplasty in most patients.

Case

A 45-year-old woman presents to your office for treatment of hypertension and obesity. She currently feels well, but relates that she has gained approximately 50 pounds in the past 5 years. She does not perform regular exercise. Family history reveals that her parents and two siblings are also obese. Currently her only medication is hydrochlorothiazide.

On physical examination, her blood pressure is 125/80 mm Hg, pulse 65 beats/min, weight 192 pounds, height 65 inches, and waist circumference 39 inches. The rest of her examination is unremarkable.

Results of recent laboratory studies, including thyroid-stimulating hormone level, are within normal limits.

1. Is this patient overweight or obese?
2. Using the NHLBI guidelines, what initial therapy should be recommended?
3. When should reevaluation be performed?

Case Discussion
Is This Patient Overweight or Obese?

In determining if she is overweight or obese, the first step is to determine her BMI. Using the equation given above, her BMI is calculated to be 32 kg/m^2, indicating stage I obesity. Because her waist circumference is over 35 inches, she is at high risk for comorbid conditions. Indeed, she already carries a diagnosis of hypertension.

Using the NHLBI Guidelines, What Initial Therapy Should Be Recommended?

Recommended initial therapy consists of a trial of weight loss, with a goal of losing 10% of her baseline weight over a 6 month period. Using her current weight of 192 pounds, her goal will be to lose 19 pounds over the next 6 months.

In general, patients should be counseled that a safe rate of weight loss is 1 to 2 pounds per week. In this female patient, a low-fat diet, similar to the NCEP step 1 diet, consisting of 1,000 to 1,200 kcal per day, can be recommended.

Instructing the patient on how to maintain a food diary can help her keep track of the average calories she consumes in 1 day. To keep a food diary, she should record the names and amounts of all food items and beverages ingested in a 24-hour period. The estimated number of calories consumed on a daily basis can then be calculated. Referral to a dietitian for specific education on weight loss dieting can be helpful.

The benefits of physical activity should be discussed. An initial goal of 30 to 40 minutes of activity such as brisk walking 3 to 5 days per week is a recommendation most patients can perform. Behavior modification and stress management counseling may be of benefit as well.

When Should Reevaluation Be Performed?

Her obesity should be reevaluated after 6 months of therapy. If she has met her weight loss goal of 10% of her baseline weight, then she should continue to follow with you on a regular basis for motivational support and guidance in maintaining her weight loss. If she has not met her weight loss goal, then you should evaluate if she has sufficient motivation to continue her weight loss efforts. At this point, she may be a candidate for pharmacologic therapy while continuing her diet and exercise therapy.

Suggested Reading

AACE/ACE position statement on the prevention, diagnosis, and treatment of obesity. Jacksonville, FL: American Association of Clinical Endocrinologists/American College of Endocrinology, 1997 (revised 1998).

Clinical guidelines on the identification, evaluation and treatment of overweight and obesity in adults. The evidence report. Bethesda: National Heart, Lung, and Blood Institute/National Institute of Diabetes and Digestive and Kidney Diseases, 1998. National Institutes of Health Publication No. 98-4083.

Hvizdos K M, Markham A. Orlistat: a review of its use in the management of obesity. *Drugs* 1999;58:743–760.

Luque C A, Rey J A. Sibutramine: a serotonin-norepinephrine reuptake-inhibitor for the treatment of obesity. *Ann Pharmacother* 1999;33:968–978.

18
Hypothyroidism
Clyde Watkins, Jr.

1. Identify the common causes of hypothyroidism.
2. Identify the clinical features and diagnostic criteria of hypothyroidism.
3. Define subclinical hypothyroidism.
4. Understand the treatment of hypothyroidism.

Discussion

Identify the Common Causes of Hypothyroidism.

Primary failure of the thyroid gland accounts for 90% to 95% of all cases of hypothyroidism (Table 18.1). The causes of hypothyroidism may be broadly classified as thyroprivic, a loss of thyroid tissue, or goitrous. In the United States, the majority of cases of primary thyroid failure are of thyroprivic origin although goitrous hypothyroidism is still common worldwide. Autoimmune (Hashimoto) thyroiditis is by far the most common cause of primary hypothyroidism in adults. In Hashimoto disease, antibodies are directed against thyroperoxidase, thyroglobulin, or the thyrotropin (thyroid-stimulating hormone, TSH) receptor. These antibodies either destroy the glandular tissue or block the TSH receptor, which leads to glandular failure. The effects of these circulating antibodies may not be specific to the thyroid gland. Their actions may become directed against the proteins of other endocrine organs, resulting in a variable insufficiency of the thyroid, adrenal, parathyroid, and gonadal function—a polyglandular endocrine deficiency state. Hashimoto thyroiditis also may coexist with other diseases in which circulating antibodies are found, such as type 1 diabetes, pernicious anemia, rheumatoid arthritis, systemic lupus erythematosus, autoimmune hepatitis, and Sjogren syndrome.

Iatrogenic destruction of the thyroid gland by surgery, radioactive iodine, or external beam radiation is the second most common cause of hypothyroidism in the United States. Drugs are an important cause of primary hypothyroidism. Lithium, amiodarone, sulfonamides and para-aminosalicylic acid, among other drugs, impair the thyroid's ability to regulate the uptake of iodide, leading to glandular failure.

Secondary failure of the thyroid gland is suprathyroid in origin. The thyroid gland is intrinsically normal, but does not receive sufficient stimulation by TSH. Necrosis, adjacent tumors, pituitary surgery or radiation may destroy pituitary thyrotrophs. Hypothalamic hypothyroidism is characterized by inadequate secretion of thyrotropin-releasing hormone, resulting in either a complete lack of TSH production or the meager production of TSH that is biologically inactive.

Table 18.1. Common Causes of Hypothyroidism

Primary hypothyroidism (95% of all causes)
    Hashimoto thyroiditis (most common cause overall)
    I^{131} therapy
    Surgical thyroidectomy
    External beam radiation
    Drug induced: lithium, amiodarone, sulfonamides, PAS
    Congenital enzyme defects
Secondary hypothyroidism (<5% of all causes)
    Panhypopituitarism
      Neoplasm
      Radiation
      Surgery
      Sheehan's syndrome
    Hypothalamic dysfunction

Identify the Clinical Features and Diagnostic Criteria of Hypothyroidism.

In the adult, clinical diagnosis of hypothyroidism is often difficult to make. The disease onset is slowly progressive, and the early symptoms are nonspecific. Common signs and symptoms of hypothyroidism are listed in Table 18.2.

Because hypothyroidism is considered a "great imitator," the key to diagnosis is a high degree of suspicion. Biochemical confirmation of the presence of hypothyroidism is best effected by measurement of serum TSH and free thyroxine index (FTI). The FTI is reduced in all cases of overt hypothyroidism. Once the diagnosis is established, the TSH aids in the determination of whether the cause is due to primary gland failure (elevated TSH) or secondary, involving the hypothalamic/pituitary axis (low or normal TSH). If a diagnosis of secondary hypothyroidism is made, then the possibility of deficiency of other pituitary hormones should be investigated prior to thyroid replacement.

Define Subclinical Hypothyroidism.

An elevated serum TSH level (<20 μIU/mL), a normal free thyroxine (T$_4$) measurement, and a lack of clinical signs and symptoms of overt hypothyroidism define

Table 18.2. Signs and Symptoms of Hypothyroidism

Symptoms	Signs
Weakness	Dry skin
Fatigue/lethargy	Edema
Cold intolerance	Weight gain
Constipation	Thin hair
Myalgia/arthralgia	Decreased deep tendon reflexes
Paresthesias	Vitiligo
Obstructive sleep apnea	Hypertension
Anorexia	Bradycardia
Amnesia	Carpal tunnel syndrome
Deepening of the voice	Pericardial effusion
Muscle cramps	Hearing impairment

subclinical hypothyroidism. It is estimated that this disorder occurs in 15% of patients over the age of 65 years. Moreover, subclinical hypothyroidism has a high frequency of developing into overt hypothyroidism, with the highest risk being in those over the age of 50 years, with elevations greater than 10 μIU/mL and/or the presence of circulating thyroid antibodies.

The evaluation of subclinical hypothyroidism should include a detailed history and physical examination looking for signs or symptoms of overt hypothyroidism, and a determination of the presence of circulating thyroid antibodies. Whether subclinical hypothyroidism should be treated is controversial. The American College of Physicians currently states that there is insufficient evidence to make a recommendation for or against treatment. However, treatment is supported in patients with serum TSH levels greater than 10 μIU/mL, symptomatic patients, patients with fertility problems, and patients with bipolar disorder, as well as children, adolescents, pregnant women, and women contemplating pregnancy. Patients with TSH levels of 5 to 10 μIU/mL and those with coronary artery disease symptoms should be followed and treated if there is progression of subclinical thyroid disease.

Understand the Treatment of Hypothyroidism.

Hypothyroidism is a disease that is easily treatable. The goal of therapy is to achieve a euthyroid state with TSH, T_4, and triiodothyronine (T_3) levels in the normal range. There are a number of preparations available for use as thyroid replacement, but levothyroxine is the preferred agent. Levothyroxine possesses a long half-life and slow onset of action, resulting in more stable T_3 concentrations.

The average replacement dose of levothyroxine varies mainly with age and to a lesser extent with the cause of hypothyroidism, as well as the level of physical activity. A levothyroxine dose ranging from 1.5 to 1.7 μg T_4/kg is usually sufficient to achieve symptomatic and biochemical replacement. Patients who have undergone radioactive iodine (RAI) therapy or total thyroidectomy may require a replacement dose of 2.1 μg T_4/kg. Once levothyroxine therapy is initiated, doses can be titrated higher in 3- to 4-week intervals. Replacement doses in the elderly are generally 20% to 30% lower than doses needed in middle-aged adults. During pregnancy, women's thyroid replacement needs increase by 30% to 50% and fall to baseline levels during the postpartum period. Patients with malabsorption or those taking aluminum preparations, cholestyramine, lovastatin, iron sulfate, or rifampin need higher replacement doses.

It is well established that excessive thyroid replacement has detrimental effects on cardiac function and bone mineralization; therefore, periodic monitoring to ensure adequacy of replacement is important. A combination of clinical evaluation, annual TSH measurements, and periodic T_3 measurements seems to be the consensus strategy for long-term monitoring of thyroid replacement therapy. An elevated TSH measurement indicates insufficient treatment, and an elevated T_3 indicates that treatment is excessive. Monitoring T_3 measurements is particularly important in patients with secondary hypothyroidism, where TSH production and secretion is defective.

Case

E.G., a 23-year-old Hispanic female, presented to the Urgent Care Center complaining of pain and swelling of her wrists and hands. She states that her symptoms began 6 weeks ago. Initially there was numbness and tingling involving the whole hand that now has progressed to frank pain. She reports that the pain is worse at night, often awakening her from sleep. She has taken acetaminophen with no relief. Past medical history and family history are unremarkable. Her medications include acetaminophen, which she has taken for hand pain, oral contraceptive pills, and an iron tablet daily. Review of systems is positive for a 10-pound weight gain over the past 3 months and constipation.

Physical examination reveals slight skin pallor. Her wrists and hands have 1+ pitting edema. Tinel's sign is negative, but Phalen's sign is positive. The rest of her examination is unremarkable.

Laboratory study results include hematocrit 37%, mean corpuscular volume 101, total cholesterol 240 mg/dL, aspartate transaminase (AST) 62 Iμ/L, alanine transaminase (ALT) 45 Iμ/L, TSH 88.8 μIU/mL, FTI <0.5, and T_3 <25 mg/dL; serum chemistries were within normal limits.

1. What clinical features suggest hypothyroidism?
2. How should the patient be treated?
3. Is additional evaluation needed?

Case Discussion

What Clinical Features Suggest Hypothyroidism?

The patient presents with a classic case of bilateral carpal tunnel syndrome. She denies a history of an occupation or hobbies that place her at risk for carpal tunnel syndrome. Hypothyroidism is a common cause of bilateral carpal tunnel syndrome. Other clues include constipation and a 10-pound weight gain. Other conditions to consider as a cause for carpal tunnel syndrome include pregnancy and rheumatoid arthritis.

How Should the Patient Be Treated?

Levothyroxine is the agent of choice for thyroid hormone replacement. Patients may typically start on replacement at doses of 1.5 to 1.7 μg T_4/kg. Persons with autoimmune disease typically require dosing on the lower end of the recommended limits. This is due to the presence of residual functioning thyroid tissue. E.G. should be monitored in 4-week intervals until her symptoms have resolved and TSH has normalized.

Is Additional Evaluation Needed?

It is well established that patients with autoimmune thyroid disease are at risk for developing a coexisting autoimmune disease or polyglandular endocrine deficiency failure. Macrocytosis, hypercholesterolemia, and liver enzyme abnormalities are not uncommon in cases of severe hypothyroidism. E.G.'s laboratory abnormalities are not only consistent with hypothyroidism, but are also suggestive of pernicious anemia. Antiparietal cell and antiintrinsic factor antibodies along with a vitamin B_{12} level should be obtained to rule out the concurrent presence of pernicious anemia.

Suggested Reading

Dillmann W. Endocrine and reproductive diseases: the thyroid. In: Bennett JC, Fatourechi V. Subclinical thyroid disease. *Mayo Clin Proc* 2001;76:413–417.

Helfand M, Redfern C C. Screening for thyroid disease: an update. *Ann Intern Med* 1998;129:144–155.

Plum F, et al., ed. *Cecil textbook of medicine,* 20th ed. Philadelphia: WB Saunders, 1996:1176–1348.

Position paper. Screening for thyroid disease. *Ann Intern Med* 1998;129:141–143.

Wartofsky L. Endocrine and metabolism: diseases of the thyroid. In: Fauci AS, et al., ed. *Harrison's principles of internal medicine,* 14th ed. New York: McGraw-Hill, 1998:1260–1262.

19

"Solitary" Thyroid Nodule

Inginia Genao

1. What are some risk factors and physical findings suggestive of thyroid malignancy in patients with a solitary nodule?
2. Formulate a differential diagnosis.
3. What is your diagnostic approach?
4. What are the treatment options?

Discussion

What Are Some Risk Factors and Physical Findings Suggestive of Thyroid Malignancy in Patients with a Solitary Thyroid Nodule?

Thyroid malignancy is diagnosed most frequently in children and in adults less than 30 or greater than 60 years of age. The incidence of thyroid malignancy is greater in males versus females. A family history of thyroid cancer or multiple endocrine neoplasia (MEN) syndromes increases the risk for malignancy. Exposure to external irradiation in infancy or childhood also increases risk. Symptoms of local invasion, history of rapid tumor growth, and cervical lymphadenopathy raise the suspicion of malignancy. Any solitary nodule or dominant lesion within a multinodular gland should be evaluated to rule out malignancy.

Formulate a Differential Diagnosis.

As one assesses carefully the solitary thyroid nodule, it is important to consider benign and malignant etiologies (Table 19.1).

Colloid (Adenomatous) Nodules

- Dominant nodules within glands that are often found to be multinodular on imaging or surgery
- Mostly hypofunctioning
- Cytologically have abundant colloid and benign follicular cells

Table 19.1. Etiologies of Thyroid Nodules

Benign	Malignant
Colloid (adenomatous) nodules	Papillary carcinoma
Hashimoto thyroiditis	Follicular carcinoma
Cysts	Medullary carcinoma
Follicular adenomas (macrofollicular)	Primary thyroid lymphoma
Laryngocele	Metastatic carcinoma

Follicular Adenomas

- Classified according to size and presence of follicles
- Macrofollicular—-most common form; resemble normal thyroid tissue
- Microfollicular—-share architectural features of follicular carcinoma and about 5% prove to be malignant; when detected, usually reported as indeterminate or suspicious

Thyroid Cysts

- Mostly form from degenerating benign adenomas.
- Approximately 15% to 25% of all thyroid nodules are cystic.
- About 15% are necrotic papillary cancers.
- Both benign and malignant lesions may have hemorrhagic fluid.
- Often yield insufficient number of cells for diagnosis.
- More likely to be malignant if they reaccumulate after aspiration.

Papillary Carcinoma

- Most common of thyroid cancers and best prognosis

Medullary Carcinoma

- Most aggressive of thyroid cancers
- May present as part of the MEN syndrome

What Is Your Diagnostic Approach?

The best approach in evaluating a thyroid nodule is still controversial. Clinical palpation is not a precise tool for assessing abnormality of the thyroid gland, and its reliability is influenced by the size and location of the nodule, size and shape of the neck, and experience of the examiner. When a single nodule is palpated on physical examination, there is about a 50% chance of ultrasonography showing other nodules, usually smaller in size. These thyroid nodules found incidentally are appropriately called incidentalomas. Autopsy data show that most of the incidentalomas examined histologically are benign. Therefore, given the low likelihood of incidentalomas being malignant, it is not recommended to screen with imaging studies for thyroid nodules. But what is the best approach to rule out malignancy once the nodule is detected on physical examination? Let us review the different diagnostic options.

Blood Tests

- Thyroid-stimulating hormone level should be assessed to identify patients with unsuspected thyrotoxicosis. If it is decreased, suspect a hyperfunctioning nodule and proceed with thyroid scan. If it is normal, proceed with fine-needle aspiration (FNA). If it is increased, consider Hashimoto thyroiditis, but thyroid cancer can coexist. Most experts recommend proceeding with FNA.
- Serum calcitonin should be assessed only when medullary thyroid cancer is suspected.
- Radiography of the neck/chest is performed to detect retrosternal goiter or distortion of airway.

Ultrasonography

- Ultrasonographic findings such as microcalcifications, irregular margins, and a hyperechoic pattern can be associated with malignancy.
- Capable of detecting nodules as small as 0.3 mm in diameter, but the clinical significance of these lesions is doubtful.
- Discriminates cystic from solid lesions. Cystic nodules constitute 15% to 25% of all thyroid nodules with a malignancy rate of about 17%.
- Indicated when cystic nodules do not disappear completely or when they recur after aspiration.
- Useful for follow-up (distinguishes nodular growth from intranodular hemorrhage).

Radionuclide Scanning

- Cannot reliably distinguish malignant from benign nodules.
- The finding of a "hot" nodule is usually benign, but more than 80% of nodules are "cold" and only 20% of these are found to be malignant.
- Valuable in identifying autonomously functioning thyroid tissue.
- Of some value in patients with indeterminate FNA results (increased uptake is almost always benign).

Fine-Needle Aspiration Biopsy

- The initial test recommended by most experts.
- Safe and inexpensive office procedure.
- There is a 90% to 97% chance of an experienced clinician obtaining an adequate thyroid nodule sample.
- Ultrasonographically guided FNA is helpful in nodules with extensive cystic degeneration or if the nodule is difficult to aspirate with palpation alone.
- Cytologic diagnostic accuracy is 70% to 97% (influenced by the surgeon's and cytopathologist's skill).
- There is a 0 to 6% false-positive rate (usually due to Hashimoto thyroiditis).
- There is a 0.7% to 6% false-negative rate (usually due to sampling error or misdiagnosis on a nodule less than 1 cm or greater than 4 cm in diameter; this can be minimized by using ultrasonographically guided biopsy).
- Leads to a better selection of patients for surgery.

There is no effective noninvasive method to identify malignant lesions when an FNA yields indeterminate results. FNA is limited in the evaluation of follicular nodules, because histology is required to distinguish between benign follicular adenoma and follicular carcinoma. Most of these lesions are hypofunctional. It is recommended to proceed with surgery if there is high clinical suspicion. A radionuclide study may be helpful if it is a hot nodule (the combination of indeterminate FNA biopsy, low clinical suspicion and hyperfunctioning nodule is almost always benign). Proceed with surgery if it is a cold nodule. For cases with inadequate cytologic findings, a repeat FNA is recommended.

What Are the Treatment Options?

Treatment is based on the cytopathology findings because most experts proceed to FNA once a nodule is palpated on physical examination.

Nonfunctioning Benign/Macrofollicular Thyroid Nodules

- Thyroxine suppression therapy is a controversial therapy sometimes used to shrink nodules and inhibit growth.
- Most nodules do not decrease in size.
- May precipitate tachyarrythmias and osteoporosis.
- Appropriate level of thyrotropin suppression is not known.

Autonomously Functioning Thyroid Nodules

- Thyroid suppression therapy is not indicated in euthyroid patients given the risk of inducing hypothyroidism.
- Most of these nodules remain stable over 1 to 15 years of follow-up.
- About 5% of patients per year become hyperthyroid.
- Radioiodine or surgery may be indicated in subclinical or overt hyperthyroidism.

Cystic Nodules

- All need to be aspirated
- May be cured by aspiration alone
- If there is no recurrence and the cytology of aspirated fluid is negative, most likely the cystic nodule is benign and no further workup is necessary; if there is recurrence, consider surgical removal if there is a risk for malignancy.

Malignant or Indeterminate with High Clinical Suspicion Thyroid Nodule

The primary mode of therapy for patients with well-differentiated thyroid carcinoma (papillary and follicular) is surgery. The extent of surgery depends on tumor size, metastasis, and extrathyroidal extension. Radioiodine can be used for ablation of residual thyroid tissue. Radioiodine is recommended for all patients over 45 years of age with differentiated carcinoma, primary tumor equal to or greater than

1.5 cm in diameter, or extrathyroidal disease. All patients should receive thyroid hormone therapy to prevent hypothyroidism and to decrease the risk of tumor growth secondary to TSH stimulation. Adjuvant radiation is controversial at this point.

Chemotherapy may be beneficial in patients with progressive disease not responding to the above treatment modalities.

For the undifferentiated thyroid tumors (anaplastic thyroid carcinomas), surgery is rarely indicated due to the aggressive nature of the disease and advanced disease at the time of presentation. If the tumor is localized to the thyroid gland, surgery plus adjuvant therapy is recommended.

For patients with medullary thyroid carcinoma, total thyroidectomy is the initial treatment modality.

Case

A 25-year-old woman arrives with her husband. She has no significant past medical history (PMH) and takes no medications, and has come to see you for a complete physical examination before conceiving her second child. Findings at physical examination are completely normal, with the exception of a soft, mobile, nontender, 2×3 cm nodule over the lower left side of the thyroid. There is no lymphadenopathy.

She denies any history of head or neck irradiation, hoarseness, dysphagia, odynophagia, dyspnea, unintentional weight loss, change in skin or hair texture, or other symptoms of thyroid disease.

No one in her family has had cancer. You inform the patient and her husband of the nodule and they become very anxious and ask the following questions:

1. What is the probability that this is cancer?
2. What diagnostic tests should be performed now?
3. Should we get pregnant now or wait until this is over?

Case Discussion
What Is the Probability that This Is Cancer?

It is common for patients to equate mass or nodule with cancer. Time is needed to answer their questions and to offer reassurance. Thyroid nodules are about four times more common in women than in men, and of all thyroid nodules, 5% to 6.5% are malignant, with the rest being benign colloid nodules. Colloid nodules are composed of irregularly enlarged follicles containing abundant colloid. This patient's only risk factor for thyroid cancer is her age. The risk for thyroid cancer in this patient is low.

What Diagnostic Tests Should Be Performed Now?

As with all medical decisions, this decision should be made jointly with the patient given that at this point you cannot rule out malignancy. Both the patient and her husband are very anxious and concerned about cancer. They indicate that they would like to pursue further diagnostic studies. TSH should be measured and FNA performed accordingly.

Should We Get Pregnant Now or Wait Until This Is Over?

The patient should be advised to postpone pregnancy given that pregnancy imposes limitations on the diagnosis and potential treatment. This patient had a normal TSH level, and ultrasonographically guided FNA was performed. Ultrasonography revealed a 1 × 2 cm nodule along with smaller cystic and solid nodules. The dominant nodule was aspirated, and the cytologic diagnosis was papillary carcinoma. She underwent total thyroidectomy followed by iodine 131 therapy and is currently on thyroid hormone replacement therapy.

Suggested Reading

Bennedbaek F N, Perrild H, Hegedus L. Diagnosis and treatment of the solitary thyroid nodule. Results of a European survey. *Clin Endocrinol* 1999;50.

Hermus A R, Huysmans D A. Drug therapy: treatment of benign nodular thyroid disease. *N Engl J Med* 1998;338.

Mazzaferri E L. Current concepts: management of a solitary thyroid nodule. *N Engl J Med* 1993;328.

Ridgway E C. Medical treatment of benign thyroid nodules: have we found a benefit? *Ann Intern Med* 1998;128.

Tan G H, Gharib H. Thyroid incidentalomas: management approaches to nonpalpable nodules discovered incidentally on thyroid imaging. *Ann Intern Med* 1997;26.

20
Osteoporosis
Janice G. Farrehi

Discussion
How Are Osteoporosis and Osteopenia Defined?

The World Health Organization (WHO) panel has developed a working definition of osteoporosis and osteopenia (Table 20.1).

What Are the Risk Factors and Secondary Causes of Osteoporosis?

Existing risk factors for osteoporosis and known secondary causes may help to identify patients who require further evaluation. Many of these factors have limited use once a bone mineral density (BMD) measurement is made, because BMD is the single best predictor of the risk of fracture. Regardless, the risk factors listed in Table 20.2 may predict low BMD.

Other secondary causes include malabsorption of calcium or vitamin D, renal calcium leak, vitamin D deficiency, acromegaly, Cushing syndrome, hyperparathyroidism, hyperprolactinemia, hyperthyroidism, hypogonadism, hepatic disease, multiple myeloma, renal insufficiency, systemic mastocytosis, and prolonged immobilization.

Although osteoporosis is less common in men, fractures in men constitute at least one fourth of all osteopenic-related fractures. A secondary cause is usually found in men with osteoporosis.

Case

A 69-year-old white woman presents for follow-up of low back pain. She was evaluated in an urgent care center 1 month earlier and is concerned because her back radiographs showed "thinning of her bones." Past medical history includes hypertension. Medications include hydrochlorothiazide 25 mg per day. Gynecologic history reveals that she is nulliparous and went through menopause at 49 years of age. She

Table 20.1. Definitions of Osteopenia and Osteoporosis

	Bone Mineral Density	Fragility Fractures
Normal bone mass	≤1.0 SD below the mean for peak bone mass	Absent
Low bone mass (osteopenia)	>1.0 and <2.5 SD below the mean for peak bone mass	Absent
Osteoporosis	≥2.5 SD below the mean for peak bone mass	Absent
Severe osteoporosis	≥2.5 SD below the mean for peak bone mass	At least one

SD, standard deviation.
Adapted from World Health Organization, Geneva. Assessment of fracture risk and its application to screening for postmenopausal osteoporosis: report of a WHO study group. Technical Report Series 843, 1994; with permission.

did not take hormones at that time. Family history is significant for breast cancer in her sister at 65 years of age. She smokes one pack of cigarettes per day and denies alcohol use and routine exercise. Physical examination shows a thin female. Blood pressure is 122/68 mm Hg, pulse is 72 beats/min, height is 64 inches, and weight is 125 pounds. Results of a complete physical examination are unremarkable.

1. What tests should you consider ordering for this patient?
2. What are her options for the prevention and treatment of osteoporosis?

Case Discussion

What Tests Should You Consider Ordering for This Patient?

Quantitative assessment of BMD is important in determining fracture risk and in confirming the suspected diagnosis of osteoporosis. Standard radiographs do not generally indicate osteoporosis until 30% to 40% of bone mass is lost. An overpenetrated film can falsely give the appearance of osteoporosis in a patient with a normal BMD. Although there are a variety of methods to assess BMD, dual-energy x-ray absorptiometry is the most commonly used. BMD can be measured at the spine, hip, or wrist. Results are given per square meter and are used to determine the T score and Z score.

Table 20.2. Risk Factors for Osteoporosis

Age
Caucasian or Asian ethnicity
Sedentary life-style
Smoking
Low body weight (<127 pounds)
Family history of osteoporosis
Excessive alcohol intake
Prolonged calcium-deficient diet
Nulliparity
Long-term use of medicines (glucocorticoids, antiseizure medicines, excessive thyroxine, heparin)
Estrogen-deficient states

Modified from AACE clinical practice guidelines for the prevention and treatment of postmenopausal osteoporosis. *Endocr Practice* 1996;2:157–171; with permission.

The T score compares the subject's BMD with the predicted mean peak BMD (in an average 30-year-old of the same sex) and expresses the difference in standard deviation.

The Z score compares the subject's BMD with mean for age-matched, sex-matched, and ethnic-matched controls and expresses the differences in standard deviation. A Z score of less than -2 may suggest a secondary cause of osteoporosis.

Although recommendations for ordering BMD vary, all patients at risk in whom treatment decisions would be altered based on results should be offered the test. A complete blood count, calcium, phosphate, liver enzymes, alkaline phosphatase, creatinine, electrolytes, urinalysis, including urine pH, and TSH may be ordered for evaluation of secondary causes.

Other tests should be ordered only if the history, physical examination, or Z score suggests a secondary cause.

What Are Her Options for the Prevention and Treatment of Osteoporosis?

This patient should be counseled on preventive measures, including adequate calcium intake (1,000–1,500 mg/day), sufficient vitamin D intake (400 IU/day), regular weight-bearing exercise, and avoidance of tobacco.

Regarding options for treatment, the American Association of Clinical Endocrinologists recommends pharmacologic therapy for patients with a T score of less than -2.5. Some organizations have recommended a T score of 2.0 as a threshold for pharmacology treatment. If this patient's BMD meets criteria for pharmacologic treatment, the following options could be considered.

Hormone Replacement Therapy

Hormone replacement therapy (HRT) has been shown to reduce the rate of bone loss in numerous controlled clinical trials in postmenopausal women. Randomized trials on fracture risk are limited, but observational studies of women receiving HRT suggest a 50% to 80% decrease in vertebral fractures and 25% decrease in nonvertebral fractures over 5 years of use.

A number of trials have shown that the combination of estrogen and progesterone given continuously or sequentially is as effective as estrogen alone in reducing postmenopausal osteoporosis. Transdermal estrogen also decreases the vertebral fracture rate in postmenopausal osteoporosis. In one randomized trial, low-dose estrogen (0.3 mg/day) combined with medroxyprogesterone (2.5 mg/day) compared with placebo also increased BMD at the spine. Fracture data do not exist for the low-dose regimen.

Contraindications to HRT include pregnancy, personal history of breast cancer, first-degree relative with breast cancer, active or chronic liver disease, recent vascular thrombosis, and undiagnosed vaginal bleeding. Other possible contraindications include known coronary atherosclerotic disease, gallbladder disease, and severe migraines. Pretreatment assessment should include complete history, physical, pelvic examination, Papanicolaou smear, and mammography.

Bisphosphonates can inhibit bone resorption and mineralization and represent an alternative to HRT. Both alendronate and risedronate have been approved by the U.S.

Food and Drug Administration for the prevention and treatment of postmenopausal and glucocorticoid-induced osteoporosis. Fracture data are similar, although slightly less efficacious than for HRT, but are based on randomized trials for hip, spine, and wrist. Patients can experience gastrointestinal side effects, and both drugs should be taken with 5 to 8 ounces of water at least half an hour before the first food, beverage, or medication of the day. Patients should not lie down after 30 minutes after taking either drug. The dose of alendronate for prevention is 5 mg per day and for the treatment of osteoporosis is 10 mg per day. A 70 mg weekly dose is available for patient convenience of administration. The dose of risedronate is 5 mg per day.

Calcitonin is yet another choice for women who are not candidates or choose not to take HRT or bisphosphonates. Calcitonin is not as effective in preventing nonvertebral fractures or in preventing steroid-induced osteoporosis. It does have mild analgesic properties and can be used in the setting of acute compression fractures. It is available in nasal spray (200 IU/day) or injection (100 IU/day).

Raloxifene is a final alternative that is a selective estrogen receptor modulator. It is approved for prevention and treatment of postmenopausal osteoporosis. It has been shown to significantly decrease the risk of vertebral fractures. Raloxifene, like HRT, decreases low-density lipoprotein and increases the risk for venous thromboembolism. Unlike estrogen, it does not increase high-density lipoprotein or stimulate the endometrium, and may confer a protective effect on the risk of breast cancer. The dose of raloxifene is 60 mg per day.

Future directions for the prevention and treatment of osteoporosis include newer selective estrogen receptor modulators and statin lipid lowering drugs. The latter have been shown to decrease fracture risk in nonrandomized trials. The use of percutaneous vertebroplasty in patients with painful vertebral fractures involves the injection of "surgical" cement into vertebra.

This patient could be offered a bisphosphonate, raloxifene, or calcitonin. Given her family history of breast cancer, HRT should probably be avoided. Raloxifene is a reasonable alternative, especially given the potential to decrease her risk for breast cancer. Alternatively, a bisphosphonate would avoid hormonal risks and has excellent fracture data, provided she can follow the administration recommendations. Calcitonin is not as efficacious as the above mentioned choices and should be reserved for intolerance of the other options. Physical therapy and balance training also may be offered to prevent falls.

Once therapy has begun, the patient should be monitored for side effects and BMD may be reassessed in 1 or 2 years to determine the efficacy of the regimen dose.

Suggested Reading

AACE clinical practice guidelines for the prevention and treatment of postmenopausal osteoporosis. *Endocr Practice* 1996;2:157–171.

American Association of Clinical Endocrinologists. Available at: www.aace.com.

Bracker M, Watts N. How to get the most out of bone densitometry. *Postgrad Med J* 1998;104:77–86.

Eastell T R. Treatment of postmenopausal osteoporosis. *N Engl J Med* 1998;338:736–746.

Lambing C L. Osteoporosis prevention, detection, and treatment. A mandate for primary care physicians. *Postgrad Med J* 2000;107:37–48.

Osteoporosis: review of the evidence for prevention, diagnosis, and treatment and cost-effectiveness analysis. *Osteoporosis Int* 1998;8(suppl):7–80.

National Institute of Health (Osteoporosis and Related Bone Diseases). Available at: www.osteo.org.

National Osteoporosis Foundation. Available at: www.nof.org.

V
Gastroenterology

21

Acute Diarrhea

John Evans
Shanthi V. Sitaraman

1. What is the natural history of adult acute diarrhea?
2. What red flags in the history and physical examination indicate the need for aggressive management?
3. When is laboratory testing indicated, and what should you order it?
4. What are the typical presentations of the most common pathogens?
5. What is the treatment of acute diarrhea?

Discussion

What Is the Natural History of Adult Acute Diarrhea?

In the United States an estimated 99 million adults per year experience an episode of acute diarrhea, and approximately 8 million a year seek medical attention. Typically most cases are self-limited resolve within 48 hours and do not require medical evaluation. Acute diarrhea is defined as more frequent, looser than normal stools for less than 2 to 3 weeks; it is objectively defined by 250 g or more of stool output per day. Acute and chronic diarrhea are clinically distinguished by time span; chronic diarrhea has a duration of at least 1 month. Acute diarrhea is often associated with other gastrointestinal symptoms, including passage of bloody stool (dysentery), abdominal bloating, nausea, vomiting, and abdominal pain.

What Red Flags in the History and Physical Examination Indicate the Need for Aggressive Management?

The history and physical examination are key aspects in determining the etiology of acute diarrhea. While taking the patient's history, the clinician should focus on some key aspects of the history and physical examination. Important components of the history include the onset of symptoms (e.g., after a suspicious meal), a history of new medication or antibiotic use, exposure to sick contacts, recent travel, and potential exposure to contaminated water (e.g., camping trips, use of well water). The presence of comorbid conditions, including human immunodeficiency virus risk factors or immunosuppression, could impact the differential diagnosis, workup, and management. Key components of the clinical assessment include the presence or absence of a fever, frequency and consistency of stools, and presence of blood in the stools.

In the adult, the following findings are red flags that should prompt a patient to seek medical attention and are helpful in directing the workup and treatment plan:

- Diarrhea in the elderly or immunocompromised patient (including acquired immunodeficiency patients, transplant patients, and those on chemotherapy or high-dose steroids)
- Duration of illness greater than 48 hours
- Diarrhea accompanied by severe abdominal pain
- Diarrhea associated with fever (temperature >38.0°C or 100.5°F)
- Blood in the stool
- More than six unformed stools a day
- Profuse watery diarrhea with dehydration

The physical examination will impact the physician's management decisions. Along with the abdominal examination and stool guaiac, special attention should be directed to the patient's vital signs and volume status. Signs of dehydration include orthostatic hypotension, poor skin turgor, and dry mucus membranes. The abdominal examination should focus on the presence or absence of bowel sounds, peritoneal signs, and distention. A rectal examination including stool guaiac should be performed on all patients. Inpatient observation should be considered for patients with the following symptoms:

- Cannot adequately hydrate themselves
- Have bloody diarrhea
- Have significant abdominal pain or a worrisome abdomen on examination
- Are immunocompromised or elderly

When Is Laboratory Testing Indicated, and When Should You Order It?

Tests to consider in the workup of diarrhea include those designed to determine its cause and those that determine the severity of electrolyte or other metabolic disturbance. In patients with red flags, you may consider basic chemistries and stool analysis to look for evidence of inflammation or infection. The presence of red or white blood cells in the stool generally signifies an inflammatory or infectious colitis. In a patient with fever, abdominal pain, or bloody stools, a stool culture for bacterial pathogens is reasonable. Because organisms are continually shed in the stool, a stool culture has very high sensitivity. If the stool is bloody, the laboratory should be told to test for *Escherichia coli* 0157:H7. Ischemic colitis should be considered, especially in the elderly population. *Clostridium difficile* toxin should be considered in patients who have recently used antibiotics or have recently been hospitalized. Studies for ova and parasites are not helpful and should not be routinely ordered unless infection with *Giardia lamblia* is suspected, the patient is homosexual, or the patient is immunosuppressed. In experienced hands and in select patients, office flexible sigmoidoscopy and biopsy may be appropriate and can be useful in expediting the diagnosis.

What Are the Typical Presentations of the Most Common Pathogens?

Acute diarrhea is usually pathogen related; therefore, determining the time course from the exposure (e.g., ingestion of a food-borne or water-borne pathogen) to the onset of symptoms can help in the diagnosis. Incubation times of less than 6 hours after exposure indicate ingestion of a preformed toxin such as that contained in *Staphylococcus aureus* or *Bacillus cereus*. Incubation times of 8 to 14 hours between ingestion and onset on symptoms are seen in *Clostridium perfringens* toxin exposure. Viral etiologies should be suspected when vomiting is the major component of symptoms and incubation times are greater than 14 hours. Adults can and do become infected with rotavirus and Norwalk virus, usually contracted from infants via fecal-oral transmission. *Giardia lamblia* is a parasite that causes a prolonged watery diarrhea lasting more than two 2 weeks. Bloody stools are associated with the following organisms: *Shigella, Salmonella, E. coli, Campylobacter,* and *Entamoeba hystolytica* (Table 21.1).

What Is the Treatment of Acute Diarrhea?

Treatment involves aggressive rehydration with electrolyte replacement if necessary, symptomatic relief, and occasionally antibiotics. The World Health Organization advises oral rehydration when possible and suggests the following regimen: half a teaspoon salt, half a teaspoon baking soda, and 4 tablespoons sugar mixed in 1 liter of water. Loperamide hydrochlorite (generic), 4 mg orally once, then 2 mg after each loose stool to a maximum of 16 mg/day is the treatment of choice in re-

Table 21.1. Typical Presentations of Common Pathogens

Scenario	Likely Organisms	Treatment	
Fever, bloody stools, with or without abdominal pain	*Shigella, Salmonella, Campylobacter, Entamoeba histolytica,* enterohemorrhagic *Escherichia coli*	*Shigella*	If acquired in U.S. then Bactrim DS b.i.d. for 3 days. If acquired elsewhere, Cipro 500 mg b.i.d. for 3–5 days
		Salmonella	If healthy host, no treatment, but for severe disease, Bactrim DS b.i.d. for 5–7 days or Cipro 500 mg b.i.d. for 5–7 days
		Campylobacter	Erythromycin 500 mg b.i.d. for 5–7 days
		Entamoeba	Cipro 500 mg for 5–7 days
		E. coli	Cipro 500 mg for 5–7 days
Onset of symptoms <6 hours from a meal	*Staphylococcus aureus, Bacillus cereus*	Supportive therapy only	
Onset of symptoms 8–14 h from a meal	*Clostridium perfringens*	Supportive therapy only	
Onset of symptoms >14 h with vomiting as a major component	Viruses: Rota and Norwalk	Supportive therapy only	

lieving the symptoms of diarrhea, and should only be started after an infectious or inflammatory cause has been ruled out. Its use is discouraged in patients with febrile dysentery because it may prolong the course of the disease, a phenomenon that has not been seen in patients with nondysenteric diarrhea. Another antimotility drug that may provide symptomatic relief is Lomotil (Searle), a combination of 2.5 mg of diphenoxylate hydrochloride and 0.025 mg atropine sulfate. The dosage is two tablets four times daily. Kaopectate is a stool bulker and does not decrease the amount of stools.

The use of empiric antibiotics is somewhat controversial and is reserved for three specific indications: (a) patients with dysentery or moderate to severe traveler's diarrhea; (b) patients with fecal leukocytes or blood in their stools and a fever; and (c) patients with suspected *Giardia* infection with 2 to 4 weeks of diarrhea and no signs of dysentery.

The controversy of antibiotic use in the treatment of acute diarrhea stems from the observations that, in most cases, antibiotics minimally impact the disease course and can prolong the shedding of the organism in the stool. Some recent studies have shown that early antibiotic treatment of enterohemorrhagic *E. coli* may increase the risks of progressing to the hemolytic uremic syndrome.

Case

A 23-year-old female medical student is brought to the emergency room after experiencing 36 hours of nausea and vomiting accompanied by diarrhea. Her symptoms began with nausea, followed by vomiting food contents, then bile. She has been unable to hold anything down. Her last meal was breakfast the day before, consisting of orange juice and a granola bar. Diarrhea began soon after the vomiting and is described as watery with no blood or fat, and an estimated 12 bowel movements in the past day. She reports bloating and mild cramping, but no fever and no abdominal pain. There is no recent history of travel. A friend and her 6-month-old child had visited 2 days earlier, and the medical student recalls changing the infant's diaper. Her past medical history is significant for asthma, well controlled on a steroid inhaler. Her family history is negative. She is allergic to shellfish. She is not sexually active, does not drink alcohol, and does not smoke. Her review of systems reveals her last menstrual period to be 3 weeks ago. On physical examination she is ill-appearing with a temperature of 36.6°C, pulse of 75 beats/min and blood pressure of 110/70 mm Hg while supine, and pulse of 104 beats/min and blood pressure of 100/60 mm Hg while standing. She has dry mucous membranes, clear lung examination, and a rapid, regular heart rhythm with a II/VI systolic flow murmur at the apex. Her abdomen has normoactive bowel sounds, and is soft and nontender without distention. She has no organomegaly and refuses a rectal examination.

1. What aspects of her history help you make the diagnosis?
2. How does the physical examination help you?
3. What laboratory tests would be helpful?
4. Should this patient be admitted to the hospital?
5. Should she receive antibiotics?
6. What is the likely cause of her diarrhea?

Case Discussion

What Aspects of Her History Help You Make the Diagnosis?

Her diarrhea is nonbloody and vomiting is a prominent feature. Mild abdominal discomfort is not unexpected after continued vomiting. It is important to note the absence of subjective fevers—many prudent patients take their own temperatures. Her symptoms began after a meal consisting of orange juice and granola bars, food items are not typically implicated in food-borne illnesses. The importance of the exposure to the small child should not be overlooked. Fecal-oral transmission of rotavirus can occur in the most prudent patients despite diligent hand washing.

How Does the Physical Examination Help You?

The patient is volume depleted as evidenced by orthostatic hypotension and dry mucous membranes. It's not uncommon for a young woman to have a flow murmur accentuated by her dehydration. Her abdominal examination is benign and gives few clues. Because she is young, has no reproducible abdominal pain, is afebrile, and denies hematochezia, it is not vital that she acquiesce to a rectal examination. Her stool is frequent enough that it can be sent for serial guaiacs. Were this patient immunocompromised or elderly, the physician would need to be more adamant about performing a rectal examination because the differential diagnosis is more complex.

What Laboratory Tests Would Be Helpful?

Because she is significantly volume contracted, she may have electrolyte abnormalities, and one would anticipate an acid–base disorder to coincide. Getting serum chemistries would be reasonable. Any woman of reproductive age reporting nausea and vomiting also should undergo a pregnancy test. She is afebrile with minimal abdominal pain and no bloody stools or signs of dysentery. The lack of evidence of an intestinal wall–invading organism and lack of travel history suggest that stool studies would be of little help.

Should This Patient Be Admitted to the Hospital?

Because the patient is unable to maintain adequate oral hydration and is already significantly volume depleted, intravenous fluids should be started immediately (rather than waiting for laboratory test results to return). She should be observed in an emergency setting until she shows evidence that she can take oral hydration or until she is admitted.

Should She Receive Antibiotics?

This patient should not receive antibiotics. Although she has a fairly severe diarrhea, she meets no criteria for empiric antibiotics.

What Is the Likely Cause of Her Diarrhea?

The most likely cause of her diarrhea is viral. Vomiting is a large component of her symptoms, she has no travel history, and she has no signs or symptoms of a bacterial pathogen. She was most likely exposed to rotavirus while changing the infant's diaper.

References

DuPont H. Guidelines on acute infectious diarrhea in adults. *Am J Gastroenterol* 1997;92:1962–1974.

Friedman L, Isselbacher K. Diarrhea and constipation. *Harrison's Principles of Internal Medicine,* 14th ed. New York: McGraw-Hill, 1999:236–244.

Kroser J, Metz D. Evaluation of the adult patient with diarrhea. *Office Practice* 1996;23:629–640.

Wong, et al. The risk of hemolytic uremic syndrome after antibiotic treatment of *E. coli* 0157:H7 infections. *N Engl J Med* 2000;342:1930–1936.

22

Gastroesophageal Reflux Disease

Marc D. Rosenberg

1. What is the underlying mechanism of gastroesophageal reflux disease and how is it defined?
2. What is the common clinical presentation of gastroesophageal reflux disease?
3. What are some atypical presentations of gastroesophageal reflux disease?
4. What life-style modifications should be made for gastroesophageal reflux disease, and do they work?
5. What medicines and treatment strategies are available for gastroesophageal reflux disease?
6. What alarming features are associated with gastroesophageal reflux disease?
7. What are the long-term risks of gastroesophageal reflux disease?
8. What treatments are available for gastroesophageal reflux disease?
9. When should further testing be considered?
10. What are the long-term risks of gastroesophageal reflux disease?

Discussion

What Is the Underlying Mechanism of Gastroesophageal Reflux Disease (GERD) and How Is It Defined?

The underlying mechanism of GERD is the reflux of acid either due to overproduction in the stomach or an abnormally relaxed lower esophageal sphincter. Although all patients have some degree of physiologic reflux, the definition of GERD describes those patients who have symptoms related to their reflux or evidence of mucosal injury related to reflux.

What Is the Common Clinical Presentation of Gastroesophageal Reflux Disease?

The most common clinical presentation of GERD is that of a patient complaining of intermittent burning substernal chest pain or heartburn. Symptoms frequently occur after eating or when the patient is supine and may result in disturbance of sleep.

Heartburn symptoms are often relieved with over the counter antacids or histamine (H_2) receptor antagonists. In addition, patients may complain of regurgitation or dysphagia.

What Are Some Atypical Presentations of Gastroesophageal Reflux Disease?

Wheezing and shortness of breath, which may be difficult to differentiate from asthma, may be a solitary complaint. It is thought that wheezing may occur as the result of aspiration of acid or vagal stimulation by the presence of acid in the esophagus. In addition, patients may present with hoarseness due to acid-induced irritation of the larynx, cough, sore throat, or globus hystericus.

What Alarming Features Are Associated with Gastroesophageal Reflux Disease?

Alarming features of GERD include weight loss and dysphagia. Weight loss is particularly disconcerting because it is often a presenting symptom of malignancy. When dysphagia occurs in a patient previously diagnosed with GERD, esophageal stricture must be ruled out and evaluated. These can both be evaluated via esophagogastroduodenoscopy or with an upper gastrointestinal series plus fluoroscopy while a barium tablet is swallowed.

What Life-Style Modifications Should Be Made for Gastroesophageal Reflux Disease, and Do They Work?

Life-style modifications involve behavioral changes (nonmedical, nonsurgical) that can improve the symptoms of GERD. They are of great value because they are inexpensive and if implemented can produce significant improvement in symptoms. They include elevating the head of the bed 6 inches or placing a wedge under the mattress, refraining from eating long before lying down, weight loss, avoidance of alcohol, and smoking cessation. Intake of fatty foods, colas, teas and coffee should be reduced because they stimulate acid production. In addition, discontinuing certain medications such as calcium channel blockers, anticholinergics, β agonists, and theophylline may reduce symptoms.

What Medicines and Treatment Strategies Are Available for Gastroesophageal Reflux Disease?

Available medicines for the treatment of GERD include antacids, H_2 receptor antagonists (cimetidine, ranitidine, famotidine and nizatidine), mucosal protectants (sucralfate), prokinetics (metoclopramide) and proton pump inhibitors (omeprazole, esomeprazole, and lansoprazole).

The step-up approach involves starting with an H_2 blocker at a standard dose for 1 to 4 weeks and then increasing the dose if there is no relief of symptoms. Subsequently stepping up to a standard dose of a proton pump inhibitor in place of an H_2 blocker is indicated in patients with persistent symptoms. Successful treatment is defined as control of symptoms. Therapy should be continued at the effective dose for 2 to 3 months, at which point the drug should be discontinued. If the patient is on a proton pump inhibitor, the dose should be tapered down because parietal cell hyperplasia with abrupt cessation has been described and may result in rapid recurrence of symptoms.

The step down approach involves starting with a standard proton pump inhibitor dose and if successful, stepping down to an H_2 blocker. If the proton pump fails, then endoscopy should be performed early.

Additional therapies include surgical fundoplication and interventional endoscopy. Further discussion is beyond the scope of this text.

When Should Further Testing Be Considered?

Further diagnostic testing should be sought if patients do not respond to appropriate therapy, have chronic symptoms, have symptoms suggesting complicated disease, (i.e., dysphagia, evidence of gastrointestinal blood loss or weight loss), or atypical symptoms (cough, shortness of breath, hoarseness, or chest pain). Furthermore, patients who have long-standing disease that requires chronic medical therapy should undergo endoscopic screening for Barrett esophagus.

What Are the Long-Term Risks of Gastroesophageal Reflux Disease?

The major risk of long-term acid exposure of the esophageal mucosa is the development of Barrett esophagus and possible progression to esophageal adenocarcinoma. Barrett esophagus is defined as the replacement of the normal squamous epithelium of the distal esophagus by metaplastic columnar epithelium. Patients with Barrett esophagus should be screened on a regular basis (although the interval is controversial) for the development of dysplasia.

The other major risk of chronic reflux is the development of esophageal stricture, which is usually heralded by the development of dysphagia.

Case

A 29-year-old white man presents to your office with the complaint of frequent episodes of heartburn. His symptoms typically occur in the evening and awaken him from sleep. The symptoms resolve after taking antacids. Typically, he eats dinner at 8 P.M. and consumes two cocktails or glasses of wine before he goes to sleep at 10 P.M. His symptoms have begun occurring more frequently and now even occur during the day. He notes that in the morning he has an awful taste in his mouth. Of note, he recently has been diagnosed with asthma.

1. How should he be treated?
2. Does he need to be referred for endoscopy?
3. What are the indications for repeat endoscopy?

Case Discussion

How Should He Be Treated?

This patient should first be treated with life-style modifications consisting of eating meals longer before bedtime, and limiting alcohol intake, particularly in the evening time. In addition, because his symptoms are also occurring more frequently during the daytime, he would likely benefit from starting an H_2 blocker. Doing so also may improve his asthmatic symptoms.

Does He Need to Be Referred for Endoscopy?

At this point it would be premature to refer for esophagogastroduodenoscopy. If a trial similar to the above recommendations is successful, and symptoms do not return after a trial without medication, then no further workup is necessary. However, if symptoms recur or the patient requires chronic therapy and is changed to a proton pump inhibitor or alarm symptoms or signs occur, then endoscopy should be performed to rule out esophagitis, Barrett esophagus, strictures, and confirm the diagnosis. In addition, if symptoms continue with a normal endoscopy, pH monitoring with or without esophageal manometry studies (particularly if dysphagia is present) would be indicated.

What Are the Indications for Repeat Endoscopy?

The indications for future endoscopy are symptoms that are refractory to medical management, development of alarm symptoms at any time, and long-standing disease. If during any endoscopy Barrett esophagus is diagnosed, the patient should have routine surveillance. The frequency of surveillance is controversial, although most clinicians agree that repeat endoscopy should be performed every 2 to 3 years with surveillance biopsies.

Suggested Reading

De Vault K R, Castell D. Updated guidelines for the diagnosis and treatment of gastroesophageal reflux disease. *Am J Gastroenterol* 1999;94:1434–1442.

Kahrilas P. Gastroesophageal reflux disease and its complications. In: Sleisenger, Fordtran, eds. *Gastrointestinal and liver disease,* 6th ed. Philadelphia: W. B. Saunders Company, 1998:498–527.

Kahrilas P. Medical management of gastroesophageal reflux disease. *Up to Date* 2000;8.

Katz P O. Treatment of gastroesophageal reflux disease: use of algorithms to aid in management. *Am J Gastroenterol* 1999;94(suppl):3–10.

Orlando R. Reflux esophagitis. In: Yamada et al., eds. *Textbook of Gastroenterology,* 3rd ed. Philadelphia: Lippincott Williams & Wilkins, 1999:1235–1263.

23
Peptic Ulcer Disease
Rahul Verma

1. What are the symptoms of acid dyspepsia and what is the differential diagnosis?
2. What are the different etiologic associations of peptic ulcer disease?
3. When should a patient be referred directly for endoscopy?

Discussion

What Are the Symptoms of Acid Dyspepsia and What Is the Differential Diagnosis?

The differential diagnosis of dyspepsia includes acid dyspepsia, functional dyspepsia, gastroesophageal reflux disease (GERD), and irritable bowel syndrome. Dyspepsia is characterized as chronic or recurrent upper abdominal pain or discomfort. The classic symptoms of peptic ulcer disease are referred to as acid dyspepsia. The symptoms are characterized as epigastric burning that improves with eating, and is worse 1 to 2 hours after meals. The discomfort is often nocturnal. Functional (nonulcer) dyspepsia is described as dyspepsia in which no definite structural or biochemical explanation for the symptoms are found after clinically appropriate investigations have been taken.

Gastroesophageal reflux disease can be differentiated fairly easily on the basis of symptoms. GERD is described as heartburn, regurgitation, or both. It can occur after large or fatty meals, and is aggravated by recumbency. The management is fairly well described.

Symptoms of irritable bowel syndrome include crampy abdominal pain with alternating diarrhea and constipation. Symptoms are intermittent and exacerbated by high-fat meals and stress. Treatment modalities include fiber, antispasmodics, anticholinergics, and antidepressants.

What Are the Different Etiologic Associations of Peptic Ulcer Disease?

Peptic ulcer disease has many etiologic associations. With the recent delineation of the association of *Helicobacter pylori* and peptic ulcer disease, it is speculated that *H. pylori* is the leading cause of peptic ulcer disease. Recent literature reports that greater than 90% of duodenal and greater than 75% of gastric ulcers are associated with *H. pylori*. There is a 30% prevalence in the general population, with the majority of these infections being asymptomatic.

The second most common association with peptic ulcers is the use of non-steroidal antiinflammatory drugs (NSAIDs). It is estimated that 10% to 20% of patients taking NSAIDs develop dyspepsia. Twenty percent of the users of these commonly prescribed medications develop ulcers. NSAIDs increase the risk of ulcer complication by four- to sixfold.

Gastric cancer is an important and clinically significant cause of peptic ulcer disease. It lends itself to close surveillance in those with dyspepsia. Other disease associations of peptic ulcer disease include stress, Zollinger-Ellison syndrome, mastocytosis, hypercalcemia, and some viral illnesses such as herpes simplex and cytomegalovirus.

When Should a Patient Be Referred Directly for Endoscopy?

Endoscopy is considered the gold standard test in excluding gastroduodenal ulcers, reflux esophagitis, and upper gastrointestinal cancers. The role of endoscopy has changed with increased understanding of the link between *H. pylori* with peptic ulcer disease and gastrointestinal cancers. In patients over 45 years of age with dyspepsia, endoscopy is indicated because the incidence of cancer increases after this age. Regardless of age, alarm features such as recurrent vomiting, dysphagia, evidence of anemia, evidence of gastrointestinal bleeding, or an abdominal mass are also indications for referral for endoscopy.

Case

A 50-year-old man with a history of coronary artery disease and osteoarthritis presents to the clinic complaining of 3 weeks of epigastric abdominal pain. The pain is described as burning and occurs about 2 hours after eating. He also reports some bloating as well. He denies any weight loss.

His most recent myocardial infarction occurred about 2 years earlier. He is currently taking atenolol, aspirin, lisinopril, and an over-the-counter pain medication for his arthritis.

On physical examination his blood pressure is 129/83 mm Hg with a heart rate of 84 beats/min and no evidence of orthostasis. He appears in no apparent distress, and his abdominal examination is significant for no epigastric tenderness and normoactive bowel sounds. The guaiac examination is negative. Other aspects of the physical examination are normal.

1. What are the more likely etiologic agents of this patient's dyspepsia?
2. What is the next step in the management of this patient's symptoms?
3. What are the proposed mechanisms of injury to the gastrointestinal tract with NSAIDs?
4. What are the factors that increase the risk of NSAID-induced ulcers?
5. Is there a synergistic role of *H. pylori* and NSAIDs in inducing ulcers?
6. Are cyclooxygenase type 2 inhibitors superior in controlling pain symptoms and preventing NSAID-related gastrointestinal complications?

7. Do histamine receptor antagonists have a role in the management of NSAID-related dyspepsia?
8. What are the current recommendations in the management of NSAID-related ulcers?
9. Which patients should be tested for *H. pylori*?
10. Is *H. pylori* linked with gastrointestinal malignancies, and if so, which ones?
11. What are the tests available for testing *H. pylori* and what is their reliability?
12. What are the current recommendations in treating *H. pylori* with regard to the agents used and duration of therapy?
13. What are important considerations in patients who are refractory to the treatment of peptic ulcer disease?

Discussion

What Are the More Likely Etiologic Agents of This Patient's Dyspepsia?

The features of this patient's symptoms are most consistent with acid dyspepsia. Other syndromes such as GERD or irritable bowel syndrome are less likely, based on the symptoms. The etiologic agents most likely to be associated with this patient's dyspepsia are *H. pylori* and NSAIDs.

The patient is taking an aspirin each day, but also gives a history of taking over-the-counter pain medications. A more detailed history should be obtained to attempt to identify the possibility of over-the-counter NSAID use.

What Is the Next Step in the Management of This Patient's Symptoms?

Although the patient has no evidence of alarm features, endoscopy is indicated (Fig. 23.1). This is based on the increased prevalence of gastric malignancies in patients over 45 years of age. The role of an upper gastrointestinal series is less defined in the era of *H. pylori*. The relationship of *H. pylori* to malignancy lends itself to the need for biopsy. Endoscopy is not recommended in patients with NSAID-related dyspepsia who are under 45 years of age, unless there is evidence of alarm features.

What Are the Proposed Mechanisms of Injury to the Gastrointestinal Tract with NSAIDs?

Nonsteroidal antiinflammatory drugs have toxic effects on the gastroduodenal mucosa via direct effects on the mucosal lining, as well as systemic effects through a reduction of prostaglandin synthesis. Prostaglandins are gastroprotective by inhibiting acid secretion, promoting bicarbonate secretion, and increasing gastric mucus production. Enhanced safety profiles of some NSAIDs occur by altering the acidic nature of the medications, thus lessening the direct toxic effect.

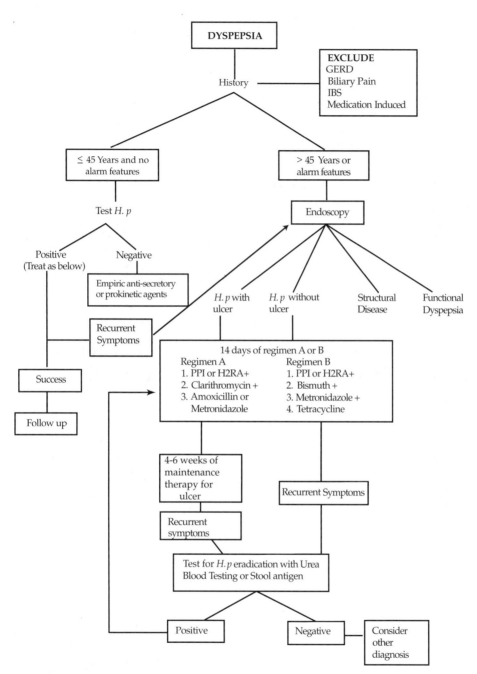

Figure 23.1. The evaluation of dyspepsia. *H.p., Helicobacter pylori*; PPI, proton pump inhibitor; H₂RA, histamine receptor antagonist. (Adapted from American Gastroenterological Association Medical Position Statement. Evaluation of dyspepsia. *Gastroenterology* 1998;114:579–581, Peterson W L, Fendrick A M, Cave D R, et al. *Helicobacter pylori*–related disease. *Arch Intern Med* 2000; 160:1285–1291; with permission.)

What Are the Factors That Increase the Risk of NSAID-Induced Ulcers?

Factors that are established as increasing the risk of NSAID-associated ulcers are advanced age, history of ulcer, systemic illness, concomitant steroid use, concomitant use of anticoagulants, use of higher doses of NSAIDs, and prolonged NSAID use. Factors that have not been well established, but are felt to be associated with peptic ulcer disease, are tobacco use, alcohol use, and coffee.

Is There a Synergistic Role of *H. pylori* and NSAIDs in Inducing Ulcers?

Although 90% of gastroduodenal ulcers are associated with *H. pylori* or NSAIDs, the mechanisms of injury are different. There is currently no synergistic mechanism suspected, and each acts independently to cause gastroduodenal injury. Studies indicate that *H. pylori* does not increase the severity of NSAID-related ulcers. Other studies indicate that in patients using NSAIDs, eradication of *H. pylori* did not reduce the recurrence rate of ulcers.

Are Cyclooxygenase Type 2 Inhibitors Superior in Controlling Pain Symptoms and Preventing NSAID-Related Gastrointestinal Complications?

By inhibiting the cyclooxygenase enzymes, NSAIDs inhibit the formation of the gastroprotective prostaglandins. There are two cyclooxygenase enzymes: cyclooxygenase type 1 (COX-1) and COX-2. The COX-2 enzyme is associated with inflammation, whereas COX-1 is associated with homeostasis of the organs, such as gastric integrity. Thus, the COX-2 inhibitors are theorized to be more gastroprotective because they exhibit little effect on the COX-1 enzyme. In studies published comparing the efficacy and safety of traditional NSAIDs and COX-2 inhibitors, the degree of symptom control is similar. However, the COX-2 inhibitors are associated with a much lower incidence of gastrointestinal complications. The COX-2 inhibitors are quite costly and are therefore recommended to be second-line choices to traditional NSAIDs, unless the patient is a high-risk candidate for NSAID-related gastroduodenal injury.

Do Histamine Receptor Antagonists Have a Role in the Management of NSAID-Related Dyspepsia?

Histamine (H_2) receptor antagonists are recommended for the management of NSAID-related dyspepsia. However, their routine use in asymptomatic patients is associated with an increased risk of gastrointestinal complications. This increased risk is theorized to be secondary to the masking of symptoms of gastrointestinal complications. Based on randomized controlled trials, there is no role for H_2 receptor antagonists in preventing NSAID-related gastropathy. Either a proton pump inhibitor or misoprostol is recommended for prophylaxis of NSAID-related gastropathy.

What Are the Current Recommendations in the Management of NSAID-Related Ulcers?

If the patient has an NSAID-related ulcer and the NSAID is discontinued, the use of either an H$_2$ receptor antagonist or proton pump inhibitor is recommended. If the NSAID will be continued, then a proton pump inhibitor is recommended.

Which Patients Should Be Tested for *H. pylori*?

The clinical and cost benefit of treating *H. pylori* in patients with ulcers is well documented. It is therefore recommended that *H. pylori* be treated in any patient with documented duodenal or gastric ulcer. *H. pylori* testing also should be performed in patients with a history of ulcer who currently are receiving antisecretory agents. The role of testing *H. pylori* in patients with NSAID-related gastropathy is controversial, but treatment is recommended in patients with *H. pylori* infection.

Testing should be performed in young patients with dyspepsia. *H. pylori* should be eradicated in any patient with mucosa-related lymphoid tissue lymphoma. Despite its association with gastric cancer, routine screening is generally not recommended.

Is *H. pylori* Linked with Gastrointestinal Malignancies, and If So, Which Ones?

Helicobacter pylori has been associated with mucosa-associated lymphoid tissue lymphoma, and its treatment may be associated with regression. In addition, there may be up to a ninefold increased incidence of gastric adenocarcinoma.

What Are the Tests Available for Testing *H. pylori* and What Is Their Reliability?

The different methods of testing for *H. pylori* and their reported sensitivities and specificities are reported in Table 23.1. Eradication should be documented 4 weeks after treatment.

Table 23.1. Methods of Testing for *Helicobacter pylori*

Test	Sensitivity	Specificity	Comment
Serologic testing	80%	90%	Test is an IgG antibody and remains positive for 6–12 mo after treatment; noninvasive
Urea breath testing	90%	99%	False negative can occur[a]; can be used for primary diagnosis or follow-up testing
Stool antigen	80%–100%		Possible role in follow-up testing
Biopsy	80%–100%	99%	False negative may occur[a]; invasive
Rapid urease test	80%–95%	95%–100%	False negative may occur[a]; invasive

[a]False negative may occur in patients using proton pump inhibitors, histamine receptor antagonists, bismuth, and antimicrobials.

What Are the Current Recommendations in Treating *H. pylori* with Regard to the Agents Used and Duration of Therapy?

Currently two regimens are recommended for the eradication of *H. pylori*. A three-drug regimen includes the use of a proton pump inhibitor or H_2 receptor antagonist, clarithromycin, and either amoxicillin or metronidazole. A four-drug regimen includes an H_2 receptor antagonist, bismuth, metronidazole, and tetracycline. The duration of therapy is 10 to 14 days for the three-drug regimen and 14 days for the four-drug regimen. Maintenance therapy should be given to patients with newly diagnosed ulcers for 4 weeks with either a proton pump inhibitor or H_2RA.

What Are Important Considerations in Patients Who Are Refractory to the Treatment of Peptic Ulcer Disease?

For recurrent ulcers, incomplete eradication of *H. pylori* should be suspected. Compliance with *H. pylori* medications should be questioned. An alternative regimen should involve changing from the three-drug to the four-drug protocol or vice versa.

After eradication of *H. pylori* has been ensured, other causes for ulcer disease should be suspected.

Suggested Reading

American Gastroenterological Association Medical Position Statement. Evaluation of dyspepsia. *Gastroenterology* 1998;114:579–581.

Capell S, et al. Diagnosis and treatment of nonsteroidal anti-inflammatory drug–associated upper gastrointestinal toxicity. *Gastroenterol Clin* 2000;29:97–124.

Consensus Statement. Medical management of peptic ulcer disease. *JAMA* 1996;275:622–629.

NIH Consensus Conference. *Helicobacter pylori* in peptic ulcer disease. *JAMA* 1994;272:65–69.

Peterson W L, Fendrick A M, Cave D R, et al. *Helicobacter pylori*–related disease. *Arch Intern Med* 2000;160:1285–1291.

Wolfe M, et al. Gastrointestinal toxicity of nonsteroidal anti-inflammatory drugs. *N Engl J Med* 1999;340:1888–1899.

24
Viral Hepatitis

Atul V. Marathe
Ira C. Marathe

1. What viruses cause hepatitis?
2. How is viral hepatitis transmitted?
3. What are the clinical features of viral hepatitis?
4. What are the laboratory findings in viral hepatitis?
5. How is the diagnosis made?

Discussion
What Viruses Cause Hepatitis?

Hepatitis is a nonspecific inflammation of the liver characterized by elevated serum aminotransferase levels. There are at least five viruses (hepatitis A through E) known to cause hepatitis. Clinical hepatitis is classified as acute or chronic. Acute hepatitis is defined as self-limited liver injury of less than 6 months duration, whereas chronic hepatitis is defined as continued inflammatory response of greater than 6 months duration. Over 90% of acute hepatitis in the United States is due to hepatitis A, B, or C. Hepatitis A and E present as only acute disease, whereas hepatitis B, C, and D may manifest in both acute and chronic forms.

Hepatitis A virus (HAV) is the most common cause of acute viral hepatitis, accounting for almost 50% of the cases in the United States. It is usually self-limited, but may lead to fulminant hepatic failure. Hepatitis A never causes chronic disease.

Hepatitis B virus (HBV) accounts for about 30% of acute hepatitis in the United States. It is the most common chronic infectious disease in the world. About 5% of infected adults, 20% of infected children, and 90% of infected neonates become chronically infected. Chronic HBV is a major cause of cirrhosis and hepatocellular carcinoma.

Hepatitis C virus (HCV) accounts for about 15% to 20% of acute hepatitis in the United States. Up to 85% of those infected develop chronic disease. About 20% of patients with chronic HCV develop cirrhosis. HCV is now the most common indication for liver transplantation in the United States.

The rare hepatitis D virus (HDV) accounts for less than 2% of acute hepatitis in the United States. Also called delta agent, it is a defective RNA virus that requires the presence of HBV to cause clinical disease. This may occur as a coinfection, which is simultaneous HBV and HDV infection, or superinfection, which is HDV infection in a chronic HBV carrier. Infection may be chronic or acute, and tends to be more severe than HBV alone.

Hepatitis E virus (HEV) is very similar to HAV and is rarely seen in the United States. Cases in the United States are usually seen in people who have recently traveled to developing countries that are considered endemic areas for this virus. Like HAV, HEV never causes chronic disease, but can rarely cause fulminant hepatic failure. For unclear reasons, HEV in pregnancy is more frequently associated with a fulminant course, causing death in 5% to 25% of cases.

There are also other viruses rarely associated with hepatitis, such as cytomegalovirus (CMV), Epstein-Barr virus (EBV), herpes simplex virus (HSV), and varicella zoster virus (VZV).

How Is Viral Hepatitis Transmitted?

Hepatitis A virus is transmitted via the fecal-oral route, usually from person to person or by contaminated food or water. It has been associated with the consumption of raw or partially cooked shellfish or seafood. Outbreaks after ingestion of fruits and vegetables have been linked to contamination by food handlers. Transmission by blood is uncommon, although there have been several reported cases. Casual contact, kissing, and sharing eating utensils are not thought to be sources of transmission.

Hepatitis B virus is transmitted through exchange of blood or body fluids. The most common routes of transmission are sexual contact, including receptive anal intercourse or heterosexual promiscuity, contaminated needles used in intravenous drug abuse, and vertical transmission from infected mother to child.

Hepatitis C virus is transmitted predominantly through percutaneous and mucosal exposure. Intravenous drug abuse accounts for about 60% of new cases. The role of sexual transmission is controversial, because transmission is not common between monogamous sexual partners. Perinatal transmission is also infrequent. Up to 40% of patients with acute disease deny having any exposure to a recognized risk factor in the previous 6 months, such as intravenous drug abuse, intranasal cocaine use, body piercing, tattoos, or history of sexually transmitted disease.

Hepatitis D virus is spread in a similar manner to HBV, because it requires its presence for infectivity.

Hepatitis E virus, like HAV, is spread via the fecal-oral route, particularly through contaminated drinking water.

What Are the Clinical Features of Viral Hepatitis?

Viral hepatitis has no specific or pathognomonic clinical features. Its onset may be abrupt or insidious. It frequently presents as an influenza-type illness. Although some symptoms occur more commonly in one type of viral hepatitis than another, there is a significant amount of overlap of symptoms, such that the type of hepatitis cannot be diagnosed by clinical presentation alone. Therefore, serologic testing is needed to make a diagnosis.

In general, there is usually a preicteric phase followed by an icteric phase. In the preicteric phase, there may be generalized malaise, anorexia, low-grade fever, nausea, vomiting, diarrhea, vague abdominal pain, right upper quadrant pain, and, occasionally, a change in the sense of taste. The duration of these symptoms is variable and sometimes may last for several weeks. In many patients this is the only manifestation of the disease. Patients who do go on to the icteric phase find that their urine darkens, their stools become lighter colored, and they become jaundiced. At this point, the majority of the systemic manifestations usually resolve. Right upper quadrant pain and anorexia frequently continue, and fatigue often worsens.

The physical examination is not usually very helpful. Patients may have mild cervical lymphadenopathy, an enlarged tender liver, and splenomegaly. If ascites, spider angiomas, gynecomastia, or palmar erythema are seen, chronic underlying liver disease must be considered. Spider angiomata, however, is occasionally seen in acute HAV.

What Are the Laboratory Findings in Viral Hepatitis?

In acute hepatitis, serum alanine aminotransferase (ALT) and aspartate aminotransferase (AST) levels are usually elevated eightfold and range between 1,000 and 3,000 IU/L. They usually return to normal within 4 to 8 weeks. Bilirubin starts to increase slightly after AST and ALT increase, to 5 to 10 mg/dL, and rarely up to 20 mg/dL. Bilirubin may remain elevated up to 5 months. Alkaline phosphatase is usually only slightly elevated. The white blood cell (WBC) count is normal or slightly low, often with atypical lymphocytes.

How Is the Diagnosis Made?

The mainstay of the diagnosis of viral hepatitis is serologic testing. The diagnosis of HAV is made by finding immunoglobulin M anti-HAV (HAV IgM) in the serum during the acute or convalescent phase of the disease. This antibody persists for 3 to 6 months after the acute phase. Immunoglobulin G anti-HAV (HAV IgG) is also produced in the convalescent phase. Commercially available tests can measure HAV IgM and total anti-HAV (IgG and IgM). Total antibody to HAV without elevation of IgM indicates prior exposure.

The viral genome of HBV contains four separate regions that encode distinct proteins, or antigens. Detection of three of these antigens—surface antigen (HBsAg), core antigen (HBcAg), and "e" antigen (HBeAg)—are used in the diagnosis of HBV. Acute hepatitis B is confirmed by the presence of HBsAg, but it cannot be excluded by its absence. HBsAg can be detected as early as 6 days after exposure, and symptoms usually occur 4 weeks thereafter. There is a gap between the disappearance of HBsAg and the appearance of hepatitis B surface antibody (HBsAb). This is referred to as the window period, when infected individuals would be both HBsAg and HBsAb negative. During this period, immunoglobulin IgG or IgM to HBcAg (HBcAb) will be present (Fig. 24.1). Thus, acute hepatitis B can only be excluded by the absence of HBcAb. Antibody to HBsAg (HBsAb) is seen after resolution of acute infection and is also seen after immunization. The presence of HbeAg and HBV DNA indicates ongoing viral replication and infectivity. It is normally detectable for only 4 to 6 weeks, but its presence after 2 months indicates that chronic infection is likely. There are two subsets of patients with chronic hepatitis B: carriers and those with hepatitis B infection. Hepatitis B carriers have low viral load, normal liver enzymes, and are HBsAg positive, HBeAb positive, but HBeAg and HBV DNA negative. Patients with chronic hepatitis B infection have high circulating levels of virus, elevated liver enzymes, and are HBsAg positive, HBeAb negative, and HBeAg positive. This differentiation is important because carriers do not

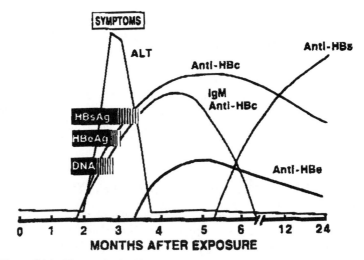

Figure 24.1. The serologic, biochemical, and clinical course of acute hepatitis.

require antiviral therapy and can be followed by their primary care physicians with repeat serologic testing and liver enzymes every 6 to 12 months.

Anti-HCV antibodies (HCVAb) arise 4 to 6 weeks after symptoms, but may not be positive for several months, and thus have little confirmatory value during acute disease. An acute presentation of hepatitis C is unusual; it usually presents as a chronic infection. A positive HCVAb test must be confirmed with either HCV RNA by polymerase chain reaction (PCR) or recombinant immunoblot assay because, depending on the pretest probability, the false-positive rate can be up to 30%.

The viral genome for HDV is very small, with only one protein being coded, hepatitis delta antigen (HDAg). Immunoglobulin IgM to HDV is present in less than 50% of patients with acute HDV infection. Immunoglobulin IgG to HDV becomes present 1 to 4 months after acute infection. The only available assay for the diagnosis of HDV in the United States is the radioimmunoassay test for total antibody, HDVAb (both IgM and IgG). This should be ordered 30 to 40 days after the onset of symptoms. The presence of HDVAb with HBsAg and HBcIgM (indicating acute hepatitis B) suggests coinfection. The absence of HBcIgM suggests superinfection.

Hepatitis E virus is diagnosed by identifying immunoglobulin IgM to HEV or HEV RNA by PCR in serum or stool.

Case

A 28-year-old white woman with no significant past medical history presents with 10 days of fatigue, headache, nausea, and anorexia. Two days ago, her husband noticed that her eyes had turned yellow. She denied the use of any medications, including over-the-counter and herbal preparations. She is married, without children, works in an office as an accountant, and eats out frequently at restaurants. She has no significant family history of liver disease. She drinks alcohol rarely and denies intravenous drug abuse or tobacco use. Her husband of 5 years was recently diagnosed with hepatitis C. Her physical examination is normal except for icteric sclera. She has no stigmata of chronic liver disease. Her laboratory values are as follows:

AST 1,040 µ/L, ALT 1,100 µ/L, alkaline phosphatase 120 U/L, bilirubin 8.6 mg/dL, international normalized ratio 1.1, albumin 4.8 g/dL, WBC count 5,000µ/L with normal differential, hematocrit 40%, platelets 250,000.

1. How is the diagnosis made?
2. How can the spread of hepatitis be prevented?
3. What is the management and treatment of viral hepatitis?

Case Discussion
How Is the Diagnosis Made?

This patient's presentation is consistent with acute hepatitis, which can be drug induced, alcoholic, autoimmune, or viral. She does not have clinical or biochemical features consistent with obstructive biliary tract disease. The history has excluded alcohol- and drug-induced hepatitis. Autoimmune hepatitis is excluded by testing for antinuclear antibody, anti–double-stranded DNA, anti–smooth muscle antibody, and anti–liver kidney antibody. Testing for viral etiologies is performed with HAV IgM, HBsAg, HBc IgM, and HCVAb. If HBsAg is positive, then HDVAb also should be ordered. If the patient had recently traveled to a developing country, then HEVAb also should be ordered.

Because this patient eats out often, HAV is high on the differential diagnosis list. HBV is less likely, because she is in a monogamous relationship and has no other risk factors. Because her husband has HCV, she is at slight risk for acquiring HCV. However, transmission from sexual intimacy is rarely seen in monogamous couples. It could be transmitted by sharing toothbrushes or razor blades. Additionally, acute illness from HCV is uncommon. In fact, some experts believe that it never presents acutely, and only occurs in the chronic form.

If all of the above serologies are negative, other rare causes of viral hepatitis must be considered, such as HSV, VZV, EBV, and CMV. These can occasionally cause serious infections, leading to fulminant hepatic failure. There are also a group of viruses not detectable by currently available assays, called non–A through E hepatitis.

This patient was found to have acute hepatitis A, likely acquired from eating in a restaurant.

How Can the Spread of Hepatitis Be Prevented?

Hepatitis A virus is spread by fecal-oral transmission, especially within the home. HAV is excreted in the stool for 1 to 2 weeks before, and at least 1 week after, the onset of illness. Human immunoglobulin with IgG anti-HAV is used for postexposure household contacts. This may not be effective if given more than 2 weeks after exposure. HAV vaccine is administered in two doses, approximately 6 months apart. The first dose may be given 2 to 4 weeks prior to travel to an endemic region. If given less than 2 weeks before travel, immunoglobulin is also needed. Other candidates for the HAV vaccine include patients with known chronic liver disease and patients at risk for viral hepatitis, such as intravenous drug abusers, male homosexuals, food handlers, primate handlers, and day-care workers.

Hepatitis B virus is present in all body secretions, so household contacts of patients with hepatitis B should take precautions. HBV immune globulin (HBIG) is a plasma-derived product with high titers of HBsAb. It is indicated for infants born to mothers positive for HBsAg or unknown status, sexual contacts, and after parenteral exposure. There are two types of HBV vaccine available: one with deactivated virus, and one from recombinant DNA. The recombinant vaccine is the one used in the United States. This vaccine is recommended for all infants and children, household contacts, health-care workers, illnesses requiring frequent blood products, and people with multiple sex partners. It also should be given to unvaccinated individuals for prophylaxis after exposure and those previously vaccinated but found to have low titers.

Patterns of HCV transmission have changed. Prior to the onset of testing of donated blood in 1992, this virus was commonly transmitted through blood transfusion. Fortunately, this is now rare. HCV is transmitted percutaneously, through needlestick, tattooing, body piercing, and particularly intravenous drug abuse. It is felt that nearly 75% of new intravenous drug abusers will become positive within 1 year after beginning drug use. Household contacts should avoid sharing any item that may be contaminated with blood, and the patient should cover all breaks in the skin. There is no evidence that coughing, sneezing, or casual contact transmits HCV. Currently, there is no vaccine for HCV. All patients with HCV should receive HAV and HBV vaccinations.

What Is the Management and Treatment of Viral Hepatitis?

The treatment of acute viral hepatitis (A through E) is supportive. Most patients can be treated at home. Vigorous physical activity should be avoided. Most patients feel better within a few weeks, but patients with acute hepatitis B may continue to be ill for up to 2 months. Only those patients who have severe nausea and vomiting, cannot tolerate oral intake, have a prothrombin time of more than 3 seconds above normal, or have evidence of acute liver failure need to be hospitalized. Acute liver failure is characterized by massive hepatic necrosis with mental status changes and impairment of liver function. These patients need urgent evaluation by a hepatologist and possible transfer to a liver transplant center.

Chronic carriers of HBV (i.e., those with a low viral load, normal liver enzymes, and who are HBsAg positive, HBeAb positive, but HBeAg and HBV DNA negative) can be followed by their primary care physicians, but patients with chronic HBV infection (i.e., those with high circulating levels of virus, elevated liver enzymes, and who are HBsAg positive, HBeAb negative, and HBeAg positive) should be referred to a hepatologist for treatment. Two drugs have been approved for the treatment of HBV: α-interferon and lamivudine. Alpha-interferon is the only drug that has been found to have lasting beneficial effect in the treatment of HBV. The overall response rate, defined as a sustained elimination of HBeAg and HBV DNA, is still only 30% to 40% with α-interferon. Candidates for treatment are patients with persistent elevations in aminotransferases, serum HBsAg, HBeAg, HBV DNA, and histologic evidence of inflammation on liver biopsy. Alpha-interferon is difficult for many patients to tolerate due to its side effects, such as fevers, chills, headaches, weakness, depression, bone marrow suppression, and muscle soreness.

Lamivudine is considered first-line therapy in more advanced liver disease or early cirrhosis. HBeAg clearance is seen in 15% to 20% of patients treated with lamivudine. There is some concern that long-term use of lamivudine is associated with the development of viral resistance. Combination therapy does not appear to confer any significant therapeutic advantage.

Liver transplantation for liver failure from HBV is a controversial topic. Patients with acute liver failure from acute hepatitis B are candidates for transplantation and have a 5-year recurrence rate of 18%. Patients with chronic HBV who lack HBeAg or HBV DNA, the markers of replication, are transplantation candidates for end-stage liver disease. Patients with chronic HBV with cirrhosis, who are positive for HBeAg or HBV DNA, are more likely to have recurrence of infection, often with accelerated disease in the new graft. Advanced cirrhosis may occur as early as 7 months, and development of hepatocellular carcinoma can occur in less than 2 years. However, with the administration of long-term HBIG, the rate of recurrence and long-term survival has improved.

The current recommended therapy for chronic HCV is the combination of α-interferon and ribavirin. Therapy is recommended for all patients with chronic HCV with elevated serum amino transferases, detectable HCV RNA, and a liver biopsy showing some degree of fibrosis or moderate to severe inflammation. Contraindications to therapy are advanced or decompensated cirrhosis, severe psychiatric illness, bone marrow disease, significant cardiovascular disease, and a history of organ transplantation other than of the liver. The response rate is close to 40%. Current studies are exploring longer acting interferons that are modified by polyethylene glycol. These longer acting "pegylated" formulations avoid some of the peaks and troughs and side effects of the current formulation. So far, the studies are promising. Patients with HCV, as with any chronic liver disease, should abstain from any alcohol use.

Patients with end-stage liver disease from chronic HCV are also eligible for liver transplantation. Approximately 90% of patients undergoing transplantation for liver disease secondary to chronic HCV develop recurrent infection in the transplanted graft. Unlike HBV, most patients with recurrent HCV have mild disease and rarely develop liver failure.

Suggested Reading

Bader T F. *Viral hepatitis: practical evaluation & treatment,* 3rd ed. Seattle: Hogrefe & Huber, 2000.

Regev A, Schiff E R. Hepatology: a century of progress, viral hepatitis A, B, and C. *Clin Liver Dis* 2000;4:47–66.

Viral hepatitis: an epidemic in the making? New approaches to the prevention, diagnosis and treatment of viral hepatitis. www.gastro.org/viral-hep.html.

Younossi Z M, ed. Viral hepatitis guide for practicing physicians. *Cleve Clin J Med* 2000;67(suppl 1).

25
Ascites

Michael D. Koplon

1. Discuss the diagnostic approach and evaluation of a patient with suspected ascites.
2. Discuss the management approach to cirrhosis-related ascites.
3. Discuss the options for management of resistant ascites.

Discussion

Discuss the Diagnostic Approach and Evaluation of a Patient with Suspected Ascites.

Ascites is the pathologic accumulation of fluid in the peritoneal cavity. Eighty percent of patients in the United States with ascites have cirrhosis. Nonhepatic causes of ascites include peritoneal carcinomatosis, tuberculosis, heart failure, dialysis, pancreatic disease, and myxedema.

Approximately 3 million Americans have cirrhosis. Cirrhosis is the 11th leading cause of death in the United States. Within 10 years after the diagnosis of compensated cirrhosis, approximately 58% of patients will have developed ascites. Approximately 50% of patients with ascites succumb to death within 2 years. This poor prognostic sign has led to the inclusion of ascites as one of the indications for initiating an evaluation for liver transplantation.

Successful treatment of ascites depends on an accurate diagnosis regarding the cause of ascites formation. Patients who have a cause for ascites formation other than cirrhosis do not usually respond to treatment with diuretics and salt restriction.

The diagnostic approach consists of the history, physical examination, and examination of ascitic fluid obtained by paracentesis.

History

Question the patient about risk factors for liver disease: alcohol use, intravenous and recreational drug use, transfusions, homosexuality, acupuncture, tattoos, ear piercing, country of origin, family history, history of jaundice or hepatitis, history of heart failure, cancer, and tuberculosis.

Physical Examination

Look for shifting dullness (must have approximately 1,500 mL of fluid to detect dullness), fluid wave, and signs of chronic liver disease. The overall accuracy of the physical examination for the detection of nonobvious ascites was only 58% in one series. In obese patients, it is often difficult to determine fluid from fat. Ultrasonography can detect as little as 100 mL of fluid.

Ascitic Fluid Analysis

Ascitic fluid analysis is the most rapid and cost-effective method of diagnosing the cause of ascites and should be performed in all patients with new-onset ascites. Bleeding is sufficiently uncommon to preclude the need for prophylactic fresh frozen plasma (FFP) or platelets.

1. Initial fluid analysis should include a cell count, differential, and ratio of ascitic fluid to albumin. Measure the albumin concentration of serum and ascitic fluid specimens and subtract the albumin concentration of the ascitic fluid value from the serum value.
2. The serum ascites albumin gradient has been proven in prospective studies to categorize ascites better than the total protein-based exudate/transudate concept.
3. With approximately 97% accuracy, a serum to ascites albumin gradient of 1.1 g/dL or greater indicates that the patient has ascites induced by portal hypertension.
4. Other tests, such as smears and culture for tuberculosis and cytologic tests, are usually reserved for situations in which the initial fluid is found to have a predominance of lymphocytic cells with a serum to ascites ratio of less than 1.1 g/dL, or if tuberculosis or cancer is suspected clinically.

The cell count provides immediate information about bacterial infection. Patients with an absolute neutrophil count of greater than or equal to 250 cells/μl should be presumed to be infected and should be started on empiric antibiotics. Recent studies have shown increased sensitivity with direct bedside inoculation of blood culture bottles with ascitic fluid.

Radiologic Evaluation

Most people advocate an initial imaging study of the liver to search for causes of ascites and possible concomitant hepatocellular carcinoma (especially because hepatitis B and C and alcoholic cirrhosis are important risk factors). Imaging cannot distinguish between benign and malignant ascites, but it may detect simultaneously the presence of a solid tumor in the abdomen. Ultrasonography, computed tomography (CT), and magnetic resonance imaging all have good diagnostic accuracy in detecting liver metastases and other hepatic tumors. CT and transvaginal ultrasonography provide reasonable accuracy in the diagnosis of ovarian cancer. CT is the most useful investigation in the diagnosis of pancreatic cancer. Ultrasonography is probably the most cost-effective initial screening choice, with further studies performed depending on clinical suspicion and ascitic fluid analysis.

Discuss the Management Approach to Cirrhosis-Related Ascites.

Treat the underlying cause of cirrhosis. Improvement in the reversible component of alcoholic liver disease can reduce portal pressure and decrease sodium retention. Patients with decompensated cirrhosis due to autoimmune hepatitis also may have a reversible component with steroid therapy or azathioprine.

Avoid the use of nonsteroidal antiinflammatory drugs. These agents inhibit the synthesis of renal prostaglandins, leading to renal vasoconstriction, a lesser response to diuretics, and the possible precipitation of acute renal failure.

The development of ascites in a patient with portal hypertension is the consequence of avid renal retention of sodium and water. The removal of ascites and edema require the induction of a negative sodium balance. The most important treatments of patients with ascites and cirrhosis are the restriction of dietary sodium intake and the use of oral diuretics. An 88 mEq (2,000 mg) per day sodium diet is the most practical and successful regimen. However, only about 15% of patients lose weight and have a reduction in the volume of ascitic fluid with sodium restriction alone. It is sodium restriction, not fluid restriction, that results in weight loss. Only severe hyponatremia (serum sodium of <120 mEq/L) warrants fluid restriction in the cirrhotic patient.

As liver function deteriorates, urinary sodium excretion decreases progressively. Thus, the induction of a negative sodium balance requires the combination of sodium restriction and diuretics. According to a multicenter randomized controlled trial, this combination is effective at controlling ascites in 90% of patients with cirrhosis.

One of the goals of diuretic treatment is to increase the urinary excretion of sodium so that it is greater than 78 mmol/day. Twenty-four–hour urine collections can be helpful in assessing the response to diuretic therapy. Urinary excretion of sodium in excess of dietary intake is a predictor of weight loss. A negative sodium balance with a weight loss of 0.5 kg per day is a reasonable goal. Excess sodium intake should be suspected when the urinary excretion of sodium exceeds 88 mmol/day, but the patient still does not lose weight.

Randomized controlled trials have shown that the combination of spironolactone and furosemide is the most effective regimen for ascites control. Furosemide alone is less effective, and results in more hypokalemia than spironolactone alone or the combination of the two agents. The best starting dose has been shown to be single morning doses of oral spironolactone and furosemide, beginning with 100 mg of spironolactone and 40 mg of furosemide. If weight loss and natriuresis are inadequate on the lower doses, both diuretics may be increased simultaneously, maintaining the 100 mg to 40 mg ratio. In general, this ratio maintains normal levels of potassium. Maximum doses are 400 mg/day of spironolactone and 160 mg/day of furosemide.

In the outpatient clinic, body weight, orthostatic symptoms, serum electrolytes, urea, and creatinine are monitored. A 24-hour urine test should be performed if the patient is not adequately losing weight to assist with management decisions. Patients who are excreting more than 78 mmol/day and are still not losing weight should be further counseled about sodium restriction. Patients who do not lose weight and who excrete less than 78 mmol/day should be given a higher dose of diuretics.

Discuss the Options for Management of Resistant Ascites.

Refractory ascites is defined as fluid overload that is nonresponsive to a sodium-restricted diet and high-dose combination diuretic therapy. Several randomized trials have shown that only 10% of cirrhotic ascites is refractory to this standard therapy.

Options for refractory patients include the following:

1. Serial therapeutic paracenteses
2. Liver transplantation
3. Peritoneovenous shunt
4. Transjugular intrahepatic portasystemic stent or shunt (TIPS)

Serial therapeutic paracenteses should be performed as needed, approximately every 2 weeks. Postparacentesis albumin infusion is expensive and has not been shown to decrease morbidity or mortality. It appears unnecessary for paracenteses of 5 L or less.

Liver transplantation should be considered in any acceptable patient, because the 2-year survival rate of patients with cirrhosis and ascites is only 50%. The 12-month survival rate of patients with ascites refractory to medical therapy is only 25%.

Case

A 52-year-old white man presents to your office complaining of increasing abdominal girth and progressive dyspnea on exertion and shortness of breath. The patient has noticed over the past month that his waistline has gradually increased to the point that he can no longer button his pants. At the same time, he reports new two-pillow orthopnea and dyspnea on exertion when walking approximately four blocks. He denies any symptoms of chest pain, chronic cough, nausea, vomiting, or diarrhea. On further questioning, the patient remembers an episode of nausea and vomiting with associated jaundice approximately 3 years earlier and was told he had an episode of hepatitis. These symptoms resolved after about 2 weeks and he has been in reasonably good health until the past few months. The patient also admits to heavy alcohol use in the past, but has tapered back to only three to four beers a day.

Physical examination reveals a generally ill-appearing man in no acute distress. Vital signs include a blood pressure of 135/80 mm Hg, pulse of 90 beats/min, and temperature of 99.3°F. Scleral icterus is noted, as are several spider angiomas on his skin. Chest examination reveals clear lung fields and mild gynecomastia. The abdomen is distended and nontender with shifting dullness and a positive fluid wave. Extremity examination reveals 1+ pretibial pitting edema.

Pertinent laboratory results are as follows: aspartate aminotransferase 65 U/L, alanine aminotransferase 34 U/L, international normalized ratio 1.34, platelets 88,000, total bilirubin 2.7 mg/dL, direct bilirubin 2.0 mg/dL, hematocrit 36.8%, and albumin 3.0 g/dL.

1. What is the most likely cause of this patient's ascites based on history?
2. What further diagnostic laboratory studies would you order?
3. What is the best management approach for this patient?

Case Discussion

What Is the Most Likely Cause of the Patient's Ascites Based on History?

Alcohol cirrhosis.

What Further Diagnostic Laboratory Studies Would You Order?

Ascitic fluid analysis is the most rapid and cost effective method of diagnosing the cause of ascites and should be obtained in all patients with new-onset ascites. With approximately 97% accuracy, a serum ascites albumin gradient of 1.1 g/dL or greater indicates that the patient has portal hypertension.

Screening for hepatitis should be performed, as should CT of the abdomen to evaluate the architecture of the liver and to rule out cancer or masses.

What Is the Best Management Approach for This Patient?

Alcohol abstinence is advised. Improvement in any reversible component of alcoholic liver disease can reduce portal pressure and decrease sodium retention.

Sodium restriction in combination with diuretics also is advised. In this patient, we could start diuretic therapy with 100 mg spironolactone and 40 mg furosemide per day. The dose of both diuretics can be increased simultaneously, maintaining the 100 mg to 40 mg ratio, if weight loss and natriuresis are inadequate on the lower doses.

The patient also should be referred for liver transplantation if he abstains from alcohol, because the 2-year survival rate of patients with cirrhosis and ascites is only 50%.

Suggested Reading

Gines P, Arroyo V, et al. Comparison of paracentesis and diuretics in the treatment of cirrhotics with tense ascites; results of a randomized study. *Gastroenterology* 1987;93:234.

Position and Policy Statement. American Gastroenterological Association policy statement on the use of medical practice guidelines by managed care organizations. *Gastroenterology* 1995;108:925.

Runyon B A. Care of patients with ascites. *N Engl J Med* 1994;330:337–342.

Runyon B A, Montano A A, et al. The serum-ascites albumin gradient is superior to the exudate-transudate concept in the differential diagnosis of ascites. *Ann Intern Med* 1992;117:215.

Watanahe A. Management of ascites. A review. *Am J Med* 1997;28:21–30.

26
Hemorrhoids

Gregory Diamonti

1. What is the anatomy and pathophysiology associated with hemorrhoids?
2. How are hemorrhoids diagnosed?
3. How do hemorrhoids typically present?
4. What treatments are available for hemorrhoids?

Discussion

What Is the Anatomy and Pathophysiology Associated with Hemorrhoids?

Hemorrhoids represent a dilation of a normal plexus of veins, which is formed by the superior and inferior hemorrhoidal veins. This plexus is located in the submucosa of the lower rectum. Hemorrhoids are defined anatomically based on their site of origin. Internal hemorrhoids originate above the dentate (pectinate) line and are covered by simple columnar rectal epithelium. Internal hemorrhoids are graded according to their degree of prolapse. Grade I hemorrhoids do not prolapse out of the anus, but may be seen with anoscopy. Grade II hemorrhoids prolapse with defecation, but reduce spontaneously. Grade III hemorrhoids must be reduced with assistance (i.e., digital rectal examination). Grade IV hemorrhoids are irreducible.

External hemorrhoids are located below the dentate line. They are covered with stratified squamous epithelium and have somatic sensory innervation. This explains why external hemorrhoids can be painful. Often, both internal and external hemorrhoids may coexist in a patient.

The exact pathogenesis of hemorrhoids is not well known, but three predominant theories exist. The first theory proposes that the connective tissue that anchors the hemorrhoids to the underlying tissue deteriorates. This leads to "sliding" of the hemorrhoids into the anal canal, with resulting symptoms. Advancing age or conditions that increase pelvic venous pressure may hasten this process.

Another theory is that hemorrhoids arise from increased tone and hypertrophy of the anal sphincter. It is hypothesized that defecation pushes the hemorrhoidal plexus against the internal anal sphincter and causes them to enlarge.

The third theory proposes that symptoms are the result of actual swelling of the hemorrhoidal cushions. It is important to realize portal hypertension is not a predisposing factor for the development of hemorrhoids. It is also debated whether chronic constipation can lead to the formation of hemorrhoids.

How Are Hemorrhoids Diagnosed?

A complete history is important for the diagnosis of hemorrhoids. Although hemorrhoids are common, they may be confused with other, sometimes more serious, conditions. A physical examination should consist of careful inspection of the perianal area and a digital rectal examination. Examination with an anoscope, if available, is also helpful. External examination may reveal external skin tags, which may be confused with hemorrhoids. These are areas of redundant tissue, which may be the result of previously thrombosed external hemorrhoids. External hemorrhoids or prolapsed internal hemorrhoids also can be seen with inspection of the perianal area. Internal hemorrhoids are not usually palpated on digital rectal examination unless they are prolapsed or thrombosed.

Hemorrhoids also may be visualized during endoscopy, especially when the instrument is retroflexed in the rectum.

How Do Hemorrhoids Typically Present?

Rectal bleeding is a common presenting symptom of internal hemorrhoids. Internal hemorrhoids commonly bleed, due to local trauma from defecation. The bleeding is usually bright red, seen on the toilet paper or coating the stool. Blood also may drip from the anus after defecation. The bleeding is seldom to the point of hemodynamic instability, and does not present as melena. Bleeding hemorrhoids may rarely be the source of an iron deficiency anemia, but this is after a complete workup reveals no other accountable lesions. Internal hemorrhoids also may prolapse and result in a palpable external mass. They occasionally cause mild incontinence or wetness from drainage. Patients may complain of mild rectal discomfort, but severe pain is unusual unless the hemorrhoids prolapse and become strangulated.

External hemorrhoids may present with severe pain, secondary to thrombosis. The pain usually peaks within the first 48 to 72 hours. Importantly, the clots in external hemorrhoids are not at risk for propagating and causing a thromboembolic event. Thrombosed external hemorrhoids can infrequently bleed when the clot erodes through the overlying skin. External hemorrhoids also may interfere with anal hygiene.

What Treatments Are Available for Hemorrhoids?

In most cases, initial treatment of hemorrhoids should be conservative. This consists of a high-fiber diet (20–30 g/day). Commercial fiber supplements may be necessary in some patients. Fluid intake also should be liberalized. These interventions are aimed at formation of soft, bulky, regular stools. Hemorrhoidal irritation and pruritus may be treated with sitz baths, hydrocortisone preparations, and local analgesics. Proper anal hygiene is also important.

A number of minimally invasive therapies are available for treating hemorrhoids. Most of these have been used to treat internal hemorrhoids. They are usually indicated when conservative treatment fails for grade I to grade III hemorrhoids:

- Injection sclerotherapy
- Rubber band ligation
- Infrared coagulation

- Laser therapy
- Electrocoagulation
- Cryotherapy

The choice of therapy should be based on availability and local expertise. All the available treatments have advantages and disadvantages. Rubber band ligation is the most commonly performed. A recent meta-analysis concluded that rubber band ligation should be the initial treatment mode for grade I to III hemorrhoids. Dilation of the internal anal sphincter also has been tried, but is not generally accepted.

Surgical treatment is indicated for failure of minimally invasive treatments or for grade IV hemorrhoids. The most common surgical procedure performed is a closed hemorrhoidectomy. Surgical intervention is also necessary for strangulated internal hemorrhoids, which are at risk for gangrene.

Surgical excision of a thrombosed external hemorrhoid may be performed within the first 48 hours of its occurrence. After this period of time the clot has organized and cannot be evacuated. Alternative treatment to thrombectomy consists of sitz baths, stool softeners, and analgesics.

Case

A 35-year-old man with no previous medical history presents to your clinic complaining of a 2-week history of intermittent rectal bleeding. He only sees blood on the toilet paper when he wipes after a bowel movement. There is no pain associated with the bleeding. He states that he had similar symptoms a month ago, which resolved without any intervention. He denies any constitutional symptoms. He does not drink or smoke. He notes no significant family history. On physical examination, his pulse is 80 beats/min and his blood pressure is 130/85 mm Hg. Abdominal examination results are unremarkable. There are no external perianal lesions. The digital rectal examination reveals good sphincter tone, no tenderness, and no masses palpated. There is a small amount of red blood on the glove upon withdrawal and some brown stool.

1. What would your initial workup consist of?
2. Is a surgical referral necessary at this time?
3. What further studies are indicated?

Case Discussion
What Would Your Initial Workup Be?

The patient's chief complaint is rectal bleeding. His vital signs indicate that he is stable, but it would also be a good idea to perform orthostatics to better estimate volume status. In addition, obtaining a complete blood count, platelet count, and prothrombin time/partial thromboplastin time would be useful. If the patient were anemic, it would suggest that the degree of bleeding is more substantial, and would broaden your differential diagnosis. It would also be important to know if the patient is coagulopathic or thrombocytopenic because this may affect your further workup and treatment.

Is a Surgical Referral Necessary at This Time?

The most likely diagnosis at this time is bleeding internal hemorrhoids. Assuming the patient is hemodynamically stable, a surgical consult would not be necessary at this point. If the patient presented with an acutely thrombosed external hemorrhoid, or strangulated prolapsed hemorrhoids, a surgeon should be called immediately. Beginning conservative treatment at this time would be reasonable, and the patient's response can be monitored.

What Further Studies Are Indicated?

This patient should be referred for an endoscopic evaluation to rule out any other lesions that could account for the rectal bleeding. Any patient with rectal bleeding who is above average risk for colon cancer should have a full colonoscopy performed. For most other patients under 40 years of age, who are not at increased risk for colon cancer, a flexible sigmoidoscopy is an adequate evaluation. This would be an appropriate evaluation for this patient.

Suggested Reading

Anonymous. Surgical management of hemorrhoids. Patient Care Committee of the Society for Surgery of the Alimentary Tract (SSAT). *J Gastrointest Surg* 1999;3:214–215.

Barnett J L. Anorectal diseases. In: Yamada T, ed. *Textbook of gastroenterology,* 3rd ed. Philadelphia: Lippincott Williams & Wilkins, 1999.

Hussain J N. Hemorrhoids. *Primary Care Clin Office Practice* 1999;26:35–51.

MacRae H M, Mcleod R S. Comparison of hemorrhoidal treatment modalities. A meta-analysis. *Dis Colon Rectum* 1995;38:687–694.

Pfenninger J L, Surrell J. Nonsurgical treatment options for internal hemorrhoids. *Am Family Physician* 52:821–834.

VI

General Medicine/Health Maintenance and Prevention

27
Breast Cancer Screening and Prevention
Alexia M. Torke

1. Why should we screen for breast cancer?
2. How should we screen for breast cancer?
3. Who is at increased risk of developing breast cancer?
4. Can a woman reduce the risk of getting breast cancer?

Discussion
Why Should We Screen for Breast Cancer?

Breast cancer screening is widely accepted as standard practice for women. The decision to screen for breast cancer is based on several factors. First, the disease is sufficiently common in the population to justify the cost of screening. Breast cancer is the most common cancer in women, and the second leading cause of cancer death in women. Second, effective screening tools are available for early detection. The combination of mammography and the clinical breast examination (CBE) has been shown to lead to early detection of breast cancer, and has led to reductions in breast cancer mortality. Finally, effective therapy is available, and early diagnosis leads to improved outcomes compared with later diagnosis.

How Should We Screen for Breast Cancer?
Mammography

There are eight randomized controlled trials that have evaluated screening mammography. Overall, these studies showed a reduction in mortality from breast cancer in women 50 to 70 years of age. The reduction in risk has been shown to be from 15% to 30%. If 1,000 women were screened for breast cancer for 10 years, 2 to 4 lives would be saved. Mammography in younger and older women is more controversial. In 1997, the National Institutes of Health released their Consensus Statement on breast cancer screening in women 40 to 49 years of age. This statement concluded that the data did not support universal screening for women in this age group. Many others have argued that certain controlled studies and meta-analyses do show a mortality benefit when the follow-up period is longer than 10 years. It is

Table 27.1. Screening Recommendations

National Cancer Institute
 Mammography every one or two years beginning at age 40
American Cancer Society
 Mammography annually, beginning at age 40
 CBE every 3 yr from ages 20 to 39 and annually thereafter
 BSE monthly after age 20
American College of Radiology
 Mammography annually beginning at age 40
 CBE annually
 BSE monthly
American College of Preventive Medicine
 Mammography every 1–2 years from ages 50 to 69
 For women 70 and older, continue treatment if health status permits breast cancer treatment
U.S. Preventive Services Task Force
 Mammography every 1 or 2 years from ages 50 to 69
 CBE in conjunction with mammography from ages 50 to 69
 No recommendation for BSE

CBE, clinical breast examination; BSE, breast self-examination.

not clear, however, whether significant differences became apparent because some of the women who started screening at younger ages reached their fifties when their cancers were diagnosed. In summary, there is no clear consensus among experts on the issue of whether to screen women in their forties.

Another controversial topic is whether there is an age at which women should stop undergoing mammography. One randomized trial included women 40 to 74 years of age, and found a reduction in mortality for these women overall. They were not able to show a significant reduction for women in the subgroup 70 to 74 years of age, although there were not enough women in this group to draw conclusions from the data. Other studies provide indirect evidence from statistical modeling that screening women over 70 years of age would reduce cancer mortality. The decision about when to stop mammography must be based on a woman's individual risk factors, comorbidities, and her own views about screening. In general, breast cancer screening should only be recommended in women who have a life expectancy of 8 to 10 years or more.

Based on the above information, national organizations have made recommendations for screening mammography (Table 27.1). All recommend regular (annual or biennial) mammograms for women 50 to 69 years of age. There is variability in the recommended age at which to begin regular mammograms, ranging from 40 to 50 years, as well as the age at which to stop, if any. This decision should be discussed between a woman and her physician. None of the national organizations recommend routine mammography before 40 years of age, even to establish a baseline. It is important to note that universal screening recommendations should be modified for women who are at increased risk for breast cancer based on family history, personal history of precancerous lesions, or other risk factors.

Clinical Breast Examination

No randomized controlled trials have compared the CBE with a program of no screening. However, several major breast cancer screening trials combined CBE and mammography in their screening protocols. These studies showed that some cancers can be detected by CBE that cannot be seen on mammography, ranging from 3.4% to 45%. The evidence to date suggests that CBE is a useful adjunct to mammography, but there is not clear evidence that CBE should be used as a single screening test. Most national organizations recommend annual CBE. Some recommend beginning at age 40 or 50 years, while other groups recommend CBE for all women.

The technique of the CBE involves several parts: observation, palpation of the breast, and lymph node palpation. First, both breasts should be observed simultaneously with the woman in the seated position. Look for symmetry of breast contour, skin changes such as dimpling, and asymmetry or inversion of the nipples. The breasts can then be observed in three different positions: with the hands above the head; with hands on the waist and the patient pressing inward to tense the pectoralis muscles; and with the patient leaning forward from the waist. Look for asymmetry of movement, skin changes such as dimpling, and asymmetry or inversion of the nipples.

The axillae can then be observed and palpated with the patient still seated. For women with large breasts, each breast also can be palpated between the examiner's hands at this time.

Next, each breast should be palpated in a systematic fashion with the patient lying flat. In women with large breasts, different positions can be used to maximally flatten the breast tissue against the chest wall. To examine the medial portion of the breast, the patient should bring her elbow up to the level of her shoulder, and for the lateral side, she should roll onto her opposite hip and place her arm on her forehead. Each breast should be examined in turn. The anatomic area of the breast extends from the clavicle, to the center of the sternum, to the mid-axillary line, to the fold below the breast. Several patterns have been recommended to ensure that all breast tissue is palpated. One study found that the vertical strip method (or lawnmower technique) was more thorough than other patterns. The breast should be palpated using the pads of the fingers, making small circles. At each location, three circles should be made with different levels of pressure, to examine superficial, intermediate, and deep tissue levels. The nipple should then be evaluated by compression between the thumb and finger in an effort to expel any secretions.

The lymph node examination can be conducted in the seated position, with the patient's arms resting at her side, or with the patient lying supine, with her arm supported by the examiner. The lymph node examination should include the anterior and posterior pectoral nodes, the brachial nodes, located high in the axilla, and the supra and infraclavicular nodes on the chest wall.

Barton et al. have pointed out that most cancers detected with CBE are found by palpation rather than inspection. They recommend that clinicians focus on palpation for asymptomatic women, using the vertical strip method.

Breast Self-Examination

Breast self-examination (BSE) is widely recommended by physicians. However, there is no clear evidence that BSE reduces mortality. Two large randomized controlled trials failed to show a difference. Data from the Breast Cancer Detection Demonstration Project was used to estimate the sensitivity of BSE. They estimated that the overall sensitivity was 26%, compared with an estimated sensitivity of 75%

for mammography plus CBE. Future studies evaluating the additive benefit of BSE are needed. At this time, despite little clear evidence of mortality benefit, many national organizations recommend that women perform BSE monthly.

Who Is at Increased Risk of Developing Breast Cancer?

The most important risk factors for developing breast cancer are female sex and age. A woman's risk at birth of developing breast cancer at any point in her life is 1 in 8. This risk is 1 in 235 for women from birth to age 39 years, but increases to 1 in 15 for women when they are between the ages of 60 and 79 years. A number of additional risk factors for breast cancer have been identified (Table 27.2). A personal history of breast cancer increases the risk to 1% per year. Presence of the BRCA1 or BRCA2 genes carry a lifetime risk of 50% or more for developing breast cancer. Lobular carcinoma in situ, a precancerous lesion, increases the risk 8- to 11-fold. It is important to note, however, that 75% of women with breast cancer have none of the risk factors listed in Table 27.2.

Can a Woman Reduce the Risk of Getting Breast Cancer?

Screening programs aim to detect breast cancer in its early stages, but do not reduce the risk of developing the disease. Possible targets for risk reduction include drug therapy, surgery, and life-style modification. In 1998, three articles were published that evaluated the effects of tamoxifen, a nonsteroidal antiestrogen, on the risk of developing breast cancer. The largest trial, the National Surgical Adjuvant Breast and Bowel Project (NSABP), evaluated tamoxifen therapy in 13,388 subjects who took the drug for 5 years. Subjects were women 35 years and older with a 5-year predicted risk of breast cancer of at least 1.66%. This study found a significant reduction in breast cancer in women who took tamoxifen, with an absolute risk reduction of 1.7% over 5 years. However, two smaller studies conducted in Europe did

Table 27.2. Breast Cancer Risk Factors

Family history
Genetic abnormalities (BRCA1 and BRCA2)
Other breast lesions
   Ductal hyperplasia
   Atypical ductal and lobular hyperplasia
   Sclerosing adenosis
   Lobular carcinoma *in situ*
Personal history of breast cancer
Early menarche
Later age at first pregnancy
High-dose radiation exposure
Exogenous hormone use (controversial)
Alcohol
High-fat diet
Obesity

not find a significant difference in breast cancer occurrence with tamoxifen. There were methodologic differences between the studies that may explain these differences. Based on these data, the U.S. Food and Drug Administration approved tamoxifen for use in the prevention of breast cancer for women at high risk. The investigators in the NSABP used the Gail model to assess a woman's risk of breast cancer based on her risk factors. Tables have also been published that allow calculation of the risk:benefit ratio of tamoxifen for an individual woman. Tamoxifen does have some serious side effects, including a slightly increased risk of endometrial cancer and thromboembolic events, as well as menopausal symptoms such as hot flashes.

Based on the current evidence and the risk of serious side effects, many clinicians would only recommend tamoxifen as chemoprophylaxis for women at very high risk. This decision must be individualized based on a woman's own concern about breast cancer and her risk for side effects. There is no evidence that more than 5 years of tamoxifen is beneficial. There is also evidence that raloxifene, a selective estrogen receptor modifier (SERM), reduces breast cancer risk. A trial is underway comparing tamoxifen with raloxifene.

There is some evidence that bilateral mastectomy significantly reduces the incidence of breast cancer in high-risk women. Mastectomy cannot remove all breast tissue, so the risk is not completely eliminated. Quality of life may be seriously affected due to both the physical and psychological affects of the surgery. Because of the irreversible nature of this procedure, a woman must carefully consider the decision to undergo prophylactic mastectomy.

There is some evidence from observational data that increased fat intake, obesity, and decreased exercise may be associated with breast cancer. Alcohol intake increases the risk in a dose-related fashion. No randomized controlled trial to date has proven whether life-style modification can reduce breast cancer risk. The Women's Health Initiative will evaluate whether dietary modification can reduce the risk.

Case

A 45-year-old woman comes to clinic. She has a past medical history of hypertension for which she takes hydrochlorothiazide. She is otherwise healthy and feels well today. She is 5 feet 4 inches tall and weighs 200 pounds (body mass index of 34). She is African American. Her menses are regular, occurring once every 30 days. They began when she was 11 years old. She performs monthly BSE and has not found any suspicious lumps. She notes that a friend has been getting mammograms since her 40th birthday and wants to know if she should have been getting them too. Her mother had breast cancer diagnosed at age 67 years. She does not know of any other cancer in the family. She has three healthy children, the oldest of whom was born when she was 23 years old.

1. What are her risk factors for breast cancer?
2. What breast cancer screening tests are appropriate for this patient?
3. Is there anything she can do to reduce her risk of breast cancer?

Case Discussion

What Are Her Risk Factors for Breast Cancer?

Her risk factors include obesity, early menses, and a family history of breast cancer in a first-degree relative.

What Breast Cancer Screening Tests Are Appropriate for This Patient?

She and her physician should discuss whether to begin mammography and CBE now or wait until she is 50 years of age. Her additional risk factors may justify screening now. The decision also depends on her personal preferences for screening. She should continue to perform BSE each month.

Is There Anything She Can Do to Reduce Her Risk of Breast Cancer?

Weight loss and decreased fat intake may have an impact on her breast cancer risk. Her risk factors would not justify treatment with tamoxifen at this time.

Suggested Reading

Barton M B, Harris R, Fletcher S. Does this patient have breast cancer? The screening clinical breast exam: should it be done? How? *JAMA* 1999;282:1270–1280.

Gail M H, Costantino J P, Bryant J, et al. Weighing the risks and benefits of tamoxifen treatment for preventing breast cancer. *J Natl Cancer Inst* 1999;91:1829–1846.

Greenlee R T, Taylor M, Bolden S, et al. Cancer statistics, 2000. *CA* 2000;50:7–31.

Harris R, Leininger L. Clinical strategies for breast cancer screening: weighing and using the evidence. *Ann Intern Med* 1995;122,539–547.

NIH consensus statement. Breast cancer screening for women ages 40–49. *J Natl Cancer Inst* 1997;89:1015–1020.

O'Malley M S, Fletcher S W. Screening for breast cancer with breast self-examination. *JAMA* 1987;257:2197–2203.

Overmoyer B. Breast cancer screening. *Med Clin North Am* 1999;83:1443–1466.

Pazdur R, Coia L R, Hoskins WJ, et al. *Cancer management: a multidisciplinary approach.* Huntington, NY: PRR, 1998.

Saunders K J, Pilgrim C A, Pennypacker H S. Increased proficiency of search in breast self-examination. *Cancer* 1986;58:2531–2537.

Tabar L, Fagerberg G, Duffy S, et al. Update of the Swedish two-county program of mammographic screening for breast cancer. *Radiol Clin North Am* 1992;20:187–210.

Willms J L, Schneiderman H, Algranati P S. *Physical diagnosis: bedside evaluation of diagnosis and function.* Baltimore: Williams & Wilkins, 1994.

28
Cervical Cancer Screening

Lisa B. Bernstein

1. What factors increase a woman's risk for cervical cancer?
2. What are the current guidelines for cervical cancer screening, including age of onset, frequency of screening and cessation of testing?
3. What is the proper procedure for performing a Papanicolaou smear?

Discussion

What Factors Increase a Woman's Risk for Cervical Cancer?

Epidemiologic evidence suggests that cervical cancer behaves like a sexually transmitted disease. In the 1960s, research began focusing on the human papillomavirus (HPV) as the sexually transmitted etiologic agent of this disease. HPV types 16, 18, 58, 52, and 31 are considered high risk types for progression to squamous cell carcinoma, whereas types 18, 16, and 45 are those most commonly associated with adenocarcinoma. All recent epidemiologic studies have shown a stronger association between progression to invasive cervical cancer in patients with high-risk HPV types or multiple types of HPV.

The greatest risk factor for cervical cancer is previous dysplasia on a cervical smear. Because of the association with a sexually transmitted agent, risk is higher for women with multiple partners or women whose sexual partners are promiscuous, thereby increasing possible exposure to HPV. In addition, women whose first sexual intercourse was at an early age may have a higher likelihood of exposure. Low socioeconomic status and oral contraceptive use have been implicated due to their possible relation to sexual behavior. No studies have shown consistent increased risk with any particular age at menarche or menopause, age at first pregnancy or live birth, or number of deliveries. Most studies demonstrate a two-fold higher risk among smokers, but they do not control for HPV status. There is also an increased prevalence of cervical cancer in human immunodeficiency virus (HIV)-positive women.

What Are the Current Guidelines for Cervical Cancer Screening, Including Age of Onset, Frequency of Screening, and Cessation of Testing?

The incidence of invasive cervical cancer has decreased significantly over the past 40 years due to organized early detection programs. The overall 5-year survival rate of cervical cancer is 67%, whereas the survival rate among women with localized disease is 90% and for women with appropriately treated preinvasive lesions almost 100%. Only one third of the eligible women are screened for cervical cancer yearly. Eight percent of women age 45 or older and 15% of women age 65 or older have never had a Papanicolaou (Pap) smear. Half of the women diagnosed with cervical cancer in the United States have never been screened, and more than 60% have not had a Pap smear in the past 5 years. Women never having a Pap smear are more likely to belong to a minority group, be elderly, live in a rural area, and live below the poverty level. Any health-care encounter should be viewed as an opportunity to provide screening with Pap smears in order to promote early diagnosis of cervical cancer and its precursors and thereby improve the likelihood of survival. Although type-specific HPV testing to identify women at risk for cervical cancer may be useful in the future, its clinical utility is currently unclear, so such testing is not recommended.

A consensus recommendation was adopted by the American Cancer Society, National Cancer Institute, American College of Obstetricians and Gynecologists (ACOG), American Medical Association, and American Academy of Family Physicians that states that all women should begin undergoing Pap smears at age 18 or onset of sexual intercourse. Thereafter, smears should be obtained annually, and after three or more annual smears have been normal, Pap testing may be performed less frequently at the discretion of the physician, but not less frequently than every 3 years. No consensus recommendation regarding cessation of screening was made, but the U.S. Preventive Services Task Force (USPSTF) suggests that regular testing may be discontinued after age 65 if previous screening is normal. The American College of Physicians recommends screening women ages 66 to 75 every 3 years if they have not been screened in the 10 years before age 66. Women who have never engaged in sexual intercourse are not at risk for cervical cancer and therefore do not require screening.

In 1995, ACOG determined guidelines calling for cervical smears to be obtained more frequently than every 3 years if a patient has one or more of these high-risk factors: multiple partners, promiscuous partners, early initiation of intercourse, partners who had previous partners with cervical cancer, current or prior HPV or condyloma, herpes simplex virus, HIV, history of sexually transmitted diseases, an immunosuppressed state, substance abuse (including alcohol and tobacco), low socioeconomic status, or a history of dysplasia or cervical cancer.

What Is the Proper Procedure for Performing a Pap Smear?

The cervix is composed of dense connective tissue with an opening called the endocervical canal, which is lined with columnar epithelium. This area extends to the outer ectocervix, which is covered with squamous epithelium. The point where these two areas meet is termed the squamocolumnar junction, a dynamic point that changes in response to hormonal state. When the columnar cells of the endocervix are exposed to the more acidic vaginal pH, they are converted to squamous epithelium, which is called squamous metaplasia. The area between the original junction and the new physiological squamocolumnar junction is the transformation zone, an area particularly susceptible to oncogenic factors, and thus where cancerous lesions are likely to arise.

One of the primary causes of false-negative Pap smears is sampling error. To enhance the likelihood of an adequate sample, the patient should not use a douche or lubricant for 24 hours prior to the examination, but such use should not preclude performing the Pap smear. Avoid heavy menses, but if the patient has abnormal vaginal bleeding, do not delay the examination. If there is obvious inflammation, postpone a routine Pap smear until the cause is treated.

The Pap smear is performed before the pelvic examination and involves placing a speculum in the vagina and visualizing the entire cervix, looking for visible lesions. Two samples are collected. First, the ectocervix and adjacent vagina are sampled with a wooden Ayre spatula rotated no more than 360 degrees, with moderate pressure on the cervix. Once the cells are transferred to a slide, they should be fixed within 10 seconds in alcohol solution or Spray-Cyte. Next, the endocervix should be sampled using a cytobrush placed in the cervix and turned one half to two full turns. Again, the cells should be transferred to a slide and fixed immediately.

Case

A 58-year-old obese African-American woman comes to your medical clinic for the first time. Her past medical and surgical history is significant for only essential hypertension, osteoarthritis, and a cesarean section at age 28. She takes a diuretic and acetaminophen occasionally for pain. She has never smoked and only drinks socially. She has been married for 35 years and is monogamous with three healthy adult children. She underwent menopause at age 50 and has not had a period for 7 years. Her review of systems and physical examination are unremarkable.

Because it is her first visit, you question her on her routine health maintenance and discover that she has not had a Pap smear or pelvic examination in several years. She assures you that all of her previous Pap smears were normal and she denies any vaginal complaints. She wants to know if she really needs to undergo a gynecologic examination at this time.

1. Does this patient need a Pap smear now?
2. Are there any circumstances that would preclude you from doing a Pap smear at this time?
3. Would your recommendations for cervical cancer screening change if this patient had undergone a hysterectomy?
4. What would you recommend if she were HIV positive?

Case Discussion

Does This Patient Need a Pap Smear Now?

Because this woman is under age 65 and has not had a gynecologic examination in several years, she definitely should have a Pap smear at some point in the near future. Because this is her first visit and you are still getting to know each other as doctor and patient, if you believe the patient to be compliant with follow-up, you can schedule an appointment for a Pap smear and pelvic examination soon. For patients who are unreliable, you should take advantage of the opportunity of having them in your office and perform the examination at that time.

Are There Any Circumstances That Would Preclude You from Doing a Pap Smear at This Time?

Because sampling error is one of the main causes of false-negative Pap smears, you obviously want to optimize the adequacy of your sample. This patient is no longer menstruating, which omits blood as a cause of sampling error, although if she were having abnormal vaginal bleeding you would definitely do the Pap smear today. If she has obvious vaginal erythema or discharge, indicating a possible inflammatory vaginitis, a wet prep should be done and the patient should be treated accordingly prior to returning for a Pap smear. You may still do the smear if the patient douched or used vaginal lubricant recently, although this should be noted on the laboratory form accompanying the sample.

Would Your Recommendations for Cervical Cancer Screening Change if This Patient Had Undergone a Hysterectomy?

If this patient had previously undergone a hysterectomy, the recommendations for screening would differ based on whether the procedure was performed for benign disease (e.g., fibroids) versus cervical dysplasia or carcinoma. Women who have undergone supracervical hysterectomies (the cervix is preserved) and those with a history of cervical dysplasia or cancer should continue to be screened following routine guidelines. However, there is still uncertainty of what to do for the approximately 30% of women who undergo hysterectomy for benign disease. Once the cervix has been removed, Pap smears are performed by scraping the vaginal cuff, using the rationale that this procedure may pick up vaginal cancers or cervical cancers in residual cervical tissue. The American Cancer Society and the National Cancer Institute recommend Pap smears be continued at intervals of 3 to 5 years depending on the reason for hysterectomy. In contrast, ACOG only recommends continued screening if there is a history of dysplasia or carcinoma *in situ*. The USPSTF feels that there are insufficient data to recommend routine screening of patients who underwent hysterectomy for benign disease because the burden of suffering for vaginal cancer is low and there is a lack of mortality data suggesting that this inefficient form of random sampling of vaginal tissue alters the history of the disease. In a study done at Charity Hospital in New Orleans and published in the *New England Journal of Medicine* in 1996, the probability of finding an abnormal Pap smear in a population of high-risk women after total abdominal hysterectomy for benign disease was 1.1%, and the positive predictive value for detecting vaginal cancer was 0%.

What Would You Recommend if She Were HIV Positive?

Women who are immunocompromised have a higher rate of persistent infection with HPV. In addition, the prevalence of invasive cervical cancer is higher for HIV positive women, especially among African-Americans and Hispanics. This finding resulted in the inclusion of invasive cervical cancer in the revision by the Centers for Disease Control and Prevention of the surveillance case definition of acquired immunodeficiency syndrome in 1993. These women should have a pelvic examination and Pap smear as part of their initial evaluation. A Pap smear should be obtained twice in the first year after diagnosis of HIV infection and, if the results are normal, annually thereafter. If the results of the Pap smear are abnormal, follow-up is the same as for HIV negative women. HIV infection is not an indication for colposcopy in women who have normal Pap smears.

Suggested Reading

Appleby J. Management of the abnormal Papanicolaou smear. *Med Clin North Am* 1995;79:345–360.

Centers for Disease Control and Prevention. 1993 Revised classification system for HIV infection and expanded surveillance case definition for AIDS among adolescents and adults. *MMWR* 1992;41.

Centers for Disease Control and Prevention. Guidelines for treatment of sexually transmitted diseases. *MMWR* 1998;47;1–118.

Goodman A. Screening for cervical cancer. *Up To Date* 1999;7.

National Institutes of Health. Cervical cancer. *NIH Consensus Statement* 1996;14:1–38.

Pearce K, et al. Cytopathological findings on vaginal Papanicolaou smears after hysterectomy for benign gynecologic disease. *N Engl J Med* 1996;335:1559–1562.

U.S. Preventive Services Task Force. Screening for cervical cancer. In: *Guide to clinical preventive services,* 2nd ed. Baltimore: Williams & Wilkins, 1996:105-117.

29
Colorectal Cancer Screening

Murtaza Cassoobhoy

1. Why screen for colorectal cancer?
2. Who should be screened for colorectal cancer?
3. What are the current recommendations for screening in average risk patients?

Discussion
Why Screen for Colorectal Cancer?

Colorectal cancer is the second leading cause of death from cancer in the United States, and approximately 150,000 new cases are diagnosed each year. Colorectal cancer is unique among cancers because the majority of cancerous lesions arise from adenomatous polyps, which are the precursor lesions. It is estimated that it takes about 10 years for an adenomatous polyp that is less than 1 cm in diameter to transform into an invasive cancer. This provides an excellent opportunity to intervene by screening. Various screening tests have been shown to decrease the incidence of colorectal cancer by detection and removal of polyps and to improve survival by detection of early stage cancers.

Who Should Be Screened for Colorectal Cancer?

Everybody over the age of 50 years should be screened for colorectal cancer. If they are asymptomatic and do not have a personal or family history of colorectal cancer or polyps, they are considered to be at average risk for developing colorectal cancer. Their lifetime risk of developing colorectal cancer is about 6%, and this group constitutes 75% of all colorectal cancers diagnosed.

Patients with a family history of a first-degree relative with colorectal cancer are at an increased risk, and screening should begin at 40 years of age. Approximately 15% to 20% of all colorectal cancers are diagnosed in this group.

Patients that fall into even higher risk groups need to undergo surveillance examinations of their colon:

- Patients in a family with familial adenomatous polyposis (FAP). This group constitutes 1% of all colorectal cancers and screening should begin at 10 to 12 years of age.
- Patients with a family history of hereditary nonpolyposis colorectal cancer. The Amsterdam Criteria are used to diagnose this condition, and patients must have

all three of the following findings: (a) three relatives with colorectal cancer (two of them must be first-degree relatives of the third); (b) colorectal cancer cases must span two generations; and (c) one case must be diagnosed under the age of 50 years.

Modification of these criteria is now favored that allows substitution of endometrial, ovarian, pancreatic, gastric, small bowel, and urinary tract cancers for colorectal cancer. These patients constitute about 5% of all colorectal cancer and screening should begin at 20 to 25 years of age:

- Patients with a history of adenomatous polyps should have a repeat colonoscopy 3 years after the last abnormal examination.
- Patients with a history of colorectal cancer should have a repeat colonoscopy 3 years after the resection if they had a complete examination preoperatively. If they were unable to have a complete examination before the resection, it should be performed 1 year after surgery.
- Patients with inflammatory bowel disease should have colonoscopy every 1 to 2 years after 8 years of disease in patients with pancolitis, or after 15 years in those with left-sided colitis.

What Are the Current Screening Recommendations in Average-Risk Patients?

Multiple societies and consensus panels have guidelines for colorectal cancer screening. The most widely endorsed guidelines are those of the Agency for Health Care Policy and Research-GI Consortium that were developed by a multidisciplinary group in 1997. They recommend fecal occult blood testing (FOBT) every year and flexible sigmoidoscopy every 5 years. Combining these two screening modalities corrects the limitations of the individual tests. There has been more evidence supporting the use of a screening colonoscopy every 10 years since these guidelines were published, and the American College of Gastroenterology currently recommends this as the preferred screening strategy in average risk patients. Colonoscopy has the advantage of evaluating the entire colon (as opposed to flexible sigmoidoscopy) especially since isolated proximal polyps and cancers are becoming more common. It appears to be cost effective and a ten-year interval should allow more patient compliance. However, currently colonoscopies are performed only by gastroenterologists, making it less widely available than sigmoidoscopy.

Case

A 55-year-old man comes to your medical clinic to establish himself with a primary care physician for routine medical care. He has had hypertension for many years and takes atenolol and hydrochlorathiazide for treatment. He is concerned about "getting" colon cancer because his father was diagnosed with it a few months ago at age 77 years. He has no other history of cancer in the family. He has not had any weight loss or gastrointestinal symptoms.

On physical examination he has a blood pressure of 124/70 mm Hg and a 2/6 holosystolic murmur at the apex radiating into the axilla. Digital rectal examination reveals a normal prostate, with no masses palpable in the rectal vault and brown stool. The remainder of his examination is unremarkable.

You order a FOBT and a complete blood count.

1. How would you explain the fecal occult blood test to your patient? What foods does he need to avoid?
2. What are the advantages and limitations of fecal occult blood testing?
3. How many positive fecal occult blood test results are needed to pursue further workup? What is the workup?
4. Does your patient need antibiotic prophylaxis before the flexible sigmoidoscopy?
5. What are the advantages and limitations of flexible sigmoidoscopy as a screening study for colorectal cancer?
6. What is a positive flexible sigmoidoscopy?
7. When does he need to be evaluated again?

Case Discussion

How Would You Explain the Fecal Occult Blood Test to Your Patient? What Foods Does He Need to Avoid?

The patient should take samples of stool from two different sites using a wooden applicator and thinly smear them on the two windows in the card. He then should repeat the procedure for the next two bowel movements and return the cards either in person or by mail within 4 days.

Consumption of foods containing peroxidases such as rare red meat, turnips, and horseradish can produce a false-positive result. Aspirin and other nonsteroidal anti-inflammatory drugs can cause gastric irritation and occult bleeding. Vitamin C can produce a false-negative result by interfering with the reaction. Iron supplements do not directly interfere with the test, but by turning the stools dark, they make it difficult to interpret the blue color change of a positive test. These foods should be avoided for 2 days prior to collecting the samples.

What Are the Advantages and Limitations of Fecal Occult Blood Testing?

The advantages of FOBT are that it is easy to use and inexpensive, and it has been shown in multiple randomized control trials to decrease mortality from colorectal cancer.

The limitations of FOBT are that usually only large polyps (>2 cm) bleed, so the test is aimed mainly at detecting cancer after it develops rather than finding precancerous lesions. FOBT also has a high false-positive rate because bleeding from any location in the gastrointestinal tract will turn the test positive, so many patients are subjected to the discomfort and cost of further testing unnecessarily. Rehydration of the specimens, which is recommended, improves sensitivity but decreases specificity, resulting in more false-positive results.

How Many Positive Fecal Occult Blood Test Results Are Needed to Pursue Further Workup? What Is the Workup?

Any one positive of the six samples tested on the three cards requires further workup.

The best choice for workup of a positive FOBT is a colonoscopy. It is very accurate and safe, and polypectomy or biopsy of a suspicious lesion can be performed. An alternative is double-contrast barium enema, which also can examine the entire colon and has relatively high sensitivity and specificity for large polyps (>1 cm). However, a positive barium enema requires a colonoscopy for further evaluation.

Your patient returns for a follow-up visit. His hematocrit is normal and results of FOBT are negative. You recommend flexible sigmoidoscopy and he agrees.

Does Your Patient Need Antibiotic Prophylaxis Before the Flexible Sigmoidoscopy?

No. Currently antibiotic prophylaxis prior to a flexible sigmoidoscopy is only recommended for patients with prosthetic heart valves, a history of endocarditis, systemic-pulmonary shunts, or synthetic vascular grafts. Prophylaxis is not necessary for rheumatic valvular dysfunction, acquired valvular disease, hypertrophic cardiomyopathy, mitral valve prolapse with mitral regurgitation, pacemakers, cirrhosis with ascites, prosthetic joints, and immunocompromised patients. Some patients with these conditions may request antibiotics before the procedure because they are used to receiving them before other invasive procedures.

What Are the Advantages and Limitations of Flexible Sigmoidoscopy as a Screening Study for Colorectal Cancer?

Flexible sigmoidoscopy allows direct visualization of the distal colon. Lesions can be examined via biopsy and the patient does not have to be sedated. However, it only allows an examination of the left side of the colon and so can miss polyps or cancer in the proximal and transverse colon. There has been a documented increase in the incidence of colorectal cancer in the proximal colon over the past few years.

What Is a Positive Flexible Sigmoidoscopy?

A polyp greater than 1 cm in diameter or a lesion that is very suspicious for cancer constitutes a positive flexible sigmoidoscopy result and the patient should be referred for colonoscopy. A polyp less than 1 cm in diameter should be submitted for biopsy. If it is found to be adenomatous, the patient should be referred for a colonoscopy. Hyperplastic polyps do not need further work-up.

Flexible sigmoidoscopy on this patient reveals a 1.5-cm polyp in the sigmoid colon. He is referred for colonoscopy and a polypectomy is done. No other polyps are seen.

When Does He Need to Be Evaluated Again?

Because the patient has a large (>1 cm) polyp, he now falls under the increased risk category and will require surveillance rather than screening. The next examination of his colon should be a colonoscopy 3 years after the polypectomy. If that colonoscopy is negative, the interval can be increased to every 5 years.

Suggested Reading

Rex D K, Johnson D A, Lieberman, D A, et al. Colorectal cancer prevention 2000: screening recommendations of the American College of Gastroenterology. *Am J Gastroenterol* 2000;95:868–877.

Winawer S J, Fletcher R H, Miller L, et al. Colorectal cancer screening: clinical guidelines and rationale. *Gastroenterology* 1997;112:594–642.

30
Prostate Cancer Screening
Erica Brownfield

1. What is the epidemiology of prostate cancer?
2. Who is at risk for prostate cancer?
3. What are the available screening tests for prostate cancer?
4. What are the controversies regarding screening?
5. What group of patients appears most likely to benefit from prostate cancer screening?
6. What are the current recommendations of various groups on screening?

Discussion
What Is the Epidemiology of Prostate Cancer?

Prostate cancer is the most common visceral malignancy and the second leading cause of cancer death in men. In 1998, there were approximately 184,500 new cases and 39,200 deaths from prostate cancer. The lifetime risk for clinical prostate cancer is approximately 10% among U.S. men. The median age of diagnosis is 69 years for African-American men and 71 years for white men. The incidence of prostate cancer has increased with screening; however, the mortality rates have remained stable until the past 2 years, when the first decrease in mortality was reported.

It is well known that prostate cancer can be found on autopsy in approximately 30% to 50% of asymptomatic men over age 50. The vast majority of these autopsy cancers are microscopic, too small to lead to an elevated serum prostate-specific antigen (PSA) level or a prostate nodule. Prostate cancers clinically detectable by elevated PSA or digital rectal examination (DRE) have a broad spectrum of biologic behavior, ranging from slow to virulent growth.

The approach to prostate cancer detection and treatment has been a challenging problem for the medical community and public. Much of the controversy that exists regarding prostate cancer screening is due to the lack of data derived from carefully controlled prospective clinical trials demonstrating a mortality benefit from screening and treatment. Part of the controversy also stems from the dilemma of using invasive treatments in the subset of individuals who will not see a morbidity or mortality benefit.

Who Is at Risk for Prostate Cancer?

Defined risk factors for prostate cancer include (a) increasing age, (b) African-American descent, and (c) family history of prostate cancer (particularly first-degree relative with prostate cancer diagnosed before age 60). There are no consistent environmental, behavioral, or dietary risk factors amenable to primary prevention measures. Two recent studies suggest that dietary saturated fat consumption may increase cancer risk. Although an initial report suggested prior vasectomy increases future risk of prostate cancer, several subsequent studies and a consensus panel have concluded there is no association.

What Are the Available Screening Tests for Prostate Cancer?

The current screening tests available and widely used for prostate cancer screening are the digital rectal examination (DRE) and the serum PSA. If one or both of these two tests yields positive results, the next step is transrectal ultrasonography with needle biopsy of the prostate. It is difficult to accurately measure the quality of the DRE and PSA as screening tests because prostate biopsy (the gold standard) is not routinely done on patients who screen negatively. Moreover, prostate biopsy as a gold standard has imperfect sensitivity.

Digital rectal examination involves palpating the posterior and lateral aspects of the prostate gland. It can be done during an office visit and is inexpensive. The DRE is not very accurate; the sensitivity is estimated at 55% to 68%, and some studies suggest 18% to 22%. There is high interobserver variability even among urologists.

In men over age 50 who undergo one screening DRE, 2% to 3% are found to have induration, marked asymmetry, or nodularity of the prostate. Such findings increase the odds of harboring a clinically significant (>0.5 mL) intracapsular tumor by twofold and odds of having extracapsular involvement by three- to ninefold. Even so, DRE has not been shown to decrease a patient's chance of dying of prostate cancer or to improve future quality of life.

Prostate-specific antigen is a glycoprotein that functions as a kallikrein-like serine protease. It is secreted by epithelial cells into prostatic ducts and seminal fluid. PSA is specific for prostatic tissue but not prostate cancer. Many disease processes or procedures [e.g., benign prostatic hyperplasia (BPH), prostatitis, acute urinary retention, malignancy, perineal trauma, prostate biopsy, or surgery] can cause the breakdown of barriers interposed between prostatic lumen and capillary blood, causing leakage of PSA into the bloodstream. DRE does not increase PSA to a clinically important degree.

There is some controversy regarding PSA "cutoff" levels that should promote diagnostic workup for prostate cancer. The normal range for PSA varies among age groups and race and should be interpreted as such. This strategy will likely decrease the number of biopsies in older men and may increase the cancer detection rate in younger men. Regardless of patient age, however, the probability of prostate cancer increases as PSA levels increase over 4 ng/mL. There is a 25% probability of cancer with PSA levels between 4 and 10 ng/mL and a greater than 50% probability for PSA values of over 10 ng/mL.

Although using DRE and PSA in combination may increase sensitivity, the use of both has not been shown to decrease disease-specific morbidity and mortality. Combining DRE and PSA results in as many as 15% of men in their fifties and 40% of men in their seventies requiring further evaluation with prostate biopsy.

What Are the Controversies Regarding Screening?

The main question in prostate cancer screening is whether screening can identify patients with aggressive disease who might benefit from early treatment. Currently there are no prospective, randomized, controlled clinical trials demonstrating that screening for prostate cancer decreases morbidity and mortality. Indirect evidence that screening may improve outcomes includes the decrease in prostate cancer mortality reported over the past 2 years, 10 years after widespread use of PSA for screening.

Survival is longer among those diagnosed with early-stage prostate cancer, and screening efforts have led to a greater proportion of tumors being detected at earlier stages. However, any perceived benefit may be due to lead-time bias (patients live longer from time of diagnosis because they are diagnosed earlier) and length bias (screening detects more slowly growing disease that is less dangerous and looks more curable). Both biases can produce an apparent survival benefit even when screening is ineffective.

The efficacy of treatment for the potentially curable, localized (intracapsular) disease is unproven, and extracapsular cancers are often incurable. In addition, there is evidence that the survival among older patients with low-grade, early-stage cancer may be good even without treatment.

Strong evidence of a positive treatment effect remains important before widespread screening tests are incorporated into medical practice. Do we screen now and stop later if trials prove screening is ineffective or does more harm than good? Or do we not screen now and start later if trials prove screening does more good than harm? Proponents of prostate cancer screening note that 30% to 40% of prostate cancers detected in men with no previous screening are early stage, potentially curable tumors, whereas 70% to 85% of cancers among PSA-screened individuals are at an early stage. Although this does not necessarily mean that outcomes with screening will be better, some screening enthusiasts believe the epidemiologic importance of a cancer in and of itself provides justification for screening pending definitive evidence of effectiveness. Opponents of screening note that PSA screening may subject many asymptomatic men to such harms as worry due to an abnormal test, discomfort from biopsies, risks of aggressive treatment (e.g., incontinence, impotence, and death), for an uncertain benefit. Furthermore, discussing prostate cancer screening with patients may detract from the time needed to educate them about unequivocally beneficial interventions such as blood pressure control.

What Group of Patients Appears Most Likely to Benefit from Prostate Cancer Screening?

Men who appear most likely to benefit from prostate cancer screening, according to the American College of Physicians and the American Urologic Association (AUA), are asymptomatic younger men (ages 50–69) with a life expectancy of 10 years or greater. Unfortunately, the primary care provider most often screens older men with significant comorbidity or with symptoms of BPH. These men are likely to have an elevated PSA due to age or the presence of BPH, and are more likely to have prostate cancer detected on biopsy. Aggressive treatment in these patients is often inappropriate.

What Are the Current Recommendations of Various Groups on Screening?

- U.S. Preventative Services Task Force and National Cancer Institute
  - Routine screening not recommended; patients who request screening should be given objective information about the risks and benefits of screening and treatment.
  - If screening is to be done, it should consist of DRE and PSA in men with greater than 10 years of life expectancy.
  - Insufficient evidence regarding the optimal interval of screening or use of PSA density, velocity, age-adjusted reference ranges.
- American College of Physicians
  - Routine screening not recommended; pros and cons of testing should be discussed and an individualized decision made about screening.
  - Men between 50 and 69 years are most likely to benefit from screening.
- American Cancer Society and American Urology Association
  - PSA should be offered annually for men age 50 and over, age 40 and over for African American men or men with two or more first-degree relatives with prostate cancer. [Of note, before 1997 this recommendation was that these men "should undergo" PSA screening.]

Case

A 77-year-old white man with a history of osteoarthritis presents for a periodic health check-up. He has been feeling well, but on review of systems admits to "occasional" frequency and nocturia. Recently, a poker buddy of his died from prostate cancer and he asks if he should be tested. His rectal examination is notable for a slightly enlarged prostate.

1. Would you recommend prostate-specific antigen testing in this patient?
2. What are the potential benefits and harms of prostate-specific antigen testing in this patient?
3. What type of counseling should you provide to this patient?

Case Discussion

Would You Recommend Prostate-Specific Antigen Testing in This Patient?

There are many issues that arise in this patient. The patient presents to you with fear of prostate cancer given his friend's death. Also, the patient reports lower urinary tract symptoms (frequency and nocturia), so the term *screening* does not apply to him because screening, by definition, is performed in asymptomatic individuals. The most appropriate approach to this patient is workup of his lower urinary tract symptoms, which may include a urinalysis, DRE (which is reported as consistent with BPH), and PSA testing.

If the patient were asymptomatic and wishes to discuss screening, one should provide the necessary counseling and proceed with PSA testing if desired by the patient. His age of 77 years is a factor to consider when discussing prostate cancer screening. If his life expectancy is less than 10 years, most experts would not favor screening.

What Are the Potential Benefits and Harms of Prostate-Specific Antigen Testing in This Patient?

Potential benefits may arise if the PSA is normal. A normal PSA may help allay any fears the patient has over prostate cancer due to his friend's death. An elevated PSA is likely to lead the recommendation to examine the prostate via biopsy and undergo treatment if cancer is detected. The potential side effects and impact on quality of life of the biopsy and treatment should be discussed with the patient, as should the uncertain benefit of treatment.

What Type of Counseling Should You Provide to This Patient?

Given the above discussion, this patient should be counseled on the pros and cons of PSA testing. He should be educated about the causes of PSA elevation, likely causes of his symptoms, and the use of the AUA symptom index score. He should also be educated on the invasiveness of prostatic biopsies, as well as the treatment options for prostate cancer and their side effects. If he still chooses to be tested, at least it will be on an informed basis.

Suggested Reading

American College of Physicians. Early detection of prostate cancer. III. Screening for prostate cancer. *Ann Intern Med* 1997;126:480–484.

Brawer M. Prostate-specific antigen: current status. *CA* 1999;49:264–281.

Coley C et al. Early detection of prostate cancer. I. Prior probability and effectiveness of tests. *Ann Intern Med* 1997;126:394–406.

Coley C et al. Early detection of prostate cancer. II. Estimating the risks, benefits, and costs. *Ann Intern Med* 1997;126:468–479.

Collins M, Barry M. Controversies in prostate cancer screening: analogies to the early lung cancer screening debate. *JAMA* 1996:276:1976–1979.

Garnick M. Measurement of prostate specific antigen. *Up to Date* 2000;8:1.

Garnick M. Screening for prostate cancer. *Up to Date* 2000;8:1.

Godley P. Prostate cancer screening: promise and peril—a review. *Cancer Detect Prev* 1999;23:316–324.

Meyer F, Fradet Y. Clinical basics: prostate cancer: 4. screening. *CMAJ-JAMC* 1998;159:968–972.

31
Physical Activity for Coronary Artery Disease Prevention

Elizabeth J. Tong
Terry A. Jacobson

1. What are the current recommendations for physical activity?
2. Which patients need cardiac evaluation prior to exercise?
3. How do you recommend an exercise prescription?

Discussion

What Are the Current Recommendations for Physical Activity?

The major guidelines for health-care professionals on physical activity and exercise are published by the American College of Sports Medicine (ACSM) and the American Heart Association (AHA). The new guidelines represent a paradigm shift because they emphasize physical activity rather than just physical fitness. Physical activity is any body movement that produces energy expenditure, whereas exercise is a subset of physical activity in which planned, structured, and repetitive body movements are used to improve or maintain physical fitness. A more detailed glossary of exercise terms is found in Table 31.1.

Increasing physical activity is a national public health goal. Americans have become more sedentary over the past 20 years, and physical inactivity is now recognized as a major risk factor for the development of coronary artery disease (CAD). There is a clear morbidity and mortality benefit to being physically active, and exercise is just one way of attaining physical activity.

The importance of physical activity has advanced from basic intuition to a mainstay in the primary and secondary prevention of cardiovascular disease as well as many other chronic diseases. Physical activity has been shown to decrease all-cause mortality among active versus sedentary adults, decrease the incidence of coronary artery disease (CAD), reduce the recurrence of coronary events, improve glucose tolerance, improve cholesterol profiles, improve blood pressure, reduce joint stiffness, improve psychological function, increase bone density, and improve immune function. The benefits of physical activity occur in a dose-dependent manner ac-

Table 31.1. Glossary of Terms

Exercise (exercise training). Planned, structured, and repetitive bodily movement done to improve or maintain one or more components of physical fitness.

Kilocalorie (kcal). A measurement of energy. 1 kilocalorie = 1,000 calories = 4,184 joules = 4.184 kilojoules.

Maximal heart rate reserve. The difference between maximum heart rate and resting heart rate.[a]

Maximal oxygen uptake (VO₂ max). The maximal capacity for oxygen consumption by the body during maximal exertion. It is also known as aerobic power, maximal oxygen consumption, and cardiorespiratory endurance capacity.[a]

Maximal heart rate (HR max). The highest heart rate value attainable during an all-out effort to the point of exhaustion.

Metabolic equivalent (MET). A unit used to estimate the metabolic cost (oxygen consumption) of physical activity. One MET equals the resting metabolic rate of approximately $3.5 \text{ mL O}_2 \times \text{kg}^{-1} \times \text{min}^{-1}$.

Physical activity. Bodily movement that is produced by the contraction of skeletal muscle and that substantially increases energy expenditure.

Physical fitness. A set of attributes that people have or achieve that relates to the ability to perform physical activity.

Relative perceived exertion (RPE). A person's subjective assessment of how hard he or she is working. The Borg scale is a numerical scale for rating perceived exertion.[a]

Resistance training. Training designed to increase strength, power, and muscle endurance.[a]

Resting heart rate. The heart rate at rest, averaging 60 to 80 beats/min.[a]

---

[a]From Wilmore J H, Costill D L. *Physiology of sport and exercise.* Champaign, IL: Human Kinetics, 1994.

Adapted from the U.S. Department of Health and Human Services. *Physical activity and health: a report of the surgeon general.* Atlanta, GA: U.S. Department of Health and Human Services, Centers for Disease Control and Prevention, National Center for Chronic Disease Prevention and Health Promotion, 1996; with permission.

---

cording to the total time spent in physical activity and the intensity level. Patients should be counseled to adopt a more active life-style by taking advantage of opportunities during their daily routine (park farther away from destination, take stairs instead of elevator, lift light-weight objects while talking on the phone or during free time at home, or become more active in housework and yard work).

The current recommendations for physical activity for all Americans are as follows (Table 31.2). The ACSM and AHA recommend an accumulation of at least 30 minutes of moderate intensity physical activity at least 5 days per week. The AHA also recommends resistance training (or training designed to increase strength or power) performed at a moderate to high intensity for a minimum of 2 days per week. The prior exercise guidelines suggested fitness benefits only if patients exercised at more vigorous intensities for 20 to 60 minutes three or more times per week. Current research indicates a health benefit from an accumulation of 30 minutes of short 5- to 10-minute bursts of moderate-intensity activity throughout the

Table 31.2. New and Old Guidelines for Exercise from ACSM and AHA

	Old Guideline	New ACSM Guideline	New AHA Guideline
Frequency	≥3 days/wk	Most if not all days/wk	Most days of week
Intensity	Moderate to vigorous[a]	Moderate[b]	Moderate[c]
Time	20–60 min/session	Accumulate 30 min/day	Accumulate 30 min/day

[a]60%–90% of maximum heart rate or 50%–85% maximal oxygen uptake.
[b]3–6 METS or 4–7 kcal/min.
[c]60%–75% of maximal oxygen uptake.
ACSM, American College of Sports Medicine; AHA, American Heart Association.

Table 31.3. Examples of Common Physical Activities for Healthy U.S. Adults by Intensity of Effort Required

Light (<3.0 METs or <4 kcal/min)	Moderate (3–6 METs or 4–7 kcal/min)	Hard/Vigorous (>6 METs or >7 kcal/min)
Walking, slowly (strolling) (1–2 mph)	Walking, briskly (3–4 mph)	Walking, briskly uphill or with a load
Cycling, stationary (<50 W)	Cycling for pleasure or transportation (≤10 mph)	Cycling, fast or racing (>10 mph)
Swimming, slow treading	Swimming, moderate effort	Swimming, fast treading or crawl
Conditioning exercise, light stretching	Conditioning exercise, general calisthenics	Conditioning exercise, stair ergometer, ski machine
—	Racket sports, table tennis	Racket sports, singles tennis, racquetball
Golf, power cart	Golf, pulling cart/carry clubs	—
Bowling	—	—
Fishing, sitting	Fishing, standing/casting	Fishing in stream
Boating, power	Canoeing, leisurely (2–3.9 mph)	Canoeing, rapidly (≥4 mph)
Home care, carpet sweeping	Home care, general cleaning	Moving furniture
Mowing lawn, riding mower	Mowing lawn, power mower	Mowing lawn, hand mower
Home repair, carpentry	Home repair, painting	—

Reprinted from *JAMA* 1995;273:402–407; with permission.

day. A list of moderate-intensity activities is provided in Table 31.3 and includes brisk walking, gardening, and doing home repairs.

The risks associated with exercise are few and include musculoskeletal injury and sudden cardiac death. However, a physician must realize from a population perspective that the benefits of a moderate physical activity recommendation in all of their sedentary patients without cardiovascular disease clearly outweighs the risks. A history and physical examination is important to screen patients for cardiac disease prior to the start of an exercise program.

Which Patients Need Cardiac Evaluation Prior to Exercise?

Exercise is associated with a low risk of sudden cardiac death. The main factors that increase the cardiac risk are age, presence of heart disease, and the exercise intensity. These risk factors are reflected in the ACSM guidelines for exercise stress testing (Table 31.4). Persons with evidence of heart disease such as unstable angina, uncontrolled heart failure, valvular disease, or uncontrolled arrhythmia should not exercise without medical supervision. Health-care professionals can safely encourage physical activities that are moderate in intensity for most patients. The AHA recommends a recent (within 6–12 months) physical examination for all people planning to start a moderate-intensity exercise program.

How Do You Recommend an Exercise Prescription?

An exercise prescription is an individualized plan for exercise. Patients interested in an exercise program to help achieve their daily physical activity goal may benefit from an exercise prescription. The five components of an exercise prescription are the type of exercise recommended, its frequency, intensity, and length of total time, as well as a plan for the progression over time. The prescription should be written

Table 31.4. American College of Sports Medicine Recommendations for Exercise Testing Prior to Participation

	Low Risk[a]	Moderate Risk[b]	High Risk[c]
Moderate exercise[d]	Not necessary	Not necessary	Recommended
Vigorous exercise[e]	Not necessary	Recommended	Recommended

[a]Men under 45 years of age and women under 55 years of age who have no symptoms and have no more than one cardiovascular risk factor (family history, cigarette smoking, hypertension, hypercholesterolemia, diabetes mellitus, obesity, sedentary life-style).
[b]Men 45 years of age or older and women 55 years of age and older or have two or more cardiovascular disease risk factors.
[c]Men and women with symptoms of cardiovascular disease or known cardiovascular, pulmonary, or metabolic disease.
[d]Intensity 40%–60% of maximal oxygen uptake.
[e]Intensity greater than 60% maximal oxygen uptake.
Reprinted by permission from American College of Sports Medicine. *ACSM's guidelines for exercise testing and prescription,* 6th ed. Philadelphia: Lippincott Williams & Wilkins, 2000.

down and followed up at subsequent medical encounters. Emphasize to all patients that exercise should be started slowly with a warm-up period (5–10 minutes of stretching and slowly progressive activity) to protect muscles from injury, increase tendon flexibility, and improve joint range of motion. Each exercise session should end with a cool-down period (5–10 minutes of diminishing activity and stretching) to bring heart rate, blood pressure, plasma catecholamines, and lactic acid levels to baseline and reduce the incidence of cardiovascular complications.

The type of exercise must be individually prescribed according to personal interest and health status. In the United States, walking is the most preferred initial exercise or physical activity. The risk of injury must be considered in sedentary individuals starting higher intensity or high-impact activities.

Duration (frequency and time) of exercise is also important. The total amount of energy expenditure needed to gain benefit has been suggested to be 700 kcal/week, with activities of more than 2,000 kcal/week not providing any additional benefit. Time spent at an activity or distance achieved is another way of measuring activity in conjunction with intensity. A deconditioned individual may need to start out at as little as 5 minutes per session, but the goal for an exercise program is 20 to 60 minutes per session. The frequency should be three to five exercise sessions per week. The rate of progression should not be more than 5 minutes per week.

The intensity of exercise can be estimated using heart rate or a patient-perceived rating of their exertion like the Borg scale of perceived exertion (Table 31.5). Heart rate is the most commonly used method and can be easily taught to exercise participants. If medications that affect heart rate are taken, then the patient rating scale method can be used. On a scale of 6 to 20 (very, very light to very, very hard), a Borg rating of 12 to 16 is considered moderate intensity. Heart rate is another way to assess intensity. Maximum heart rate is calculated as 220 minus age in years or is measured during an exercise stress test. The maximum heart rate can be used to set the range of target heart rate during exercise (50%–70% of heart rate reserve). The formula for target heart rate is as follows:

[(Maximum heart rate − resting heart rate) × 0.50 to 0.70)] + (resting heart rate)

The target heart rate should be achieved after 5 to 10 minutes of performing the physical activity. The activity can be increased according to exertion required to achieve target heart rate.

Table 31.5. Classification of Physical Activity Intensity Based on Physical Activity Lasting up to 60 Minutes

Relative Intensity	% HRR	% HR max	RPE[a]
Intensity			
Very light	<20	<35	<10
Light	20–39	35–54	10–11
Moderate	40–59	55–69	12–13
Hard	60–84	70–89	14–16
Very hard	≥85	≥90	17–19
Maximal	100	100	20

[a]Borg rating of perceived exertion, scale of 6 to 20.
HRR, heart rate reserve; HR max, maximal heart rate; RPE, relative perceived exertion.
Adapted from Pollock M L, Gaesser G A, Butcher J D, et al. The recommended quantity and quality of exercise for developing and maintaining cardiorespiratory and muscular fitness, and flexibility in healthy adults. *Med Sci Sports Exerc* 1998;30:975–991; with permission.

Resistance training may be completed on the same day or may be alternated with days of dynamic exercise. The prescription for resistance training in individuals free of heart disease should start at 2 days per week and move up to 3 days per week for additional improvement. It is recommended that a single set (10–12 repetitions or lifts) of 8 to 10 exercises for arms, shoulders, chest, trunk, back, hips, and legs, including the front and back of the major muscle groups (e.g., arms include both biceps and triceps) be performed each session. This means using free weights or weight-lifting machines at 50% (±10%) of maximum single-repetition weight. The starting weight should be easily lifted with moderate effort (Borg scale rating of 13–15 out of 6–20). The proper technique consists of a slow 2-second rise and 4-second fall of the weight for each repetition along with an inspiration and expiration (no breath holding). A workout as just described should last approximately 20 to 30 minutes. The rate of progression should not exceed an increase of 5% of maximum single-repetition weight per session.

Case

A 38-year-old African-American man comes to your office for an annual examination and is interested in joining a health club facility. He has no complaints and denies having chest pain, palpitations, or shortness of breath. His past medical history is significant only for hypertension and tobacco abuse. He has smoked a pack of cigarettes per day for the past 5 years. He works a desk job as an Internet website designer and lives with his wife and two children. His current physical activity consists only of walking to and from the parking lot to his office and some weekend yard work (30 minutes per week). He has no family history of premature CAD. His only medication is hydrochlorothiazide for hypertension. His vital signs are blood pressure 120/80 mm Hg, pulse 82 beats/min, respiration 14 breaths/min, temperature 36.7°C, height 5 feet 8 inches, and weight 260 pounds. Generally, he is a well-developed overweight black male in no acute distress. His cardiovascular examination shows normal S$_1$/S$_2$, and no murmurs, rubs, or gallops. The rest of the physical examination is also within normal limits.

Laboratory results are as follows: total cholesterol 205 mg/dL, low-density lipoprotein (LDL) cholesterol 141 mg/dL, high-density lipoprotein cholesterol 40 mg/dL, triglycerides 120 mg/dL, and glucose 85 mg/dL.

1. Would you perform an exercise stress test on this individual prior to exercise?
2. What kind of exercise prescription is appropriate for this patient?

Case Discussion

Would You Perform an Exercise Stress Test on This Individual Prior to Exercise?

Being under 40 years of age, this patient is at moderate risk, but he is a current smoker with hypertension, sedentary life-style, and slightly elevated lipids (LDL cholesterol 141 mg/dL). His blood pressure is currently under control. He does not have a family history of premature CAD or diabetes. If the patient plans on engaging in a moderate-intensity activity, there is no need for a stress test. However, if the patient is considering more vigorous exertion, an exercise stress test may be considered, but is not absolutely necessary. Clinical judgment is required when recommending vigorous exercise to patients with significant risk factors for CAD. Because the patient is overweight and mainly sedentary, you should advise him not to start out with vigorous exercise due to risk of injury.

What Kind of Exercise Prescription Is Appropriate for This Patient?

Counsel the patient on increasing physical activity during the day and then set an exercise prescription. The patient should select an appropriate type of exercise that uses dynamic muscle groups. The patient elected to get an exercise stress test (which was normal) and had a maximum heart rate of 182 beats/min, which was the same as predicted (220 − age). You calculate his target heart rate range to be 132 to 152 beats/min ($[(182 − 82) \times 0.50$ to $0.70] + 82$). You suggest he start out at 20 minutes of exercise on a treadmill 3 to 5 days per week with a warm-up and cool-down period. You counsel him to increase the duration no more than 5 minutes per week. He returns to the clinic after 8 weeks, happy with his exercise program and ready to begin resistance training. You add 2 days per week of moderate-intensity weight training at his health club using 8 to 10 machines (arms, shoulders, chest, trunk, back, hips, and legs). You start out with one set of 10 to 12 repetitions for each exercise.

Suggested Reading

American College of Sports Medicine. *ACSM's guidelines for exercise testing and prescription,* 6th ed. Philadelphia: Lippincott Williams & Wilkins, 2000.

Fletcher G F, Balady G, Blair S N, et al. Statement on exercise: benefits and recommendations for physical activity programs for all Americans. A statement for health professionals by the Committee on Exercise and Cardiac Rehabilitation of the Council on Clinical Cardiology, American Heart Association. *Circulation* 1996;94:857–862.

Fletcher G F, Balady G, Froelicher V F, et al. Exercise standards. A statement for healthcare professionals from the American Heart Association. Writing Group. *Circulation* 1995;91:580–615.

Pate R R, Pratt M, Blair S N, et al. Physical activity and public health. A recommendation from the Centers for Disease Control and Prevention and the American College of Sports Medicine. *JAMA* 1995;273:402–407.

Pollock M L, Franklin B A, Balady G J, et al. Resistance exercise in individuals with and without cardiovascular disease: benefits, rationale, safety, and prescription. An advisory from the Committee on Exercise, Rehabilitation, and Prevention, Council on Clinical Cardiology, American Heart Association. *Circulation* 2000;101:828–833.

32
Chronic Stress

Holly Avey
Terry A. Jacobson

1. How is chronic stress defined and diagnosed?
2. What is the prevalence of chronic stress disorders in primary care?
3. What are the physiologic effects of chronic stress?
4. What is the relaxation response?
5. What disease states are associated with chronic stress and have been shown to benefit from stress reduction techniques?
6. What are the treatment options?
7. How can a practitioner initiate a stress prescription with relaxation exercises?

Discussion
How Is Chronic Stress Defined and Diagnosed?

Stress can be defined as "the process in which environmental demands tax or exceed the adaptive capacity of an organism, resulting in psychological and biological changes that may place persons at risk for disease" (Cohen, Kessler, and Underwood Gordon, 1995). It is easy to understand how distinct life events such as death, divorce, or the loss of a job could be psychologically stressful and lead to depression or physical illness, but research shows that not all people who experience stressful life events become ill. *Perception* and *engagement* are two key factors that help to determine who will become sick as a result of stress and who will be resilient. A woman who perceives that she has adequate resources to meet the demands of a stressor will be more resilient than a woman who feels helpless, like she is out of control. A man who is engaged in an event and feels that the outcome is important may be more susceptible to the negative consequences of stress than a man who is indifferent to the outcome.

Chronic stressors may be even more physiologically damaging than major life events, because of their constant presence. In fact, mounting evidence suggests that people do not psychologically habituate to chronic stressors. These stressors include events or conditions such as marital/relationship stress, workplace stress, environmental stress from poor living or working conditions, financial stress, discrimination, and physical stress from disability or disease. Again, the events themselves do not necessarily result in disease—it depends upon the person's perception of the events and how important the events are to him or her.

Table 32.1. Stress Warning Signals

Physical Symptoms	Behavioral Symptoms	Emotional Symptoms	Cognitive Symptoms	Spiritual Symptoms	Relational Symptoms
Headaches	Excess smoking	Crying	Trouble thinking	Emptiness	Isolation
Indigestion	Bossiness	Nervousness	clearly	Loss of meaning	Intolerance
Stomachaches	Compulsive gum	Boredom	Forgetfulness	Doubt	Resentment
Sweaty palms	chewing	Ready to explode	Lack of creativity	Unforgiving	Loneliness
Sleep difficulties	Critical of others	Feeling powerless	Memory loss	Martyrdom	Lashing out
Dizziness	Grinding teeth at	Easily upset	Loss of sense of	Looking for magic	Hiding
Back pain	night	Overwhelming	humor	Loss of direction	Clamming up
Tight muscles	Overuse of alcohol	pressure	Inability to make	Cynicism	Lowered sex
Racing heart	Compulsive eating	Anger	decisions	Apathy	drive
Restlessness	Inability to get	Loneliness	Thoughts of	Needing to	Nagging
Tiredness	things done	Unhappy for no	running away	"prove" self	Distrust
Ringing in ears		reason	Constant worry		Lack of
					intimacy
					Using people
					Fewer
					contacts

From Webster A, Wells-Federman C, Stuart E. Healthy Lifestyles Program, Mind/Body Medical Institute, 1996.

If people perceive events in their lives that are important to them as chronically stressful and beyond their control, then intervention may be appropriate. Some of the most common signs of chronic stress include changes in physical symptoms, behavior, emotions, memory, thinking, or relationships (Table 32.1).

You can also assess a patient's stress level by administering the four-item perceived stress scale developed by Cohen, Kamarck, and Mermelstein (1983). You may initiate the conversation by first asking, "Have you been under a lot of stress lately?" (very often, fairly often, sometimes, almost never, or never), then continuing with the following questions:

- In the last month how often have you felt . . .
  - that you were unable to control the important things in your life?
  - confident about your ability to handle your personal problems?
  - that things were going your way?
  - difficulties were piling up so high that you could not overcome them?

Patients who answer three or four of the questions above with one of the most extreme options should be considered at moderate to high levels of perceived stress and in need of intervention.

What Is the Prevalence of Chronic Stress Disorders in Primary Care?

Stress is an underlying factor for a wide variety, and perhaps even the majority, of health-care provider visits. In 1981, a landmark study by Cummings and Van den Bos reviewing the charts of Kaiser-Permanente patients concluded that "60% to 90% of physician visits reflect emotional distress" and somatization. A similar study published in 1989 by Kroenke and Mangelsdorff reviewed the diagnoses and treatments for the 14 most common complaints of 1,000 patients followed in an internal medicine clinic over a 3-year period. Although diagnostic testing was performed in two-thirds of the cases, an organic etiology was demonstrated in only 16% of the complaints. The authors reported, "It is probable that many of the symptoms of unknown etiology were related to psychosocial factors."

What Are the Physiological Effects of Chronic Stress?

The body's physiologic response to a perceived stressor involves the activation of the autonomic nervous system, the hypothalamic-pituitary-adrenal (HPA) axis, and the cardiovascular, metabolic, and immune systems. *Stress-related hormones* such as epinephrine, norepinephrine, and glucocorticoids are secreted, as well as glucagon, endorphins, enkephalins, prolactin, and vasopressin. Simultaneously, hormones such as estrogen, progesterone, testosterone, growth hormone, and insulin are inhibited.

Allostasis is the process by which the human body adapts to change or to stress. This process generally works well in situations related to acute stressors (i.e., the fight-or-flight response), but the body seems ill prepared to deal with *chronic* activation. The long-term effect of the physiologic response to stress has been referred to as "allostatic load." Over weeks, months, or years, chronic overactivity of stress hormones can result in pathophysiologic consequences. According to McEwen (1998), allostatic load comes in three forms:

1. Lack of adaptation. Example: the continued increase in cortisol secretions even after subjects have been habituated to a stressful event.
2. Prolonged response (inability to shut off adaptive responses after a stress is terminated). Example: the maintenance of elevated blood pressure in some individuals after experiencing a stressful event.
3. Inadequate response (impaired cortisol response leading to compensatory hyperactivity of other chemical mediators). Example: hyporesponsiveness of the HPA axis leads to the increased secretion of inflammatory cytokines (normally counterregulated by cortisol), resulting in autoimmune and inflammatory disturbances.

Two consequences of chronic stress may be reactive *depression* and *increased pain sensitivity*. Under normal circumstances, norepinephrine activates reward centers in the brain and endorphins elevate mood. However, when chronic stress consistently increases the production of these biochemicals, it causes reactive inhibition due to tissue fatigue. The resulting depletion of norepinephrine and endorphins then produces the opposite reaction: anhedonia and depression. Endorphins also work as pain killers, producing stress-induced analgesia in acute situations. However, depletion due to overactivation from chronic stress can produce hyperalgesia, contributing to chronic pain conditions.

What Is the Relaxation Response?

Specific stress management techniques that elicit the relaxation response may help to counteract the pathophysiology of chronic stress. In 1974, cardiologist Herbert Benson used the phrase *relaxation response* to describe an integrated hypothalamic response that results in generalized decreased sympathetic nervous system activity. During further study, Dr. Benson consistently showed that the physiologic changes initiated by specific relaxation guidelines are the opposite

Table 32.2. Physiologic Effects of Stress and Relaxation

Stress Response (Fight-or-Flight Response; Dr. Walter B. Cannon, 1941)	Relaxation Response (Dr. Herbert Benson, 1974)
Increase in: Heart rate Blood pressure Respiratory rate Metabolic rate	Decrease in: Heart rate Blood pressure Respiratory rate Metabolic rate

of the fight-or-flight response (i.e., decreased oxygen consumption, heart rate, arterial blood pressure, respiratory rate, and arterial blood lactate) and are different from changes reported during sleep or quiet sitting. In addition, slow α waves of the electroencephalogram increase in intensity during relaxation. Repeated elicitation of the relaxation response results in reduced norepinephrine end-organ responsivity, suggesting there may be long-lasting benefits to regular relaxation practice (Table 32.2).

What Disease States Are Associated with Chronic Stress and Have Been Shown to Benefit from Stress Reduction Techniques?

Infectious and Immune-Mediated Diseases

Although recent research suggests that acute psychological and physical stressors actually temporarily enhance the immune system, chronic stressors (those that last for 60 minutes or more) produce the opposite response and can suppress immune function. Stress has been associated with greater severity and duration of infectious diseases as well as immune-mediated diseases such as asthma, rheumatoid arthritis, multiple sclerosis, inflammatory bowel disease, and cancer. In the first prospective study of its kind, Cohen, Tyrell, and Smith (1991) demonstrated that psychological stress was associated in a dose-response manner to rates of infections in acute respiratory illnesses. There is now significant research showing that psychological stress can downregulate various aspects of the cellular immune response and disrupt the bidirectional communication links between the central nervous system and the immune system. A randomized clinical trial with patients who had immune-mediated rheumatoid arthritis (Bradley et al., 1987) measured the effects of a psychological intervention and social support program on the patients' pain behavior, disease activity, and trait anxiety. Compared with the control program, the intervention produced significant decreases in disease activity and pain. The investigators stated that the relaxation training may have been the most important component of the psychological intervention.

Cardiovascular Disease

An extensive body of evidence from both animal and human studies reveals that chronic psychosocial stress can lead to exacerbation and acceleration of coronary artery atherosclerosis as well as to hypercortisolemia. Acute stress also has been shown to trigger myocardial ischemia, promote arrhythmogenesis, stimulate platelet function, increase blood viscosity, and cause coronary vasoconstriction in the presence of underlying atherosclerosis (Fig. 32.1). A recent review by Rozanski et al. (1999) concluded that present studies "provide clear and convincing evidence that psychosocial factors contribute significantly to the pathogenesis and expression of coronary artery disease."

Hypertension

Stress has been shown to increase blood pressure and heart rate. Studies reviewing the impact of stress reduction techniques on hypertension have been inconsistent in their findings. Although a few studies have found no difference from controls, many studies have shown that stress management can reduce hypertension. Some studies have found that stress management does not reduce hypertension to the same extent as pharmacotherapy, but is a useful adjunct. Despite these inconsistencies, the evidence does not preclude the use of stress management as an adjunctive treatment for hypertension.

Chronic Pain

A 1996 National Institutes of Health (NIH) Technology Assessment Panel "found strong evidence for the use of relaxation techniques in reducing chronic pain in a va-

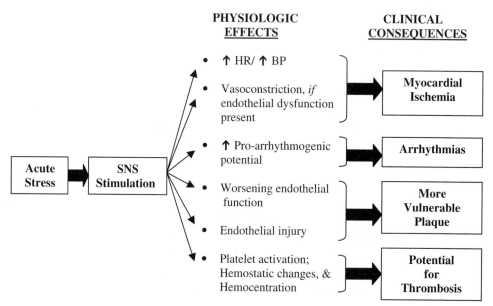

Figure 32.1. Acute stress produces sympathetic nervous system (SNS) stimulation, which leads to a range of effects such as heart rate and blood pressure stimulation, endothelial injury, impaired endothelial functioning, and hemostatic changes. Clinical consequences include development of myocardial ischemia, cardiac arrhythmias, and vulnerable coronary plaques. These changes set the stage for acute myocardial infarction and sudden cardiac death. From Rozanski A, Blumenthal J A, Kaplan J. Circulation © 1999. Used with permission.

riety of medical conditions," including tension headaches, low back pain, rheumatoid arthritis, osteoarthritis, irritable bowel syndrome, and pain associated with cancer. The panel concluded, "Although relatively good evidence exists for the efficacy of several behavioral and relaxation interventions in the treatment of chronic pain, the data are insufficient to conclude that one technique is usually more effective than another for a given condition. For any given individual patient, however, one approach may indeed be more appropriate than another." Some examples include a meta-analysis on treatments for recurrent tension headaches (Bogaards and ter Kuile, 1994), which revealed that relaxation therapy was superior to placebo treatment in studies using headache diaries, whereas pharmacologic therapy was not.

Insomnia

The HPA axis, which plays an important role in sleep-wake regulation, also alters the sleep-wake cycle secondary to exposure to acute or chronic stressors. The same 1996 NIH Technology Assessment Panel that reviewed behavioral and relaxation approaches to chronic pain concluded that relaxation was effective in alleviating insomnia, and the most pronounced improvements were in sleep latency and time of awakening after sleep onset.

Somatization Disorders

The very definition of somatization is "the experience of physical symptoms in response to emotional distress" (Servan-Schreiber, Kolb, and Tabas, 1999). One prospective study of primary care patients experiencing physical symptoms with a psychosocial component (e.g., palpitations, gastrointestinal disturbances, headaches, malaise, sleep disorders) investigated the effectiveness of two group behavioral medicine interventions. Both interventions focused on the mind/body relationship and used relaxation-response training. Patients in the behavioral medicine groups showed significantly greater reductions in clinic visits and in discomfort from physical and psychological symptoms compared with controls.

Psychiatric Disorders

See section on Anxiety Disorders in Chapter 79.

What Are the Treatment Options?

Patients assessed to have moderate to high levels of perceived stress may be instructed in the elicitation of the relaxation response (see stress prescription below) or referred to a mental health provider or health educator for stress management instruction and guidance. In addition, there are many books, audiotapes, and websites that may be recommended to patients.

It is important to pay special attention to the stress levels of patients with cardiovascular disease or cardiovascular disease risk factors (e.g., hypertension), impaired immune systems, chronic pain, psychiatric diseases, insomnia, or multiple medical symptoms, because these patients are most likely to benefit physiologically from relaxation exercises.

How Can a Practitioner Initiate a Stress Prescription with Relaxation Exercises?

When guiding a patient in how to elicit the relaxation response, there are two simple steps to remember: (1) repetition of a simple mental focus (breath, word, short phrase), and (2) passive mental attitude toward other thoughts, feelings, and sensations.

A variety of techniques can elicit the relaxation response, including diaphragmatic breathing, meditation, progressive muscle relaxation, imagery/visualization, mindfulness (focusing awareness on the present moment), and yoga stretching.

Instruct your patients to practice their relaxation routine once or twice per day for 10 to 20 minutes in a place that is free of distractions (if possible) such as phone, family, and pets. Practicing in the same place and at the same time every day helps to make it a habitual pattern. Relaxation practice works well after physical exercise, but should not be done on a full or empty stomach. Possible contraindications to relaxation-response training include psychosis and severe depression (due to the inability to concentrate).

Other techniques that are helpful in reducing stress include physical activity, cognitive behavior therapy (changing the way you think), and writing about stressful life events (journaling) or expressing these emotions in some other creative way (painting, dance, music, etc.) (Table 32.3).

Case

A 56-year-old postmenopausal black woman with hypertension and osteoarthritis presents to your office complaining of several months of an increase in headaches, difficulty sleeping, and daily arthritis pain. She continues to function at a high level at work and home, but wonders if she can continue to function this way because she feels like a "mess." Upon further questioning, she reports that her stress and symptoms have been going on for many months, and that she is overwhelmed by new responsibilities at work and at home with a new grandchild. She worries that her increased headache pain may be something more severe like a "tumor," but she was extensively examined 1 year ago via computed tomography by a neurologist, who diagnosed "tension" headaches. Her daughter reports that she seems more anxious and irritable than usual. Current medications include estrogen, progesterone, amlodipine, hydrochlorothiazide, and multivitamin.

Physical examination reveals an obese, slightly anxious woman. Vital signs show a blood pressure of 155/95 mm Hg, pulse 88 beats/min, and respirations 16 breaths/min. The remainder of the physical examination is unremarkable. Results of laboratory studies are as follows: complete blood count within normal limits, serum chemistries within normal limits, and thyroid-stimulating hormone (TSH) 1.0 μIU/mL.

1. What organic etiologies of her symptoms need to be ruled out first?
2. Of the symptoms reported by the patient, which ones may be due to stress? Also, is there evidence that stress can result in elevated blood pressure and heart rate as seen in this patient?
3. You diagnose the patient with chronic stress. What is your first line of therapy?

Table 32.3. Instructions for Relaxation Techniques

Diaphragmatic Breathing (Belly Breathing)	Focused Meditation
Sit in a comfortable chair. Loosen your belt or any restrictive clothing. Place your hands just below your belly button. Close your eyes. Think of a balloon inside your belly. Each time you breathe in, picture the balloon filling with air. Your hands will gently rise. Each time you breathe out, picture the balloon shrinking. Your hands will gently settle lower down. Focus on how your breathing sounds and feels as you become more and more relaxed.	Sit in a comfortable position and close your eyes. Relax your muscles and focus on your breathing. Focus your attention on your breath, a word, a phrase, or a prayer (examples: relax, peace, one). If other thoughts come into your mind, don't just observe them from a distance and let them pass by. Return your attention to the focus of your meditation.
Mindfulness Meditation	Progressive Muscle Relaxation

Sit in a comfortable position and close your eyes.
Relax your muscles and focus on your breathing.
When thoughts come into your mind, don't try to make them go away. Instead, focus all of your attention on that thought.
Don't judge the thought. Just observe it from a distance.
Imagine that the thought belongs to someone else and you are studying it.
Pay attention to the thought until it goes away.
When the next thought comes into your mind, focus all of your attention on that thought.
Soon, you may find that your mind becomes quiet. Not as many thoughts enter your mind.
	Sit in a comfortable chair or lie down on your back.
	Tense your muscle to the point of pressure, but not pain.
	Hold for 5 seconds and notice what the tight muscle feels like.
	Breathe out and let the muscle go completely limp.
	Feel the difference between muscles that are tight and the ones that are relaxed.
	Go through your body tensing and relaxing each muscle group twice.
	Muscles to relax:
	  Head and face
	  Neck and throat
	  Chest, back, and shoulders
	  Hands and arms
	  Stomach and buttocks
	  Legs and feet
	  Your whole body

4. What specific recommendations can a primary care physician make to patients to help relieve their stress?

Case Discussion

What Organic Etiologies of Her Symptoms Need to Be Ruled Out First?

After ruling out organic etiologies of her symptoms with laboratory studies and physical examination, you question her about depression. She does not seem to have significant signs such as dysthymia, depressed mood, anhedonia, weight change, or decrease in function at work or home. She does not appear to have a psychiatric disorder as defined by the *Diagnostic and Statistical Manual of Mental Disorders* (4th edition), such as generalized anxiety disorder, an acute stress disorder, or posttraumatic stress disorder. You rule out substance abuse with illicit drugs or excessive use of alcohol or caffeine. You also consider hypothyroidism, which is common in elderly women, but her TSH level is normal. Although some of her symptoms might also be postmenopausal changes, she has been on hor-

Table 32.4. Patient Education Resources

Resource Centers

Mind/Body Medical Institute
Beth Israel Deaconess Medical Center
Division of Behavioral Medicine
Tel. 617-432-1525
Web: http://www.mindbody.harvard.edu/

Center for Mindfulness in Medicine, Health Care, and Society
University of Massachusetts Medical Center
55 Lake Avenue North
Tel. 508-856-2656
Web: http://www.umassmed.edu/cfm/

Transcendental Meditation Program
Maharishi University of Management
Tel. 1-888-532-7686
Web: http://www.mum.edu/tm_program/welcome.html

Health Journeys
The Guided Imagery Resource Center
Tel. 1-800-800-8661
Web: http://www.healthjourneys.com

Books

Benson, Herbert and Stuart, Eileen M. *The wellness book. The comprehensive guide to maintaining health and treating stress-related illness.* New York: Simon & Schuster, 1993.
Kabat-Zinn, Jon. *Wherever you go there you are. Mindfulness meditation in everyday life.* New York: Hyperion, 1994.
Pennebaker, James W. *Opening up. The healing power of expressing emotions.* New York: Guilford, 1990.
Seligman, Martin E P. *Learned optimism. How to change your life and your mind.* New York: Pocket Books, 1998.
Sobel, David S and Ornstein, Robert. *The healthy mind healthy body handbook.* New York: Patient Education Media, 1996.

mone replacement therapy for 2 years without complaints. You start to consider that her increased symptoms might be due to the chronic stresses in her life.

Of the Symptoms Reported by the Patient, Which Ones May Be Due to Stress? Also, Is There Evidence That Stress Can Result in Elevated Blood Pressure and Heart Rate as Seen in This Patient?

Symptoms reported by the patient that may be caused or exacerbated by chronic stress include tension headaches, insomnia, anxiety, arthritis pain, hypertension, irritability, and feeling overwhelmed and worried. Elevation in blood pressure and heart rate are classic symptoms of the fight-or-flight response involving activation of the sympathetic nervous system. Lack of adaptation or prolonged response versions of allostatic load from chronic stress may result in continued elevation of these readings.

You Diagnose the Patient with Chronic Stress. What Is Your First Line of Therapy?

The first line of therapy is psychological assessment and stress reduction counseling. Pharmacotherapy with an anxiolytic agent or selective serotonin reuptake inhibitor is not considered first-line therapy. You initiate supportive counseling and recommend that the patient see a health professional skilled in stress reduction, psychology, or psychiatry. In addition, consider prescribing the relaxation response or referring to a stress reduction program. You can also recommend several patient education resources (Table 32.4). As part of a team, you can help the patient cope with her stress and deal with her stress-related symptoms.

What Specific Recommendations Can a Primary Care Physician Make to Patients to Help Relieve Their Stress?

A primary care physician can initiate stress reduction by teaching several proven techniques to reduce stress, such as deep breathing, meditation, or progressive muscle relaxation.

Suggested Reading

Bogaards M C, ter Kuile M M. Treatment of recurrent tension headache: a meta-analytic review. *Clin J Pain* 1994;10:174–190.

Bradley L A, Young L D, Anderson K O, et al. Effects of psychological therapy on pain behavior of rheumatoid arthritis patients. Treatment outcome and six-month followup. *Arthritis Rheumatism* 1987;30:1105–1114.

Cohen S, Kamarck T, Mermelstein R. A global measure of perceived stress. *J Health Social Behav* 1983;24:385–396.

Cohen S, Kessler R C, Gordon L U. *Measuring stress: a guide for health and social scientists.* New York: Oxford University Press, 1995.

Cohen S, Tyrell D A, Smith A P. Psychological stress and susceptibility to the common cold. *N Engl J Med* 1991;325:606–612.

Cummings N A, VandenBos G R. The twenty years Kaiser-Permanente experience with psychotherapy and medical utilization: implications for national health policy and national health insurance. *Health Policy Q* 1981;1:159–175.

Glaser R, Rabin B, Chesney M, et al. Stress-induced immunomodulation: implications for infectious diseases? *JAMA* 1999;281:2268–2270.

Hellman C J, Budd M, Borysenko J, et al. A study of the effectiveness of two group behavioral medicine interventions for patients with psychosomatic complaints. *Behav Med* 1990;16:165–173.

Hoffman J W, Benson H, Arns P A, et al. Reduced sympathetic nervous system responsivity associated with the relaxation response. *Science* 1982;215:190–192.

Kroenke K, Mangelsdorff A D. Common symptoms in ambulatory care: incidence, evaluation, therapy, and outcome. *Am J Med* 1989;86:262–266.

Linden W, Chambers L. Clinical effectiveness of non-drug treatment for hypertension: a meta-analysis. *Ann Behav Med* 1994;16:35–45.

McEwen B S. Protective and damaging effects of stress mediators. *N Engl J Med* 1998;338:171–179.

NIH Technology Assessment Panel on Integration of Behavioral and Relaxation Approaches into the Treatment of Chronic Pain and Insomnia. Integration of behavioral and relaxation approaches into the treatment of chronic pain and insomnia. *JAMA* 1996;276:313–318.

Rozanski A, Blumenthal J A, Kaplan J. Impact of psychological factors on the pathogenesis of cardiovascular disease and implications for therapy. *Circulation* 1999;99:2192–2217.

Sapolsky R. *Why zebras don't get ulcers. An updated guide to stress, stress-related diseases, and coping,* 4th ed. New York: WH Freeman, 1999.

Servan-Schreiber D, Kolb R, Tabas G. The somatizing patient. *Primary Care Clin Office Pract* 1999;26:225–242.

33

Treating Tobacco Use and Dependence

Sunil Kripalani

1. What is the magnitude of tobacco abuse in the United States?
2. What are the effects of tobacco smoke on the cardiovascular system and other organs?
3. What general strategy is recommended for physicians to help their patients quit smoking?
4. How can physicians effectively counsel patients to quit smoking?
5. What is the role of pharmacotherapy in smoking cessation?

Discussion

What Is the Magnitude of Tobacco Abuse in the United States?

Almost 25% of Americans smoke, and tobacco use is responsible for more than 400,000 deaths annually in the United States. Exposure to second-hand, or environmental smoke may contribute to another 50,000 deaths. Approximately 40% of these deaths are from cardiovascular causes, including myocardial infarction and stroke. The remainder are due to various forms of cancer and chronic lung disease. These statistics make smoking the leading preventable cause of death in our society, responsible for one in six deaths. Tobacco abuse is estimated to cost the U.S. economy nearly $100 billion annually, including indirect costs such as lost wages and productivity.

What Are the Effects of Tobacco Smoke on the Cardiovascular System and Other Organs?

Tobacco smoke contains more than 4,000 adverse chemicals; at least 63 of these are known carcinogens. Smoking cigarettes creates up to a tenfold increase in the risk of certain cancers affecting the lung, oral cavity, larynx, and esophagus. Cancers of the stomach, pancreas, bladder, kidney, and cervix are also more common in cigarette smokers. People who use cigars have a significantly higher risk of developing cancer of the oral cavity, larynx, esophagus, and lung. Carcinogens mix with the

Table 33.1. When Smokers Quit

20 minutes	Blood pressure and pulse return to normal
8 hours	Carbon monoxide level in blood returns to normal
	Oxygen level in blood increases to normal
24 hours	Risk of myocardial infarction decreases
48 hours	Senses of smell and taste start to improve
2 weeks to 3 months	Circulation improves
	Lung function improves
1 to 9 months	Respiratory symptoms (coughing, congestion, etc.) decrease
	Cilia regrow
	Energy level increases
1 year	Excess risk of coronary disease decreases by 50%
5 years	Death rate from lung cancer decreases by almost 50%
	Excess risk of oral and esophageal cancer decreases by 50%
	Stroke risk decreases
10 years	Death rate from lung cancer is similar to that of nonsmokers
15 years	Risk of coronary disease decreases to that of a nonsmoker

From the American Cancer Society. Available at http://www.cancer.org/tobacco/quitting.html.

saliva, so cancer rates rise even if the cigar user does not inhale. Exposure to second-hand smoke from either cigarettes or cigars increases the risk of cancer, heart disease, and respiratory symptoms and infections.

Effects on the cardiovascular system are mediated primarily through nicotine and carbon monoxide. Nicotine is an adrenergic agonist that elevates catecholamine levels and increases myocardial demand by raising both heart rate and blood pressure. Carbon monoxide interferes with the binding of oxygen to hemoglobin, reducing the delivery of oxygen to the myocardium and other tissues. Smoking also accelerates atherogenesis, adversely affects the lipid profile, and promotes a thrombogenic state by increasing platelet reactivity and fibrinogen levels. Importantly, these effects are all reversible with smoking cessation. The excess risk of coronary disease decreases by 50% at 1 year and returns to baseline at 15 years. Risk of death from lung cancer declines by 50% at 5 years of cessation (Table 33.1).

What General Strategy Is Recommended for Physicians to Help Their Patients Quit Smoking?

Each year, at least 70% of smokers visit a physician's office, creating a number of opportunities for intervention. Many of these visits are prompted by smoking-related complaints, raising a "teachable moment" that can help motivate cessation. Measures to promote smoking cessation do not have to be time consuming, and they do not have to work for every patient in order to have a large public health impact. If physicians attain only a 5% success rate in their efforts, an additional 2 million smokers will quit each year. The following strategy outlines brief interventions that can be used in any outpatient encounter.

Remember the five A's: ask, advise, assess, assist, and arrange. *Ask* each patient if he or she smokes, and chart smoking as a fifth vital sign. *Advise* all smokers to quit in a clear, strong, and personalized manner. Simply doing this doubles the chance that the patient will quit smoking in the next year. *Assess* each patient's willingness to quit smoking. *Assist* in the quit attempt by setting a quit date, providing appropriate counseling, and offering pharmacologic therapy. *Arrange* for follow-up to congratulate success and help prevent relapse (Table 33.2).

Table 33.2. The "Five A" Strategy for Smoking Cessation

Step 1. Ask: Systematically identify all tobacco users at every visit.
 Take smoking status as a fifth vital sign.
Step 2. Advise: Strongly urge all smokers to quit.
 Use a clear, strong, and personalized approach.
 Encourage clinic staff to reinforce the cessation message.
Step 3. Assess: Determine which smokers are ready to make a quit attempt.
 For those unwilling to quit at this time, provide a motivational intervention.
Step 4. Assist: Aid the patient in quitting.
 Set a quit date and help the patient prepare for quitting.
 Offer pharmacologic therapy.
 Give advice on how to make the attempt more successful.
 Provide educational materials.
Step 5. Arrange: Schedule follow-up contact.
 Contact the patient soon after the quit date to congratulate success and avoid relapse.
 Use relapses as a learning tool for the next quit attempt, not as a sign of failure.

Adapted from Fiore M C, Bailey W C, Cohen S J, et al. *Treating tobacco use and dependence.* Clinical Practice Guideline. Rockville, MD: U.S. Department of Health and Human Services. Public Health Service, June 2000.

How Can Physicians Effectively Counsel Patients to Quit Smoking?

The stages of change model can help you determine your patients' readiness to quit and provide them with appropriate counseling. Ask if they intend to quit smoking in the next 6 months, in the next month, or if they have tried to quit in the past year. Individuals who do not intend to quit in the next 6 months are in the *precontemplation* stage. Appropriate counseling for this group includes general information about the unhealthy effects of smoking and the benefits of cessation, with the goal of moving them into the next stage, in which they think about quitting. Most smokers fall into the *contemplation* stage and intend to quit smoking in the next 6 months. These individuals frequently need to build confidence in their ability to quit and will benefit from specific advice about how to overcome their barriers to cessation. In the *preparation stage,* smokers are taking steps toward quitting, such as cutting down on the number of cigarettes. They may intend to quit in the next month and should be encouraged to take action. Patients in the *action* stage are ready to quit in the next month, and they have often tried to quit in the past year. You can help them by setting a quit date and again reviewing methods to overcome their personal barriers to cessation. The final stage, *maintenance,* is important for reviewing the benefits of abstinence, such as improved taste for food, reduced respiratory symptoms, and greater social acceptance. If relapse occurs, it should not be seen as a sign of failure. Rather, it is an opportunity to learn about the individual's barriers to cessation and improve the chances of future attempts.

What Is the Role of Pharmacotherapy in Smoking Cessation?

Evidence suggests that cigar smokers have much less nicotine dependence than do cigarette smokers. Hence, nicotine replacement therapy (NRT) and other pharmacologic aids are established only for the cessation of cigarette smoking. Multiple clinical trials have demonstrated that NRT doubles the quit rate compared with placebo.

Four forms of NRT are approved by the U.S. Food and Drug Administration (FDA): patch, gum, inhaler, and nasal spray. The nicotine patch and gum can be purchased without a prescription. Different brands of patches cost $3 to $4 per day; the gum costs $2 to $8 dollars per day, depending on the number of pieces used at $0.40 to $0.55 per piece. Individuals must quit smoking when they begin NRT. There are few data regarding the use of these products in smokers who smoke fewer than 10 cigarettes per day.

Most experts recommend the patch because it is easy to use. Nicoderm (Glaxo-SmithKline, Research Triangle Park, NC) and Habitrol (Ciba-Geigy; Summit, NJ) patches come in strengths of 21, 14, and 7 mg. Nicotrol patches are sold only in the 15-mg strength. All of these should be used for 6 to 8 weeks and tapered per package instructions. The 21-mg patches contain more nicotine than a pack of cigarettes and should not be used by those who smoke one pack per day or less. It is important to wear a new patch every day, rotating sites to minimize skin irritation.

Nicotine gum (Nicorette: GlaxoSmithKline; Research Triangle Park, NC) works more effectively when used on a scheduled basis, rather than as needed. Smokers should use one to two pieces every 1 to 2 hours for 6 weeks, then taper for an additional 6 weeks. Light smokers should use the 2-mg, rather than the 4-mg, dose. To use the gum, chew until a peppery taste emerges, then park it between the cheek and gums, chewing and parking intermittently for a total of 30 minutes. For better absorption, avoid eating and drinking anything except water for 15 minutes before and during use.

The nicotine nasal spray and nicotine inhaler are additional options, available by prescription only (Nicotrol: Pharmacia; Peapack, NJ). The spray is the most rapid means of nicotine delivery and is given one to two times per hour for 3 months. Although most users experience nasal and throat irritation initially, tolerance to the side effects usually develops within 1 week. The nicotine inhaler, a plastic rod with a nicotine plug, bears some resemblance to cigarettes. It delivers its medication locally to the buccal mucosa, with pharmacokinetics similar to that of nicotine gum.

Bupropion (Zyban: GlaxoSmithKline: Research Triangle Park, NC) is an antidepressant approved by the FDA for smoking cessation. When used for 7 weeks, it doubles the quit rate at 1 year. Although most guidelines recommend using 150 mg twice a day, this dose was no more effective than 150 mg daily in a randomized, controlled trial. Zyban should be started 1 week before the quit date to allow for a therapeutic level, and must be used with caution in patients who have a seizure disorder. Therapy costs $3.00 to $3.50 per day.

Case

Mrs. M is a 58-year-old woman who presents to your medical clinic for a new patient visit. She has a history of seizures, which are well controlled on phenytoin. She smokes one pack per day, but at the insistence of her daughter, does not smoke around her two young grandchildren. She has tried giving up cigarettes several times, but she usually starts smoking again after taking several puffs of her husband's cigarettes. Mrs. M works 5 to 6 hours a day in housekeeping at a nearby hotel and notes that she has had to cut back her hours because of fatigue. She also takes a short break every 30 to 40 minutes when her left shoulder starts hurting. This pain has been present for 6 to 8 months and is often accompanied by mild shortness of breath; both resolve with a few minutes of rest. On examination, she appears comfortable, apart from occasional coughing. You smell cigarette smoke on her clothes and see a yellowish discoloration to the fingertips of her right hand. Her blood pressure is 154/92 mm Hg. The remainder of the examination is unremarkable, including shoulders.

1. What are the "teachable moments" in this encounter?
2. How should you counsel Mrs. M about smoking cessation?
3. Should you offer her pharmacologic therapy? If so, what type?

Case Discussion

What Are the "Teachable Moments" in This Encounter?

The smell of cigarette smoke, yellowish skin discoloration, and periodic cough all provide opportunities to discuss the patient's tobacco use. These would be helpful clues to her smoking status if she had not volunteered that information.

There are also a few teachable moments that could help motivate her to quit. First, the cough could be related to smoking, and as a smoker she has a higher risk of respiratory symptoms and pneumococcal disease. Second, her elevated blood pressure may be due to a recent cigarette, or it could represent hypertension that would be a cardiovascular risk factor, in addition to smoking and postmenopausal age. Next, the shoulder pain might represent angina. Smoking will worsen any existing coronary disease and raise the risk of myocardial infarction two- to sixfold. Finally, not being able to spend as much time around her grandchildren is another potential motivator to quit, especially because they also have a higher rate of respiratory infections when exposed to second-hand smoke.

How Should You Counsel Mrs. M about Smoking Cessation?

Because Mrs. M has already tried quitting, she remains in the action stage and should have enough motivation for another quit attempt. It would still be appropriate to briefly reinforce the importance of smoking cessation, taking advantage of the teachable moments listed above. However, the focus of your smoking intervention should be to set a quit date, perhaps the date of her daughter's or a grandchild's birthday, or the first of the month. You can also discuss her previous attempts to quit smoking and try to tackle her personal barriers to cessation, such as availability of her husband's cigarettes.

Should You Offer Her Pharmacologic Therapy? If So, What Type?

Absolutely. Given her history of seizures, bupropion is relatively contraindicated, although it only caused problems at higher doses in clinical trials. The patient's possible coronary disease raises a concern about the safety of NRT. Although few definitive data are available, a large observational study and three smaller experimental trials did not show any increased risk of acute coronary events in patients using

NRT. A likely explanation is that the nicotine levels are no higher with NRT than with cigarette smoking, and NRT does not include the carbon monoxide or the 4,000 other harmful chemicals found in cigarette smoke. For these reasons, it is considered safe in patients with stable coronary disease. Until more information is available, it should be used cautiously in patients with unstable heart disease, such as those with myocardial infarction in the past 4 weeks, worsening angina, or serious arrhythmias. Either the nicotine patch or gum is appropriate and should be started at a dose of 11 to 15 mg for the patch, or 2 mg for the gum.

If physicians attain only a 5% success rate in their cessation efforts, an additional 2 million smokers will quit each year.

Suggested Reading

Agency for Health Care Policy and Research Smoking Cessation Clinical Practice Guideline. *JAMA* 1996;275:1270–1280.

Baker F, Ainsworth S R, Dye J T, et al. Health risks associated with cigar smoking. *JAMA* 2000;284:735–740.

Benowitz N L, Gourlay S G. Cardiovascular toxicity of nicotine: implications for nicotine replacement therapy. *J Am Coll Cardiol* 1997;29:1422–1431.

He J, Vupputuri S, Allen K, et al. Passive smoking and the risk of coronary heart disease—a meta-analysis of epidemiologic studies. *N Engl J Med* 1999;340:920–926.

Hughes J R, Goldstein M G, Hurt R D, et al. Recent advances in the pharmacotherapy of smoking. *JAMA* 1999;281:72–76.

Hurt R D, Sachs D P L, Glover E D, et al. A comparison of sustained-release bupropion and placebo for smoking cessation. *N Engl J Med* 1997;337:1195–1202.

Prochaska J O, Goldstein M G. Process of smoking cessation: implications for clinicians. *Clin Chest Med* 1991;12:727–735.

Rigotti N A, Pasternak R C. Cigarette smoking and coronary heart disease: risks and management. *Cardiol Clin* 1996;14:51–68.

U.S. Department of Health and Human Services. The health benefits of smoking cessation: a report of the Surgeon General. Atlanta, GA: U.S. Department of Health and Human Services, Public Health Service, Centers for Disease Control and Prevention, Center for Chronic Disease Prevention and Health Promotion, Office on Smoking and Health, 1990. DHHS publication CDC 90-8416.

U.S. Public Health Service. A clinical practice guideline for treating tobacco use and dependence. *JAMA* 2000;283:3244–3254.

34
Red Eye
Erica Brownfield

1. What is the differential diagnosis of red eye? Which are common?
2. What are key elements of the history in a patient with red eye?
3. How does one examine a patient with red eye?
4. What warrants emergent/urgent referral to an ophthalmologist?
5. Are there causes of red eye a primary care physician can treat?

Discussion
What Is the Differential Diagnosis of Red Eye? Which Are Common?

Red eye is a common complaint in the outpatient setting. Although general internists are often not formally trained in ophthalmology, they should be able to diagnose common causes of red eye and recognize when referral to a specialist is indicated. The differential diagnosis of red eye is large, and will be classified based on eye anatomy.

Conjunctiva

- Conjunctivitis: inflammation of the conjunctiva; affected eye often stuck shut in the morning
  - Bacterial: usual pathogens include *Staphylococcus aureus, Streptococcus pneumoniae, Hemophilus influenzae,* and *Moraxella*; highly contagious; typically unilateral but can be bilateral; purulent discharge throughout the day
  - Viral: usual pathogen is adenovirus; highly contagious; watery, stringy discharge; clinical course parallels viral syndrome; patients have grittiness, burning, irritation
  - Allergic: bilateral usually; watery discharge, itchy eyes; patients may have a history of allergies
  - Nonspecific: usually secondary to transient mechanical or chemical insult
- Subconjunctival hemorrhage: extravasated blood (sharply demarcated area of injection resulting from rupture of small subconjunctival vessels); typically an episode of trauma, coughing, vomiting, straining
- Episcleritis: usually a benign inflammation of superficial episcleral vessels

Cornea

- Corneal abrasion: localized loss of epithelium from cornea; typically caused by a foreign body, finger nails, contact lens; patients can have sudden pain and foreign body sensation
- Foreign body
- Contact lens overwear
- Infectious keratitis: can be caused by bacteria, herpes simplex; perilimbal ciliary flush is characteristic

Uveal Tract

- Uveitis: inflammation of the uveal tract, including iris, ciliary body, choroid; typically patients have pain, photophobia, redness and ciliary flush
- Iritis: typically idiopathic but can be associated with systemic and ocular diseases (ankylosing spondylitis, sarcoidosis, juvenile rheumatoid arthritis, lupus, Behcet disease, tuberculosis); can also be secondary to trauma

Intraocular

Acute closure glaucoma is an ocular emergency that presents as a painful, red eye with prominent ciliary flush and a mid-dilated and fixed pupil.

Eyelid/Lashes

- Blepharitis: inflammation involving the structures of the lid margin; typically have scaling and crusting; many patients have associated seborrhea
- Hordeoleum (stye): acute staphylococcal infection of the meibomian glands or of the glands of Zeis or Moll around the lashes
- Chalazion: sterile granulomatous inflammation of the meibomian gland

What Are Key Elements of the History in a Patient with Red Eye?

In all patients with red eye, the following questions should be asked:

- *Is there pain?* A painful red eye is characteristic of acute closure glaucoma, uveitis/iritis, or corneal injury.
- *Is vision affected?* If vision is affected, one needs to consider acute closure glaucoma, uveitis/iritis, or corneal injury as possible causes of red eye.
- *Is there photophobia?* Photophobia is generally present in uveitis/iritis, corneal processes, infectious keratitis, and sometimes in glaucoma or viral conjunctivitis.
- *Is there a foreign body sensation?* Foreign body sensation is the cardinal symptom of an active corneal process. Occasionally patients with viral or allergic conjunctivitis can complain of foreign body sensation.
- *Is there discharge that continues throughout the day?* Bacterial conjunctivitis and keratitis present with a mucopurulent discharge; viral conjunctivitis can have a mucoid discharge.
- *Was there trauma?*

• *Does the patient wear contact lens?* Contact lens wearers are at higher risk for *Pseudomonas* infection.

How Does One Examine a Patient with Red Eye?
General Assessment

A lot can be learned by simply observing the patient. Is the patient wearing sunglasses or blocking the light from the eye (photophobia)? Does the patient have rhinorrhea or congestion (suggesting allergies or viral syndrome)? Does the patient have trouble keeping the eye open (suggesting corneal involvement)? Is the patient in obvious distress with malaise and headache (suggesting acute closure glaucoma)?

Measurement of Visual Acuity

Each eye should be tested separately. The standard is the Snellen acuity measured at 20 feet. However, it is appropriate to perform a crude estimate of visual acuity by having the patient hold a card or book at a comfortable distance and measure vision. It is helpful if patients can only distinguish light, forms, or large versus small print.

Penlight Examination

Is the pupil reactive to light? In acute closure glaucoma, the pupil is mid-dilated and fixed. *Is the pupil pinpoint?* Corneal abrasions, uveitis/iritis, and infectious keratitis contract the pupils. *Is there purulent discharge?* Purulent discharge suggests bacterial conjunctivitis or keratitis. *What is the pattern of redness?* If there is diffuse injection of the conjunctiva, think conjunctivitis. If injection is most marked at the limbus (ciliary flush), think of uveitis/iritis, infectious keratitis, or angle closure glaucoma. *Is there a white spot or opacity on the cornea?* Think infectious keratitis. *Is there hypopyon (layer of white cells in the anterior chamber)?* This is indicative of infectious keratitis. *Is there hyphema (layer of red cells in anterior chamber)?* This is indicative of significant blunt or penetrating trauma.

Fundus Examination

Examination of the fundus usually is not helpful in the evaluation of red eye.

Fluorescein Dye

Fluorescein dye is used to confirm a corneal process. Bacterial and herpes simplex keratitis pick up stain; foreign bodies do not pick up stain.

What Warrants Emergent/Urgent Referral to an Ophthalmologist?

In general, one should refer patients to an ophthalmologist if vision is affected, pupil is unreactive, there is objective foreign body sensation, photophobia or corneal opacity is present (Table 34.1).

Table 34.1.

Emergent (Same Day)	Urgent (1–2 Days)
Acute closure glaucoma	Uveitis/iritis
Hyphema	Viral keratitis
Hypopyon	Foreign body (if present after 1 day)
Bacterial keratitis	

Are There Causes of Red Eye That a Primary Care Physician Can Treat?

Some of the most common causes of red eye can be managed by a primary care physician. A general rule to remember: if you have any questions or concerns about patients, consult an ophthalmologist (Table 34.2).

Case

A 67-year-old man calls your office with 1 to 2 days of right eye pain. He states he has never had anything like this before, he has trouble reading, and the light bothers his eye. He thinks he may have gotten some particles in his eye while gardening, but he is not sure. His medical history includes sarcoidosis and coronary artery disease. His medications include aspirin, atenolol, lisinopril, vitamin E, and simvastatin. He wants to know if he should try to irrigate his eye or if he needs to make an appointment to see you.

1. What advice should you give to the patient over the phone?
2. What are the red flags in his history that prompt evaluation and referral?

Table 34.2. Common Causes of Red Eye and Treatment

Condition	Treatment
Bacterial conjunctivitis	First line: erythromycin ointment, sulfa drops
	Alternative: bacitracin, polysporin, fluoroquinolones
	Stop wearing contact lens until healed
	Throw out contact lens case
	Return to work/school once discharge gone or have received 24 hours of topical therapy
Viral conjunctivitis	Symptom relief: naphazoline
	Same return to work/school as above
Allergic conjunctivitis	Symptom relief: naphazoline
	Olopatadine
	Cromolyn ophthalmic
Subconjunctival hemorrhage	Self-limiting, reassurance
Corneal abrasion	Topical antibiotics can help prevent infections
	Eye patch that prevents lid motion for 1–2 days
	Avoid eye intensive activities (reading, TV)
	Short-acting cycloplegic agents
	Close daily follow up
Foreign bodies	Vigorous irrigation
	If not removed, can use cotton swab carefully
Blepharitis	Warm compresses
	Diluted Johnson's baby shampoo washes
Hordeolum	Warm compresses

3. The patient comes to your office; what is the appropriate evaluation?
4. What can you do to manage this patient?

Case Discussion

What Advice Should You Give to the Patient over the Phone?

This patient should be advised to seek medical attention. If he is unable to get to your office, he needs to go to the closest facility where a physician can evaluate his eye and determine the likely cause.

What Are the Red Flags in His History That Prompt Evaluation and Referral?

The patient complains of pain, photophobia, and visual disturbance. The last two are indications for referral to an ophthalmologist. Given the patient has a history of sarcoidosis, he is at risk for uveal tract disease. His age also places him at higher risk for glaucoma. Both should trigger concern in a physician talking to him over the phone. Finally, if the patient has a foreign body sensation, he needs to be referred to a specialist.

The Patient Comes to Your Office; What Is the Appropriate Evaluation?

You need to rule out uveal tract disease, glaucoma, and foreign body. Therefore, you need to inspect the eye to determine if ciliary flush is present, and perform a general assessment for photophobia, pain, and objective foreign body sensation. You need to perform a penlight examination and measure visual acuity.

On examination, the patient is in obvious distress, wearing sunglasses. He appears ill and complains of nausea. He has ciliary flush and has a mid-dilated fixed pupil. There is no obvious foreign body. Even though uveitis/iritis also involves a ciliary flush, you are convinced he has acute closure glaucoma with the general discomfort and unreactive pupil. The acute angle closure glaucoma could be secondary to sarcoidosis-induced uveitis/iritis.

What Can You Do to Manage This Patient?

This patient must be seen by an ophthalmologist today because he is at high risk for permanent vision loss. The specialist may ask you to initiate therapy upon his arrival and may recommend measures to decrease aqueous humor production and lower intraocular pressure (e.g., acetazolamide 500 mg orally or intravenously followed by 250 mg every four hours with or without topical β-adrenergic antagonists). Constriction of the pupil, which may improve the flow of aqueous humor, might be accomplished with topical pilocarpine 2% one drop every 5 minutes for the first 2 hours.

Suggested Reading

Beaty L, Herting R. Ophthalmology: the red eye. In: *University of Iowa family practice handbook*, 3rd ed, Chapter 12. Mosby, 1997. Also at: http://www.vh.org/provides/clinref/FPHandbook/FPContents.htm/.

Jacobs D. Evaluation of the red eye. *Up to Date* 2000;8.

Jacobs D. Conjunctivitis. *Up to Date* 2000;8.

Steinert R. Evaluation of the red eye. In: Goroll A, May A, Mulley A, eds. *Primary care medicine: office evaluation and management of the adult practice,* 3rd ed. J. P. Lippincott Company, Philadelphia, PA. 1995:956–960.

35

Insomnia

Jada Bussey-Jones

1. What are the prevalence and implications of insomnia?
2. What are the important historical and clinical features of insomnia?
3. What laboratory tests are available to evaluate insomnia?
4. What are the principles of behavioral therapy for insomnia treatment?
5. What are the available pharmacologic options and when should they be used?
6. How do you treat insomnia related to circadian rhythm disorders?

Discussion

What Are the Prevalence and Implications of Insomnia?

Insomnia, the complaint of unsatisfactory sleep quantity or quality, is a symptom rather than a disease. Traditionally, insomnia is divided into four categories: difficulty falling asleep, mid-sleep awakenings, early morning awakenings, and non-restorative sleep.

In the United States, approximately one third of adults report occasional difficulties with sleeping; about 10% report their sleep problems are chronic and serious. Insomnia complaints are about 1.3 times more common in women than in men. Also, patients over 65 years of age are 1.5 times more likely to complain about insomnia than are those under 65. There is also a higher prevalence of insomnia among persons of lower socioeconomic status, in divorced, widowed, or separated individuals, and in those with recent stress, depression, and drug or alcohol abuse.

The consequences of insomnia are varied. Although most people with insomnia complain about impairment in daytime function, mood, memory, or ability to concentrate, it is hard to objectively measure impairment. Insomniacs are more likely to drop out of difficult jobs and to receive fewer promotions. They often seek out ineffective and potentially harmful treatments such as over-the-counter (OTC) medications and alcohol (40% have tried OTC medications or alcohol for their insomnia). Roth et al. estimated the overall economic costs of insomnia in the United States to be about $35 billion. This includes direct cost of medical care as well as the costs to society (e.g., decreased work productivity).

What Are the Important Historical and Clinical Features of Insomnia?

The first step in the assessment of patients with sleep difficulty is a careful evaluation of the sleep history. This should include a careful review of sleep habits, drug and alcohol consumption, medical, psychiatric, and neurologic illness, and family history. Interviewing a bed partner (or caregiver) can complement the patient's subjective impressions and may provide additional information regarding drug or alcohol use and psychological stressors.

Sleep History

The patient should be questioned about the entire 24 hours rather than just the events at sleep onset or during the night. Key questions in the sleep history include the following:

- What is the chronology of the onset of insomnia? Sudden onset suggests life stressors or a change in sleep environment.
- Is the insomnia transient, intermittent, or persistent? Persistent insomnia may be related to a primary sleep disorder or medical, neurologic, or psychiatric disease.
- Do sleep difficulties involve initiation or maintenance of sleep? Sleep apnea rarely causes difficulty in initiating sleep.
- Is the patient preoccupied with bedtime rituals (suggesting psychophysiologic insomnia)?
- Do symptoms occur at sleep onset (e.g., paresthesias and uncontrollable limb movements of restless leg syndrome) or during sleep (e.g., repeated awakenings due to snoring, paroxysmal nocturnal dyspnea (PND), frequent urination, or apneic periods).
- Are there daytime symptoms (e.g., daytime fatigue, irritability, or lack of concentration)?

Medical problems that can impair sleep include chronic lung disease [chronic obstructive pulmonary disease (COPD)/asthma], heart disease (congestive heart failure, nocturnal angina), gastrointestinal illnesses (peptic ulcer disease and reflux esophagitis), allergies, neurodegenerative diseases, restless leg syndrome, and pain. A family history of insomnia may suggest certain primary sleep disorders. For example, a positive family history is found in about one third of patients with idiopathic restless leg syndrome.

The patient should be asked about use of alcohol, caffeine, tobacco, and other drugs that can directly cause insomnia:

- Alcohol. Alcohol may help in sleep onset but arouses patients after a few hours, and therefore should be avoided.
- Caffeine. Also a stimulant, as little as 150 mg of caffeine (the equivalent of one to two cups of coffee) has been shown to disturb the quality of sleep by increasing sleep latency and reducing sleep time.
- Nicotine. This may act as a stimulant and impair sleep.
- Central nervous system stimulants. These drugs have a profound impact on sleep quality and architecture. Pemoline, methylphenidate, and amphetamine all disturb sleep by increasing the latency to sleep onset and by increasing the wakeful-

ness during the sleep period. Many OTC decongestants contain ephedrine or pseudoephedrine, which are similar in chemical structure to the above stimulants. Although these agents have not been specifically studied, it is likely that they also disturb sleep.

- Theophylline. Methylxanthines disturb sleep quality in healthy normals by delaying sleep time and increasing wake time during the sleep period. In patients with COPD and asthma, however, the drug has no harmful effect. It is likely that the therapeutic effect of the drug on breathing counteracts any direct negative effect of the drug on sleep.
- Beta blockers. These medications have been associated with complaints of insomnia, hallucinations, and nightmares. Objective studies have shown that they increase the number of awakenings and the amount of wake time during the sleep period, and they suppress rapid eye movement (REM) sleep. These effects on sleep seem to be limited to lipophilic agents (e.g., propranolol and metoprolol). Hydrophilic agents, like atenolol and sotalol, do not appear to have similar effects.
- Corticosteroids. The effect of these medications on sleep has not been studied extensively. However, one early study observed disruption of sleep in healthy normal individuals.

Sleep Log

The sleep history is greatly facilitated when the patient keeps a log. A log kept for a 2-week period gives valuable information on sleep hygiene and patterns of sleep. The log should note when the patient tries to sleep, the duration and character of sleep, when the patient ends the night by getting out of bed, and the time of use of medications or substances that can affect sleep (e.g., caffeine). The patient should be encouraged to document time in bed engaging in nonsleep activities, sleeping aids used, and daytime functioning.

Physical Examination

The examination should be directed toward medical disorders (listed above) that may impact sleep.

What Laboratory Tests Are Available to Evaluate Insomnia?

Polysomnography

The indications for polysomnography (PSG) are somewhat controversial. Insomnia is primarily a clinical syndrome, and the American Sleep Disorders Association Standards of Practice Committee Guidelines do not suggest PSG in routine evaluations. It may be useful in the following situations:

- A sleep-related breathing disorder (sleep apnea) or periodic limb movement disorder is suspected.
- Insomnia has been present for more than 6 months, and medical, neurologic, and psychiatric causes have been excluded.
- Insomnia has not responded to behavioral or pharmacologic treatment.

Actigraphy

This is a recently developed technique that uses an activity monitor (a wristwatch-sized motion detector worn on the nondominant wrist) to record activities during sleep and waking. This is useful in circadian sleep disorders and is helpful in addition to sleep log.

Multiple Sleep Latency Test

This is helpful in documenting pathologic sleepiness.

Neuroimaging

This is rarely helpful in the diagnosis of sleep disorders, unless a specific neurologic deficit is found.

Other Laboratory Tests

A wide variety of tests may be helpful to evaluate medical conditions that may cause insomnia and should be guided by your history and physical examination. In patients suspected of having a psychiatric cause for insomnia, neuropsychiatric testing may be helpful.

What Are the Principles of Behavioral Therapy for Insomnia Treatment?

Sleep Hygiene

- Sleep only as much as you need to feel rested.
- Keep a regular sleep schedule.
- Avoid forcing sleep.
- Exercise regularly for at least 20 minutes, preferably 4 to 5 hours before bedtime.
- Avoid caffeinated beverages after lunch.
- Avoid alcohol near bedtime.
- Avoid smoking, especially in the evening.
- Do not go to bed hungry.
- Adjust bedroom environment.
- Deal with your worries before bedtime.
- Eliminate the bedroom clock—looking at the bedroom clock can cause arousal and frustration.

Relaxation

Many patients with insomnia seem to be hyperaroused and may respond to relaxation therapy. This involves progressive muscle relaxation and biofeedback to reduce somatic arousal. One small study of several different relaxation procedures found a 42% improvement in self-reported sleep after 1 year.

Stimulus Control Therapy

Stimulus control therapy may be beneficial in patients with chronic insomnia when the patients' expectations of poor sleep becomes a perpetuating factor itself. As night approaches, a mounting dread may become a self-fulfilling prophecy. The patient may additionally attempt to cope by sleeping late, taking daytime naps, staying in bed longer, going to bed earlier, taking caffeine to improve daytime performance, and drinking alcohol to induce sleep—all actions that perpetuate or exacerbate the problem.

Stimulus control therapy is based on the concept that sleep is under partial control of the stimuli that surround it. In a good sleeper, those stimuli (e.g., the bedroom environment) are associated with relaxation and encourage sleep. In poor sleepers, the same stimuli become associated with arousal or even anxiety. Bootzin's stimulus control therapy tries to change these associations.

The following six steps should be explained to the patient:

1. Lie down, intending to go to sleep only when you are sleepy.
2. Do not use your bed for anything except sleep. Sexual activity is the only exception. On such occasion, follow these instructions afterwards.
3. If you find yourself unable to sleep easily, get up and go to another room. Stay up as long as necessary and return to the bedroom only when you feel like you can fall asleep. The goal is to associate your bed with falling asleep quickly.
4. Repeat step 3 as often as necessary.
5. Set the alarm and get up at the same time every morning, no matter how you slept. That helps maintain circadian cycling.
6. No naps during the day.

Of all the behavioral techniques available today, the Bootzin technique is the best researched. In all studies comparing that therapy to any other behavioral treatment of insomnia, stimulus control has always been found either equal or superior to the other technique (reported to improve insomnia complaints in approximately 50% over 1 year). Behavioral therapy may be more time consuming than hypnotic agents in the short run, but over time they will be more cost effective than frequent visits and prescriptions.

Cognitive Therapies

Most patients have erroneous beliefs and attitudes about their sleep. Unless the beliefs are addressed, insomnia treatment is unlikely to be successful. Patients commonly attribute insomnia to their personal failings. Patients also may have unrealistic expectations, believing that they need 8 hours of sleep, or the more sleep they get, the healthier they will be. Patients also may have cognitive distortions (e.g., remembering only the bad nights, either sleep is excellent or awful).

Cognitive therapy attempts to restructure these faulty thoughts. The goal is to attempt to decatastrophize insomnia and replace the maladaptive thoughts with more functional ones. In a patient who used to think, "My insomnia will lead to a disaster tomorrow," direct him to think, "My insomnia is a miserable condition, but I know from past experience that I can get by tomorrow in spite of it." This type of counseling often requires expertise. Simply telling the patient that his thinking is wrong will lead nowhere.

Sleep Restriction Therapy

This therapy may improve sleep efficiency by restricting the total time in bed for sleep. First, examine the sleep logs and then restrict bedtime hours to the total hours of actual sleep reported on the logs (although never less than 4.5 hours in bed). The typical approach is to keep the wake-up time constant and to delay the time to bed (e.g., if a patient is allotted 5 hours of bed time and wakes at 7 A.M., bedtime would be no earlier than 2 A.M.). As sleep improves, the patient's time in bed can be increased by 15 to 30 minutes.

What Are the Available Pharmacologic Options and When Should They Be Used?

Whenever a specific cause for insomnia is found, that cause is treated first. When disease-specific treatments have already been used, but insomnia persists in some form, pharmacologic treatment may be considered.

Acute Insomnia

The goal is to determine the cause to prevent the acute insomnia from developing into a chronic insomnia. Once that cause is identified and addressed, hypnotic agents are the treatment of choice. Acute insomniacs are expected to sleep well again within a few days or weeks, making the question of drug tolerance, addiction, and withdrawal less important. Additionally, behavioral techniques often take weeks to become effective, making them less useful for acute insomnia.

Chronic Insomnia

The longer insomnia lasts, the more important behavioral therapies become. This is because the more chronic the insomnia, the more important the various learned perpetuating factors. Issues of drug tolerance and rebound also become more important, making sedatives less appropriate for chronic than acute insomnia.

Both nonpharmacologic and pharmacologic therapies may be useful in the management of idiopathic insomnia. One trial randomized 78 patients with idiopathic insomnia to treatment with cognitive-behavioral therapy, pharmacotherapy with temazepam, both interventions, or neither intervention. The three active treatment arms had better results than the placebo arm after 3 months of therapy, and there was a trend toward better outcomes with the use of combination of cognitive-behavioral and pharmacologic therapies. The use of behavioral therapy was associated with more sustained improvements in sleep over the 24-month period.

Benzodiazepines

The mechanism of action of benzodiazepines in facilitating sleep is unclear. They often produce subjective improvement in the quality and quantity of sleep rather than appreciable objective improvement in polysomnographic studies. The main concern when prescribing these agents is the development of tolerance and the possibility of rebound insomnia when the agent is withdrawn. The selection of a specific agent should be based primarily on the half-life. If sleep onset is the problem, agents with shorter half-lives (e.g., aprazolam and triazolam) should be prescribed. If mid-sleep awakenings are the issue, then intermediate-acting agents are preferred (e.g., temazepam, lorazepam). Drugs with longer elimination half-lives may induce prolonged daytime somnolence.

Newer Nonbenzodiazepine Hypnotic Agents

The first imidazopyridine used in the United States was zolpidem (Ambien), which has a mean elimination half-life of 2.5 hours. It is therefore a good choice for problems with sleep onset. Another agent that is soon to be released (Zaleplon) has an elimination half-life of 1 hour. This will be useful for sleep onset and mid-sleep awakenings. These agents act at the benzodiazepine receptor but differ in structure. These newer agents are less likely to produce tolerance or rebound when the drug is discontinued.

Antidepressants

Many antidepressant medications have sedative properties (e.g., amitriptyline, trazadone) because of central anticholinergic or antihistamine activities. These agents are most useful in the management of patients in whom depression and insomnia coexist. They are generally of limited use in nondepressed patients because tolerance to the sedative effects develops rapidly.

Antihistamines

Many OTC sleep aids contain sedating antihistamines such as diphenhydramine. These medications are generally not helpful in the management of chronic insomnia.

Melatonin

Melatonin is an indole-amine secreted by the pineal gland at night. It is clearly implicated in the regulation of the sleep/wake cycle. Data regarding the efficacy and safety of melatonin are minimal, but the hormone does not appear to be a potent hypnotic for most patients with chronic insomnia. Elderly patients with low melatonin levels have benefited from this therapy, as have individuals affected by jet lag.

How Do You Treat Insomnia Related to Circadian Rhythm Disorders?

Circadian rhythm disorders cause insomnia because of lack of synchronization between the individual's internal clock and the external schedule. Examples include individuals with delayed sleep phase syndrome (DSPS), who are "night owls" and have a life-long pattern of feeling at their best in the evening and their worst in the morning. They tend to wake later in the mornings and "sleep in" on the weekends to compensate. In contrast, many elderly individuals have advanced sleep phase syndrome (ASPS)—going to bed much earlier in the evening and waking at 2 or 3 A.M. The problem is not in the quality or quantity of sleep, but in the timing.

Chronotherapy

This refers to the intentional delay of sleep onset by 2 or 3 hours on successive days until the desired bedtime has been achieved. After this, the patient strictly enforces the sleep/wake schedule. One study showed a high success rate, but there is a tendency to return to the original sleep habits after a period of time.

Phototherapy

Exposure to bright light on awakening is effective in altering sleep onset and synchronizing body temperature rhythm in patients with DSPS. The patient sits in front of 10,000 lux light for 30 minutes upon awakening; in addition, room lighting should be markedly reduced in the evening. Response generally requires 2 weeks. Many patients frequently require indefinite treatment to maintain synchronization. In patients with ASPS, bright light exposure in the evening has been successful in delaying sleep onset.

Case

A 42-year-old female accountant complains of difficulty falling asleep, frequent nocturnal awakenings, and daytime lethargy. These problems followed a miscarriage 1 year ago. She denies depressed mood but does admit to intrusive thoughts at night when attempting to fall asleep. Additionally, she has used OTC diphenhydramine and alcohol to "help her sleep." She attempts to cope during the day by drinking three to four cups of coffee, taking naps, and sleeping late on the weekends to "catch up."

Her medical history includes hypertension, asthma, and obesity. In addition to alcohol use, she smokes one pack of cigarettes daily but denies recreational drug use. She takes albuterol, theophylline, propranolol, and recently completed a course of prednisone.

On physical examination her blood pressure is 140/74 mm Hg and her weight is 202 pounds. The remainder of her examination is within normal limits.

1. What is the likely precipitating event that initiated this patient's insomnia?
2. What are factors that may have perpetuated or contributed to her sleeping difficulty?
3. What treatment options would you pursue?

Case Discussion

What Is the Likely Precipitating Event That Initiated This Patient's Insomnia?

You should be concerned about depression or other psychiatric disorders as the initiating problem for insomnia in this patient.

What Are the Factors That May Have Perpetuated or Contributed to Her Sleeping Difficulty?

In many cases of chronic insomnia, the impact of the precipitating factor has resolved, and the sleep disturbance has taken on a life of its own. She has several factors that could have perpetuated her insomnia (poor sleep hygiene). Her daily medications (β blockers and albuterol) could be contributing. Corticosteroids and theophylline are less likely to be significant factors. Her comorbid conditions may play a role, and nocturnal asthma or central sleep apnea should be considered.

What Treatment Options Would You Pursue?

Treatment of this patient will require a team approach (you and the patient) that will be long term. Sedative medications are unlikely to be useful in this case. Review sleep hygiene; limiting time in bed, alcohol, tobacco, and caffeine should be attempted first. The patient should be instructed to keep a sleep log and her progress followed closely. Psychotherapy may be indicated.

Suggested Reading

Gillin J C, Byerle W F. The diagnosis and management of insomnia. *N Engl J Med* 1990;332:239–248.

Kupfer D J, Reynolds C F III. Management of insomnia. *N Engl J Med* 1997;336:341.

Morin C M, Stone J, Trinkle D, et al. Nonpharmacological interventions for insomnia: a meta-analysis of treatment efficacy. *Am J Psychiatry* 1994;151:1172–1180.

Roberts J E, Reme C E, Dillon J, et al. Exposure to bright light and the concurrent use of photosensitizing drugs. *N Engl J Med* 1992;326:1500–1501.

Spielman A J, Nunes J, Glovinsky P B. Sleep disorders I. *Neurol Clin* 1996;14:3.

36
Herbal Supplements

Naveen V. Narahari
Laura J. Martin

1. Why are herbal supplements important?
2. What are herbal supplements?
3. Are there guidelines involving the definition and uses of herbal supplements?
4. What information do clinical trials provide concerning St. John's wort, saw palmetto, ginseng, and ginkgo biloba?
5. What are some other important herbal supplements in the outpatient setting?

Discussion
Why Are Herbal Supplements Important?

The use of herbal medications transcend time and culture. They influence the delivery of health care regardless of the impact of Western medicine. Although rationale is not necessary, we should point to ethnocentric medicine, historical use, prescription cost, and failure of the conventional health paradigm as reasons for the most recent surge in the use of alternative medicine. Recent inquiry into this subject by Eisenberg shows that the prevalence of herbal supplement use has increased 25% from 1990, with approximately 15 million adults spending nearly $27 billion on herbal supplements in 1997. Indeed, with no gender, income, or age predilection, and with one in five, patients taking prescription medication also using herbal supplements, it becomes increasingly important to understand the role of herbals in the health-care setting.

What Are Herbal Supplements?

Many of the medications that we use today are derived from plant matter. Companies either use an ethnobotanical approach utilizing local shamans, healers, and botanists, or random analysis en masse of plants to isolate medicinal compounds. Pharmaceutical companies are held to stringent standards in product isolation, testing, and production. These standards are not applied to the companies marketing herbal medicines and supplements. Subsequently, there are many herbal "cures" that have been propagated.

Are There Guidelines Involving the Definition and Uses of Herbal Supplements?

The World Health Organization (WHO) published a definition of herbal supplements in 1991. A prerequisite for classifying an herb as a supplement is a documented history of years of use of the herb for a specific medical disorder, with particular reference to countries where the herb has a long track record of use. The WHO also requires submission of toxicity and abuse data. More recently, the German E monographs have assumed the role of assessing herbal medications. The German Commission, established in 1978 by the German government, has reviewed the use of popular phytomedications by using information based on human clinical trials, commercial information, and historical/traditional use information. Modern criticisms of the German E monographs include lack of information regarding botanical constituents, pharmacology, standards of isolation, or citations of primary sources of information. Additionally, many herbs were thought to have been ushered into the monographs with "grandfather clauses" or commercial bias. The text, however, attempts to stratify herbal medicines with information on botanical properties when available, and subsequent clinical data. Recent English translation by the American Botanical Society will further promote debate regarding the use of this classification system.

In the United States, the 103rd Congress passed the Dietary Supplement Health and Education Act in 1994. This legislation dictated that the U.S. Food and Drug Administration (FDA) could not regulate dietary supplements as food additives or pharmacologic drugs. Physicians are therefore asked to give counsel with limited information and quality assurance. However, much more investment in research dollars is presently being allocated by Congress to the National Center for Complementary and Alternative Medicine (established 1994) to study these issues.

What Information Do Clinical Trials Provide Concerning St. John's Wort, Saw Palmetto, Ginseng, and Ginkgo Biloba?

The following passages are meant to highlight a few of the most popular herbal medications. When possible both pharmacological and clinical data is supplied.

St. John's Wort (Hypericum perforatum)

The active ingredient in St. John's wort is hypericin. Its mechanism of action is via serotonin reuptake inhibition. It has additionally been shown to have mild monoamine oxidase inhibition. The half-life of hypericin is 24 to 48 hours.

Primary use for St. John's wort has been for symptoms of mild depression. It is prescribed four times as often as prescription antidepressants in Germany. There are no absolute contraindications other than allergy. However, it should not be dosed along with other selective serotonin reuptake inhibitors because of the risk of developing a serotonergic syndrome. This syndrome results from excess central nervous syndrome serotonin levels and can cause agitation, confusion, hyperreflexia, autonomic instability, fever, and tremor. It is also recommended to avoid concomitant use of monoamine oxidase inhibitors. Another major side effect, seen in fair-skinned people, is a photosensitivity reaction consisting of a rash with raised erythematous, pruritic skin lesions. Clinicians also should be aware of the possible side effect of a neuropathy secondary to demyelination induced by sun exposure. Minor side effects include dry mouth and mild dizziness.

Randomized controlled studies have shown *Hypericum perforatum* to be efficacious in treating mild depression. A meta-analysis of 23 randomized studies was published in the *British Medical Journal* in 1996. The meta-analysis included 1,757 outpatients with depression. Fifteen studies were placebo controlled, whereas eight studies compared *Hypericum* with another antidepressant medication. The majority of trials included were 4 to 8 weeks in duration. Results showed *Hypericum* to be significantly superior to placebo and equally effective as the antidepressant medications studied. Side effects were noted to occur in 19.8% of patients on *Hypericum* and in 52.8% of patients on standard antidepressants.

Saw Palmetto (Serenoa repens)

The active ingredients in saw palmetto are sitosterols. The sitosterols inhibit testosterone 5α-reductase in high concentrations. Saw palmetto is thought to work in a similar manner as finasteride in decreasing prostate size.

An isolate of the ripe berries of the saw palmetto dwarf palm tree, the primary use of sitosterols have been for the treatment of symptoms related to benign prostatic hypertrophy. The side effect profile includes headache, gastrointestinal upset, hypertension, and impotence. However, reports of these complaints are uncommon. It is contraindicated in patients who develop an allergic reaction. There are no noted drug–herb interactions.

Eighteen randomized controlled trials involving 2,939 men were reviewed in the *Journal of the American Medical Association* in 1998. The average study duration was 9 weeks, with a range of 4 to 48 weeks. Men receiving *Serenoa repens* had a significant reduction of urinary tract symptom scores and improvement in nocturia and peak urine flow scores as compared with placebo. In comparison with the finasteride group, men taking *Serenoa repens* had similar improvement in urinary symptom scores and peak urine flow. Erectile dysfunction was more frequent with finasteride (4.9%) than with *Serenoa repens* (1.1%).

Ginseng (Panax ginseng, Panax quinquefolius, Elentherococcus senticosus)

The active ingredients in ginseng are ginsenosides (triterpene saponins) and panaxans. Panaxans (glycans) have been found to have hypoglycemic effects in mice. It is hypothesized that the active ingredients affect an increase in adrenal steroid genesis by the pituitary gland and produce immunostimulatory effects. It is also thought to have estrogenic effects.

Ginseng is used widely around the world. Of the forms mentioned above, *Panax ginseng* is found in China and Korea, whereas the quinquefolius variant is found in the United States. The last species, *Elentherococcus senticosus,* found in Siberia, is not truly ginseng, although it possesses the same active ingredients. Ginseng has been used to increase the body's ability to fight off toxins and provide normal body function in times of stress. Other uses include blood glucose control in diabetics, treatment of fatigue, and postmenopausal symptom management. Potential side effects include insomnia, headache, and increased blood pressure. There have been cases described of uterine bleeding secondary to estrogenic effects. Contraindications include allergy and pregnancy. Caution is urged in using ginseng alone to treat diabetes. A drug–herb interaction has been noted with anticoagulation therapy, resulting in an increased international normalized ratio (INR) secondary to herbal antiplatelet activity. There has been at least one reported interaction with phenelzine. Ginseng supplements can be taken as raw root, tea, wine mixture, or tablet.

A double-blind placebo-controlled study was published in *Diabetes Care* in 1995 involving 36 type II diabetics who were treated for 8 weeks with ginseng or placebo. A 200-mg dose of ginseng was found to improve Hgb A1C and reduce fasting blood sugar, while placebo did not alter fasting blood glucose. The ginseng therapy also was found to elevate mood. A review of 16 trials on the health claims of ginseng was published in the *European Journal of Clinical Pharmacology* in 1999. This review concluded, based on the data reviewed, that the efficacy of ginseng root extract in producing immunostimulatory effects, improvement in blood sugar in type II diabetes mellitus, and improvement in cognitive function could not be established beyond reasonable doubt. More rigorous investigations to assess efficacy and safety were considered warranted given ginseng's widespread use around the world.

Ginkgo biloba

The active ingredients in *Ginkgo biloba* are ginkosides (flavonoids, terpenoids, organic acids). These active ingredients are thought to be free-radical scavengers and therefore may prevent cell damage. They are also thought to have less defined circulatory effects.

Common uses are for limiting and reversing cognitive decline as in Alzheimer dementia. *Ginkgo biloba* is approved in Germany for treatment of dementia. *Ginkgo* is thought to improve cerebral and peripheral circulation. This herb is also used for sexual dysfunction. Its side effect profile includes mild gastrointestinal upset and headache. There are four reports of spontaneous bleeding events in patients. Contraindications include concurrent anticoagulation therapy and allergy. Caution should be given for increased risk of bleeding if taken with salicylates.

A meta-analysis of eight placebo-controlled trials published in *Lancet* in 1992 suggests efficacy for cerebral insufficiency. Patient symptoms that were monitored included memory changes, dizziness, tinnitus, headache, and emotional instability with anxiety. A randomized controlled trial published in the *Journal of the American Medical Association* in 1997 looked at an extract of *Ginkgo biloba* (Egb 761) in the treatment of dementia. Outpatients (n = 202) were randomized to the *Ginkgo* extract or placebo over a 52-week period. The population was diverse with regard to the extent of dementia and etiology (Alzheimer versus multiinfarct dementia). The mean age was 69 years, and results of the Mini-Mental Status examination ranged from 9 to 26. Objective evaluation with the Alzheimer's Disease Assessment Scale–Cognitive subscale (ADAS-Cog) score revealed a 1.4-point improvement with patients taking *Ginkgo*. Geriatric Evaluation by Relative's Rating Instrument (GERRI) showed a 0.14-point improvement compared with the placebo group. An overall trend suggested improvement in attention and overall function with *Ginkgo* extract.

Evidence for improvement of sexual dysfunction comes from an open-label trial of 37 patients with drug-induced sexual dysfunction. Over a 4-week period of administration, 86% of the sample reported improvement. *Gingko* also has been used for impotence secondary to arterial insufficiency, but no controlled trials have been conducted to date.

What Are Some Other Important Herbal Supplements in the Outpatient Setting?

Echinacea purpurea

Echinacea purpurea is thought to have immunostimulatory effects on a short-term basis. It is used in the treatment and prevention of upper respiratory infections. Side effects are noted to include rash, pruritus, and dizziness. Long-term effects on the immune system are not known. There is a question of hepatotoxicity with long-term use. It is contraindicated with allergy. There are no reported drug–herb interactions. It is dosed orally with 300 to 400 mg of dried extract three times daily or 2 to 3 mL of tincture three times daily. There is inconclusive evidence at this time regarding efficacy of *Echinacea* supplements.

Kava Kava (Piper methysticum)

Kava kava is thought to have sedative effects. It is used for anxiety and as a muscle relaxant. Significant side effects include extrapyramidal effects and reported kava dermopathy (South Pacific) involving papules/plaques and subsequent sebaceous gland destruction. A drug–herb interaction has been reported with anticonvulsant medications, resulting in an increased sedative effect. There also have been reports of prolonged anesthetic effect after surgery and with concomitant use of benzodiazepines. It is taken orally in the form of suspension, tincture, or tablets. Most evidence is anecdotal with respect to the overall efficacy and safety of kava extract.

Feverfew (Tanacetum parthenium, Chrysanthemum parthenium)

Feverfew is thought to inhibit prostaglandin synthesis. It is used for migraine prophylaxis, insect repellent, as an antipruritic agent, and for its antiinflammatory properties for arthritis. Side effects include mouth ulcers if the leaves are taken raw. Concurrent use of anticoagulant medication has resulted in supertherapeutic INRs in patients. Dosage varies because the herb may be applied to skin as a paste, taken as fresh leaves in food, or as a drink infusion.

Ginger (Zingiber officinale)

Ginger is known for its antiemetic properties. It is used to treat nausea. It may prolong bleeding time and should be avoided in individuals on anticoagulation medication. It is dosed orally by tablet or tea.

Valerian (Valeriana officinalis)

Valerian is considered to have sedative properties. It is used for the treatment of insomnia and anxiety. Potential side effects include fatigue, tremor, headache, and paradoxic insomnia. It is not advisable to be taken with other hypnotics (barbiturates and benzodiazepines). It can be taken orally as a tablet (400 mg) at night or as tea. There is inconclusive evidence regarding the efficacy of valerian.

Garlic (Allium sativum)

The active ingredient in garlic is allicin. For further discussion on the use of garlic for medicinal purposes, the reader is referred to Chapter 10.

Ephedra (Ma Huang)

The active ingredients in ephedra are ephedrine-containing alkaloids. A common ingredient in herbal phen-fen, this herb has been used for natural weight loss in combination with St. John's wort. It is also used for heightened sexual awareness as "herbal ecstasy" and as treatment for asthma. Nearly 800 adverse reactions have been reported. These side effects range from insomnia, nervousness, and tremor to tachycardia, hypertension, myocardial infarction, stroke, and death. Seizures have also been observed with use. The FDA presently suggests dosage limitation to less than 24 mg/day. However, effects have been seen even at 1- to 5-mg doses. Patients with neurologic, cardiovascular, or endocrine comorbidities should be counseled against use. Administration with other pseudoephedrine-containing compounds is also discouraged.

Case

A 60-year-old woman presents to your office for routine follow-up for her hypertension, atrial fibrillation, and mild depression. She has complaints of insomnia, poor appetite, fatigue, and trouble concentrating. She relates no suicidal ideation. You prescribed sertraline 50 mg a day at her last visit four weeks ago. She also takes a thiazide diuretic for hypertension. She has been therapeutic on her coumadin (INR 2.2) for her atrial fibrillation. At this visit she adds that she has a sensation of cotton mouth and occasional dizziness. She has checked her blood pressure and it has been normal. On further questioning, she admits to, on the advise of her neighbor, taking St. John's wort along with the sertraline. On examination, this fair-skinned woman has a blood pressure of 130/85 mm Hg and pulse of 75 beats/min. She has clear lungs fields and irregularly irregular heart sounds. There is no peripheral edema. Neurologic exam is nonfocal. Laboratory results show a normal complete blood count, and normal creatinine and sodium measurements.

1. What is the drug interaction in this case?
2. Does the patient need to know any other effects of St. John's wort?
3. Which medication should she take?
4. Does she need counseling on other herbal medications?

Discussion

What Is the Drug Interaction in This Case?

When serotonin reuptake inhibitors are started, patients should be informed that it usually takes 4 to 6 weeks to experience full therapeutic effects. In this case, the patient chose to start taking St. John's wort to "supplement" the sertraline given by her physician. The dry mouth and dizziness are probably related to a syndrome of serotonergic excess resulting from the combination of sertraline and St. John's wort. Although mild at this presentation, more severe forms with confusion can occur.

Does the Patient Need to Know Any Other Effects of St. John's Wort?

It was remarked that the patient was quite fair skinned. As such, if it were opted to continue the St. John's wort instead of the sertraline, she would need to protect herself from the phototoxic effects of the herbal supplement with sunscreen and protective clothing.

Which Medication Should She Take?

This decision will need to be mutual between the patient and the physician. Of course, severity of depression is a major factor in choosing between the antidepressants. The patient's attempt to "supplement" her antidepressant might indicate that her symptoms are limiting. However, if the symptoms do not affect overall function and she wishes a "natural" remedy, then she could choose to discontinue the sertraline. Her depression should continue to be reassessed at 4- to 6-week intervals.

Does She Need Counseling on Other Herbal Medications?

In this case the physician appropriately continued questioning to include alternative and complementary therapies, which in this case led to the diagnosis. She has already shown that she is willing to try herbal supplements. As such she should be cautioned to avoid those supplements that have been shown to interact with anticoagulation therapy. Additionally, she should be encouraged to bring any medication, prescribed or otherwise, for review with her physician.

Suggested Reading

Blumenthal M, Busse W R, et al., eds. *The complete German commission E monographs: therapeutic guide to herbal medicines,* 1st ed. Austin, TX: American Botanical Council; Boston: Integrative Medicine Communications, 1998.

Eisenberg D M, et al. Trends in alternative medicine use in the United States: results of a follow up national survey. *JAMA* 1998;280:1569–1575.

Kleijnen J, Knipschild P. Ginkgo biloba. *Lancet* 1992;340:1136–1139.

LeBars P L, Katz M M, Berman N, et al. A placebo-controlled double-blinded, randomized trial of an extract of *Ginkgo biloba* for dementia. *JAMA* 1997;278:1827–1832.

Linde K, Ramirez G, et al. St. John's wort for depression—an overview and meta-analysis of randomized clinical trials. *BMJ* 1996;313:253–258.

Mar C, Bent S. An evidence-based review of the 10 most commonly used herbs. *West J Med* 1999;171:168–171.

Miller L G. Herbal medicinals. Selected clinical considerations focusing on known or potential drug–herb interaction. *Arch Intern Med* 1998;158:2200–2211.

Planta M. Prevalence of the use of herbal products in a low-income population. *Fam Med* 2000; 32:252–257.

Wilt T J, Ishani A, et al. Saw palmetto extracts for treatment of benign prostatic hyperplasia. *JAMA* 1998;280:1604–1609.

37

Using Cost-Effectiveness Evaluations in Primary Care

Kimberly Rask

1. What are cost-effectiveness evaluations and why are they relevant to primary care practitioners?
2. What costs should be measured?
3. What kinds of interventions are cost-effective?

Discussion

What Are Cost-Effectiveness Evaluations and Why Are They Relevant to Primary Care Practitioners?

Clinicians make many decisions about the care of individual patients but can also be asked to participate in decisions for large groups of patients, for example, whether or not to add a new medication to the hospital formulary. When making decisions for groups of patients, clinicians need to weigh the benefits and risks of treatment and assess whether or not these benefits will be worth the health-care resources (or costs) required. Cost-effectiveness analysis (CEA) compares the costs and outcomes of alternative treatments. CEAs evaluate a health intervention by asking, "How much health benefit do we get for our money?"

Cost effectiveness is expressed as a ratio, where the numerator quantifies the cost and the denominator quantifies the health outcome, for example, dollars per year of life saved. Costs are usually measured in dollars, whereas health benefits can be measured in many different ways. Cost effectiveness is the difference in cost between two interventions divided by the difference in health benefit that is gained.

$$\text{Cost effectiveness of treatment A relative to treatment B} = \frac{(\text{costs of treatment A} - \text{costs of treatment B})}{(\text{health benefit of treatment A} - \text{health benefit of treatment B})}$$

What Costs Should Be Measured?

It is important to include all costs and benefits relevant to the clinical question. Patients may be responsible for a sizable proportion of their health-care bills. High

Table 37.1. Examples of Costs that Are Commonly Measured

Direct Medical	Direct Nonmedical	Productivity
Physician visits	Caregiver costs	Work loss
Medications	Transportation	
Hospitalizations		

patient costs are likely to discourage compliance and decrease treatment effectiveness.

Most published CEAs will account for direct medical and nonmedical costs. These include the costs such as physician's time, nursing time, and medications. Future costs that are directly attributable to the treatment also must be included. For example, studies evaluating the cost effectiveness of tissue type plasminogen activator (t-PA) in the treatment of acute myocardial infarction must include the increased risk of hemorrhagic strokes associated with t-PA (Table 37.1).

What Kinds of Interventions Are Cost Effective?

Because cost effectiveness is a ratio of costs balanced against health outcomes, interventions that have low costs or interventions with high health benefits will generally be more cost effective. Interventions are also likely to be more cost effective if they (a) prevent a common condition that is otherwise costly to treat, (b) have a positive impact quickly, and (c) do not need to be readministered frequently.

There is no value or threshold that defines a treatment as absolutely cost effective. Instead, cost-effectiveness ratios can be used to compare different interventions (Table 37.2). A reasonable rule of thumb is that interventions that cost $50,000 or less per quality-adjusted life year (QALY) are generally considered cost effective, and those that cost more than $100,000 per QALY are not. Whether interventions costing between $50,000 and $100,000 per QALY are considered cost effective is debated.

Case

You practice in a publicly funded clinic serving predominantly low-income and uninsured patients. As part of a quality improvement project for the clinic, you were asked to review the management of hyperlipidemic patients. You find that few hyperlipidemic patients are on lipid-lowering therapy and even fewer are at target

Table 37.2. Examples of Cost per QALY for Different Medical Interventions ($ for 1991)

CABG for left main disease	$8,100
CABG for two vessel disease	$37,400
HCTZ for hypertension	$24,900
Mammogram over age 50	$50,000
Mammogram under age 50	$220,400
Hip replacement for osteoarthritis	$8,700
Pneumovax	$6,100

QALY, quality-adjusted life year; CABG, coronary artery bypass graft; HCTZ, hydrochlorthiazide.

low-density lipoprotein levels according to National Cholesterol Education Program guidelines.

The clinic does provide some medications to patients at a reduced price. However, the clinic receives a fixed pharmacy budget each year, and based on that budget, a formulary committee selects which medications to provide to patients and at what cost. In preliminary discussions, you find that the pharmacy budget will preclude offering subsidized medications to all hyperlipidemic patients. The formulary committee asks whether there are subgroups of patients who would most benefit from lipid-lowering therapy and how can they use their limited budget to offer the maximum health benefit to the patients that they serve.

In a literature search you find two articles that evaluate the relative cost effectiveness of lipid-lowering therapies based on patient characteristics. One study reviews the clinical efficacy of statins and the potential health benefits of targeting selected patient populations. The authors identified the elderly, diabetic patients and patients with left ventricular hypertrophy as groups with the highest absolute risk for coronary heart disease (CHD).

The second study performed economic simulations based on published data from clinical trials. The efficacy of dietary counseling and statin drugs were evaluated for both primary and secondary prevention. Intervention costs included the costs of medications, physician visits, and patient travel. Medication costs were calculated by using the average wholesale prices of pravastatin and simvastatin. The cost effectiveness of dietary and statin therapy was evaluated by gender, age, smoking status, high-density lipoprotein level, and diastolic blood pressure. Selected cost-effectiveness ratios are shown in Table 37.3. For example, the cost effectiveness of treating hypertensive women between the ages of 55–64 with statin therapy is $120,000 per QALY. Treating the same group of women with diet therapy is less costly, only $20,000 per QALY.

Table 37.3. Primary Prevention with Statin if LDL >160, Nonsmoker, Normotensive ($ per QALY)

Age (yr)	35–44	55–64	75–84
Men	$390,000	$170,000	$180,000
Women	$960,000	$220,000	$180,000

Primary Prevention with Statin if LDL >190, Smoker, Hypertensive ($ per QALY)

Age (yr)	35–44	55–64	75–84
Men	$54,000	$59,000	$66,000
Women	$190,000	$120,000	$62,000

Primary Prevention with Diet if LDL >190, Smoker, Hypertensive ($ per QALY)

Age (yr)	35–44	55–64	75–84
Men	$6,700	$9,500	$1,900
Women	$46,000	$20,000	$8,200

Secondary Prevention with Simvastatin ($ per QALY)

Age (yr)	35–44	55–64	75–84
Men	$4,500	$3,900	$9,900
Women	$40,000	$8,400	$11,000

QALY, quality-adjusted life year.

1. How can the cost-effectiveness evaluations help target drug therapy for your patients?
2. What special considerations affect the applicability of these findings to your patient population?

Case Discussion

How Can the Cost-Effectiveness Evaluations Help Target Drug Therapy for Your Patients?

In a low-risk population, a preventive intervention will be cost effective only if it is very inexpensive (Table 37.3). Compare the first part of the table (low risk) with the second part (high risk) and the second part (statin) with the third part (diet). The cost effectiveness of lipid treatment is markedly affected by (a) patient characteristics (the lipid profile and other risk factors) and (b) treatment costs (statin vs. diet). Table 37.3 shows that statins generally became more cost effective as the number of risk factors increased. Based on the cost-effectiveness ratios, statin therapy for secondary prevention should be a high priority, regardless of patient age or gender.

Based on these findings, you recommend that the clinic make subsidized statin prescriptions available to patients with known CHD. You could also recommend emphasizing smoking cessation, hypertension control, and dietary counseling while reserving statin therapy for primary prevention in patients with multiple risk factors who remain hyperlipidemic.

What Special Considerations Affect the Applicability of These Findings to Your Patient Population?

Out-of-pocket costs of treatment may be prohibitive for your patients even if treatment is cost effective from a societal perspective. Other strategies to minimize patient out-of-pocket costs include promoting healthy diets, exercise, and smoking cessation. Maximize statin effectiveness by promoting compliance. The clinic also might consider other lipid-lowering agents (e.g., niacin) that are less expensive but also may be poorly tolerated.

A chart review can be used to identify what proportion of clinic patients fall into the higher risk groups, allowing an estimate of the financial impact to the clinic of subsidizing treatment for those groups. The investigators reported that drug costs represent approximately 90% of the costs associated with primary prevention with a statin. The clinic might pursue volume purchases of a single brand and negotiate price discounts. The ability to obtain free medications through pharmaceutically sponsored programs for indigent patients might change your treatment recommendations.

Suggested Reading

Drummond M F, Richardson W S, O'Brien B J, et al., for the Evidence-Based Medicine Working Group. Users' guides to the medical literature. XIII: How to use an article on economic analysis of clinical practice. A: Are the results of the study valid? *JAMA* 1997;277:1552–1557.

Jacobson T A, Schein J R, Williamson A, et al. Maximizing the cost-effectiveness of lipid-lowering therapy. *Arch Intern Med* 1998;158:1977–1989.

O'Brien B J, Heyland D, Richardson W S, et al., for the Evidence-Based Medicine Working Group. Users' guides to the medical literature. XIII: How to use an article on economic analysis of clinical practice. B: What are the results and will they help me in caring for my patients? *JAMA* 1997;277:1802–1806.

Prosser L A, Stinnett A A, Goldman P A, et al. Cost-effectiveness of cholesterol lowering therapies according to selected patient characteristics. *Ann Intern Med* 2000;132:769–779.

38

Laboratory Toxicity Monitoring of Chronic Medications

Lisa M. Woolard
Timothy A. Briscoe
Clyde Watkins, Jr.

1. What is the appropriate laboratory toxicity monitoring for commonly prescribed cardiovascular agents?
2. What is the appropriate laboratory toxicity monitoring for commonly prescribed hyperlipidemic agents?
3. What is the appropriate laboratory toxicity monitoring for commonly prescribed endocrine agents?
4. What is the appropriate laboratory toxicity monitoring for commonly prescribed central nervous system agents?
5. When should plasma level monitoring of commonly prescribed medications be obtained?

Discussion

What Is the Appropriate Laboratory Monitoring for Commonly Prescribed Cardiovascular Agents?

Table 38.1 lists the recommended monitoring parameters for selected cardiovascular medications.

Amiodarone

Perform baseline and periodic liver function tests (LFTs) secondary to potential for liver dysfunction. Because amiodarone can inhibit the conversion of thyroxine (T_4) to triiodothyronine and is a potential source of iodine, amiodarone can cause hypo- or hyperthyroidism. Monitor thyroid function tests (TFTs) at baseline and periodically thereafter, particularly in the elderly and patients with existing thyroid dysfunction. In addition, antiarrhythmics such as amiodarone may be ineffective or

Table 38.1. Laboratory Toxicity Monitoring for Commonly Prescribed Cardiovascular Agents

Medication	Toxicity	Monitoring
Amiodarone	Liver dysfunction, hypo- or hyperthyroidism, arrhythmias in hypokalemia	Baseline and periodic LFTs, TFTs, and potassium
ACE inhibitors/ARBs	Hypotension, renal insufficiency, hyperkalemia	Na^+, K^+, Scr, BUN within 1 wk of initiation or increase in stable dose and every 3–6 mo thereafter
Diuretics	Electrolyte deficiencies	Na^+, Cl^-, K^+, Mg^{2+}, Scr, BUN, and HCO_3 within 1–2 wk of initiation and periodically based on history and concurrent medications
Hydralazine	Lupus syndrome	Baseline CBC and ANA titers. Positive ANA titers on follow-up may not predict lupus. Discontinue if symptoms occur.
Methyldopa	Hemolytic anemia, hepatitis	Coomb test and CBC at baseline, 6 and 12 mo. LFTs at baseline, 1 and 3 mo.
Quinidine	Blood dyscrasias, hepatoxicity, toxicity in hypokalemia	Baseline liver LFTs and repeat in the first 4 to 8 wk of therapy. Obtain baseline and periodic blood counts and potassium levels.

LFT, liver function test; TFT, thyroid function test; ACE inhibitor, angiotensin-converting enzyme inhibitor; ARB, angiotensin receptor blocker; Scr, serum creatinine; BUN, blood urea nitrogen; CBC, complete blood count; ANA, antinuclear antibody; D/C,   .

arrhythmogenic in the presence of hypokalemia. Monitor serum potassium and magnesium at baseline and periodically, particularly in patients taking agents that affect electrolyte balance (e.g., diuretics, glucocorticoids, etc.).

Angiotensin-Converting Enzyme Inhibitors and Angiotensin Receptor Blockers

Angiotensin-converting enzyme (ACE) inhibitors and angiotensin receptor blockers (ARBs) can cause significant hypotension and renal insufficiency in sodium-depleted or volume-depleted patients. Renal insufficiency may develop in the presence of bilateral renal artery stenosis. In addition, these agents can cause an increase in serum potassium levels secondary to their effects on the aldosterone system. A serum chemistry that includes sodium (Na^+), potassium (K^+), serum creatinine (Scr), and blood urea nitrogen (BUN) should be performed at baseline. The serum chemistry should be repeated within 1 week. If stable, the serum chemistry should be repeated periodically (i.e., every 3–6 months) or within 1 week of an increase in dose of the ACE inhibitor/ARB or diuretic (if used concomitantly). Particular care is warranted in patients with existing renal insufficiency and congestive heart failure (CHF). It may be prudent to monitor these patients more closely.

Diuretics

Significant electrolyte deficiencies may occur with the use of diuretics. Obtain baseline Na^+, Cl^-, K^+, Mg^{2+}, Scr, BUN, and HCO_3. Laboratory studies should be repeated within 1 to 2 weeks after initiating diuretic therapy. If stable, the recommendation for periodic laboratory monitoring will vary depending on the patient's medical history and concurrent medications.

Potassium should be monitored more regularly in patients taking potassium-sparing diuretics in combination with potassium supplements or ACE inhibitors. Hypokalemia and hypomagnesemia from a diuretic may result in digoxin toxicity and arrhythmias. Serum creatinine should be monitored more frequently in patients taking a nonsteroidal antiinflammatory drug or an ACE inhibitor/ARB in combination with a diuretic secondary to potential for dehydration and subsequent reduced renal perfusion leading to renal insufficiency.

Diuretics may increase serum uric acid levels. Regular monitoring may be warranted in patients with gout. Although diuretics may increase plasma glucose levels within the first month, the levels will usually normalize over time.

Hydralazine

Immunologic reactions, which present as a hydralazine-induced lupus syndrome, may occur. Higher doses, longer duration of therapy, and genetics contribute. It appears to occur more commonly in whites and women versus blacks and men. Obtain baseline complete blood count (CBC) and antinuclear antibody (ANA) titers. Periodic monitoring also may be warranted. However, many patients who develop positive ANA titers may not develop the syndrome. Discontinuation of the drug may not be necessary until clinical features of lupus exist (i.e., arthralgia, arthritis, and fever).

Methyldopa

Obtain a direct Coomb test and CBC at baseline and after 6 and 12 months to monitor for reversible hemolytic anemia. A positive Coomb test result may occur without the development of hemolytic anemia. Discontinue methyldopa only if anemia is present. The Coomb test result may remain positive for up to a year after discontinuation of the drug. Hepatic dysfunction should be monitored within the first month and then after 3 months secondary to the potential for reversible hepatitis.

Quinidine

Hepatotoxicity and blood dyscrasias including thrombocytopenia, anemia, and agranulocytosis can occur with the use of quinidine. Like digoxin, quinidine can cause arrhythmias in the presence of hypokalemia. In addition, quinidine can markedly increase digoxin levels. Monitor digoxin levels initially and periodically when given in combination with quinidine. Monitor baseline liver function and repeat in the first 4 to 8 weeks of therapy. Obtain baseline and periodic blood counts and potassium levels (particularly when given in conjunction with a diuretic).

What Is the Appropriate Laboratory Toxicity Monitoring for Commonly Prescribed Hyperlipidemic Agents?

Table 38.2 lists the recommended monitoring parameters for selected hyperlipidemic medications.

Table 38.2. Laboratory Toxicity Monitoring for Commonly Prescribed
Hyperlipidemic Agents

Gemfibrozil	Blood dyscrasias, hepatic dysfunction	Obtain baseline CBCs and LFTs and monitor Q 3–6 mo
Niacin	Hepatotoxicity, hyperglycemia, hyperuricemia	LFTs, glucose, uric acid at baseline 6 wk after stable dose then every 3 mo for the first year then every 6–12 mo
HMG reductase inhibitors	LFT abnormalities	LFTs at baseline, 6 and 12 wk after initiation or increase in dose and then semiannually (varies from statin to statin)

CBC, complete blood count; LFT, liver function test; HMG, 3-hydroxy-3-methylglutaryl-coenzyme A.

Fibric Acid Derivatives

Gemfibrozil, fenofibrate, and clofibrate have the potential to cause hepatic dysfunction and blood dyscrasias. Therefore, monitor baseline CBC and LFTs. Follow-up CBCs and LFTs should be performed every 3 to 6 months.

Niacin

Niacin may cause hepatotoxicity, hyperglycemia, and hyperuricemia. Obtain baseline LFTs, fasting glucose, and uric acid. Repeat all laboratory tests 4 to 6 weeks after stabilized dosage, and every 3 months for the first year, then every 6 to 12 months.

3-hydroxy-3-methylglutaryl-coenzyme A Reductase Inhibitors (Statins)

Statins can potentially cause increases in LFTs. The recommendations for monitoring LFTs vary from statin to statin. For cerivastatin and lovastatin, obtain baseline LFTs at 6 and 12 weeks after initiation or increase in dose, then twice yearly thereafter. For atorvastatin, fluvastatin, and pravastatin, obtain baseline LFTs at 12 weeks after initiation of therapy or increase in dose, then semiannually thereafter. For simvastatin, obtain baseline LFTs, then semiannually for the first year or until 1 year after the last increase in dose. In patients taking 80 mg of simvastatin, obtain additional LFTs 3 months after increasing to this dose. Although the recommendations differ, the incidence of LFT abnormalities is similar among the statins.

What Is the Appropriate Laboratory Monitoring for Commonly Prescribed Endocrine Agents?

Table 38.3 lists the recommended monitoring parameters for selected endocrine medications.

Estrogen

The metabolic effects of estrogen may result in glucose intolerance and hypertriglyceridemia. Obtain baseline cholesterol, triglyceride, and glucose. Repeat laboratory tests at yearly physicals.

Table 38.3. Laboratory Toxicity Monitoring for Commonly Prescribed Endocrine Agents

Estrogens	Hyperglycemia, hypertriglyceridemia, liver dysfunction	Cholesterol profile and glucose at baseline and at yearly physicals
Levothyroxine	Hyperthyroidism	TSH at baseline, then 6 weeks, then with dose increases at least 3 weeks apart. Check annually once stable.
Propylthiouracil/methimazole	Hypothyroidism, agranulocytosis, liver dysfunction, hypoprothrombinemia (PTU)	Free T_4/T_4 index and TSH monthly until euthyroid, then every 3–6 mo. Obtain CBC with differential occasionally (especially in the first 3 mo). Monitor LFTs. Monitor prothrombin time periodically for PTU.
Glucocorticoids	Endocrine and electrolyte abnormalities	Monitor Na^+, K^+, glucose, Ca^{2+}, lipids, and CBC at baseline and periodically (every 6–12 mo).
Thiazolidinedione (glitazones)	Potential liver dysfunction	Monitor LFTs at baseline and every 2 mo for 1 yr then periodically thereafter.
Allopurinol	Bone marrow suppression and liver dysfunction	CBCs with platelets and LFTs at baseline and periodically thereafter. Adjust dose in renal insufficiency.
Colchicine	Bone marrow suppression	CBCs and platelets at baseline and periodically thereafter. Adjust dose in renal insufficiency.
Metformin	Lactic acidosis in renal or liver insufficiency	Perform baseline LFTs and Scr and monitor periodically (every 6–12 mo).

TSH, thyroid-stimulating hormone; T_4, thyroxine; CBC, complete blood count; PTU, propylthiouracil; LFT, liver function test; Scr, serum creatinine.

Levothyroxine

After initiating levothyroxine, thyroid-stimulating hormone (TSH) should be measured after 6 weeks to ensure steady state has been achieved. Once steady state has been achieved, the dosage may be titrated every 3 weeks. Once TSH is normal on two consecutive laboratory tests performed 6 to 8 weeks apart and patient is stable, check TSH annually. A trough level should be obtained (i.e., at least 10 hours after tablet ingestion) to avoid transient peaks.

Methimazole/Propylthiouracil

Monitor free T_4 or T_4 index and TSH monthly until euthyroid, then every 3 to 6 months. Obtain CBC with differential occasionally (especially in the first 3 months) to assess for agranulocytosis. LFTs also should be obtained secondary to potential for hepatotoxicity. Propylthiouracil may cause hypoprothrombinemia and bleeding. Prothrombin times should be monitored during therapy, especially before surgical procedures.

Glucocorticoids (Dexamethasone, Methylprednisolone, Prednisone)

With long-term therapy, endocrine (hyperglycemia and hyperlipidemia) and electrolyte disturbances (hypocalcemia, increased sodium retention, hypokalemia, and metabolic alkalosis) can occur with glucocorticoids. Monitoring of Na$^+$, K$^+$, serum glucose, Ca^{2+}, lipids, and CBC should be performed periodically (every 6–12 months). More frequent monitoring may be required in high-risk patients (i.e., diabetics, elderly, etc.)

Metformin

Although metformin does not cause significant renal or liver abnormalities, lactic acidosis may occur in the presence of renal or liver dysfunction. Perform baseline LFTs and Scr and monitor periodically (every 6–12 months). Metformin is contraindicated in patients with liver dysfunction and patients with Scr greater than 1.4 mg/dL for females and 1.5 mg/dL for males.

Thiazolidinediones (Pioglitazone, Rosiglitazone)

Troglitazone, an insulin-sensitizing agent, was pulled from the market on March 21, 2000, secondary to reports of liver failure and death. Because pioglitazone and rosiglitazone are in the same class, the U.S. Food and Drug Administration has required patients to have LFT checks every other month for the first year of therapy and periodically thereafter.

Allopurinol

Bone marrow suppression and liver dysfunction may occur. Obtain CBCs, platelet counts, and LFTs at baseline and periodically thereafter.

Colchicine

Aplastic anemia, agranulocytosis, or thrombocytopenia can occur in patients receiving long-term therapy. Obtain CBCs and platelet counts at baseline and periodically thereafter, particularly in patients with signs and symptoms of bone marrow suppression.

What Is the Appropriate Laboratory Monitoring for Commonly Prescribed Central Nervous System Agents?

Table 38.4 lists the recommended monitoring parameters for selected central nervous system (CNS) medications.

Anticonvulsants

Felbamate, carbamazepine, phenytoin, valproic acid, and ethosuximide can cause blood dyscrasias, including anemias, thrombocytopenias, and agranulocytosis. Obtain CBC and platelet counts at baseline. Periodic monitoring should be performed, particularly in the presence of symptoms of blood dyscrasias (i.e., sore throat, fever, hemorrhage, bruising, etc.) Hepatotoxicity also may occur with many of these agents. Obtain a baseline LFT before initiating therapy and continue to monitor periodically.

Table 38.4. Laboratory Monitoring for Commonly Prescribed Central Nervous System Agents

Felbamate	Aplastic anemia, liver dysfunction	LFTs should be checked every 2 wk. CBCs and platelets should also be monitored closely.
Carbamazepine	Agranulocytosis, anemia, thrombocytopenia, liver dysfunction	Obtain baseline CBC, white cell differential, and platelets and repeat every month for the first 2 mo and then yearly thereafter. Obtain baseline and periodic evaluations of LFTs.
Phenytoin	Blood dyscrasias, toxic hepatitis, hyperglycemia	Baseline CBCs and platelets at baseline and monthly for several months. Baseline and periodic evaluation of glucose and LFTs.
Lithium	Hypothyroidism, sodium depletion, glucosuria, albuminuria, renal dysfunction, leukocytosis	Perform baseline and periodic assessments of electrolytes, serum creatinine, urinalysis, CBCs, and TFTs.
Valproic acid	Thrombocytopenia, abnormal coagulation, hepatotoxicity	Baseline and periodic bleeding times, platelets, and LFTs.

LFT, liver function test; CBC, complete blood count; TFT, thyroid function test.

The definition of *periodic* varies from one agent to another. Felbamate can cause severe aplastic anemia and liver dysfunction. LFTs should be checked every 1 to 2 weeks in patients taking felbamate, and CBCs and platelet counts should be monitored closely. Felbamate should be avoided unless the patient's epilepsy is so severe that the benefits outweigh the risks.

Aplastic anemia, agranulocytosis, and liver dysfunction may occur with the use of carbamazepine. Obtain baseline CBC, white cell differential, and platelet count, and repeat every month for the first 2 months and then yearly thereafter. Obtain baseline and periodic evaluation of LFTs.

Blood dyscrasias have occurred with the use of phenytoin. Obtain baseline CBC and platelet count and repeat at monthly intervals for several months after initiation of therapy. Phenytoin also may induce toxic hepatitis and liver damage, and LFTs should be checked periodically as therapy continues. In addition, phenytoin may increase blood glucose through an inhibitory effect on insulin release. Periodic monitoring of fasting blood glucose is warranted, particularly in diabetic patients or those with a family history of diabetes.

Thrombocytopenia and abnormal coagulation parameters can occur with valproic acid, particularly at plasma concentrations that are higher than the therapeutic range (>100 μg/mL). Bleeding times and platelet counts should be determined at baseline and periodically thereafter. Surgical procedures and use of anticoagulant or antiplatelet medications (i.e., aspirin, warfarin, etc.) warrant additional monitoring. Serious or fatal hepatotoxicity may occur with the use of valproic acid. Monitor LFTs at baseline and periodically thereafter, particularly within the first 6 months of therapy. Ethosuximide also has been associated with blood dyscrasias. Periodic blood counts should be performed particularly with symptoms of infection (i.e., sore throat, infection).

Lithium

Lithium decreases reabsorption of sodium by the kidney, which may result in depletion of sodium. Lithium also may interfere with the synthesis of levothyroxine, resulting in subsequent hypothyroidism. Enlargement of the thyroid gland may occur with increased secretion of TSH. Polyuria and polydipsia consistent with nephrogenic diabetes insipidus may occur secondary to inhibition of the action of antidiuretic hormone on the kidney. Glucosuria, albuminuria, leukocytosis, and renal impairment also may occur. Perform baseline and periodic assessments of electrolytes, serum creatinine, urinalysis, CBC, and TFTs.

When Should Plasma Level Monitoring of Commonly Prescribed Medications Be Obtained?

Periodic plasma monitoring should be performed to help the clinician determine a patient's level of compliance and determine the effectiveness of a medication. Because patients respond differently to medications, plasma level monitoring also helps the clinician determine the most appropriate dosage. When symptoms of toxicity indicate excessive doses of the drug, plasma levels should be drawn for verification. Plasma levels also should be obtained when a medication known to interact with the current therapy is prescribed. Table 38.5 outlines some common drugs requiring plasma serum level monitoring.

Warfarin

Monitor international normalized ratio (INR) every 2 to 3 days when initiating therapy, then weekly. Once patients are stabilized on a dose, the INR should be monitored on a monthly basis. Patients on medications that interact with warfarin require more frequent monitoring. Consider obtaining a urinalysis, serial stool guaiacs, and hemoglobin/hematocrit levels on a yearly basis or sooner if patient symptoms indicate internal bleeding.

Case

Mrs. O is a 65-year-old widow whom you have inherited from a retired colleague. She presents today for routine care and offers no new complaints. She has a past

Table 38.5. Common Drugs Requiring Serum Level Monitoring

Medication	Therapeutic Level	Time to Sample
Carbamazepine	4–8 mg/dL	Trough levels weekly in the first month and periodically thereafter.
Digoxin	0.5–1.5 ng/L	Toxic >3 ng/L. Draw levels 6–8 h after oral dose or 4 h after IV dose. Monitor at baseline and periodically when given with quinidine.
Lithium	0.6–0.8 ng/L (0.8–1.2 ng/L in acute mania)	Draw levels 8–12 h after last dose. Obtain every 3–4 days during initiation. Once clinical condition has stabilized, obtain every 2–3 mo.
Phenobarbital	10–30 mg/L	Trough levels 2–3 wk after initiation of therapy or change in dose.
Phenytoin	10–20 mg/L	Obtain trough levels. Steady state achieved in 2–4 wk.
Quinidine	2–5 mg/L	Obtain trough levels. Steady state achieved in 24 h.
Theophylline	5–15 mg/L	Toxic >20 mg/L. Trough levels can be drawn 1–3 days after initiation or dose change then periodically thereafter.
Valproic acid	50–100 mg/L	Trough concentrations can be drawn 2–4 days after initiation or change in dose.

history of CHF, due to systolic dysfunction, type II diabetes, hypertension, hyper-cholesterolemia, and hypothyroidism. Her current medications include lisinopril 40 mg daily, digoxin 0.25 mg daily, furosemide 20 mg daily, simvastatin 20 mg daily, metformin 500 mg twice daily, glipizide 5 mg daily, levothyroxine 0.125 mg daily, and aspirin 325 mg daily. On physical examination Mrs. O has a normal blood pressure and pulse. The rest of her physical examination is unremarkable.

Laboratory results obtained within the past 2 years include hemoglobin A1C 6.5% (4 months ago), TSH 2.3 μIU/mL (8 months ago), low-density lipoprotein cholesterol 110 mg/dL (1 year ago), and high-density lipoprotein cholesterol 65 mg/dL.

1. What drug toxicities may occur given Mrs. O's current drug regimen?
2. What laboratory tests should you order and for what drugs?
3. Should you order a CPK level to monitor for myositis?

Discussion

What Drug Toxicities May Occur Given Ms. O's Current Drug Regimen?

- Renal failure (lisinopril and furosemide)
- Digoxin toxicity
- Hepatitis (simvastatin and metformin)
- Hyperthyroidism
- Lactic acidosis (not a toxicity of metformin, but patients with renal insufficiency are at increased risk)
- Electrolyte abnormalities (K^+, Mg^+, and Na^+, from furosemide, lisinopril, and digoxin)

What Laboratory Tests Should You Order and for What Drugs?

- SMA-7 (furosemide, lisinopril, metformin, and digoxin)
- Aspartate aminotransferase/alanine aminotransferase (simvastatin and metformin)
- Digoxin level

Should You Order a CPK to Monitor for Myositis?

There are no recommendations for routine monitoring of creatine phosphokinase (CPK) levels to detect myositis in patients taking human menopausal gonadotropin (HMG) reductase inhibitors. The overall risk of developing myositis due to therapy with HMG reductase inhibitors is less than 1%. However, the risk increases significantly when this class of drugs is combined with other drugs (e.g., niacin, gemfibrozil, erythromycin, cyclosporine). The current data suggest that this interaction appears to be more severe with combinations of lovastatin as opposed to other agents in this class of medications. If patients have symptoms suggestive of myositis, the current recommendation is that CPK measurements should be obtained and the medication discontinued if the values are found to be abnormal.

Suggested Reading

Anderson P, Knoben J, Troutman W. *Handbook of clinical drug data,* 9th ed. Illinois: Appleton & Lange, 1999.

McEvoy G K, Litvak K, Welsh O H, et al., eds. *AHFS drug information.* Bethesda: American Society of Health-System Pharmacists, 2001.

Murray L, Gwynned K, eds. *Physicians' desk reference,* 55th ed. Montvale, NJ: Medical Economics Company, 2001.

39
Outpatient Adverse Drug Events

Sunil Kripalani

1. What is an adverse drug event, and how common is the problem?
2. What medications are responsible for adverse drug events, and what are the most common reactions?
3. How can physicians help prevent adverse drug events?

Discussion

What Is an Adverse Drug Event, and How Common Is the Problem?

An adverse drug event is any injury that results from administration of a drug. The term includes complications arising from the medication itself (an adverse drug *reaction*) or from improper administration or noncompliance with the medication. A recent meta-analysis estimated that drug reactions were responsible for approximately 100,000 deaths in the United States in 1994, ranking them as approximately the fifth leading cause of death.

Although most attention has focused on inpatient adverse drug events and other medical errors, outpatient drug complications are also common. They may result in over 1 million hospital admissions each year, comprising nearly 5% of all admissions at an estimated cost of $47 billion annually. By comparison, the cost of all diabetes care is approximately $45 billion.

What Medications Are Responsible for Adverse Drug Events, and What Are the Most Common Reactions?

In a recent telephone survey by Gandhi and colleagues, 18% of patients taking prescription drugs noted a complication, defined as "a problem or symptom in the last year related to their prescription medications." They identified antibiotics (21%), antidepressants (13%), and nonsteroidal antiinflammatory drugs (NSAIDs; 6%) as the most frequent culprits. Common reported side effects included gastrointestinal symptoms, sleep disturbances, fatigue, mood changes, disequilibrium, headache, rash, musculoskeletal complaints, and incontinence. By contrast, physicians noted adverse events in only 3% of these patients' charts. Physicians also documented different types of complications, including allergic reactions/rashes (36%), gastrointestinal (14%), central nervous system (11%), metabolic (5%), cardiovascular (3%), bleeding (2%), and other reactions (30%). This discrepancy suggests that outpatient drug complications are frequently not reported to the physician, they are often not charted, and perceptions of the most common or important reactions may differ between patients and physicians.

How Can Physicians Help Prevent Adverse Drug Events?

Experts estimate that 10% to 30% of adverse drug events are preventable. In Gandhi's study, for example, 13% of patients had a previously documented allergy or other reaction to the causative drug. Taking an adequate medication and allergy history is therefore essential to preventing adverse drug events. Avoiding polypharmacy is also important because the incidence of adverse drug events generally increases with the number of medications. This is most problematic when medications interact, share anticholinergic side effects, or have different dosing schedules.

Physicians must realize that patients have trouble understanding complex medication regimens, or even simple ones. The National Adult Literacy Survey found that nearly 100 million Americans are functionally illiterate or have marginal literacy skills, amounting to over one third of the U.S. population. Low health literacy is a related problem, described as a diminished ability to perform the basic reading required to function in the health-care environment. In the largest study of health literacy in the United States, 42% of patients were unable to understand basic instructions on a medication bottle, such as "take one pill on an empty stomach every morning." The lowest health literacy levels are found in elderly, minority, and underserved patient populations.

Elderly patients are also susceptible to drug complications because of multiple chronic medical problems (particularly renal disease), multiple prescription medications, limited functional status, and decreased visual acuity. Physicians caring for the elderly should therefore direct special attention to potential drug interactions and side effects. One report estimated that 28% of elderly admissions were drug related, far exceeding the average of 4% to 5% cited for the general population.

Another important strategy for preventing adverse drug events is to be familiar with the side effects, contraindications, and "clinical pearls" for prescribing common medications (Table 39.1). Some of these will be illustrated in the case below.

Case

Mr. G is an 82-year-old African-American man who recently designated you as his primary care physician. His wife passed away 6 months ago, and he moved to the area at his daughter's request, so she could visit him daily. She is with him in the office today. Mr. G now lives in an apartment tower for independent seniors, where they offer regular meals but no other services. He feels depressed about the loss of his wife, has lost interest in many activities, and has trouble concentrating. His appetite is poor on some days, and he frequently skips breakfast. His knees have been bothering him for the past few months, to the point of limiting activities. He also

Table 39.1. Clinical Pearls for Common Outpatient Medications

NSAIDs cause dyspepsia in 10%–20% of patients; about 1% have a serious GI complication.

Although cyclooxygenase-2 inhibitors carry a lower risk of GI ulceration and bleeding, they have the same incidence of dyspepsia as NSAIDs.

The anticoagulant effect of warfarin can increase with amiodarone, disulfiram, cephalosporins, erythromycin, azole antifungals, levothyroxine, metronidazole, quinidine/quinine, and trimethoprim/sulfamethoxazole; it may decrease with carbamazepine and phenobarbital.

First-generation sulfonylureas (chlorpropamide, tolazamide, and tolbutamide) and glyburide have a long half-life and therefore a greater risk of prolonged hypoglycemia, especially in elderly patients or those with renal or hepatic disease.

Salicylates may potentiate the effects of insulin and sulfonylureas, leading to hypoglycemia.

Metformin is contraindicated in patients with a creatinine clearance less than 60–70 mL/min (serum creatinine ≥1.5 mg/dL in men, or ≥1.4 mg/dL in women).

To minimize side effects (flushing and GI distress), take niacin with meals; start at 100 mg t.i.d. and increase the dose each week toward a target of 500 mg t.i.d.; take a baby aspirin 30 minutes prior to each dose for the first month.

Start cholestyramine at half a scoop daily, increasing slowly to two scoops per day; take with orange juice for improved taste.

Prescribe a spacer with metered dose inhalers in order to significantly increase medication delivery to the lungs; most patients and clinicians do not know how to properly use an inhaler.

Concomitant use of sildenafil and nitrates is contraindicated; sildenafil appears to be safe in patients with stable coronary disease who do not take nitrates.

There are case reports of angioedema associated with use of ARBs; ARBs are contraindicated in patients who have developed angioedema with ACE inhibitors.

To minimize rebound hypertension while stopping oral clonidine, taper over 4 days; it is unknown whether or not to taper the patch; overlap by 2 days when switching from oral clonidine to its patch.

Taper β blockers over 2 weeks to avoid rebound hypertension.

Antihypertensives that commonly cause hypotension are doxazosin, terazosin, prazosin, and ACE inhibitors, especially in volume-depleted patients or when starting at a high dose.

Lipid-soluble drugs, such as propranolol, have more central nervous system toxicity.

Medications that cause a surprising incidence of sedation include clonidine, propranolol, metoclopramide, phenytoin, phenobarbital, benzodiazepines, tricyclic antidepressants, paroxetine, and most antihistamines.

Caution patients not to drive when taking antihistamines; their sedative effect is similar to two drinks of alcohol.

Be wary of prescribing multiple medications with anticholinergic side effects.

NSAID, nonsteroidal antiinflammatory drug; GI, gastrointestinal; t.i.d., three times daily; ARB, angiotensin receptor blocker; ACE, angiotensin-converting enzyme.

has trouble putting on his shoes in the afternoon because his feet and ankles have become swollen. He used to sleep on one pillow at night but now requires three in order to breathe comfortably. Review of systems is otherwise unremarkable. His past medical history includes myocardial infarction, hypertension, atrial fibrillation, congestive heart failure (CHF), diabetes, and osteoarthritis. His previous physician had prescribed aspirin 325 mg daily, digoxin 0.125 mg daily, captopril 25 mg three times daily, glyburide 10 mg daily, metformin 500 mg twice daily, warfarin 5 mg a day, and lasix 40 mg daily. His weight today is 60 kg, blood pressure 135/80 mm Hg, heart rate 82 beats/min (irregular), and respiration 14 breaths/min. An Accucheck reading showed a glucose of 70 mg/dL. He has mild bilateral cataracts. When you ask him to read the cover of a magazine to estimate his visual acuity, he tells you that he forgot his glasses. Other notable examination findings are mildly elevated jugular venous pulsations, a laterally displaced point of maximum impulse, soft S_3 gallop, scant bibasilar rales, 1+ pitting edema of the ankles, and bilateral knee crepitus. Recent laboratory values reveal a potassium of 5.8 mEq/L, creatinine of 1.8 mg/dL (with a baseline of 1.2mg/dL 6 months ago), glucose of 82 mg/dL, hemoglobin A1C of 6.2%, and international normalized ratio of 2.9. Electrocardiography shows atrial fibrillation and Q waves in the lateral leads.

1. What additional information would you like to know about Mr. G?
2. What risk factors does Mr. G have for experiencing a drug complication?
3. What complications may have resulted from his use of NSAIDs?
4. What changes should be made to his diabetic regimen?

Case Discussion

What Additional Information Would You Like to Know about Mr. G?

It is important to ask Mr. G if he has any drug allergies, uses any over-the-counter (OTC) medications, or takes any herbs or other alternative therapies. Because he has osteoarthritis with knee pain, you can assume that he is taking analgesics or antiinflammatory medications until proven otherwise. If he does not immediately recall taking any OTC products, you should rephrase the question, asking something like, "Do you use any other pills or herbs that you can buy at the grocery store, drug store, or convenience store?" If he still says no, it is appropriate to start naming medications in an attempt to elicit a complete history. It is surprising how many patients do not consider OTC products to be medications, and how many people assume that herbs and other alternative remedies do not have any side effects because they are "all natural." In this case, you discover that Mr. G has been taking Motrin (ibuprofen) twice a day for the past 2 months and *ginkgo biloba* to help improve his concentration.

What Risk Factors Does Mr. G Have for Experiencing a Drug Complication?

Mr. G has several risk factors predisposing him to a drug complication, including age, decreased renal function (calculated creatinine clearance = 28 mL/min), multiple medical problems, and multiple medications with a complex dosing schedule. Whenever possible, try to prescribe medications taken once per day. For example, captopril can be replaced with benazepril or lisinopril.

Dementia (or pseudodementia related to depression) appears to be another problem, as manifested by difficulty concentrating. You should administer a mini-mental status examination. Another concern is that we have no assessment of his visual acuity or literacy. When patients say they have forgotten their glasses or rely on a family member to navigate office visits, consider the possibility that they are unable to read or understand health-related information. Low literacy aids are available, such as pill boxes prepared weekly by a family member.

Of specific concern is his risk for bleeding. Aspirin and ibuprofen are well-known causes of ulcer disease, and *ginkgo biloba* has been associated with platelet dysfunction and spontaneous bleeding. Combined use with anticoagulants can be dangerous, especially in the elderly. If aspirin is necessary, switching to the 81-mg dose reduces the danger of bleeding by half. In high-risk patients taking NSAIDs, a proton pump inhibitor or misoprostol may be used for ulcer prophylaxis, but doing so adds another medication to an already complex regimen. A better alternative is to switch from ibuprofen to acetaminophen for the treatment of his osteoarthritis.

What Complications May Have Resulted from His Use of NSAIDs?

NSAID use can explain Mr. G's worsening renal function, hyperkalemia, and CHF. By inhibiting prostaglandin synthesis, NSAIDs decrease renal blood flow and glomerular filtration rate (GFR), leading to fluid retention. Patients with CHF, renal insufficiency, or cirrhosis are most susceptible to volume shifts. In fact, NSAIDs may be responsible for up to 20% of CHF hospitalizations. NSAIDs also can cause significant gastrointestinal complications, including dyspepsia, ulcers, and bleeding. This is a particular concern in patients who are elderly and taking aspirin or warfarin. It has been estimated that 16,500 NSAID-related deaths occur each year in the United States, comparable to the number of deaths from acquired immunodeficiency syndrome.

What Changes Should Be Made to His Diabetic Regimen?

The benefits of tight diabetes control must be weighed against the potential complications. Mr. G is at risk for lactic acidosis from metformin, which should not be used in patients with CHF or a GFR of less than 60 to 70 mL/min. He is also at risk of hypoglycemia due to poor appetite, unreliable oral intake, and glyburide, which has a long half-life, especially in patients with renal insufficiency. Given these potential complications, a more reasonable target is a fasting blood glucose around 130 mg/dL and hemoglobin A1C of 7.0% to 7.5%. A single medication should be adequate to achieve this goal, and potential agents include glipizide, glymeperide, repaglinide, rosiglitizone, and pioglitizone. These all carry a lower risk of inducing hypoglycemia than glyburide, particularly the latter three.

Suggested Reading

Bates D W, Spell N, Cullen D J, et al. The costs of adverse drug events in hospitalized patients. *JAMA* 1997;277:307–311.

Gandhi T K, Burstin H R, Cook E F, et al. Drug complications in outpatients. *J Gen Intern Med* 2000;15:149–154.

Health literacy. Report of the Council on Scientific Affairs. *JAMA* 1999;281:552–557.

Lazarou J, Pomeranz B H, Corey P N. Incidence of adverse drug reactions in hospitalized patients: a meta-analysis of prospective studies. *JAMA* 1998;279:1200–1205.

Miller L G. Herbal medicinals. Selected clinical considerations focusing on known or potential drug-herb interactions. *Arch Intern Med* 1998;158:2200–2211.

Wolf M M, Lichtenstein D R, Singh G. Gastrointestinal toxicity of nonsteroidal antiinflammatory drugs. *N Engl J Med* 1999;340:1888–1899.

40

End-of-Life Care

Colleen Sam

- Discussion   *249*
- Case   *252*
- Case Discussion   *252*

1. Review the cases of Karen Ann Quinlan and Nancy Cruzan, two landmark Supreme Court cases addressing end-of-life decisions.
2. Do patients have the right to refuse treatment, even life-sustaining treatment?
3. What role does the health-care proxy play in the decision-making process?
4. What are the principles of withdrawing therapy?
5. What is the Patient Self-Determination Act (1991)?

Discussion

Review the Cases of Karen Ann Quinlan and Nancy Cruzan, Two Landmark Supreme Court Cases Addressing End-of-Life Decisions.

In 1976, Karen Ann Quinlan was in a persistent vegetative state (PVS) after two periods of anoxia. Although her parents wanted to be appointed her guardians, they could not because she was already over the age of 18 years. The physicians treating her were fearful of repercussions if they terminated her life. Her parents sought court authorization to remove her from the ventilator. A New Jersey Supreme Court made a unanimous decision authorizing removal of the ventilator on the basis of Quinlan's right to privacy, which was based on common law, and the right to self-determination, which the courts decided was being exercised on her behalf by her parents.

Nancy Cruzan also was in a PVS after an automobile accident on a deserted road in Missouri in 1983. She required only tube feeding (rather than a ventilator and tube feeding) to continue to survive. Her parents firmly believed that she would not have wanted to continue tube feeding under such circumstances. This was concluded from past statements she had made to her parents. The trial judge authorized the parents to order that the tube feedings be discontinued. However, the Missouri Supreme Court reversed the decision because the consequence would have been death and the state had a legitimate interest in preserving life regardless of its quality. The right to refuse treatment was Nancy's alone and no one could exercise it for her. Her parents appealed this decision to the U.S. Supreme Court. The U.S. Supreme Court assumed that a competent person's refusal of treatment was guaranteed by the liberty clause, but at the same time the Constitution did not prohibit states from regulating how surrogates may make such decisions on behalf of patients.

Do Patients Have the Right to Refuse Treatment, Even Life-Sustaining Treatment?

Competent patients have the right to refuse treatment, even life-sustaining treatment. A competent person's right to refuse treatment is guaranteed by the liberty clause of the XIVth Amendment of the Constitution: "No State shall make or enforce any law which shall abridge the privileges or immunities of citizens of the United States; nor shall any state deprive any person of life, liberty, or property, without due process of law."

There is no requirement that a patient accept a recommendation for bypass surgery for coronary artery disease or ranitidine for peptic ulcer disease. So a patient who is approaching death, whose disease is terminal, does not lose the capacity to make decisions for himself or herself. Patients with cancer or acquired immunodeficiency syndrome are not required to accept treatment that might prolong life, nor are they required to remain hospitalized if they request to go home and die. The right of competent patients to refuse treatment has been supported consistently in the court system.

The Cruzan decision emphasized the importance of advance directives. The loss of the ability to make or express one's wishes does not terminate the individual's right to decide about his or her medical care. Advance directives allow individuals to determine their desires for medical treatment before incompetence develops. In recognition of this, most states permit naming a durable power of attorney for health care, and more than 40 states have enacted "living will" statutes. The exceptions are Alaska, which authorizes living wills only, and Michigan, New York, and Massachusetts, which have statutes authorizing the appointment of a health-care proxy (HCP) only. These statutes provide immunity to physicians and health-care providers who follow the patient's wishes as expressed in the living will. No court has overturned a terminally ill patient's written instructions for treatment, even if a living will statute did not exist.

What Role Does the Health-Care Proxy Play in the Decision-Making Process?

The goal of appointing an HCP, also called a durable power of attorney, is to simplify the process of making decisions and to make it more likely that the patient's wishes be followed. Most physicians welcome the ability to discuss the treatment options with a person chosen by the patient who has legal authority to give or withhold consent. The HCP has the same authority to make decisions that the patient would have if he or she were still competent. The HCP must make decisions that are consistent with the wishes of the patient, if these are known, and otherwise that are consistent with the patient's best interest. Only competent adults who actually execute a document can name an HCP.

Traditionally, "do not resuscitate" (DNR) orders and living wills do not apply to emergencies outside the hospital, and ambulance crews could not honor them. They are obligated to carry out a full resuscitation. During the 1990s states began passing laws to allow emergency medical teams to respect out-of-hospital DNRs for dying patients receiving care at home. Seven states and the District of Columbia do not allow out-of-hospital DNRs: Delaware, Iowa, Mississippi, Nebraska, North Dakota, Pennsylvania, and Vermont.

What Are the Principles of Withdrawing Therapy?

There is no distinction among the various forms of life-sustaining treatment; nutrition and hydration are not different from more "high-tech" types of support such as central lines or even ventilators. Gastrostomy and tube feedings have more in common with other medical procedures than the typical ways of providing nutrition. Artificial feeding can be viewed on a level with cardiopulmonary resuscitation, dialysis, or ventilation and can therefore be withheld or withdrawn.

No differentiation should be made between withholding and withdrawing treatment. The rationale is that there is little distinction between the first breath on a ventilator and the 101st, or the first tube feeding and the next. To withdraw ventilation or tube feeding is equivalent to withholding the next breath or the next feeding.

When a physician proposes a treatment course for a patient, the outcome is unknown and the benefits and risks may not be fully appreciated. For example, a patient with chronic obstructive pulmonary disease develops pneumonia and needs ventilation. It may be uncomfortable for the patient, but without it, the patient has no chance of recovery. With it, the possibility arises that the patient may survive the pneumonia but fail attempts at weaning from the ventilator. If the ethical and legal aspects of withholding and withdrawing mechanical ventilation are appreciated, then there is no reason for a physician or patient to fear starting treatment because of unwanted long-term mechanical ventilation. The treatment can always be withdrawn if its burden outweighs the benefits. The Supreme Court does not forbid either withholding or withdrawing life-sustaining treatments from competent or incompetent patients.

What Is the Patient Self-Determination Act (1991)?

This is a federal law that requires all health-care facilities that receive Medicare or Medicaid, including nursing homes, to give patients written information about their right to fill out advance directives. Patients are given the opportunity to complete the advance directives such as a living will or durable power of attorney. The law requires hospital and nursing homes to document in each person's records whether he or she has completed an advance directive. No patient will be required to do so, but it is hoped that the law will result in more informed decision making.

Most patients (75%) with terminal disease know a year before dying that the disease will kill them. The importance of discussions prior to the onset of incapacitating illness is obvious, but many physicians fail to plan with the patients. Life-sustaining techniques are mandated for hospitalized patients unless a DNR order is written. Studies have shown that as many as 70% of hospitalized patients have DNR orders written before their deaths. However, most (60%) of the orders are written within 3 days before the patient's death, suggesting that there had been little advance planning. Furthermore, in only 14% of the cases had the patient been consulted about the DNR order.

Doctors who try to resuscitate patients against their will are rarely penalized. Alaska and Utah have established penalties in legislation, but these are often not significant. Lawyers have begun to press "medical battery" claims against doctors and hospitals that do not honor living wills.

Case

Diana, a 37-year-old woman, entered the hospital to have surgery to remove her gallbladder. She appointed her best friend Elena to be her HCP "just in case anything bad happens." During the surgery, there was a power failure and the anesthesia monitoring machine malfunctioned. The back-up power system also failed, and Diana was left unconscious, in a coma, because of lack of oxygen to her brain. The physicians believe that there is nothing that can be done for Diana to wake her from the coma, but they are not sure who has the right to make treatment decisions for Diana.

1. Does Diana have the right to have her wishes about further treatment respected?
   a. No, because she is no longer competent.
   b. No, because she has appointed an HCP.
   c. Yes, because she is a competent adult.
   d. Yes, because, even though she is incompetent, she has the same rights as a competent adult.
2. What are Elena's legal obligations with respect to making treatment decisions for Diana?
   a. Elena must make whatever decision Diana would have wanted.
   b. Elena must act in Diana's best interest, regardless of what Diana might want.
   c. Elena must consent to any treatment that could prolong Diana's life, regardless of what Diana might want.
   d. Elena must go to court and ask the judge what treatment Diana should have.
3. Diana's coma progresses to a PVS. She is breathing on her own without the ventilator, but needs a feeding tube to enable her to get nutrition to survive. If Elena tells the doctor to remove the feeding tube, must the doctor comply with her request?
   a. Yes, because a feeding tube is not necessary medical treatment for a patient with PVS.
   b. Yes, because Elena is Diana's HCP, unless Elena is acting in bad faith and there is good evidence that Diana would want to keep the feeding tube.
   c. No, because removing the feeding tube would be equivalent to killing Diana.
   d. No, because a feeding tube is not medical treatment and patients cannot refuse things that are not medical treatment.

Case Discussion

Does Diana Have the Right to Have Her Wishes about Further Treatment Respected?

The patient has the same rights as a competent adult. This was decided in the Karen Quinlan case, when it was shown that the right of an incompetent patient is substantively the same as that of a competent person (answer d).

What Are Elena's Legal Obligations with Respect to Making Treatment Decisions for Diana?

Elena is the HCP and therefore she is executing substituted judgment and is expressing what she thinks the patient, Diana, would have wanted. Recall that she was appointed by the patient prior to her surgery (answer a).

If Elena Tells the Doctor to Remove the Feeding Tube, Must the Doctor Comply with Her Request?

Withdrawal of tube feeding is the same as withdrawing a ventilator. At this time the patient is in a PVS and the HCP is expressing what she believes the patient would have wanted (answer b).

Suggested Reading

Annas G J. Nancy Cruzan and the right to die. *N Engl J Med* 1990;323:670–673.
Annas G J. The health care proxy and the living will. *N Engl J Med* 1991;324:1210–1213.
Balaban R B. A physician's guide to talking about end-of-life care. *J Gen Intern Med* 2000;15:195–200.
Fairman, R P. Withdrawing life-sustaining treatment: lessons from Nancy Cruzan. *Arch Intern Med* 1992;152:25–27.
Grady D. At life's end, many patients are denied peaceful passing. *The New York Times* 2000; CXLIX(51,403):A1, A13.

VII
Gynecology

41

Interpreting Pap Smear Results

Judith R. Rudnick

1. Why do we screen for cervical cancer?
2. How are Pap smear results reported?
3. What does the term *atypical squamous cells of undetermined significance* (ASCUS) mean?
4. What are the recommendations for follow-up of an ASCUS Pap smear result?
5. What are the new Pap screening procedures?
6. What other Pap results can be seen using the Bethesda system?

Discussion

Why Do We Screen for Cervical Cancer?

Cervical cancer is a disease that lends itself to screening because there is a long pre-clinical (asymptomatic) period, and the screening is simple and inexpensive. Cervical cancer is the fourth most common type of cancer in the United States. World-wide it is the second most common cancer in women (after breast cancer). No randomized controlled clinical trials have been undertaken to document improved survival with screening for cervical cancer. However, historical studies have demonstrated a correlation between the decrease in mortality from cervical cancer and the rate of screening. Case control studies show that women with invasive cervical cancer were less likely to have been screened by Papanicolaou (Pap) smear. Data from large screening programs show that annual screening reduces the probability that a woman will develop invasive cervical cancer by 93.3%, and screening every 3 years reduces the probability by 91.2%.

Most cervical cancer is squamous cell (about 85%), whereas most of the other 15% of cases are adenocarcinoma. Squamous cell carcinoma of the cervix tends to develop at the squamocolumnar junction of the cervix. This transitional zone is near the external cervical os. In postmenopausal women, however, the junction may retract inside the endocervical canal.

How Are Pap Smear Results Reported?

Currently, all Pap smear results are reported using the Bethesda (home of the National Institutes of Health) system. The Bethesda Classification System was

Table 41.1. Traditional Classification of Papanicolaou Smear

Normal
Metaplasia
Inflammation
Minimal atypia (koilocytosis)
Mild dysplasia (CIN I)
Moderate dysplasia (CIN II)
Severe dysplasia/carcinoma *in situ* (CIN III) invasive carcinoma

CIN, cervical intraepithelial neoplasia.

Table 41.2. The 1991 Bethesda System

Adequacy of the specimen
  Satisfactory for evaluation
  Satisfactory for evaluation but limited by (specify reason)
  Unsatisfactory for evaluation (specify reason)
General categorization (optional)
  Within normal limits
  Benign cellular changes (see descriptive diagnoses)
  Epithelial cell abnormalities (see descriptive diagnoses)
Descriptive diagnoses
  Benign cellular changes
    Infection
      Trichomonas vaginalis
      Fungal organisms morphologically consistent with *Candida* species
      Predominance of coccobacilli consistent with shift in vaginal flora
      Bacteria morphologically consistent with *Actinomyces* species
      Cellular changes associated with herpes simplex virus
      Other[a]
  Reactive changes
    Reactive cellular changes associated with
      Inflammation (includes typical repair)
      Atrophy with inflammation (atrophic vaginitis)
      Radiation
      Intrauterine contraceptive device
      Other
  Epithelial cell abnormalities
    Squamous cell
      Atypical squamous cells of undetermined significance (qualify[b])
      Low-grade squamous intraepithelial lesion encompassing human papillomavirus,[a] mild
        dysplasia/CIN 1
      High-grade squamous intraepithelial lesion encompassing moderate and severe dysplasia,
        CIS/CIN 2 and CIN
      Squamous cell carcinoma
    Glandular cell
      Endometrial cells, cytologically benign, in a postmenopausal woman
      Atypical glandular cells of undetermined significance (qualify[b])
      Endocervical adenocarcinoma
      Endometrial adenocarcinoma
      Extrauterine adenocarcinoma
      Adenocarcinoma, non–organ specific
    Other malignant neoplasms (specify)
  Hormonal evaluation (applies to vaginal smears only)
    Hormonal pattern compatible with age and history
    Hormonal pattern incompatible with age and history (specify)
    Hormonal evaluation not possible due to (specify)

[a]Cellular changes of human papillomavirus previously termed koilocytotic atypia or condylomatous atypia are included in the category of low-grade squamous intraepithelial lesion.

[b]Atypical squamous or glandular cells of undetermined significance should be further qualified, if possible, as to whether a reactive or premalignant/malignant process is favored.

CIN, cervical intraepithelial neoplasia; CIS, carcinoma *in situ*.

Reprinted from Kurman R J, Henson D E, Herbst A L, et al. Interim guidelines for management of abnormal cervical cytology. *JAMA* 1994;271:1866–1869; with permission.

Table 41.3. Bethesda Classification (Modified)

Adequacy of smear
Infection type
Squamous abnormalities
Reactive (inflammatory change) epithelial cell abnormalities
Atypical type, undetermined
Squamous intraepithelial lesions
Low grade: HPV or mild dysplasia (CIN I)
High grade: moderate to severe dysplasia/carcinoma *in situ* (CIN II–III)
Glandular cells
Atypical and source
Adenocarcinoma and source

HPV, human papillomavirus; CIN, cervical intraepithelial neoplasia.

adopted in 1988, and by the early 1990s it had replaced the traditional (Papanico-laou) classification system, which reported smear results as class I through class V (Tables 41.1–41.3). The reason for this change was that the traditional system did not communicate sufficient clinical information and lacked reproducibility with histologic diagnosis (Figure 41.1). By contrast, the Bethesda system seems at times to give too much information. Instead of simply putting the results in a class, the result provides general categorizations of the results (normal or other), a descriptive diagnosis, and possibly a recommendation for further evaluation.

In the Bethesda Classification, first there is a comment on specimen adequacy: satisfactory, satisfactory but limited, or unsatisfactory. If the satisfactory but limited category is used, the reason for limitation should be given (e.g., lack of endocervical component).

Next the specimen is categorized as normal or other. If the specimen is not normal it will be described as having benign cellular changes (infection), reaction changes (inflammation, atrophy), or epithelial abnormalities. All cancerous and precancerous lesions are included in the latter category.

Three sets of terms are used to describe premalignant cellular findings:

1. *Dysplasia* is categorized as mild, moderate, severe, or carcinoma *in situ* (CIS). These descriptions were used in the traditional Pap classification.
2. *Cervical intraepithelial neoplasia* (CIN) refers to the same findings as in dysplasia, but use the terminology of histology. In this classification, CIN I is mild dysplasia, CIN II is moderate dysplasia, and CIN III is severe dysplasia and CIS.
3. Most recent is the term *squamous intraepithelial lesions*. Such abnormalities are classified into two tiers. Low-grade squamous intraepithelial lesions (LGSILs) include koilocytosis and mild dysplasia, whereas high-grade squamous intraepithelial lesions (HGSILs) include moderate dysplasia, severe dysplasia, and CIS.

What Does the Term *Atypical Squamous Cells of Undetermined Significance* Mean?

The category *atypical squamous cells of undetermined significance* (ASCUS) is used in the Bethesda system of classifying Pap smear results. It is used to describe specimens that show abnormal squamous cells that do not fit into any of the other criteria. There is also a category of atypical glandular cells of undetermined significance (AGCUS) that you may see on occasion.

What Are the Recommendations for Follow-Up of an ASCUS Pap Smear Result?

There are no evidence-based guidelines for appropriate follow-up. There are four possible strategies, each of which may be appropriate for some patients. The most common recommendation for a single ASCUS Pap smear result is to repeat the Pap smear in 4 months. If this Pap smear result is within normal limits, the smear is then repeated every 4 to 6 months until there have been three consecutive normal results. If any of these repeat smears show ASCUS, the patient is referred for colposcopy. This strategy is only appropriate for compliant patients.

Because data suggest that 35% to 49% of women will again have ASCUS on the second Pap smear, this has led to the suggestion that colposcopy should be performed on all women with an ASCUS Pap smear result. This strategy would allow earlier diagnosis of the 5% to 10% of women found to have HGSIL after an ASCUS Pap smear result.

The third management option is to perform an additional diagnostic test to help determine a woman's risk for cervical cancer. The most widely used is a test for human papillomavirus (HPV), because infection with HPV is a risk factor in the development of cervical cancer. Using this strategy, women who tested positive for HPV would be referred immediately for colposcopy, whereas those who tested negative would be followed by repeat smears. Although HPV is thought to have a causative role in the development of cervical cancer, most HPV infections do not progress to neoplasm, and they may resolve spontaneously. This strategy is also

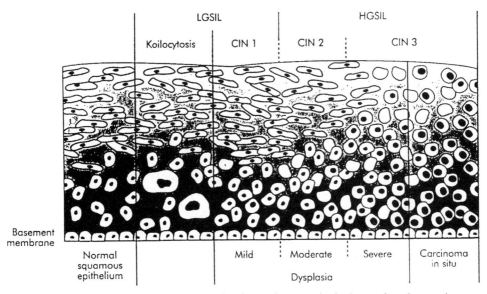

Figure 41.1. Diagram of cervical epithelium showing various terminologies used to characterize progressive degrees of cervical neoplasia.

limited because HPV tests may not be widely available, and their sensitivity and specificity are still being determined.

The fourth management strategy would be to subdivide ASCUS based on pathology. The Interim Guidelines Committee proposed that ASCUS be subdivided into three categories: ASCUS favoring reactive, unqualified ASCUS, and ASCUS favoring dysplasia. Patients with the first two types would receive repeat Pap smears, whereas patients with ASCUS favoring dysplasia would be referred for colposcopy. Unfortunately, there are no prospective studies that show the validity of these classifications. Because Pap smear results are not routinely reported this way, this strategy is largely theoretic.

What Are the New Pap Screening Procedures?
Thin Prep System

The Thin Prep System (Cytyc Corp., Boxborough, MA) is a liquid-based technique for preparing the smear. The sample is placed in a vial of liquid; it is not put on a slide until it gets to the laboratory. There it is stained and examined in the conventional way. This test costs $10 to $20 more than "old fashioned" Pap smears.

PapNet System

The PapNet System (Neuromedical Systems, Inc., Suffern, NY) is a computer-assisted technique that rescreens all slides read as normal. A computer locates the 128 most abnormal cells on every specimen. These cells are projected as a computer image to be examined by the cytotechnologist or pathologist, who then makes the final diagnosis. This technique takes up to 1 week longer than traditional methods and adds $35 to $40 to the cost.

AutoPap System

In the AutoPap System (NeoPath, Inc., Redmond, WA) a computer assigns each slide a score according to its probability of containing abnormal cells. These scores can be used several ways; for quality control, all normal results are manually reviewed. As a primary screening device, the 25% of smear results most likely to be negative are not manually reviewed, whereas all other results are. This technique adds $35 to every Pap test.

All these systems were developed to increase the sensitivity (decrease the false-negative rate) of the Pap screening test. They all result in a larger number of ASCUS and LGSILs. And although these techniques may help individual patients, they do not help in the management of the mildly abnormal Pap smear results.

What Other Pap Smear Results Can Be Seen Using the Bethesda System?

Specimen satisfactory, but limited by absence of endocervical component. This is always the result if the patient has had a hysterectomy but the cervical cuff remains. It also occurs if no cells from the transformation zone were obtained (either because of poor technique or because the transformation zone has regressed up the cervical os and was not reached by the brush). Patients with this result may be followed up at the regular interval for age assuming that they have had previous normal smear results with endocervical component or they have had a hysterectomy. In a patient who has not recently been screened, a repeat smear may be considered. There are no data on the incidence of lesions in patients rescreened for this reason.

Endometrial cells present. A postmenopausal woman with this finding should be referred to a gynecologist for further evaluation. In one study, 13.5% of patients with endometrial cells seen on Pap smear had carcinoma of the endometrium.

Within normal limits, mild to moderate inflammation. Patients may be followed at the usual interval. If there is evidence for a specific pathogen (e.g., *Trichomonas vaginalis* or yeast), the patient should be treated appropriately.

Case

A 42-year-old African-American woman comes to your medical clinic for follow-up of her high blood pressure. She had a Pap smear at her last visit 2 months ago and wants to know the results. She has had three pregnancies and three successful deliveries. Her last menstrual period was several weeks ago and she reports it as normal. Her medications are triamterene/hydrochlorothiazide and a calcium supplement. Her past medical history is significant for hypertension, but there is no history of sexually transmitted diseases. She is currently sexually active with one male partner. She does not routinely use condoms.

Her Pap smear results are as follows: the specimen was adequate, endocervical component was present, and ASCUS are present.

1. What does this result mean?
2. How should you explain these results to the patient?
3. What recommendations will you make to her for follow-up and or additional procedures?

Case Discussion
What Does This Result Mean?

This result is abnormal, with epithelial cell abnormalities. It is important to remember that these changes are part of a continuum of slight to severe atypia, which may progress to invasive cancer. However, it is not known where on this continuum our patient's results should be placed.

How Should You Explain These Results to the Patient?

Because it is unclear what our patient's Pap smear result means histologically, it is hard to know what to tell a patient. She should be told that the result is considered abnormal. It is important to stress that the results do not show any evidence of cervical cancer (foremost in a patient's mind when given an abnormal result). Having said that, you should try to answer any questions the patient might have.

What Recommendations Will You Make to Her for Follow-Up and or Additional Procedures?

This patient has three choices for follow-up: repeat Pap smear at an earlier interval (e.g., in 4–6 months), colposcopy, or additional testing to determine if colposcopy is required. There are clearcut recommendations in this case. When making a clinical recommendation to a patient, there are several factors to consider.

First, the Pap smear is a screening test; as such, abnormal results should be followed up. Otherwise, a developing cancer may not be detected. The chance that a patient with ASCUS on Pap smear will be found at colposcopy to have a more serious lesion is not completely defined. Five percent to 33% of patients (depending on study) will have a CIN lesion (either LGSIL or HGSIL) if colposcopy is performed following a Pap smear showing ASCUS. Before simply recommending colposcopy for all women with abnormal smear results, one must remember that a proportion of patients with ASCUS and LGSIL have lesions that will regress without any treatment.

Second, in making recommendations to a patient one must consider the likelihood that her lesion will progress to cancer versus the possibility of performing an unnecessary semiinvasive procedure (e.g., colposcopy).

In addition, there are racial differences in the incidence of cervical cancer. In the United States the incidence is 8.7 per 100,000 women. The incidence is twice as high for African Americans (14.3 vs. 7.9 per 100,000 women under 50; 33.6 vs. 15.8 per 100,000 women over 50). As these numbers show, cervical cancer is a disease of older women (premalignant lesions are more common in young women). Postmenopausal women who have not had regular screenings are those most likely to be diagnosed with cervical cancer by Pap smear. Thus a patient's age, previous screening history, and race should be considered when deciding whether to recommend colposcopy.

Suggested Reading

American College of Obstetrics and Gynecology Committee Opinion. New pap test screening techniques. 1998;206:1–3. Committee on Gynecologic Practice, American College of Obstetricians and Gynecologists. *International Journal of Gynecology and Obstetrics* 1998;63(3):312–314.

American Society of Colposcopy and Cervical Pathology practice guideline management guidelines for follow-up of atypical squamous cells of undetermined significance (ASCUS). *Colposcopist* 1996;27:1–9.

Herbst A L, Marshall D, Stengheuer M, et al. Intraepithelial neoplasia of the cervix. In: *Comprehensive gynecology,* 3rd ed. St. Louis: C V Mosby, 1997:801–833.

Kurman R J, Henson D, Herbst A, et al. Interim guidelines for management of abnormal cervical cytology. *JAMA* 1994;271:1886–1869.

Warner E A, Parsons A K. Screening and early diagnosis of gynecologic cancers. *Med Clin North Am* 1996;80:45–62.

42
Vaginitis

Lisa B. Bernstein

1. What is the standard diagnostic workup of a patient with vaginal discharge?
2. What are the major causes of vaginitis and how do you diagnose them?
3. What are the approved treatment options for the major causes of vaginitis, and do you treat the patient's sexual partner?
4. What are the approved treatment regimens for pregnant women?

Discussion

What Is the Standard Diagnostic Workup of a Patient with Vaginal Discharge?

The diagnosis of vaginitis begins with evaluation of the quality and quantity of discharge, presence or absence of odor, and associated signs and symptoms, although these are most often not predictive of the actual etiology of the vaginitis. As a result, diagnostic tests, such as microscopic and pH evaluation of the discharge, are also required. A sample of the discharge should be diluted in one to two drops of 0.9% normal saline solution on one slide and 10% potassium hydroxide (KOH) on another slide. The motile trichomonads of trichomoniasis or clue cells of bacterial vaginosis (BV) are usually easily identifiable on the saline wet preparation, and an inflammatory response or estrogen effect also may be noted. If there is a fishy odor noted before or after adding KOH (positive whiff test), it is likely BV (although trichomoniasis also can be accompanied by an odor). Yeast or pseudohyphae of vulvovaginal candidiasis are more easily identified using KOH. Evaluating the pH of the discharge is also helpful. Normal vaginal pH is 3.8 to 4.4. Patients with yeast infections have a normal pH, whereas those with BV and trichomoniasis have an alkaline pH. Douching and menses alter the vaginal pH.

What Are the Major Causes of Vaginitis and How Do You Diagnose Them?

Normal vaginal secretions are clear or white, homogeneous, and viscous. Vaginitis is usually characterized by vaginal discharge that may be malodorous and accompanied by vulvar irritation, pruritus, dysuria, or dyspareunia. The most frequent causes of vaginitis are BV, trichomoniasis, vulvovaginal candidiasis (VVC), and atrophic vaginitis. Other causes include other sexually transmitted diseases (STDs) such as gonorrhea, chlamydia, or herpes simplex, bacterial infections, allergies to douches or spermicides, foreign bodies or trauma, collagen vascular diseases, and vulvar neoplasms. Patients may present with multiple etiologies at one time.

In the United States, bacterial vaginosis is the most common cause of vaginitis. This condition is characterized by a reduction in the concentration of normal vaginal lactobacilli with a resultant increase in the prevalence of anaerobic bacteria. Half of the women with BV are asymptomatic. The diagnosis of BV requires the presence of three of the following: a thin, homogeneous white noninflammatory discharge (like skim milk) often adherent to the vaginal walls, presence of clue cells on microscopic examination (>20% of epithelial cells), pH of vaginal fluid more than 4.5, or a fishy odor before or after adding 10% KOH (positive whiff test).

Trichomoniasis is caused by the flagellated anaerobic protozoan *Trichomonas vaginalis*. Most men are asymptomatic, but female patients often complain of a copious, malodorous (fishy), yellow-green frothy discharge with vulvar irritation and resulting pruritus, dysuria, or dyspareunia. Physical examination may reveal punctate cervical microhemorrhages, often called the classic strawberry cervix. Motile trichomonads are identified on wet preparation, and white blood cells are usually present due to the accompanying inflammatory state. The vaginal pH is markedly elevated (almost always >5.0).

An estimated 75% of women will have at least one episode of VVC, which is usually caused by *Candida albicans* or, less frequently, by other *Candida* species, *Torulopsis* species, or other yeasts. The main symptom is intense vulvar pruritus along with a thick curdlike vaginal discharge, vulvar erythema, edema, and soreness, with possible dyspareunia and external dysuria. Predisposing factors to recurrent infection include uncontrolled diabetes mellitus, steroid use, tight-fitting clothing and synthetic underwear, antibiotic use, increased coital frequency, immunocompromised states, and use of an intrauterine device. Oral contraceptives containing higher estrogen doses (75–150 µg) also have been associated with increased likelihood of VVC. Diagnosis is suggested clinically and corroborated with a normal pH (4.0–4.7) and a wet preparation/KOH demonstrating yeasts or pseudohyphae.

Menopause is associated with a marked reduction in endogenous estrogen production. As a result, the vaginal epithelium becomes atrophied and dry, which can cause vaginal discomfort, itching, and dyspareunia, as well as urinary frequency, urgency, dysuria, and incontinence. The vaginal mucosa is often pale with decreased rugal folds. The vaginal pH increases, and vaginal fluid appears thin and grayish. Saline wet mount reveals numerous leukocytes with small round epithelial cells. Diagnosis is suggested in postmenopausal women clinically and supported with a physical examination revealing urogenital atrophy and a vaginal pH commonly higher than 5.0.

What Are the Approved Treatment Options for the Four Major Causes of Vaginitis, and Do You Treat the Patient's Sex Partner?

All symptomatic women with BV should be treated. Standard regimens with fairly equal overall cure rates are metronidazole 500 mg twice daily orally for 7 days, intravaginal metronidazole gel 0.75% twice daily for 7 days, or clindamycin cream

2% intravaginally twice daily for 7 days. Alternative regimens include the less effective metronidazole 2 g orally in a single dose, clindamycin 300 mg orally twice a
day for 7 days, and flagyl ER (750 mg) once daily for 7 days. Routine treatment of
sex partners is not recommended, and follow-up is unnecessary if symptoms resolve.

For *Trichomonas* infection, systemic treatment is essential. The recommended
regimen is metronidazole 2 g orally in a single dose; with concurrent BV, metronidazole 500 mg twice daily for 7 days should be used. Sex partners should be
treated, and patients should be counseled to avoid intercourse until therapy is completed and both they and their partner are asymptomatic. Follow-up is unnecessary
for patients who are asymptomatic after treatment.

Topical agents are the most commonly used initial treatment of uncomplicated
VVC. Recommended regimens include a variety of antifungal intravaginal creams,
tablets, or suppositories for up to 7 days. Oral fluconazole 150 mg in a single dose
should be reserved for patients with resistant or recurrent infections or an inability
to tolerate topical therapies. Vulvar care measures are also important in the treatment of VVC. Instruct the patient not to use harsh soaps or perfumes and to keep
the genital area dry. She should avoid tight clothing and frequent or prolonged
use of hot tubs. Follow-up is unnecessary unless symptoms persist or recur, and
treatment of sex partners is not recommended, except in women with recurrent
infection.

The mainstay of treatment for the acute symptoms of atrophic vaginitis is daily
estrogen replacement in the form of topical intravaginal estrogen cream for 2
weeks. If there is a contraindication to oral estrogen therapy, vaginal creams are
also contraindicated because there is considerable systemic absorption.

What Are the Approved Treatment Regimens for Pregnant Women for Each of the Major Causes?

All high-risk pregnant women with BV, regardless of whether they have symptoms,
should be treated due to risk of adverse pregnancy outcomes, such as premature
rupture of the membranes, preterm labor, and infants born with low birth weight.
The recommended therapy is metronidazole 250 mg orally three times daily for 7
days, with alternative therapies including metronidazole 2 g orally in a single dose
or clindamycin 300 mg orally twice a day for 7 days. Do not use clindamycin gel
because this has been linked to an increased risk of pre-term deliveries in two randomized trials.

Treatment for pregnant women with trichomoniasis is the same as for nonpregnant women: metronidazole 2 g in a single dose. Only topical azole therapies
should be used to treat pregnant women with vulvovaginal candidiasis, and therapy
should be continued for 7 days.

Case

A 27-year-old woman presents to your office with a chief complaint of vaginal discharge. She is concerned that she might have an STD, although her partner is
asymptomatic.

She describes a thin, yellowish discharge over the past few weeks, which is accompanied by a fishy odor and vaginal itching. She has been sexually active for 3 months with one partner and usually uses condoms. She has no other past medical history, including no STDs. Her menstrual periods, which began at age 12, have been regular, with her most recent menses ending a few days ago. She denies fevers, chills, abdominal pain, nausea, vomiting, or diarrhea and she only takes Tylenol occasionally. Physical examination of the heart, lungs, and abdomen is normal. You proceed to the pelvic examination, where you note erythema and swelling of the labia majora and minora in addition to a mildly foul-smelling thin yellowish discharge in the vaginal vault. The cervix appears mildly erythematous. There are no lesions and no inguinal lymphadenopathy.

1. What are the main causes of vaginal discharge you are considering in this patient?
2. What workup would you perform on this patient?
3. What are the treatment options for this condition? Would you treat her partner?

Case Discussion

What Are the Main Causes of Vaginal Discharge You Are Considering in This Patient?

Given the clinical symptoms and findings on physical examination, the top two diagnoses to consider are BV and trichomoniasis. You also must consider gonorrhea and chlamydia in a young sexually active patient.

What Workup Would You Perform on This Patient?

After taking a good history and performing a physical examination (including a pelvic examination), check the pH of the vaginal discharge and perform a microscopic evaluation, as well as gonorrhea and chlamydia cultures. This patient has foul-smelling yellow discharge and evidence of cervicitis. Her wet preparation reveals clue cells and motile trichomonads.

What Are the Treatment Options for This Condition? Would You Treat Her Partner?

The most effective therapy for concurrent BV and trichomoniasis is metronidazole 500 mg twice daily for 7 days. The one-time dose of metronidazole 2 g is not as effective for BV. You must treat the partner of a patient with trichomoniasis to prevent re-infection, but you would not have to treat her partner if she only had bacterial vaginosis.

Suggested Reading

Centers for Disease Control and Prevention. Guidelines for treatment of sexually transmitted diseases. *MMWR* 1998;47(No. RR-1). Also at wonder.cdc.gov/wonder/STD/STD98TG.
Fox K, Behets F. Vaginal discharge: how to pinpoint the cause. *Postgrad Med* 1995;98:87–104.

Haefner H. Current evaluation and management of vulvovaginitis. *Clin Obstet Gynecol* 1999;42: 184–195.

Pandit L, Ouslander J. Postmenopausal vaginal atrophy and atrophic vaginitis. *Am J Med Sci* 1997;314:228–231.

Reife C. Office gynecology for the primary care physician. *Med Clin North Am* 1996;80(2):299–303.

Schaaf V K, Perez-Stable E J, Borchardt K. The limited value of symptoms and signs in the diagnosis of vaginal infections. *Arch Intern Med* 1990;150:1929–1933.

Wiesenfeld H, Macio I. The infrequent use of office-based diagnostic tests for vaginitis. *Am J Obstet Gynecol* 1999;181:39–41.

43

Breast Lump Evaluation

Judith Tsui

1. What are the most common causes of breast masses in women?
2. What are some features of a breast lump that suggest a benign versus malignant diagnosis?
3. What are the various tools available to the physician for diagnosing breast cancer in a woman with a palpable breast mass? What are the relative advantages and disadvantages of each?

Discussion

What Are the Most Common Causes of Breast Masses in Women?

The four most common causes of a breast lump are fibroadenoma, macrocyst, fibrocystic change, and breast cancer. Other less common etiologies include: abscess, lipoma, hematoma, fat necrosis, thrombophlebitis, and duct ectasia. The challenge for the evaluating physician is to exclude breast cancer from other benign causes of breast mass.

What Are Some Features of a Breast Lump that Suggest a Benign Versus Malignant Diagnosis?

Features of a breast lump that suggest malignancy are size greater than 2 cm, hardness, irregular shape, fixation to the chest wall, or nonmobility upon palpation. Calculated likelihood ratios for each of these features are modest, ranging from 1.6 to 2.4, with fixed nature and size greater than 2 cm being the most predictive. In comparison, an abnormal screening mammogram carries a likelihood ratio of 26.3 for breast cancer.

Benign breast lesions also have characteristic features. Fibroadenomas are said to feel rubbery or firm. Cysts are generally described as soft and squishy, but they may feel hard, especially when located deep within the breast tissue. Fibroadenomas are more common among young women, whereas cysts are more prevalent later in life, in the perimenopausal period. Both fibroadenomas and cysts are less commonly seen in postmenopausal women. Normal breast nodularity can be mistaken for pathologic lumps. The breast is not a homogeneous structure, but is composed of multiple glands and ducts that comprise lobes, creating a heterogeneous texture. In addition, hormonal changes during the menstrual cycle induce cell proliferation as well as alter fluid retention and vascularity, which further enhance breast texture. These are generally referred to as fibrocystic changes. It is important to differentiate a single, dominant mass from physiologic nodularity or fibrocystic changes.

What Are the Various Tools Available to the Physician for Diagnosing Breast Cancer in a Woman with a Palpable Breast Mass? What Are the Relative Advantages and Disadvantages of Each?

The currently accepted modalities for investigating a dominant breast mass include mammography, ultrasonography, fine-needle aspiration (FNA), and biopsy (either open surgical or tissue core needle). Open surgical biopsy, while being the most definitive procedure for excluding the diagnosis of breast cancer, obviously is the most invasive and potentially disfiguring. Therefore, much attention has been given to finding accurate ways to diagnose or exclude breast cancer without subjecting all patients to surgical biopsies.

In women over the age of 35, a diagnostic mammogram can provide important information both by clarifying the nature of the breast mass and by excluding clinically occult lesions in either breast. However, mammograms alone should not be used to rule out breast cancer because breast cancers may be mammographically silent. Because younger women tend to have denser breast tissue, mammography in this age group is more difficult to interpret and may be less useful. In one observational study of approximately 1,900 patients younger than 40, not a single case was found where the mammography results changed the working diagnosis. As a result, some breast centers will not use diagnostic mammograms for women under the age of 35 and may rely on ultrasonography more frequently for this patient population.

The role of ultrasonography has traditionally been viewed as similar to that of needle aspiration. Its use has been primarily to distinguish between cystic and noncystic lesions. However, the current technology has improved so that ultrasonography can provide more information, even identifying benign versus malignant features in solid lesions. It can be used to evaluate palpable lesions that are occult on mammography, or as an adjunct to mammography for following clinically benign lesions. Ultrasonography also has a role in guiding FNA or biopsy to yield better sample results.

Fine-needle aspiration is a useful component of the workup for a breast lump. The advantages of performing FNA are its cost effectiveness, ability to be performed in the outpatient setting, and the immediate results it can provide. The technique involves inserting a 22-gauge needle, either alone or attached to a syringe to provide suction, into the mass in question. In the case of a cyst, fluid is obtained and the procedure becomes therapeutic as well as diagnostic. Cyst fluid that is bloody should be sent for cytology, otherwise it is assumed to be benign and should be discarded. If the mass is solid, the needle is withdrawn and reinserted many times. Its contents are then aspirated onto a slide and fixed. Although FNA can be highly sensitive and specific in some centers, its accuracy depends on the skills of the physician performing the biopsy as well as the cytopathologist reading the results. FNA results are most useful when they confirm clinical suspicion of a benign or malignant mass. Equivocal results such as "atypical" or "suspicious" require biopsy for diagnosis. FNA also has the disadvantage of being unable to differentiate between invasive ductal carcinoma and ductal carcinoma *in situ*.

Case

A 35-year-old woman presents to your clinic complaining of a breast lump that she found while examining herself in the shower a few days ago. It is nontender, but she also relates symptoms of intermittent general breast pain, usually before her period. She also is concerned that she is able to squeeze fluid from her nipple during her breast self-examination. She is nulliparous, has no prior medical history, and is not currently taking any medications. Family history is significant only for a great aunt who had breast cancer in her seventies.

1. How do you evaluate this patient's complaints during this initial visit?
2. How do you decide what workup is most appropriate to exclude breast cancer?
3. What might be some causes for this patient's mastalgia and nipple discharge? Are treatments needed or available for these symptoms?

Case Discussion

How Do You Evaluate This Patient's Complaints During This Initial Visit?

The first step in evaluating this patient's breast lump is to take a careful history. The history should include how long the mass has been present and whether any change over time has been noted. A mass that is persistent and does not vary with menstruation should be viewed with suspicion. Any other symptoms such as breast pain, skin changes, or nipple discharge should be noted. Breast pain and nipple discharge are rarely the sole presentations for breast cancer, but are less likely to be benign in the context of a palpable breast mass. The presence of a single lump (dominant mass) is also of more concern than multiple lumps that are likely to represent fibrocystic change or normal physiologic nodularity of the breast. Risk factors for breast cancer should be addressed, but should not influence the decision to work up a breast mass further. One should bear in mind that the majority of women in whom breast cancer is diagnosed have no identifiable risk factors. Strong risk factors for breast cancer are a prior history of breast cancer or a history of a breast biopsy showing atypical hyperplasia, lobular carcinoma *in situ*, or ductal carcinoma *in situ*. Other risk factors include advanced age, strong family history, and a history of prolonged estrogen exposure (early menarche, late menopause, nulliparity, or pregnancy after the age of 30 years).

The second step in her evaluation is to perform a clinical examination of the breast. There are several standardized methods for examining the breast that are detailed elsewhere. All are based on visual inspection followed by palpation. A thorough breast examination covers the entire breast boundaries (mid-axillary line, clavicle, mid-sternum, and inferior bra line) and includes palpation for axillary and supraclavicular lymphadenopathy. It is calculated that a complete examination of both breasts should take at least 6 minutes. Many normal structures (glandular nodularity, the inframammary ridge, rib edges, etc.) can be mistaken for a breast lump, and for some patients all that is needed is reassurance. In one series of young women presenting with complaint of breast mass, only approximately 30% were confirmed by a surgeon's examination.

How Do You Decide What Workup Is Most Appropriate to Exclude Breast Cancer?

In general, the workup of a breast mass should be led by the patient's age and the level of clinical suspicion. For suspected cysts, the first step is aspiration or ultrasonographic examination. If nonbloody fluid is obtained and the mass completely resolves, no further workup is needed. However, masses that do not fully resolve or recur after drainage require further investigation. Asymptomatic simple cysts that are detected by ultrasonography can be observed. Complex cysts should undergo evaluation with aspiration. Masses that are solid should be worked up with mammograms or ultrasonography and either FNA or biopsy. For women over 40 years of age with a palpable mass, a mammogram is essential. If there is any uncertainty as to the nature of the lesion on mammogram, ultrasonography may be helpful. Women who have a clinically benign appearing lump (but not a cyst) and a benign mammogram should have an FNA to ensure a benign diagnosis. This combined use of clinical breast examination, mammography, and FNA is called the triple test. Studies have shown that concordance of all three tests for a diagnosis of a benign or malignant mass has a high degree of accuracy. When there is a discrepancy between the results, or an inconclusive result, further workup or biopsy is needed to resolve the diagnosis. For women who have clinically suspicious lesions, mammography and biopsy should be directly performed because a benign FNA in the face of a suspicious breast examination would be inadequate to rule out breast cancer.

Managing breast lumps in young women can be especially challenging. Although women under age 35 have the lowest rate of breast cancer, they comprise the largest percentage of office visits for breast complaints and constitute the majority of malpractice suits. Young women who have clinically suspicious lesions should be treated in the same fashion as older women. Young women with clinically benign appearing lesions may be evaluated with a modified triple test (clinical breast examination, ultrasonography, and FNA), which has been reported to have accuracy similar to that of the triple test. For very young women (<30) who have had unsuspicious lesions for less than 1 month, observation alone is felt to be adequate by some experts.

In general, review of breast cancer cases shows that most errors in management usually occur in cases where the physician places too much confidence in a single test (e.g., not referring a woman with a palpable mass for further workup because of a normal mammogram). Management of a breast mass also may depend on the patient's wishes and her level of anxiety. Some women may want the reassurance of immediate open surgical biopsy rather than undergoing tests that may yield inconclusive results. Throughout the process, it is important that the physician maintain good communication with the patient because this has been shown to not only reduce immediate anxiety, but impact the patient's psychological well-being months later. The workup of a breast mass should be completed in a timely manner. Given that the tumor doubling time is approximately 260 days, it is reasonable to expect that the workup should be completed within a minimum of 90 days.

For the patient in this case, your workup would depend considerably on what you detected on physical examination. If no dominant mass was palpated, you might reassure the patient and encourage her to continue to do monthly breast self-examinations coupled with your yearly clinical examination. If the mass felt like a cyst, you could aspirate it in the office, or send the patient for an untrasound to confirm the presence of a cyst. If the mass was of an unclear nature but did not have suspicious features, referral for an ultrasound (because of her age) and FNA is a reasonable approach. For a frankly suspicious lesion, ordering mammography and referring for excisional biopsy is the most prudent course of action. Her only risk factor is her nulliparity; her family history of breast cancer is too remote to influence her risk.

What Might Be Some Causes for This Patient's Periodic Mastalgia and Nipple Discharge? Are Treatments Needed or Available for These Symptoms?

Breast pain is a common complaint; estimates for lifetime prevalence range from 41% to 69%. Up to one third of women report symptoms so severe as to interfere with the activities of daily living. The exact etiology for cyclic mastalgia has not been established. A hormonal cause is presumed given its association with the premenstrual phase and improvement with menopause. Elevated prolactin levels have been implicated; an increased prolactin response to thyrotropin-releasing hormone has been observed in patients with breast pain. Abnormal fatty acid profiles also have been noted in women with cyclic mastalgia and is the basis for treatment with evening primrose oil. Mastalgia can be part of a constellation of symptoms defined as premenstrual syndrome, or may be the sole complaint. Cyclic mastalgia has been defined as moderate to severe pain (>4 out of 10 on a visual analogue scale) for greater than 5 days. Medical treatment should be reserved for patients with severe symptoms for at least 6 months, because many patients' symptoms may resolve spontaneously. For mild symptoms, behavior modification such as limiting intake of caffeine may be useful. Wearing a well-fitting brassiere has been shown to improve symptoms. Evening primrose oil that is high in the essential fatty acid γ-linolenic acid has been reported to be effective. Unfortunately, at therapeutic doses (1,500 mg twice daily) the treatment can be quite costly and take up to 4 months to be effective. Oral contraceptive pills may be of some benefit, but medroxyprogesterone alone has not been shown to be effective. Medical therapies that have proven benefit are danazol, bromocriptine, and tamoxifen. However, given the multiple side effects, their use should be restricted to patients with severe intractable symptoms. Danazol has been shown to be effective even when given in the luteal phase only, thus reducing its side effects (masculinization, osteoporosis). Danazol is the only treatment for cyclical mastalgia approved by the U.S. Food and Drug Administration; it is dosed at 200 mg a day on days 14 through 28 of the menstrual cycle.

Nipple discharge is also a common breast complaint in the outpatient setting. It is rarely a presentation for breast cancer. Discharge that is unilateral, spontaneous, originates from one duct, and is serous or bloody is more likely to be pathologic. Patients with a pathologic discharge should be referred for mammography and then for nipple duct exploration. Sending nipple discharge fluid for cytology is rarely useful. Even in cases of suspicious discharge, only 10% to 15% of these are caused by breast cancer; most often they are attributed to intraductal papillomas and duct ectasia, which are both essentially benign conditions. Discharge that is mechanically expressed and bilateral is likely normal. Many women are capable of expressing discharge from their breasts with mechanical stimulation. Thus, in most cases all that is needed is reassurance and instruction not to stimulate the breasts further. Spontaneous bilateral discharge (galactorrhea) is usually caused by abnormal prolactin secretion that may be secondary to drugs (phenothiazines, opiates, etc) or prolactin-secreting tumors (pituitary adenoma).

This patient's complaint of periodic breast pain prior to menstruation is likely cyclic mastalgia secondary to hormonal changes. If her symptoms are very mild, you may just need to reassure her. If her symptoms are more severe, you would probably want to try interventions with few side effects, such as evening primrose oil and wearing a well-fitting brassiere. If she is not trying to become pregnant, you can prescribe oral contraceptive pills. If she has more severe symptoms that affect her quality of life, you may want to treat her with danazol. Her discharge is likely secondary to mechanical stimulation. If it is spontaneous or bloody you should refer her to a breast specialist. Otherwise, simply requesting that she refrain from expressing her breasts should take care of the problem. She does not take any medicines that can be blamed, nor does she have any other systemic complaints that might suggest an underlying medical cause for galactorrhea.

Suggested Reading

Barton M, Harris R, Fletcher S. Does this patient have breast cancer? *JAMA* 1999;282:1270–1280.

Hansen N, Morrow M. Breast disease. *Med Clin North Am* 1998;82:203–223.

Hindle W H et al. Clinical value of mammograms for symptomatic women 35 years of age and younger. *Am J Obstet Gynecol* 1999;180:1484–1490.

Holland P and Gately C. Drug tharpy of mastalgia. *Drugs* 1994;48:709–716.

Morrow M et al. Evaluation of breast masses in women younger than 40 years of age. *Surgery* 1998;124:634–641.

Scott S, Morrow M. Breast cancer: making the diagnosis. *Surg Clin North Am* 1999;79:991–1005.

Steinbrun B, Zera R, Rodriguez J. Mastalgia. *Postgrad Med* 1997;102:183–198.

44
Abnormal Uterine Bleeding
Linda J. Schultz

Discussion

How Do You Distinguish Between Ovulatory and Anovulatory Bleeding?

The first step in evaluating the complaint of abnormal uterine bleeding is to determine what type of bleeding has occurred, ovulatory or anovulatory. The differential diagnosis and approach to the evaluation and treatment of the bleeding can then be tailored. To review, ovulation occurs after the proliferative phase of the menstrual cycle. During this time, luteinizing hormone (LH) and follicle-stimulating hormone (FSH) increase the level of estrogen until a mid-cycle LH surge occurs, resulting in ovulation. In the second half of the cycle, the secretory phase, progesterone increases the lining of the edometrium. If pregnancy does not occur, the corpus luteum regresses and menstruation follows.

Ovulatory bleeding occurs at regular intervals and is usually preceded by premenstrual symptoms (e.g., breast tenderness, weight gain, cramping, and mood swings). Anovulatory bleeding occurs at irregular intervals. If the patient does not know the interval between her menstrual periods or reports both regular and irregular intervals, there are several different tools to help determine if the bleeding is ovulatory or anovulatory.

One tool is the daily basal body temperature chart. After ovulation, progesterone produced by the corpus luteum causes the basal body temperature to rise by roughly 0.3° to 0.6°C. Because this change is subtle, it can be seen only by careful compliance with the chart. The patient takes her temperature with a basal body thermometer at the same time each day, preferably before getting out of bed each morning, and records the measurement on the temperature chart. If a basal body chart cannot be performed, a patient can create a menstrual calendar over several months to chart the degree of menstrual regularity.

Other methods to determine if ovulation has occurred include measuring a serum progesterone level 7 days before the next expected menstrual period. If the level is greater than 9.5 n*M* (3 ng/mL), then ovulation has occurred. An endometrial biopsy also can be performed at the onset of bleeding, and if any secretory changes are found, ovulation has occurred.

How Do You Evaluate and Treat Menorrhagia?

Menorrhagia, defined as prolonged menstrual periods occurring at regular intervals, is diagnosed by a detailed menstrual history. The diagnosis is usually made based on subjective data because it is not practical to actually measure the amount of blood loss in pads or tampons. Although no pathology is found in the majority of women, possible causes of menorrhagia include an inherited coagulopathy, liver disease, hypothyroidism, and structural lesions in the uterus. These causes can be ruled out by a careful history and physical examination, including an assessment of the size and shape of the uterus. Depending on the scenario, the laboratory evaluation should include a complete blood count, including platelets, prothrombin time, partial thromboplastin time, von Willebrand antigen level, and thyroid stimulating hormone (TSH) level. Adolescents with menorrhagia or anyone with new petechiae or bruising need a coagulopathy evaluation. A hematocrit is generally the most objective measurement to follow to assess the degree of bleeding.

If the physical and laboratory findings are normal, the patient can be reassured and treated medically. If the patient has mild anemia, she also can be treated medically. There are multiple options for medical treatment, but the first line of medical treatment includes nonsteroidal antiinflammatory drugs (NSAIDs) and oral contraceptive pills (OCPs). NSAIDs have been shown to reduce bleeding by 20% to 50%. They work by altering intrauterine prostaglandins, which in turn causes vasoconstriction and increases platelet aggregation. The NSAIDs should be taken on the first day of bleeding for each cycle and continued until the bleeding stops. A second option for treatment is OCPs, which reduce bleeding by 50%. They are a good choice if the patient is interested in contraception. Another option, medroxyprogesterone, can be given every month on days 16 to 25 of the cycle, at 10 mg per day. Oral progesterone was used more in the past but now trials have shown that it is significantly less effective than danazol or intrauterine progesterone. There is also a strong trend in favor of NSAIDs over progesterone in the trials. Danazol, a synthetic steroid derived from testosterone, decreases the estrogen level. This causes atrophy of the endometrium by suppressing ovulation and inhibiting release and synthesis of LH and FSH. Danazol's androgenic side effects (e.g., hirsutism, weight gain, acne, irritability, and decreased libido) make the drug poorly tolerated. The gonadotropin releasing hormone (GnRH) analogues can be used to place the patient in a temporary menopause, but the associated increased risk for osteoporosis limits its use.

Patients should be referred to a gynecologist when they have severe anemia, a structural lesion in the uterus, or when the above medications are not tolerated or are not effective. Before proceeding to a hysterectomy, there are other options for the patient. Progesterone or levonorgestrel intrauterine devices can be inserted in the uterus. The progesterone device decreased bleeding by 65% at 1 year, whereas the levonorgestrel device decreased bleeding by 90% at 1 year. Several new surgical techniques to remove the endometrial lining have been developed to prevent or prolong the time to hysterectomy. These new techniques include laser photovaporization, electrocautery ablation with a loop or roller ball, transcervical resection of the endometrium, and radiofrequency ablation.

How Do You Evaluate and Treat Intermenstrual Bleeding?

Intermenstrual bleeding, defined as bleeding that occurs between periods, is diagnosed by a detailed menstrual history. Pregnancy must be ruled out because the bleeding could represent an ectopic pregnancy or trophoblastic disease. Other causes include OCP use, drug interactions with OCPs, uterine fibroids or polyps, vaginal or cervical lacerations, cervicitis (especially from *Trichomonas* or *Chlamydia*), and cervical or endometrial cancer. Most of these causes can be found on a careful history and pelvic examination, including a Papanicolaou (Pap) smear and cervical cultures. If the patient is postmenopausal (by history or FSH level >40 IU) or if the patient is over age 35, then an endometrial biopsy should be performed to rule out endometrial cancer.

If the pregnancy test is positive, the patient needs an immediate evaluation for a possible ectopic pregnancy or spontaneous abortion. If no etiology is found or if a structural lesion is suspected, refer to a gynecologist for a hysteroscopy to look for fibroids and polyps.

How Do You Evaluate and Treat Anovulatory Bleeding?

Anovulatory bleeding occurs at irregular intervals. The differential diagnosis is extensive and includes pregnancy, menopause, and several medications or drugs (e.g., OCPs, tricyclic antidepressants, metoclopramide, and heroin). Several endocrinopathies such as hypothyroidism, hypercorticolism, hyperprolactinemia, and hyperandrogenism can interfere with ovulation, as can chronic hepatic and renal disease. Polycystic ovarian syndrome is a common cause of anovulation. Vigorous exercise, strict dieting, and stressful life situations can all temporarily interrupt ovulation. A careful history and physical examination focusing on the above conditions can rule out many of these diseases. The laboratory evaluation should include a pregnancy test, complete blood count, TSH, and prolactin level.

If no abnormality is found, then the patient should be treated for dysfunctional uterine bleeding, defined as anovulatory bleeding unrelated to any structural or systemic disease after a normal history, physical, and laboratory evaluation. Dysfunctional uterine bleeding is most common at adolescence and during the perimenopausal period. When deciding how to further evaluate and treat dysfunctional uterine bleeding, it helps to divide the patients by age group.

The adolescent can have several years of anovulatory bleeding prior to ovulatory bleeding. This occurs because the hypothalamic-pituitary-ovarian axis is immature and there is no mid-cycle surge of LH. Without the LH surge there is continuous estrogen stimulation to the endometrium. When the estrogen level decreases spontaneously, there is heavy and prolonged bleeding, usually at intervals of 22 to 45 days. Treatment options include OCPs or progesterone alone. OCPs are continued for 3 to 6 months then stopped to watch for ovulatory bleeding to occur. Medroxy-progesterone can be given at 10 mg per day for 10 to 12 days of the cycle each month. It should be tried for 3 to 6 months then stopped, and the patient monitored for ovulatory bleeding. If anovulatory bleeding continues despite this treatment, then refer to a gynecologist.

During a woman's reproductive years, a few episodes of anovulatory bleeding can occur, but they are usually followed by ovulatory cycles that restart and continue. Some women have chronic anovulation. The treatment is OCPs or medroxyprogesterone in the same format as described for the adolescent. If the patient has anovulatory bleeding for more than 1 year, then an endometrial biopsy must be performed to rule out endometrial cancer from the chronic unopposed estrogen. If the biopsy results are adenomatous hyperplasia or proliferative changes, then treatment should be continued and the biopsy repeated in 3 months. If the biopsy results are atypical hyperplasia or cancer, refer to a gynecologist.

In perimenopausal women, the ovary becomes less sensitive to FSH and LH, and less estrogen is produced. The high level of estrogen needed to induce the LH surge is not reached, so there is no ovulation and no progesterone is produced. Continuous estrogen production stimulates the endometrium until it outgrows its blood supply, becomes necrotic, and sheds. Although this type of perimenopausal bleeding is common, there is still a 30% incidence of significant pathology, and an endometrial biopsy is essential to the evaluation. As before, if the biopsy reveals cancer or atypical hyperplasia, then refer the patient to a gynecologist. If the biopsy reveals proliferative changes or a combination of proliferative and secretory changes, then the bleeding can be treated with OCPs or medroxyprogesterone. OCPs can be used in this age group if the patient does not have hypertension or use tobacco. They are actually a good choice, because they will serve as birth control at a time when there may still be intermittent ovulation. OCPs can be continued up until menopause, at which time the patient can be changed over to hormone replacement therapy if appropriate. To help determine when menopause has occurred, check the FSH level on day 6 or 7 of the placebo pills; if it is greater than 40 IU/L, then ovarian failure has occurred and the patient is in menopause. Cyclic medroxyprogesterone can be used until there is no further withdrawal bleeding, at which time the patient can be changed over to hormone replacement therapy if she chooses. Hormone replacement therapy can only be used initially if the biopsy shows atrophic changes.

Postmenopausal bleeding must be evaluated to rule out endometrial cancer. The risk factors for endometrial cancer include obesity, nulliparity, early menarche/late menopause, chronic anovulation, and a history of high-dose estrogen. If the patient is not on HRT, then an endometrial biopsy should be performed and the patient should be referred if cancer or atypical hyperplasia is found. If the patient is on continuous HRT, then she can have abnormal bleeding for several months. If the bleeding continues after 6 months to a year, then an endometrial biopsy should be performed. The patient on cyclic HRT will continue to bleed regularly; therefore, an endometrial biopsy should be performed if the bleeding occurs off schedule or if the amount of bleeding changes. The most common type of endometrial biopsy is the Pipelle biopsy, which is easy to perform, well tolerated, and has a 96% to 97% sensitivity. Some studies have combined transvaginal ultrasonography with the endometrial biopsy to evaluate for endometrial cancer in perimenopausal and postmenopausal women. A thin endometrium (<5 mm by ultrasonography) has been shown to indicate a decreased risk of significant pathology. However, this is controversial because endometrial cancer has been found in endometria less than 4 mm thick, and the ultrasonographic report depends on the ability of the person performing and reading the ultrasonogram. If ultrasonography shows a thickness of less than 5 mm and the biopsy is negative for cancer, then no further evaluation is needed. If ultrasonography shows a thick endometrium and the biopsy is negative, then refer to a gynecologist for a hysteroscopy. The patient also should be referred to a gynecologist if the biopsy cannot be performed due to cervical stenosis or any other cause.

Case

The patient is a 48-year-old woman who reports that over the past 6 to 9 months her periods have been irregular and she has missed months completely. She has recorded the bleeding on a calendar and brings this to the office. She no longer has breast tenderness or bloating prior to her bleeding. She reports a past history of regular periods except for a 2-year time span of irregular bleeding, but she cannot remember what treatment, if any, she received. She does remember that her period started at the early age of 11. The patient is sexually active with one partner and has no history of sexually transmitted diseases. She has had one child without complications. She complains of fatigue and mild constipation, but denies any other problems. She also denies any recent diets or new exercise routines. The patient denies any significant past history and has no family history of breast or endometrial cancer.

Her physical examination reveals an overweight female. She has no thyromegaly. Abdominal examination shows a soft, obese, and nontender abdomen. She has a normal-appearing vulva, vagina, and cervix. The uterus is normal in size and nontender. The ovaries are of normal size and there are no adnexal masses.

1. What type of bleeding is the patient having?
2. What workup should be performed next?
3. What treatment should be started?

Case Discussion
What Type of Bleeding Is the Patient Having?

The irregularity of the bleeding, based on her calendar, and lack of premenstrual symptoms suggests anovulatory bleeding. She is also 48 years old, making anovulatory bleeding due to a perimenopausal state the most likely diagnosis.

What Workup Should Be Performed Next?

Although the differential for anovulatory bleeding is long, most of the causes can be ruled out by her history. Her physical examination is normal at this time. Laboratory test results, including a pregnancy test, complete blood count, TSH, and prolactin, are in the normal range. Results of a Pap smear performed during her pelvic examination were also normal. An endometrial biopsy should be performed in this patient because she has anovulatory bleeding and multiple risk factors for endometrial cancer, including obesity, early menarche, low parity, and a history of episodes of anovulation. An endometrial biopsy is performed, and proliferative changes are found, but the results are negative for cancer or atypical hyperplasia.

What Treatment Should Be Started?

Treatment options for her include OCPs or cyclic progesterone. You discuss the pros and cons of both treatments with her and she decides to take cyclic medroxy-progesterone. Because she has the risk factors for endometrial cancer, her pattern of bleeding will need to be followed closely for any changes.

Suggested Reading

Bayar S R, DeCherney A H. Clinical manifestations and treatment of dysfunctional uterine bleeding. *JAMA* 1993;269:1823–1828.

Stirrat G M. Choice of treatment for menorrhagia. *Lancet* 1999;353:2175–2176.

Stovall T G, Photopulos G J, et al. Pipelle endometrial sampling in patients with known endometrial carcinoma. *Obstet Gynecol* 1991;77:954–956.

Van den Bosch T, Vandendael A, et al. Combining vaginal ultrasonography and office endometrial sampling in the diagnosis of endometrial disease in postmenopausal women. *Obstet Gynecol* 1995;85:349–352.

Wathen P I, Henderson M C, Witz C A. Abnormal uterine bleeding. *Med Clin North Am* 1995;79:329–342.

45

Hormone Replacement Therapy

Joyce P. Doyle

1. How is menopause diagnosed?
2. What are the indications for hormone replacement therapy?
3. What are the contraindications for hormone replacement therapy?
4. What assessment is indicated prior to prescribing hormone replacement therapy?
5. What are options for prescribing hormone replacement therapy?
6. Is there a role for selective estrogen receptor modulators (e.g., raloxifene)?

Discussion

How Is Menopause Diagnosed?

Natural menopause occurs after the permanent cessation of ovarian follicular cell activity. It is generally defined as the absence of menses for greater than 6 months to 1 year for which there is no other cause (e.g., pregnancy). On average, menopause occurs at 51 years of age, and over 90% of women have undergone menopause by age 55. The most common associated symptoms surrounding menopause include menstrual irregularities, vasomotor symptoms such as hot flashes and day or night sweats, and vaginal dryness. Other symptoms, such as insomnia and irritability, are often attributed to menopause, but the association is less clear. Serum elevation of the pituitary hormone follicle-stimulating hormone (FSH) above 40 IU/L is consistent with estrogen deficiency and can be used to confirm menopause in women who have had a hysterectomy or whose history is atypical.

What Are the Indications for Hormone Replacement Therapy?

The only two clear indications for HRT are treatment of vasomotor symptoms related to menopause (e.g., hot flashes) and prevention of osteoporosis. HRT should not be prescribed for these or any other reason without review of its potential risks and benefits. Its use for cardioprotection has recently become highly controversial due to the results of the first randomized, placebo-controlled trial on HRT use, the Heart and Estrogen-Progestin Replacement Study (HERS). In the HERS trial, HRT was associated with increased coronary risk among women with established coronary disease. This is in conflict with multiple observational studies in which women who used HRT had a 35% to 55% lower cardiovascular risk than nonusers. One frequently cited explanation for these contradictory results is that the observational (nonrandomized) studies are biased in favor of HRT because healthier women are more likely to use HRT and lead healthful life-styles.

Although estrogen may favorably affect the overall lipid profile by lowering the low-density lipoprotein (LDL) cholesterol fraction and increasing the high-density lipoprotein (HDL) fraction, HRT is not an accepted treatment for dyslipidemia. Drugs with documented effectiveness (e.g., statins) should be used. The addition of a progestin to estrogen blunts some of estrogen's beneficial effect on LDL and HDL.

Estrogen elevates triglycerides and should be avoided in patients with hypertriglyceridemia. Preliminary data suggest HRT may have a protective effect against Alzheimer dementia and colorectal cancer. Further study in this area is needed.

What Are the Contraindications to Hormone Replacement Therapy?

The following are contraindications to HRT based on the 1997 recommendation of the American College of Obstetrics and Gynecology (ACOG):

- Known or suspected pregnancy
- Unexplained vaginal bleeding
- Active or chronic liver disease
- Recent vascular thrombosis with or without embolus
- Current therapy for carcinoma of the breast or endometrium

In 1999, the American College of Cardiology and American Heart Association added the following recommendations:

- Do not initiate HRT in older postmenopausal women with confirmed coronary heart disease
- In women with existing coronary heart disease who have been taking HRT longer than 1 year, it is reasonable to continue, pending further data.

Relative contraindications to HRT use include:

- Gallbladder disease
- Hypertriglyceridemia
- Migraine headaches
- Seizure disorder
- Personal history of thromboembolic disease
- Family history of breast cancer or uterine leiomyomas

What Assessment Is Indicated Prior to Prescribing Hormone Replacement Therapy?

Prior to prescribing HRT, the provider must confirm that the history or other findings are consistent with menopause (e.g., FSH > 40 IU/L). After an assessment of absolute and relative contraindications, a discussion of the risks and benefits of HRT must occur. A physical examination should include a breast and pelvic examination, and mammography results should be negative for evidence of malignancy.

What Are Options for Prescribing Hormone Replacement Therapy?

The basics of HRT include prescribing estrogen daily. In women with an intact uterus, a progestin must be added to prevent endometrial hyperplasia, a precursor to endometrial cancer. When adding a progestin, there are two major options: continuous daily or cyclic (days 1 to 14 each month). The major consideration for choosing a progestin regimen is withdrawal bleeding. When a daily progestin is used, bleeding will be unpredictable for the first 6 months of use. In women who have recently entered menopause, the bleeding can be heavy. Use of a cyclic progestin regimen will lead to predictable bleeding once per month, similar to menses, beginning day 6 of the cycle.

What Is the Role of the Selective Estrogen Receptor Modulators (e.g., Raloxifene)?

Raloxifene belongs to a new category of drugs called selective estrogen receptor modulators (SERMS). Raloxifene has estrogenic effects on bone and lipids, and an anti-estrogen effect on breast and uterine tissue, and may be protective against breast and endometrial cancer. It has recently been approved for use in osteoporosis prevention because it appears to increase bone mineral density in the spine, hip, and total body, although less so than estrogen or alendronate. Raloxifene decreases LDL cholesterol with no change in HDL cholesterol or triglycerides. A large clinical trial is underway to see if it decreases cardiovascular morbidity and mortality. Raloxifene may provoke menopausal symptoms, due to its antiestrogen effect, and imparts a small but significant increased risk for venous thromboembolism, due to its estrogenic effects.

Case

A 50-year-old white woman presents to your office for a health maintenance examination. She has no known medical problem, but had a hysterectomy 10 years ago for fibroids. She offers no complaints, has no drug allergies, and takes no medications. She has never smoked, and drinks one alcoholic beverage weekly. Her mother died of a myocardial infarction at age 75, and her father died from prostate cancer. On physical examination she weighs 124 pounds and is 5 feet 7 inches tall. Blood pressure is 138/68 mm Hg, pulse rate is 70 beats/min. The rest of her examination is unremarkable, other than for a midline pelvic scar. On further questioning she reports some recent irritability and hot flashes for the past 4 months and wonders if she is going through menopause. She has heard about hormone replacement and wants to know if she should consider it.

1. Has this patient begun menopause?
2. How do you systematically counsel a patient regarding hormone replacement therapy?
3. How would you prescribe hormone replacement therapy in this patient?

Case Discussion

Has This Patient Begun Menopause?

The patient's age and clinical history of vasomotor symptoms are suggestive of menopause. Because she has had a hysterectomy, absence of menses does not assist you in making the diagnosis. To confirm menopause you could order a serum FSH level. A value of greater than 40 IU/L is consistent with menopause. In her case, the FSH level was 52 IU/L, consistent with menopause.

How Do You Systematically Counsel a Patient Regarding Hormone Replacement Therapy?

Counseling a patient on the risks and benefits of HRT is complex. A systematic approach is best, and the use of patient education materials may help. Factors that will assist you and the patient in deciding whether to begin HRT include the severity of her menopausal symptoms and her risk for osteoporosis. A family history of bony fractures, loss of height, or kyphoscoliosis would be helpful, but you can assume this patient is already at high risk for osteoporosis because she is white and thin. Table 45.1 lists the risks and benefits of HRT, which should be reviewed with the patient.

Table 45.1. Postmenopausal Hormone Replacement Therapy

Benefits	
Menopausal symptoms (e.g., hot flashes)	Very effective
Osteoporosis	Decreases fracture risk with long-term use
Cholesterol	Decreases LDL, increases HDL
Heart disease	May prevent heart disease by up to 50%
Alzheimer dementia	May prevent by up to 30%
Colorectal cancer	May reduce by up to 60%
Risks	
Heart disease	May be dangerous to start HRT in women with existing heart disease
Triglycerides	Increases triglycerides
Breast cancer	<5 years of use: no clear increased risk
	≥5 years of use: may be 30% increased risk
Uterine cancer	Two- to tenfold increase with unopposed estrogen
	No increased risk with use of a progestin
Venous thromboembolism	Threefold increase overall, higher risk in older women (1 in 250 per year)
Gallbladder disease	Increased by 40% in older women
Common side effects	
Estrogen	Breast tenderness, nausea, headaches
Progesterone	Depressed mood, irritability

LDL, low-density lipoprotein; HDL, high-density lipoprotein; HRT, hormone replacement therapy.

How Would You Prescribe Hormone Replacement Therapy in This Patient?

Because this patient does not have an intact uterus, she could begin daily estrogen at hormone replacement dosages. She does not need the addition of a progestin. If her menopausal symptoms are severe, you may double the dose temporarily and then return to the standard dosage.

How Would You Prescribe HRT if She Had Not Had a Hysterectomy?

If she had an intact uterus, because she is recently menopausal the addition of a cyclic progesterone (days 1 to 12 or 14) generally would be preferable. She is likely to have heavy, erratic bleeding with a daily progestin.

Suggested Reading

Col N F, Eckman M H, Karas R H, et al. Patient-specific decisions about hormone replacement therapy in post menopausal women. *JAMA* 1997;277:1140–1147.

Hulley S, Grady D, Bush T, et al. Randomized trial of estrogen plus progestin for secondary prevention of coronary heart disease in post menopausal women. *JAMA* 1998;280:605–613.

Mosca L, Grundy S M, Judelson D, et al. AHA/ACC scientific statement: consensus panel statement. Guide to preventive cardiology for women. *J Am Col Cardiol* 1993;33:1751–1755.

Khovidhunkit W, Shoback D M. Clinical effects of raloxifene hydrochloride in women. *Ann Intern Med* 1999;130:431–439.

McNagny S E. Prescribing hormone replacement therapy for menopausal symptoms. *Ann Intern Med* 1999;131:605–616.

National Women's Health Information Center website: www.4woman.org.

46
Contraception

Susan Borys

1. What are the various types of contraception that are currently available in the United States, and how are they categorized?
2. How are contraception failure rates reported and what are typical rates for each method?
3. Discuss the mechanism of action, as well as the health benefits and health risks, of each hormonal method of contraception.

Discussion

What Are the Various Types of Contraception Currently Available in the United States and How Are They Categorized?

Methods of contraception can be categorized as reversible and irreversible. Reversible methods can further be categorized as episodic and continual. Episodic contraceptive methods are used only during coitus and include condoms, spermicides, sponges, diaphragms, and cervical caps. Continual contraception includes oral contraceptives (combination or progestin only), levonorgestrel subdermal implants, injectable medroxyprogesterone acetate, and intrauterine devices (IUDs). Irreversible methods of contraception are the most prevalent methods chosen by couples in the United States (39%) and include tubal sterilization and vasectomy.

Withdrawal, or coitus interruptus, is still widely practiced in this country, especially among teenagers in their first year of becoming sexually active. Periodic abstinence, or the rhythm method, is practiced among couples of certain religious groups.

How Are Contraception Failure Rates Reported and What Are Typical Rates for Each Method?

Failure rates are reported as the number of accidental births per 100 couples in their first year of contraception use. The perfect use failure rate is failure inherent in the contraceptive alone if used perfectly. The typical use failure rate takes into account inaccuracies in the patients' uses. The reported failure rates for each method are outlined in Table 46.1.

Table 46.1. Contraceptive Failure Rates

Method	Perfect Use Failure	Typical Use Failure
No method	85%	85%
Periodic abstinence	9%	20%
Withdrawal	4%	18%
Spermicide alone	6%	21%
Male condom (latex)	3%	12%
Female condom	5%	21%
Sponge	11% (20% if parous)	18% (28% if parous)
Diaphragm + spermicide	6%	18%
Cervical cap + spermicide	11% (26% if parous)	18%
IUD	0.6%–1.5%	0.8%–2%
Oral contraceptive (combined)	0.1%	3%
Oral progesterone	0.5%	3%
Injectable progesterone	0.3%	0.3%
Levonorgestrel implants	0.04%	0.04%
Tubal ligation	0.2%	0.4%
Vasectomy	0.1%	0.15%

Adapted from Choice of contraception. *Med Lett* 1995;37:9–12; with permission.

Discuss the Mechanism of Action as Well as the Health Benefits and Health Risks of Each Hormonal Method of Contraception.

Combination oral contraceptive pills (OCPs) are the second most commonly used form of contraception (27%). OCPs work by suppressing pituitary gonadotropin secretion and preventing ovulation. The progestin component of OCPs causes changes in the cervical mucus and endometrium that enhance the antifertility effect of the OCPs should ovulation occur. There are substantial benefits to the use of these formulations apart from that of contraception. Women taking OCPs report more predictable and regular periods as well as reduced symptoms of dysmenorrhea and premenstrual dysphoria. A reduction in the amount and length of flow of menses leads to an increase in iron stores in women with iron deficiency associated with menorrhagia. OCPs also can prevent endometrial hyperplasia in women with abnormal bleeding caused by chronic anovulation. Benign breast disease, including fibroadenoma and cystic changes, occur less frequently with the use of OCPs. The incidence of pelvic inflammatory disease is reduced by OCP use, probably owing to its effects on cervical mucus and to decreased retrograde menstruation. Because OCPs prevent ovulation, ectopic pregnancies are rare and occur 500-fold less often than in women using no contraceptive method. Worldwide studies have consistently found that OCP use is associated with an approximately 40% reduced risk of malignant as well as borderline epithelial ovarian cancer. The protective effect increases with duration of use, so that women who have used OCPs for a decade or more experience an 80% risk reduction. The protection appears to last up to 19 years after discontinuation of the pill. The use of OCPs for 1 year or more also has been associated with a 50% reduced risk of endometrial adenocarcinoma. This protection appears to persist up to 12 years following discontinuation.

Oral contraceptive pills are also associated with side effects and certain health risks. Estrogenic side effects of OCPs are nausea, bloating, and breast tenderness.

Increased weight, acne, depression, and fatigue are possible progestin side effects. Some women have reported an increased incidence of migraine headaches while on OCPs. In addition, an increase in blood pressure has been noted, especially in the first 3 months of contraceptive use. Altered lipid metabolism can occur. Although estrogen increases high-density lipoprotein (HDL) cholesterol, the overall effect may be increased low-density lipoprotein (LDL) cholesterol and a lower HDL cholesterol owing to the progestin component. In obese women, marked increases in triglycerides have been noted. Although the risk for venous thromboembolism has been a much debated topic, especially in newer generation OCPs, combination OCPs with ethinyl estradiol levels of less than 50 μg are thought to pose only a slightly increased risk of venous thromboembolism regardless of the progestin chosen. Another area of controversy is that of OCP use and risk of cervical and breast cancers. There may be an increase in the risk of cervical cancer in current users and within 10 years after use ceases. The risk of breast cancer in younger women also may be slightly increased as well.

Depot medroxyprogesterone acetate (DMPA) (Depo-Provera, Pharmacia & Upjohn, Peapack, NJ) is the only injectable contraceptive in the United States and is gaining in popularity. It is given as an injection of 150 mg of medroxyprogesterone every 3 months. The initial injection is usually given within 5 days of the onset of menses. Its mechanism of action is to inhibit the secretion of gonadotropins, which in turn prevents follicular maturation and ovulation. The health benefits of DMPA include an even greater reduction of endometrial cancer than is found with OCP use. Also noted is a reduced seizure frequency in women with seizure disorders. Like OCPs, DMPA is associated with decreased premenstrual symptoms and a reduced risk of pelvic inflammatory disease. Although bleeding abnormalities with DMPA are common at initiation of therapy, amenorrhea with resultant increased iron stores usually ensues. The irregular and unpredictable menstrual bleeding is the most troublesome side effect of DMPA, and patients should be counseled on this prior to starting this medication. Headaches, bloating, fatigue, reduced libido, and weight gain are other potential side effects. Depression is a reported side effect of DMPA that has recently been disputed. The most noteworthy health risk of DMPA is that of decreased bone density. This does tend to be reversible with discontinuation, however. Rare hypospadias in male fetuses and low-birth-weight infants are risks of DMPA use during pregnancy.

Levonorgestrel subdermal implants (Norplant System, Wyeth-Ayerst, Philadelphia, PA) are composed of six Silastic capsules containing 36 mg of crystalline levonorgestrel that is steadily diffused into the circulation. Circulating progestin levels are sufficient to prevent ovulation in most women using implants. In some women, however, ovulatory activity continues to occur, especially in later years of Levonorgestral subdermal implant use. These women may still get what they perceive as a normal menstrual flow. Luteal insufficiency and impaired oocyte maturation, as well as hostile cervical mucus, usually prevents fertilization in these cases. These women do have an increased pregnancy rate and should have a pregnancy test should they become amenorrheal. Side effects and health risks include initial menstrual irregularities, headaches, and rare idiopathic intracranial hypertension. Some women using these implants develop ovarian cysts. These can cause abdominal discomfort but are usually asymptomatic. Local skin damage and keloid formation may cause pain with removal of implants. One potential benefit of using Levonorgestral subdermal implants is that, unlike DMPA, return to fertility is rapid. Reestablishment of fertility may take up to 18 months with DMPA.

Case

A 22-year-old woman presents for a routine Papanicolaou smear and pelvic examination. She will be getting married soon and wishes to discuss contraception. She has no major illnesses, but does have mild acne. Her gynecologic history reveals that she had menarche at age 12 years. She currently menstruates every 25 to 35 days, and her periods last 5 to 7 days. She admits to premenstrual dysphoria, breast tenderness, fluid retention, and moderate cramping with menses. She also occasionally gets headaches with her periods. She has one partner and has never been pregnant. She has never used contraception other than condoms or withdrawal. She has been considering oral contraception but is concerned about cancer. She is on no medications except for multivitamins. Her social history is significant for tobacco use of three to four cigarettes per day. Results of her physical examination, including pelvic examination, are normal. Her urine pregnancy test result is negative.

1. How would you choose an oral contraceptive pill and what specific advice would you give this patient prior to starting these?
2. Suppose the patient returns to your office in 3 months with complaints of "breakthrough bleeding." How would you manage this?
3. What is "emergency contraception" and is it appropriate for this patient?

Case Discussion

How Would You Choose an Oral Contraceptive Pill and What Specific Advice Would You Give This Patient Prior to Starting These?

Because this patient has no contraindication to estrogen (breast cancer, breast-feeding, heavy smoker, smoker or diabetic patient over the age of 35, diabetic patient with vascular disease, known risk or history of thromboembolism, hypertension, headaches exacerbated by estrogen, or active liver disease), she can be prescribed a combination OCP. Combination OCPs usually contain 20 to 50 μg of estradiol or mestranol. There are several progestins that are used in these preparations. Norgestimate and desogestrel are newer generation progestins and are least androgenic. Monophasic OCPs have a constant dose of estrogen and progestins. Phasic OCPs alter the dose of the estrogen, or more commonly the progestin, in hopes of lowering the cumulative metabolic effects over the course of the 21-day cycle of active pills. There are many formulations of oral contraceptive pills from which to choose, and physician or patient familiarity as well as cost usually play a role in this choice. The formulations come in 21-day packs or in 28-day packs that include seven inert pills.

In recommending an initial OCP, however, the physician should choose the most effective pill with the least potential for side effects. Nausea, breast soreness and fluid retention are estrogen side effects. Because this patient experiences some of these symptoms, consider starting a preparation containing a lower estrogen dose. Increasing weight, acne, depression, and fatigue are progestational side effects. Third-generation progestins, norgestimate, and desogestrel have lower relative binding affinities to androgen receptors as well as a greater ability to lower free testosterone when compared with older progestins and thus exhibit less of these androgenic side effects.

When choosing the right pill for this patient, her acne and her headaches also should be taken into consideration. All combination OCPs probably are beneficial for treating acne and hirsutism. Preparations containing newer generation progestins, however, are considered the best choice for this purpose. A formulation containing one of these agents would probably be a good initial choice for this patient. Oral contraceptive pills may decrease the frequency of headaches, but they also can increase their frequency or not affect them at all. This information should be reviewed with this patient, and she should be encouraged to report any change in her headache pattern.

The advice given to this patient prior to starting her OCPs is important to their success. There are several ways she can initiate therapy. OCPs could be initiated on the first day of her menses or the first Sunday after her menses begin. If the Sunday method is chosen, condoms need to be used for the first week. The delayed start regimen may result in less breakthrough bleeding and thus improved compliance.

Compliance is critical to ensure efficacy. The patient should be encouraged to establish a regular routine to take the pill at the same time each day (e.g., when brushing her teeth). The 28-day pack can be prescribed so that she could continue this routine during the pill-free week. This too may help compliance. She should be encouraged to always have a back-up method of contraception available. Potential side effects should be discussed, especially that of breakthrough bleeding. The patient can be instructed that if she experiences breakthrough bleeding, she should note when in her cycle it occurs. If a woman misses a dose, she should follow the directions given with her pack of pills. That is, she should take a pill as soon as she remembers. For one missed dose, taking two pills in 1 day is all that is necessary. If two pills are missed during the first 2 weeks of the cycle, the patient should take two pills a day for 2 days and use a back-up method of contraception for a week. If the patient misses two doses in week 3 or if she misses more than two doses that month, she should throw out the rest of her pack and start a new pack that day. If she is a Sunday starter, she can take pills from her current pack until Sunday. At that point, she can start the new pack. She should use another form of contraception such as condoms for the next 7 days. The patient may not menstruate that month. If two menstrual cycles are missed, a pregnancy test should be performed.

Although this patient is not considered a heavy smoker, she should be encouraged to discontinue tobacco use. There is some evidence that OCPs may be less effective in smokers. Smokers also may have increased breakthrough bleeding.

The Patient Returns to Your Office in 3 Months with Complaints of Breakthrough Bleeding. How Would You Manage This?

Breakthrough bleeding is common with low-dose combination OCPs and is the most frequent medical reason that women discontinue their use. It occurs most commonly during the first cycles of use because the patient's endometrium is adjusting to a lower amount of estrogen and progestin than was present prior to their use. Generally, the hormonal preparation is not changed during the first 3 or 4 months that it occurs. The patient should be instructed to use a back-up method of contraception, however, because bleeding may signify incomplete efficacy of the pill.

Because missed pills are the most common reason for breakthrough bleeding, the first question to this patient should be that of compliance. Also, inquire whether she started a new medication or antibiotic that may have interacted with the OCP. If no immediate reason for breakthrough bleeding can be ascertained, a consideration to change the hormonal preparation can be made at this time. A pregnancy test also should be performed.

If the bleeding occurs within the first 10 days or is mild and continues from the previous cycle, it is due to insufficient estrogen activity. This type of bleeding is often associated with a failure to menstruate during the pill-free interval. To manage this, the estrogen component can be increased. Usually no more than 35 μg of estrogen is needed.

If the bleeding occurs on day 11 or later, it is usually due to insufficient potency or dose of the progestin component. Heavy menses and menstrual cramps may accompany this type of bleeding. Progestins that are more androgenic usually induce less breakthrough bleeding. Switching to a different OCP with a more androgenic progestin, such as levonorgestrel, may provide improved cycle control without raising overall progestin or estrogen doses.

If the patient continues to have breakthrough bleeding after an appropriate change in her regimen, an evaluation for other causes should be considered. Other reasons for breakthrough bleeding are drug interactions (ampicillin, tetracycline, seizure medications, and certain antifungal medications), infection (especially *Chlamydia*), endometriosis, and an insensitivity of the endometrium to the OCP (this can occur after many months of use). Referral to a gynecologist also should be considered at this point.

What Is "Emergency Contraception" and Is It Appropriate in This Patient?

Emergency contraception is a method of preventing pregnancy after unprotected sexual intercourse. It is not as effective as primary contraception and is not intended to be used as a first-line contraceptive method. To be successful, emergency contraception must be used within 72 hours after coitus. Thus, this patient should be made aware of this option beforehand, so that she will be prepared should the need arise. She also should be informed about the lesser efficacy of emergency contraception and encouraged to comply with her primary contraceptive method.

The most commonly prescribed method of emergency contraception consists of four tablets of an oral contraceptive containing 50 μg of ethinyl estradiol. These can be taken as two doses of two tablets each, usually 12 hours apart. Because the incidence of accompanying nausea and vomiting is high, an antiemetic can be prescribed with this regimen. The patient also should be made aware of these side effects.

Controversy with emergency contraception use has arisen due to the belief that its mechanism is to prevent implantation of a fertilized ovum and thus act as an abortifacient. The main mechanism of the hormonal method of emergency contraception is now considered to be prevention or delay of ovulation or prevention of fertilization. This information may be helpful to this patient if she had such concerns about its use.

Suggested Reading

Abramowicz M, ed. Choice of contraception. *Med Lett* 1995;37:9–12.
Dickey R P. *Managing contraceptive pill patients,* 9th ed. EMIS, 1998:66–72.
Hewitt G. Update on adolescent contraception. *Adolesc Gynecol* 2000;27:143–162.
Kaunitz A M. Contraception. *Med Clin North Am* 1995;79:1377–1409.

47
Preconception Counseling
Lisa B. Bernstein

1. What is preconception counseling and why is it important for primary care physicians?
2. What are the general recommendations for screening of women contemplating pregnancy?
3. What behavioral modifications should be recommended in the preconception period?
4. What are the guidelines for prescribing medications for women contemplating pregnancy?

Discussion

What Is Preconception Counseling and Why Is It Important for Primary Care Physicians?

Ideally, the counseling of any woman contemplating pregnancy should begin before conception. This task is often difficult because approximately 50% of pregnancies in the United States are not planned, and the majority of women do not enter prenatal care until after organogenesis is complete. Approximately 15% of women entering prenatal care have other medical conditions. The primary care provider often has a unique advantage over obstetricians by seeing patients before conception. The U.S. Public Health Service recommends a specific preconception visit to a physician for all women of childbearing age, but any office visit by a woman of reproductive age should be considered an opportunity to dispense preconception care.

During a preconception visit, the physician and patient can identify psychosocial, medical, behavioral, and genetic problems that may affect a pregnancy or be affected by it. The physician should fully assess the woman's baseline medical conditions and determine the likelihood that pregnancy may affect the mother's health, or conversely, that the mother's medical condition will affect her fetus. In addition, the patient's prescription, over-the-counter, and herbal medications should be reviewed and her regimen changed, if needed, to minimize teratogenicity. In some cases the physician may want to instruct the patient to delay pregnancy and use appropriate birth control methods until her medical conditions are optimally controlled, or in extreme situations, to avoid pregnancy altogether. The patient's provider also should discuss the physical and emotional changes she may experience with pregnancy and stress the importance of enrolling in early prenatal care. By addressing these issues before conception, the physician and patient can intervene early to lessen or eliminate the risks to the mother and fetus during pregnancy.

What Are the General Recommendations for Screening of Women Contemplating Pregnancy?

The preconception period is a good time to determine the patient's serologic status for many conditions that may impact the outcome of a pregnancy. If the patient is not immune to rubella, she should receive the rubella vaccine and delay pregnancy for 3 months. She also may be screened for toxoplasmosis, varicella, cytomegalovirus, and hepatitis B virus. If she is determined to be at increased risk, a human immunodeficiency virus (HIV) test and tuberculosis screening should be performed.

In addition to serologic testing, carrier screening for genetic disorders may be offered to members of specific populations at high risk for a particular disease. For instance, African Americans should be screened for sickle cell anemia and Ashkenazi Jews should undergo testing for Tay-Sach disease, Fanconi anemia, Canavan disease, Gaucher disease, and Niemann-Pick disease. Couples from the Mediterranean should be screened for both α- and β-thalassemia. Women with cystic fibrosis in their family should consider undergoing DNA analysis. In addition, older women concerned about chromosomal abnormalities or women with a history of recurrent poor pregnancy outcomes should be referred for genetic counseling.

What Behavioral Modifications Should Be Recommended in the Preconception Period?

The preconception visit should include counseling to promote healthy behaviors and thus minimize the risk to the developing fetus. As a result of several prospective trials demonstrating the protective effect of folic acid supplementation in the prevention of neural tube defects, the U.S. Public Health Service recommends preconceptional folic acid supplementation to all women of childbearing age. Folic acid must be present before day 28 of organogenesis in order to positively affect the spinal cord. Women planning a pregnancy should begin taking 0.4 to 0.8 mg of folic acid daily 1 month before conception and continue at least through the first trimester. Women who have previously given birth to babies with neural tube defects should take 4 mg per day of folate.

During pregnancy women should continue to wear safety belts while in motor vehicles to minimize maternal and fetal mortality in the event of an accident. Mild to moderate exercise in pregnancy is beneficial, although the patient should remain hydrated and avoid any activity that increases the possibility of abdominal trauma. A work and environmental history should be obtained to minimize exposure to chemicals, such as some anesthetic gases, that may cause a poor pregnancy outcome. Women should be educated to avoid contact with cat feces and not eat raw meat to minimize exposure to and infection with *Toxoplasma gondii*. They should also avoid excessive heat exposure in the first trimester, which may increase the risk for neural tube defects.

A thorough social history, including whether the patient smokes, drinks alcohol, or uses illicit drugs, should be obtained at the preconception visit if it has not been obtained before. There is a possible increased risk for spontaneous abortion with high caffeine consumption, so the physician should counsel patients to minimize caffeine intake during pregnancy.

Approximately one fourth of women of reproductive age smoke, and up to 30% of these women continue to smoke while they are pregnant. Smoking during pregnancy is associated with decreased birth weight and an increased risk of placental abruption, preterm delivery, and perinatal death. Even second-hand smoke may cause low birth weight. All patients, especially those contemplating pregnancy or who are pregnant, should be aggressively encouraged to stop smoking and to avoid second-hand smoke when possible. Extensive behavioral counseling is recommended as first-line therapy for treating pregnant smokers. The risk:benefit ratio favors consideration of pharmacologic therapy in most women who have not quit without medication. In pregnant smokers, bupropion is classified as category B and nicotine gum as category C. All other nicotine replacement products are pregnancy category D.

Maternal alcohol abuse is associated with a specific pattern of birth defects known as fetal alcohol syndrome, which includes mental retardation, prenatal and postnatal growth restriction, craniofacial abnormalities, and central nervous system disorders. In addition, alcohol consumption increases the risk for spontaneous abortion and placental abruption. Women who drink are also more likely to smoke or use drugs during pregnancy. Although there is no appreciable risk with an occasional drink taken during pregnancy, it is safest to advise female patients to avoid alcohol consumption in the immediate preconception period and throughout pregnancy.

The prevalence of cocaine use during pregnancy ranges as high as 17%. Cocaine decreases uterine blood flow and may cause fetal growth retardation and abnormalities of the genitourinary, cardiac, and central nervous systems. In addition, it may result in ophthalmologic and limb defects. As a result, all women should be screened for cocaine use and strongly encouraged to abstain during pregnancy.

What Are the Guidelines for Prescribing Medications for Women Contemplating Pregnancy?

The primary care physician should always consider potential pregnancies before prescribing drugs for women of childbearing age. In women with concurrent medical illnesses who are contemplating pregnancy, the practitioner must first understand and communicate to the patient how her conditions will affect her pregnancy and vice versa. In most cases, the better controlled the maternal medical illness is before and during pregnancy, the lower the morbidity and mortality for the mother and fetus. Although it is simple to justify pharmacologic therapy for progressive chronic or acute maternal conditions, it is less so for her acute, self-limited medical problems. For most conditions, the treatment options include no treatment, non-pharmacologic treatment, or the use of more established versus newer pharmacologic therapies. In each case, the physician must weigh the risks and benefits to the mother and the fetus of withholding treatment or using pharmacologic therapy. In general, no medication should be started unless clearly indicated, and an effective treatment should not be stopped without good reason. Few medications are absolutely contraindicated. Physicians should remember to ask about the patient's use of over-the-counter and herbal remedies as well.

Case

A 32-year-old nulliparous African-American woman is referred to you after discovering that her blood pressure was elevated on a routine health screen at work. She has no complaints today. She has no significant past medical history, and her family history is significant for hypertension in both of her parents. She smokes one or two cigarettes only when she is under stress and drinks socially. She takes no medications other than an oral contraceptive and an occasional Tylenol or Advil for a headache. On physical examination, she is 5 feet 4 inches tall and weighs 200 pounds. Her blood pressure is 144/92 mm Hg, and the remainder of her examination is normal. During the course of conversation, she tells you that she got married 3 months ago and is eager to start a family. She just completed her normal menstrual cycle yesterday and states that she is planning to discontinue her oral contraceptive pill soon.

1. What steps would you tell this patient to take in preparation for pregnancy?
2. What screening tests would you recommend for this patient?
3. How will her pregnancy affect her blood pressure, and how will her hypertension affect her pregnancy?
4. Would you treat her hypertension at this time, and are there any medications you would avoid?

Case Discussion

What Steps Would You Tell This Patient to Take in Preparation for Pregnancy?

You should advise her to take a daily multivitamin containing at least 0.4 mg of folic acid to minimize the risk of neural tube defects. You should also inform her of the risks of drinking and smoking during pregnancy and tell her to avoid alcohol and tobacco, as well as minimize or omit caffeine intake. She should be counseled to continue to wear her seatbelt and may engage in nonstrenuous exercise. She should avoid aspirin and nonsteroidal antiinflammatory agents as well as contact with cat feces or raw meat to minimize exposure to *Toxoplasma gondii*. Obese women have a higher risk of developing gestational diabetes, hypertension, and infections, as well as giving birth to infants with neural tube defects or having stillbirths. Therefore, you might suggest that this patient also try to lose some weight prior to attempting to conceive.

What Screening Tests Would You Recommend for This Patient?

Given that she is African American, you might consider screening her and her husband for sickle cell disease. In addition, she should have her rubella titer checked and undergo routine serologic testing for toxoplasmosis, varicella, cytomegalovirus, and hepatitis, as well as HIV.

How Will Her Pregnancy Affect Her Blood Pressure, and How Will Her Hypertension Affect Her Pregnancy?

This patient has mild chronic hypertension. Chronic hypertension is blood pressure equal to or greater than 140/90 mm Hg before pregnancy or diagnosed before the 20th week of gestation. The prevalence of chronic hypertension in pregnant women ranges from 1% to 5% and is classified as either mild or severe. The rates are higher in older, obese, and African-American women. Early in gestation, diastolic pressures decrease by an average of 7 to 10 mm Hg, with an increase toward the patient's prepregnancy levels in the third trimester. Pregnant women with long-standing hypertension, especially those with diastolic pressure equal to or above 110 mm Hg or with preexisting cardiovascular or renal disease, should be counseled that they are at increased risk for superimposed preeclampsia and abruptio placentae, and that their babies have an increased risk of perinatal morbidity and mortality. The risk for superimposed preeclampsia is higher in primigravid women, those with a familial predisposition, and those carrying twins. In women with mild, uncomplicated chronic hypertension during pregnancy, maternal and fetal outcomes are similar to those of women without elevated blood pressure.

Would You Treat Her Hypertension at This Time, and Are There Any Medications You Would Avoid?

Women with mild hypertension considering pregnancy should be informed that they will most likely have a favorable outcome. Studies have not definitively demonstrated the maternal or fetal benefit of treating mild hypertension during pregnancy. Due to the possible adverse effects of antihypertensive therapy on the mother or fetus, it is preferable to control mild blood pressure elevations (diastolic pressures of 90–99 mm Hg) without medication when possible. In the preconception period, the physician may encourage weight loss and exercise, which would be otherwise avoided during pregnancy. During pregnancy, restriction of activity may be effective in lowering blood pressure as well. The use of tobacco and alcohol should be discouraged.

If diastolic pressure exceeds 100 mm Hg, pharmacologic treatment should be considered to avoid hypertensive vascular damage. If possible, methyldopa should be the first-line agent for treatment of elevated blood pressure because it has been shown to be safe in long-term studies for both the mother and fetus. In reality, the only classes of antihypertensive agents that are absolutely contraindicated are the angiotensin-converting enzyme (ACE) inhibitors and angiotensin receptor blockers because they have been associated with neonatal skull hypoplasia, renal failure, and increased neonatal mortality. Thus, if a patient cannot tolerate methyldopa, she may be switched to any class of blood pressure medications other than ACE inhibitors.

Suggested Reading

Fiore M C, Bailey W C, Cohen S J, et al. *Treating tobacco use and dependence. Clinical practice guidelines.* Rockville, MD: U.S. Department of Health and Human Services. Public Health Service. June 2000.

Kuller J A, Laifer S A. Preconceptional counseling and intervention. *Arch Intern Med* 1994;154: 2273–2280.

Lee R, et al. *Medical care of the pregnant patient.* Philadelphia: American College of Physicians–American Society of Internal Medicine, 2000.

National High Blood Pressure Education Program Working Group on High Blood Pressure in Pregnancy. *Am J Obstet Gynecol* 1990;163:1689–1712.

Sibai B M. Treatment of hypertension in pregnant women. *N Engl J Med* 1996;335:257–265.

VIII
Hematology

48
Iron Deficiency Anemia

Lorenzo Di Francesco

- Discussion   *300*
- Case   *303*
- Case Discussion   *304*

1. Review the physiology of iron balance in humans (e.g., iron storage, absorption, and loss).
2. What is the typical sequence of laboratory changes in iron deficiency?
3. What is the gold standard for making the diagnosis of iron deficiency anemia? How is the reticulocyte production index defined and used? What are the role and limitations of ferritin testing?
4. What are an appropriate workup and recommended treatment for a patient diagnosed with iron deficiency anemia?

Discussion

Review the Physiology of Iron Balance in Humans (e.g., Iron Storage, Absorption, and Loss).

There are approximately 3 to 5 g of iron (Fe) found in each person, of which two thirds is found in hemoglobin. A typical Western diet contains 15 mg iron per day, of which about 10% to 15% is absorbed. The low pH of the stomach helps dissolve ingested iron and provide a proton-rich milieu for the enzymatic reduction of the ferric form (Fe^{2+}) into the ferrous form (Fe^{3+}) by ferrireductase. This ferrous form is absorbed by enterocytes in the duodenum and upper jejunum, bound to transferrin in blood, and transferred to the bone marrow, where it is stored as ferritin (accessible source) and hemosiderin (insoluble form in macrophages). In general, about 1 to 2 mg iron is lost per day in urine, feces, and sweat, or is shed with skin and gastrointestinal cells. Females may lose an additional 20 mg iron per menstrual period. Pregnancy can increase overall needs by 500 to 1,000 mg for a full-term pregnancy.

What Is the Typical Sequence of Laboratory Changes in Iron Deficiency?

A patient in persistent negative iron balance will undergo the typical sequence of laboratory changes in the development of clinical iron deficiency as presented in Table 48.1. Under normal circumstances, the bone marrow has 2+ to 3+ iron stores and 40% to 60% sideroblasts; the mean serum ferritin and transferring saturation are 100% and 35%, respectively. There are four stages of iron deficiency. Stage I,

Table 48.1. Sequential Changes in the Laboratory Diagnosis of Iron Deficiency Anemia

Stages	Normal	Stage I (Negative Balance)	Stage II (Iron Depletion)	Stage III (Defective Erythropoiesis)	Stage IV (Clinical Fe Deficiency)
BM Fe	2+ to 3+	1+	0–1+	0	0
TIBC µg/dL	330 ± 30	330–360	360	390	410
Ferritin ng/mL	100 ± 60	<25	20	10	<10
% Fe absorbed	5–15	10–15	10–15	10–20	10–20
Plasma Fe µg/dL	115 ± 50	<120	115	<60	<40
% Saturation	35 ± 15	30	30	<15	<15
% Sideroblasts	40–60	40–60	40–60	<10	<10
RBC protoporphyrin	30	30	30	100	200
Erythrocytes	Normal	Normal	Normal	Normal	Microcytic/ hypochromic anemia

BM, bone marrow; TIBC, transferrin iron binding capacity; RBC, red blood cell.

called negative iron balance, is evidenced by reduced bone marrow iron and serum ferritin. In stage II, bone marrow iron and serum ferritin are depleted, but there is no evidence of defective erythropoiesis or anemia. Stage III, a state of defective erythropoiesis, is depicted by increased red blood cell protoporphyrin levels, but without anemia. Stage IV is clinical iron deficiency with all of the previous cumulative changes (low bone marrow iron/serum ferritin, increased transferrin, low serum iron and percentage saturation) and the development of low reticulocyte production and microcytic anemia. As the severity of iron deficiency increases, there is a compensatory increase in gut absorption of iron.

What Is the Gold Standard for Making the Diagnosis of Iron Deficiency Anemia? How Is the Reticulocyte Production Index Defined and Used? What Are the Role and Limitations of Ferritin Testing?

The gold standard for diagnosing iron deficiency anemia is a bone marrow biopsy demonstrating depleted iron stores. Iron deficiency anemia is suspected in patients with or without symptoms who have a microcytic anemia with low reticulocyte production. Other possible causes of microcytic anemia include chronic inflammation, sideroblastic anemia, and thalassemia. Low reticulocyte production is defined as a reticulocyte production index (RPI) of less than 2 using the following formula:

$$\text{RPI} = \text{reticulocyte \%} \times \frac{\text{hematocrit \%}}{45\%} \div \text{maturation factor}$$

The maturation factor is 2.5 for hematocrit of 10% to 19%, 2 for hematocrit of 20% to 29%, and 1.5 for hematocrit of 30% to 39%.

The best noninvasive test for screening for iron deficiency anemia is serum ferritin. A serum ferritin value of 15 ng/mL or less has a likelihood ratio of 52, effectively ruling in the diagnosis; a serum ferritin of 100 ng/mL or greater has a likelihood ratio of 0.08, effectively ruling out iron deficiency. Most of the limitations of screening with serum ferritin relate to the fact that it is also an acute phase reactant. This poses difficulties when we are doing workup for iron deficiency on patients

Table 48.2. Screening for Iron Deficiency Anemia

Hemoglobin	Serum Ferritin	Explanation
Normal	Normal	Fe deficiency excluded
Normal	≤15	Fe storage depletion
Low	≤15	Fe deficiency anemia
Low	16–100	Fe deficiency possible
Low	>100	Fe deficiency excluded as main cause

who may have a chronic inflammatory or liver disease, both known to increase serum ferritin. At any given level of bone marrow iron, inflammatory diseases generally increase serum ferritin by about threefold, and liver disease increases ferritin by about fivefold. In patients with nondiagnostic serum ferritin levels between 15 and 45 and known or suspected chronic illness, diagnostic options include performing a bone marrow biopsy versus a trial of oral iron therapy. If the hemoglobin increases by at least 1.0 g/dL within 3 to 4 weeks of oral iron, iron deficiency is considered a significant contributor to the patients' anemia.

General guidelines for screening for iron deficiency anemia in patients with or without chronic inflammatory or liver disease are presented in Tables 48.2 and 48.3.

What Are the Appropriate Workup and Recommended Treatment for a Patient Diagnosed with Iron Deficiency Anemia?

Once a patient is found to be iron deficient, the most important step is determining the cause of the patient's iron deficiency. Major causes are broadly listed in Table 48.4.

The evaluation includes a full clinical history and physical examination, with particular emphasis on the gastrointestinal tract in elderly patients and appropriate gynecologic evaluation in younger females. All patients should have a stool guaiac to look for occult gastrointestinal bleeding. A urinalysis can be performed to look for hematuria. Base your workup on the patient's age and most likely organ system involved. Elderly iron-deficient patients with no obvious cause should undergo lower and, if necessary, upper gastrointestinal tract visualization via endoscopy. Younger females with a history of menorrhagia or menometrorrhagia should undergo a pelvic examination. Referral to a gynecologist for further evaluation may be indicated to look for organic disease such as endometrial cancer, particularly in women over 35 years of age.

Table 48.3. Interpretation of Serum Ferritin in Anemic Patients with Microcytic Anemia Who also Have Chronic Inflammatory Disease or Liver Disease

Serum Ferritin	Fe Deficiency	Response to Oral Fe
<15	Diagnostic	Yes
15–45	Possible	Possible
45–100	Rare	No
>100	Excluded	No

Table 48.4. Causes of Iron Deficiency

Inadequate absorption
  Poor bioavailability
  Antacid therapy or high gastric pH
  Excess dietary bran, tannin, phytates, or starch
  Competition from other metals (e.g., copper or lead)
  Loss or dysfunction of absorptive enterocytes
  Bowel restriction
  Celiac disease
  Inflammatory bowel disease
  Intrinsic enterocyte defects
Increased loss
  Gastrointestinal blood loss
    Epistaxis
    Varices
    Gastritis
    Ulcer
    Tumor
    Meckel diverticulum
    Parasitosis
    Milk-induced enteropathy of early childhood
    Vascular malformations
    Inflammatory bowel disease
    Diverticulosis
    Hemorrhoids
  Genitourinary blood loss
    Menorrhagia
    Cancer
    Chronic infection
  Pulmonary blood loss
    Pulmonary hemosiderosis
    Infection
  Other blood loss
    Trauma
    Excessive phlebotomy
    Large vascular malformations

Adapted from Andrews NC et al. Disorders of iron metabolism. *N Engl J Med* 1999;341:1986–1995; with permission.

In patients who are anemic, start treatment with iron replacement immediately once the diagnosis of iron deficiency anemia is made because a delay in treatment can result in a further decrease in hemoglobin. Options for iron replacement include ferrous sulfate (325 mg/65 mg elemental iron), one tablet four times daily (before meals and at bedtime), or ferrous gluconate (320 mg/36 mg elemental iron), one tablet four times daily. Both preparations are available in liquid forms if necessary. The main side effects of all ferrous medications are nausea, abdominal discomfort or pain, constipation, diarrhea, or dark stools.

Case

A 67-year-old man with osteoarthritis presents to your office complaining of fatigue and dyspnea on exertion over a 3-month period. He has no other cardiopulmonary symptoms. A physical examination reveals pale conjunctiva, a normal cardiopulmonary examination, and guaiac-negative stool test. A laboratory assessment reveals microcytic anemia with a hematocrit of 30% with normal chemistries.

1. What is the differential diagnosis of this patient's anemia?
2. What tests are necessary to support the diagnosis of iron deficiency?
3. What additional evaluations might your patient need based on his diagnosis?

Case Discussion

What Is the Differential Diagnosis of This Patient's Anemia?

Assuming this patient has a microcytic, low-production anemia, the differential diagnosis includes iron deficiency, anemia of chronic inflammation, sideroblastic anemia, and thalassemia. If the patient has had a normal hemoglobin and mean corpuscular volume in the past, thalassemia would be unlikely given that this abnormality would be genetically and phenotypically carried from birth.

What Tests Are Necessary to Support the Diagnosis of Iron Deficiency?

Serum ferritin analysis would be the single most useful noninvasive test to confirm the diagnosis of iron deficiency. If equivocal, a reticulocyte count, total iron-binding capacity, percentage transferring saturation, and serum iron level may assist with the diagnosis. This patient had a ferritin level of 12 ng/mL, effectively ruling in iron deficiency anemia.

What Additional Evaluations Might Your Patient Need Based on His Diagnosis?

Blood loss from chronic nonsteroidal antiinflammatory drug use is a distinct possibility despite being guaiac negative. However, due to his advanced age and risk of gastrointestinal malignancy, he should undergo endoscopic evaluation of the lower gastrointestinal tract followed by an assessment of the upper gastrointestinal tract, as indicated. This patient should be started on oral iron therapy.

Suggested Reading

Andrews N C, et al. Disorders of iron metabolism. *N Engl J Med* 1999;341:1986–1995.

Guyatt G H, et al. Diagnosis of iron-deficiency anemia in the elderly. *Am J Med* 1990;88:205–209.

Guyatt G H, et al. Laboratory diagnosis of iron-deficiency anemia: an overview. *J Gen Intern Med* 1992;7:145–153.

Herbert V. Anemia. In: *Clinical nutrition,* 2nd ed. St. Louis: CV Mosby 1988:593–608.

Looker A C, et al. Prevalence of iron deficiency in the United States. *JAMA* 1997;272:973–976.

Patterson C, et al. Iron deficiency anemia in the elderly: the diagnostic process. *Can Med Assoc J* 1991;144:435–440.

49

Folic Acid and Vitamin B$_{12}$ Deficiency

Yacob Ghebremeskel

1. Discuss the physiology of folic acid.
2. What are the main causes of folic acid deficiency?
3. What are the clinical manifestations of folic acid deficiency?
4. How do you treat a patient with folic acid deficiency?

Discussion

Discuss the Physiology of Folic Acid.

Folic acid is required for the transfer of one carbon unit from one compound to the other. It plays an important role in the conversion of homocysteine to methionine and deoxyuridine monophosphate to deoxythymidine monophosphate, which is essential for the synthesis of DNA. The absence of folic acid compromises this process and leads to megaloblastic changes in rapidly dividing cells. Folic acid is also involved in purine synthesis.

Primary dietary sources of folic acid are fruits and vegetables. The daily folic acid requirement is 50 to 400 μg. Pregnant and lactating women require 500 to 800 μg/day. Additional folic acid supplementation is required to prevent neural tube defects in pregnant women. The human body stores 5 to 20 mg of folic acid. Therefore, it only takes 3 to 4 months to develop folic acid deficiency for nutritional reasons. The normal serum folic acid level is 1.7 to 12.6 ng/mL. Red blood cell (RBC) folate is higher, 153 to 602 ng/mL. One third of hospitalized patients have a low serum folic acid level due to a transient decrease in their folic acid intake, but their tissue folic acid level usually stays normal. It is advisable not to check the serum folic acid level in hospitalized patients.

Folic acid in food is found in a polyglutamated form. Conjugases in the intestinal lumen convert the polyglutamates to mono- and diglutamates, which are readily absorbed in the proximal jejunum. In the serum, folic acid is transported in the form of *N*-methyltetrahydrofolate to the cells. In the cell, the *N*-methyl group is removed in a cobalamin-requiring process and then converted back into polyglutamate form, which is unable to diffuse back into the serum. Therefore, the tissue folate level is relatively constant, whereas the serum folate level fluctuates with the diet. The

RBC folate level is more reflective of tissue folate content than is the serum folate level. Vitamin B_{12} (also known as cobalamin) deficiency can falsely increase the serum folate level and decrease the RBC folate level by the above-mentioned mechanism. Sixty percent of patients with pernicious anemia have a low RBC folate level.

What Are the Main Causes of Folic Acid Deficiency?

Inadequate dietary intake is the most common cause of folate deficiency. It is usually seen in alcoholic adults and in infants who suffer from eating disorders, although patients whose diet is devoid of vegetables may develop deficiency over time.

An increased requirement for folic acid is another common problem that is usually seen in pregnancy, infancy, malignancy, chronic hemolytic anemia, chronic exfoliative skin disorders, and hemodialysis.

Malabsorption of folic acid is a rare cause of folic acid deficiency that is seen in tropical and nontropical sprue. Certain drugs such as phenytoin, barbiturates, and ethanol interfere with the enterohepatic circulation of folic acid.

Certain drugs also cause impaired metabolism of folic acid. This list of drugs includes dihydrofolate reductase inhibitors, methotrexate, pyrimethamin, trimethoprim, and pentamidine. Dihydrofolate reductase deficiency also is a rare cause of folic acid deficiency.

What Are the Clinical Manifestations of Folic Acid Deficiency?

Clinical manifestation of folic acid deficiency is similar to that of vitamin B_{12} deficiency without neurologic symptoms. Megaloblastic changes of the gastrointestinal epithelium cause sore tongue, diarrhea, and malabsorption. Megaloblastic anemia causes fatigue, dyspnea on exertion, and tachycardia, and if severe can cause high-output heart failure.

How Do You Treat a Patient with Folic Acid Deficiency?

It is important to check the serum vitamin B_{12} level before treating folic acid deficiency, because supplementation with folic acid corrects the hematologic manifestation of vitamin B_{12} deficiency without correcting the neurologic changes. That is why there is great concern regarding folic acid supplementation to cereal products. This can delay the diagnosis of vitamin B_{12} deficiency. The usual dose is 1 mg of folic acid per day orally, but higher doses of up to 5 mg may be needed in some cases, such as in patients with sickle cell disease and severe hemolytic anemia. The hematologic response is similar to that seen in the treatment of vitamin B_{12} deficiency. The duration of treatment depends on the cause of the state of deficiency. Patients should be encouraged to maintain an optimal diet containing an adequate amount of folate.

Vitamin B_{12} Deficiency

1. Discuss the physiology of vitamin B_{12}.
2. What are the main causes of vitamin B_{12} deficiency?

3. How common is vitamin B$_{12}$ deficiency?
4. What are the clinical manifestations of vitamin B$_{12}$ deficiency?
5. What tests are used to diagnose vitamin B$_{12}$ deficiency?
6. What is the treatment for vitamin B$_{12}$ deficiency?

Discussion

Discuss the Physiology of Vitamin B$_{12}$.

Humans cannot synthesize vitamin B$_{12}$ (cobalamin). Its main source in food is animal protein (e.g., milk, meat, eggs). The recommended daily requirement for cobalamin is 2 to 5 μg/day. Because the human body stores approximately 1,000 times this amount (2–5 mg), it takes 2 to 5 years to develop vitamin B$_{12}$ deficiency.

Dietary cobalamin is protein bound. In the presence of acid and pepsin in the stomach, cobalamin is freed from the food protein and binds to the R factor. The cobalamin–R factor complex travels to the duodenum, where pancreatic enzymes and the alkaline environment free the cobalamin from the complex and allow the cobalamin to quickly bind to intrinsic factor (secreted by the antrum of the stomach).

The cobalamin–intrinsic factor complex travels to the terminal ileum, where it is absorbed by an active process mediated by the specific ileal receptors in the terminal ileum. After being absorbed, cobalamin is freed from the cobalamin–intrinsic factor complex and binds to transport proteins called transcobalamins. Most of the metabolically active cobalamin is transported by transcobalamin II. Inside the cells, cobalamin is converted to methylcobalamin, essential for the synthesis of methionine and adenosylcobalamin. In the presence of methylcobalamin and methionine synthase, homocysteine is converted to methionine. Methionine is the cornerstone of DNA and myelin synthesis. Dividing cells require a constant DNA supply for cell division. In the absence of DNA synthesis, cells cannot divide but will continue to grow, leading to a condition called megaloblastosis. The lack of new myelin formation causes nerves to degenerate. Methyltetrahydrofolate (CH$_3$-THF) also plays an important role in methionine synthesis, but myelin synthesis proceeds even in the absence of CH$_3$-THF.

What Are the Main Causes of Vitamin B$_{12}$ Deficiency?

Inadequate intake, a rare cause of vitamin B$_{12}$ deficiency, is occasionally found in vegetarians. Malabsorption is the most common reason for vitamin B$_{12}$ deficiency and has several possible mechanisms: the inability to release vitamin B$_{12}$ from food, the absence of intrinsic factor, a functionally abnormal intrinsic factor, competition for vitamin B$_{12}$ in the intestine, and terminal ileum diseases.

Low gastric pH is required for the metabolism of food protein–bound vitamin B$_{12}$. In the absence of this acidic milieu, as in gastrectomy or long-term acid suppression by proton pump inhibitors or atrophic gastritis, vitamin B$_{12}$ remains bound to the food protein and unable to bind to R factor or intrinsic factor. The presence of anti–intrinsic factor antibodies in pernicious anemia and the production of functionally abnormal intrinsic factor are other gastric causes of vitamin B$_{12}$ malabsorption.

Intestinal bacterial overgrowth and fish tapeworm infestation causes vitamin B_{12} deficiency by consuming vitamin B_{12} in the intestine. There will be no vitamin B_{12} available for absorption.

Terminal ileum diseases, such as Crohn disease, intestinal resection, neoplasm, and tropical and nontropical sprue, cause vitamin B_{12} malabsorption. There is also a rare postreceptor defect that can result in selective cobalamin malabsorption.

Drugs such as p-aminosalicylic acid, colchicine, and neomycin can interfere with absorption or enterohepatic circulation of cobalamin.

Other rare causes of cobalamin malabsorption include nitrous oxide exposure (oxidizes cobalamin to an inactive form) and transcobalamin deficiency.

How Common Is Vitamin B_{12} Deficiency?

The prevalence of vitamin B_{12} deficiency increases with age. Depending on the population screened, the prevalence of vitamin B_{12} deficiency is 5% to 15%. In a sample of surviving older members of the original Framingham study cohort, the prevalence of vitamin B_{12} deficiency (serum vitamin B_{12} level < 200 µg/mL) was 12%. In one study, where elevation of serum methylmalonic acid and homocysteine levels were taken as a gold standard for diagnosing tissue vitamin B_{12} deficiency, the prevalence of vitamin B_{12} deficiency was 14.5%. The female:male ratio was 1.5:1.0. The mean age of diagnosis was 62 years.

The prevalence of pernicious anemia in persons over 65 is 1.0% to 3.0% (1.9%). The high prevalence of vitamin B_{12} deficiency in the elderly cannot be explained by pernicious anemia only, because pernicious anemia is a disease of late middle age. There is interesting evidence that many elderly patients with a normal Schilling test and no anti–intrinsic factor antibody may have malabsorption of food protein–bound cobalamin. This may explain the high prevalence of vitamin B_{12} deficiency in the elderly.

What Is the Clinical Manifestation of Vitamin B_{12} Deficiency?

The clinical manifestation of vitamin B_{12} deficiency is related to defective DNA and myelin synthesis. Megaloblastosis of the gastrointestinal epithelial cells presents with sore tongue, malabsorption, and diarrhea. This exacerbates the preexisting vitamin B_{12} deficiency. Patients with megaloblastic anemia also present with fatigue, palpitation, dyspnea on exertion, chest pain, and heart failure. In the bone marrow, 90% of the red blood cells are destroyed, resulting in jaundice and elevated lactate dehydrogenase (LDH).

Healton et al. reviewed the clinical presentations of 143 patients with known vitamin B_{12} deficiency. Paresthesias alone occurred in 33%, ataxia alone in 9%, and memory loss in 3% of the patients. Others had mixed symptoms such as insomnia, impotence, anosmia, urinary incontinence, personality changes, light-headedness, and diminished ability to taste. The classic neurologic lesion in vitamin B_{12} deficiency is subacute combined nerve degeneration. It involves both the dorsal (position and vibration sense) and lateral column (pain, pin prick, and light touch). Involvement of the peripheral nerves is still unclear.

What Tests Are Used to Diagnose Vitamin B$_{12}$ Deficiency?

The workup for vitamin B$_{12}$ deficiency is generally initiated when patients present with macrocytic anemia or neuropsychiatric complaints, but most patients with vitamin B$_{12}$ deficiency have neither. Folate supplementation to cereal foods for prevention of neural tube defects further complicates the problem because folate corrects the megaloblastic changes of B$_{12}$ deficiency without correcting the neurologic defects. Therefore, patients will be diagnosed late in their illness with possible irreversible neurologic deficit. Because of these concerns, clinicians should have high clinical suspicion for identifying vitamin B$_{12}$ deficiency, especially in high-risk patients.

In a recent study of patients with vitamin B$_{12}$ deficiency, only 29% had anemia and 64% had macrocytosis [mean corpuscular volume (MCV) > 100 fL]. This means that 36% of the patients with vitamin B$_{12}$ deficiency do not have macrocytosis. Iron deficiency, thalassemia, and folate supplementation can mask the macrocytosis of cobalamin deficiency. On the other hand, not all macrocytosis is due to B$_{12}$ deficiency. In a study of 100 patients with macrocytosis (MCV > 115 fL), only 50% had low serum cobalamin, low folic acid, or both. Other causes of megaloblastosis include myelodysplastic syndrome, zidovudine (AZT), and some chemotherapeutic agents. Causes of nonmegaloblastic macrocytosis include alcoholism, liver disease, hemolysis, hemorrhage, and cold agglutinin disease. Other findings on blood smear include ovulocytosis, poikilocytosis, and hypersegmented neutrophils (5% of the neurophils with five or more lobes). Hypersegmentation is neither sensitive nor specific for vitamin B$_{12}$ deficiency. Bone marrow biopsy has limited value in detecting the cause of megaloblastic anemia of vitamin B$_{12}$ deficiency, and in mild anemia it is inconclusive. A bone marrow biopsy commonly shows hypercellular, megaloblastic, erythroid metaplasia with giant metamyelocytes.

Elevation of LDH and unconjugated bilirubin and low platelet and white blood cell counts are commonly seen. The degree of LDH elevation correlates with the severity of the deficiency.

Serum cobalamin is a good initial screening test. Its normal value depends on the technique used. The widely used technique is an automated nonradioisotope chemiluminiscence assay. Its normal value ranges from 250 to 1,000 ng/mL. The sensitivity and specificity of the test varies from study to study because of the lack of a gold standard. Stabler et al. used elevated serum methylmalonic acid and homocysteine level as a gold standard for diagnosing vitamin B$_{12}$ deficiency and found that 90% to 95% of the patients have a serum cobalamin level of less than 200 μg/mL, whereas 5% to 10% of the patients with proven B$_{12}$ deficiency have a serum level of 200 to 300 μg/mL. It is important to know that there are other reasons for elevation of serum homocysteine or of methylmalonic acid in the serum. Renal failure, dehydration, hypothyroidism, inborn metabolic abnormalities, pyridoxine, and folate deficiencies are listed among the causes. If the pretest probability for vitamin B$_{12}$ deficiency is high, a low-normal serum cobalamin level does not exclude the possibility of tissue cobalamin deficiency. In this situation elevation of serum homocysteine and methylmalonic acid may help to clarify the clinical question. In vitamin B$_{12}$ deficiency, both methylmalonic acid and homocysteine levels are elevated, whereas in folate deficiency only homocysteine increases. Folic acid supplementation does not correct the serum methylmalonic acid level.

Anti–parietal cell antibody is present in 85% to 90% of patients with pernicious anemia and in 3% to 10% of healthy elderly individuals. Its clinical use is limited. There are two types of anti–intrinsic factor antibody. Type I blocks cobalamin from binding to intrinsic factor, and is present in 70% of patients with pernicious anemia. Type II blocks the intrinsic factor–cobalamin complex from binding to the ileal receptors. It is found in 40% of the patients with pernicious anemia. It is highly specific for pernicious anemia.

The result of a Schilling test usually does not alter management. The test has three stages. In stage I of the test, the patient is given 1 mg of radiolabeled cyanocobalamin orally and a 1,000-μg intramuscular injection of cobalamin to saturate binding proteins; then 24-hour urinary cobalamin is measured. Normal subjects excrete 10% to 35% of the oral dose. If stage I is abnormal, then proceed to stage II after 3 to 7 days. This interval is required for the clearance of radiolabeled cyanocobalamin from the initial test. In stage II, the test is repeated with exogenous intrinsic factor. In pernicious anemia the urinary cobalamin excretion will be corrected with exogenous intrinsic factor. In the presence of intestinal and pancreatic disease, the urinary cyanocobalamin level stays low. In stage III, the second test is repeated with antibiotic therapy. In the presence of intestinal bacterial overgrowth without intestinal mucosal disease, the urinary cyanocobalamin will be corrected by antibiotic therapy. The test result remains abnormal if there is intestinal disease. The presence of renal insufficiency and poor urine collection technique can influence the test results.

What Is the Treatment for Vitamin B$_{12}$ Deficiency?

The treatment of vitamin B$_{12}$ deficiency depends on the cause of the disease. For example, patients with intestinal bacterial overgrowth are treated with antibiotics. Most causes of malabsorption can be treated with high doses of oral crystalline vitamin B$_{12}$ or intramuscular vitamin B$_{12}$ injection. Studies have shown that 1% of the oral crystalline cyanocobalamin is absorbed even in the presence of pernicious anemia. In one study, 2,000 μg of crystalline cyanocobalamin given orally was as effective as the standard intramuscular injection protocol. This is a good choice for patients receiving anticoagulation therapy, where intramuscular injection is contraindicated. Standard therapy consists of 100 μg of intramuscular cobalamin every day for the first week, then 100 μg every week for 6 to 8 weeks to provide 2,000 μg in the first 6 weeks, then 100 μg every month for the rest of the patient's life. At times, 1,000 μg may be given every 2 to 4 months, but the risk of relapse is significantly higher than with the standard therapy. After appropriate treatment with vitamin B$_{12}$ supplementation, the reticulocyte count increases in 2 to 3 days and peaks at 5 to 7 days. The mean corpuscular volume starts to decrease in 3 to 4 days and completely normalizes in 25 to 78 days.

Case

A 75-year-old man presents with a chief complaint of "I can't walk straight." The patient stated that he had been having difficulty with his gait for months, but recently got worse in the past 3 weeks prior to this visit. He also reported intermittent numbness in both hands and feet. His wife stated that he has been having difficulty remembering things for several weeks. His past medical history is significant for partial gastrectomy for a bleeding gastric ulcer and osteoarthritis. His medications include acetaminophen and omeprazole.

On physical examination, he is a thin man in no acute distress. He is tachycardic, without orthostatic hypotension. His sclera are icteric. There is a yellowish discoloration of the oropharyngeal mucosa. No thyromegaly or lymphadenopathy is present, and his lungs are clear. Cardiovascular examination reveals tachycardia, normal S$_1$ and S$_2$, and II/VI systolic flow murmur. There is a supraumbilical median laparotomy scar and bowel sound present, and the abdomen is soft and nontender. There is no organomegaly. The neurologic examination reveals intact cranial nerves, 2+ deep tendon reflexes, and 5/5 muscle strength throughout. There are diminished vibration, position, and soft touch sensation in the lower extremities bilaterally. Heel-to-shin and finger-to-nose tests are normal. The Mini-mental status score is 20/30.

Laboratory data show a white blood cell count of 3,400 cells/µL with 5% hypersegmented neutrophils, hematocrit 30%, MCV 105 fL, LDH 280 IU/L, aspartate aminotransferase 34 IU/L, alkaline phosphatase 78 IU/L, total bilirubin 3.5 mg/dL, and direct bilirubin 2.4 mg/dL.

1. What is your differential diagnosis?
2. What other causes of macrocytosis do you know?
3. What further tests do you order to clarify the diagnosis?
4. What were the patient's risk factors for developing vitamin B$_{12}$ deficiency?
5. How do you treat this patient?

Case Discussion
What Is Your Differential Diagnosis?

The above clinical scenario can be summarized as a 75-year-old patient with gradual onset of jaundice, ataxia, paresthesia, and mild dementia. Laboratory tests were significant for macrocytosis, hypersegmented neutrophils, and macrolytic anemia. Folic acid deficiency can cause similar hematologic changes described above, but it does not cause neurologic deficit. Systemic vasculitides can present with hemolytic anemia, elevated MCV (secondary to reticulocytosis), paresthesias and multiinfarct dementia, but absence of fragmented red blood cells (schistocytes) associated with low haptoglobin and hemoglobinuria excludes this diagnosis. Neutrophilic hypersegmentation is also absent in extramedullary hemolytics. This patient's presentation is very typical for vitamin B$_{12}$ deficiency.

What Other Causes of Macrocytosis Do You Know?

Other causes of megaloblastosis include folate deficiency in alcoholic patients, AZT treatment in patients infected with the human immunodeficiency virus, and myelodysplastic syndrome and chemotherapeutic agents. Macrocytosis without megaloblastosis can present in patients with alcohol abuse, liver disease, drugs, reticulocytosis as in hemolysis, hemorrhage, and cold agglutinin disease.

What Further Tests Do You Order to Clarify the Diagnosis?

Determination of the serum vitamin B_{12} level is essential. If it is low (<100 fL), it will confirm the diagnosis. A low-normal level does not exclude vitamin B_{12} deficiency. Elevated serum homocysteine and methylmalonic acid levels are helpful when pretest probability is high and serum cobalamin level is low-normal. The clinical suspicion in this patient is high enough to warrant treatment and follow the normalization of methylmalonic acid or homocysteine level. Resolution of the symptoms, normalization of hematologic abnormalities, and metabolites will confirm the diagnosis. Positive antiintrinsic factor antibody would swing the diagnosis toward pernicious anemia. If the patient's serum cobalamin level normalized in a stage I Schilling test (e.g., he has malabsorption of the food protein–bound cobalamin), he will respond to oral crystalline cyanocobalamin.

What Were the Patient's Risk Factors for Developing Vitamin B_{12} Deficiency?

His risk factors for developing vitamin B_{12} deficiency include partial gastrectomy, proton pump inhibitor therapy, and older age.

How Do You Treat This Patient?

Vitamin B_{12} deficiency in this patient may be due to the inability to metabolize food-bound vitamin B_{12}. This is most likely because of decreased secretion of gastric acid or diminished production of intrinsic factor from his prior gastric surgery leading to B_{12} malabsorption. This patient can be treated with high-dose oral cyanocobalamin (2000 mm orally every day) or intramuscular cobalamin injection.

Suggested Reading

Ban-Nock T, et al. Pernicious anemia. *N Engl J Med* 1997;337:1441.

Green R, Kinsella L J. Current concepts in the diagnosis of cobalamin deficiency. *Neurology* 1995;45:1435.

Hoftbrand V. Macrocytic anemias: ABC of clinical hematology. *BMJ* 1997;314:430.

Lumley J. Periconceptual supplementation with folate and/or MVI for preventing neural tube defects. The Cochran database of systematic review.

Babior B M and Bunn H F. Megaloblastic anemias. *Harrison's textbook of medicine.* New York: John Wiley & Sons. 1998:653.

Snow C F. Laboratory diagnosis of B_{12} and folate deficiency: a guide for primary care physicians. *Arch Intern Med* 1999:1289.

Stabler S P. Diagnosis of cobalamin deficiency, relative sensitivities of serum cobalamin, methylmalonic acid and total homocysteine concentration. *Am J Hematol* 1990;34:99.

Stabler S P. Screening the older population for cobalamin deficiency. *J Am Geriatr Soc* 1995;43:1290.

50

Deep Venous Thromboses

Neil H. Winawer

- Discussion *313*
- Case *316*
- Case Discussion *316*

1. What is the differential diagnosis of unilateral lower extremity edema?
2. What factors help to narrow the differential diagnosis?
3. What are the risk factors for developing deep venous thrombosis?
4. What are the choices among diagnostic tests in the evaluation for deep venous thrombosis? What are their strengths and weaknesses?

Discussion

What Is the Differential Diagnosis of Unilateral Lower Extremity Edema?

The differential diagnosis of unilateral lower extremity edema includes the following:

- Deep venous thrombosis (DVT; proximal or calf vein)
- Ruptured Baker cyst
- Cellulitis
- Venous stasis
- Lymphedema
- Phlebitis/postphlebitic syndrome
- Muscle tear (gastrocnemius muscle)
- Partial or compete tendon rupture (Achilles, plantaris)

What Factors Help to Narrow the Differential Diagnosis?

The history and physical examination are crucial elements in the assessment of patients with lower extremity swelling. Because DVT is a potentially life-threatening disorder, much of the initial workup of lower extremity edema focuses on estimating a patient's absolute risk of developing a clot (low, moderate, or high). There have been several attempts to use a point system to categorize a patient's risk for DVT. Although accurate, these systems can be laborious and are often not used clinically. However, several important items from the history and physical can help to establish a fairly accurate pretest probability of DVT. DVTs can present either in the distal veins of the leg (calf veins) or in the more proximal portions (femoral vein). Although proximal and distal DVTs can have similar clinical presentations, edema extending above the knee suggests a proximal clot. Patients with DVT also may complain of pain along the posterior portion of the leg, most notably in the calf. Dorsiflexion of the foot may worsen this pain (Homan sign); however, this is not a highly specific finding.

Many conditions can mimic DVT. Fluid collections in the popliteal fossa (Baker cyst) can dissect or rupture, releasing their contents down into the calf. The result is unilateral lower extremity edema and pain. A Baker cyst can form in patients with a naturally occurring communication between the knee joint and the semimembranous-gastrocnemius bursa. If these patients develop a synovial effusion (as seen in rheumatoid arthritis, osteoarthritis, and other derangements of the knee), a popliteal cyst will develop. These patients typically describe knee swelling prior to the acute onset of their pain. Cellulitis of the lower extremity can also present with swelling, pain, and warmth. Clues suggesting cellulitis include evidence of a point of entry on the skin, excessive skin warmth, fever, and leukocytosis. Venous stasis also can present with unilateral lower extremity swelling, and often presents with hyperpigmentation and a characteristic dermatitis of the lower extremity. In severe cases, pressure ulcers may develop. Lower extremity lymphedema also can mimic DVT. The edema, however, is usually nonpitting secondary to the increased viscosity of lymphatic fluid. Superficial thrombophlebitis also can cause pain and edema. Often the superficial vein is easily identified. In patients with a prior history of DVT presenting with symptoms of phlebitis, distinguishing between postphlebitic syndrome and acute DVT can be difficult. A tendon rupture (Achilles/plantaris tendon) or partial muscle tear also can present with severe pain and swelling in the calf. A firm mass may be palpable in the posterior calf, representing the gastrocnemius muscle torn from its insertion. Patients with an Achilles tendon rupture typically have difficulty with plantar flexion of the foot. In these patients, applying pressure around the calf will produce a markedly diminished or absent plantar flexion response (the Thompson test).

What Are the Risk Factors for Developing DVT?

Any process resulting in venous stasis or a hypercoagulable state increases a patient's risk for developing DVT. These processes include incompetent valves in the venous system, prolonged sitting (i.e., transcontinental air travel), prolonged standing (i.e., train conductors, toll booth attendants), and medical conditions that result in prolonged bed rest. Patients with hereditary clotting disorders (protein S deficiency, etc.) and acquired clotting disorders (antiphospholipid antibody) are at high risk for DVT. The hypercoagulable state associated with malignancy also puts patients at a higher risk for clotting. Traumatic fractures and recent surgery (particularly hip/knee replacement or pelvic surgery) increase the risk for developing DVT. Medications such as estrogen, tamoxifen, and the selective estrogen receptor modulators (e.g., raloxifene) increase a patient's risk for DVT. Finally, a past medical history or family history of DVT also increases one's risk.

What Are the Choices Among Diagnostic Tests in the Evaluation of Deep Venous Thrombosis? What Are Their Strengths and Weaknesses?

Duplex ultrasonography is very sensitive and specific for proximal DVT but has poor sensitivity and specificity in the calf veins. It combines the benefits of ultrasonographic compression with the identification, measurement, and display of blood flow through Doppler technology. A transducer is placed over the venous system of the lower extremity from the thigh to the popliteal fossa. A test is considered positive if a vein demonstrates noncompressibility. Ultrasonography cannot distinguish between old and new clot, but the presence of significant collateral veins, suggests an old clot. Experienced technicians at some institutions will often comment on the patency of a patient's calf veins. There are no well-designed clinical trials looking at the utility of Doppler technology in diagnosing calf veins DVTs, although sensitivity and specificity are certainly increased with color flow imaging.

On certain occasions a Doppler ultrasonogram may be read as inconclusive or indeterminate. Usually this occurs when data from the ultrasonographic and Doppler data appear to be inconsistent. For example, sometimes a portion of a proximal vein may appear thickened or demonstrate only partial compressibility, yet the Doppler reveals normal flow. On other occasions the vein may not exhibit augmentation (an increase in blood volume in the proximal veins when the leg is compressed distally) but may reveal a normal Doppler flow pattern.

The *venogram* is considered the gold standard in the diagnosis of DVT, but considerable experience is required for adequate performance and interpretation of the test. A vein is cannulated at the dorsum of the foot, and radiocontrast dye is infused.

Often the veins are difficult to cannulate, and about 30% of tests are considered technically limited. Without careful injection of contrast medium into a dorsal foot vein, there may be nonfilling of the calf veins that is falsely attributed to thrombosis (because the vein is not filled) or interpreted as normal (because the filling defect produced by the thrombus is not seen). It is considered an invasive test and can have complications such as phlebitis, allergic reactions or renal failure.

The *nuclear venogram* has some advantages over venography (avoiding radiocontrast dye reactions) but is equally invasive and operator dependent. A radioisotope is injected into the dorsum of the foot with scanned images taken at a later time. The test is analyzed on the basis of the degree of uptake in the deep veins.

Impedance plethysmography (IPG) is noninvasive and accurate in the proximal veins, but fails to detect the majority of calf vein thrombi because most calf vein thrombi do not obstruct the main venous outflow tract. This test involves placing electrodes on the patient's calf followed by inflation of a thigh cuff to increase lower extremity venous pressure. If an occlusive thrombus is present, venous emptying will be delayed upon deflation of the cuff. This increased blood volume results in decreased electrical impedance. False negatives results may occur in patients with old clots and well-developed collateral veins. IPG also cannot distinguish between thrombotic and nonthrombotic forms of obstruction. A false-positive test result may occur if a patient is not positioned correctly (e.g., knee bent) or if the patient is not adequately relaxed (veins may be constricted by contracting muscles). False-positive results also can occur when venous outflow is impaired by elevated venous pressure, as in congestive heart failure.

Technetium 99m apcitide injection (AcuTect) is a complex of the synthetic peptide apcitide and the radionuclide technetium (^{99m}Tc). The compound binds to glycoprotein IIb/IIIa receptors found on activated platelets (based on *in vitro* and *in vivo* animal data, not confirmed clinically). The test offers a unique advantage in that it focuses on the acuity of the disease process, helping to differentiate between old and new clots. It is administered as a peripheral intravenous injection in an upper extremity, an advantage over contrast venography and nuclear venograms. Regional images are obtained of the pelvis, thighs, knees, and calves at 10 minutes and at 60 to 90 minutes. Acute DVT is indicated by asymmetric linear uptake of the tracer in a deep vein segment (greater than the corresponding contralateral deep vein segment) that persists or becomes apparent on later images. Similar to venography, the validity of the AcuTect scan is related to the quality of the images obtained. Consistent leg positioning and camera field of view are very important. Normal variant images occasionally occur and should not be confused with an abnormal test result.

D-dimer levels are sensitive to the process of fibrin formation/dissolution occurring with ongoing thrombosis. However, they are not highly specific for venous thromboembolism because they are elevated in other conditions (e.g., cancer, surgery, infectious disease). Recently new assays have been introduced that allow rapid quantitative D-dimer estimations in individual patients. These assays remain sensitive, and thus have a high negative predictive value in ruling out DVT (>90%, at a 2,000 ng/mL cutoff). The combination of compression ultrasonography with D-dimer testing (if both tests are normal) is a highly effective means of ruling out DVT. The cost effectiveness of such a strategy has yet to be determined.

Case

A 55-year-old woman with a past medical history of hypertension and osteoarthritis presents to the hospital with complaints of left leg swelling and pain for the past two days. The patient localizes her pain to the calf and states that it hurts more while walking. She denies any shortness of breath or chest pain and is otherwise asymptomatic. There is no history of surgery or trauma to the affected leg. She denies any prior history of DVT. The patient takes atenolol 25 mg daily and has been taking acetaminophen for pain control. She denies any history of tobacco use and drinks alcohol socially. She is postmenopausal and has never been on hormone replacement therapy. On examination the patient has stable vital signs. The left lower extremity is notable for 2+ pitting edema that extends from her foot toward her calf. There is no warmth or erythema. Dorsiflexion of the foot produces mild discomfort. Squeezing the calf produces pain. Plantar flexion of the foot is noted with this maneuver. The remainder of the patient's physical examination is benign.

1. Which is the preferred initial diagnostic test to evaluate for deep venous thrombosis in this patient?
2. If the patient has a calf vein deep venous thrombosis, what is the probability that it will migrate proximally?
3. What is the likelihood that a patient with a negative lower extremity Doppler test result will have a calf vein deep venous thrombosis that will migrate proximally?
4. How often does a patient need to be followed up after a first negative lower extremity ultrasonographic result?

Case Discussion

Which Is the Preferred Initial Diagnostic Test to Evaluate for Deep Venous Thrombosis in This Patient?

Duplex ultrasonography (compression ultrasound with Doppler flow imaging) is the preferred test for several reasons. As noted previously, it is noninvasive and has a sensitivity and specificity of about 97% in the proximal veins. It is important to note that in most institutions a negative Doppler test result only relates to the proximal veins (imaging usually proceeds from the proximal deep veins of the thigh to the popliteal fossa). Although it may be important to know whether or not a patient has a calf vein DVT (for purposes of workup), the data from multiple studies indicates that the incidence of calf DVTs is small. In fact, approximately 5% of patients suspected of having a first-time lower extremity DVT will have a calf vein DVT. Consequently, only a few calf vein DVTs will be missed by solely imaging the proximal veins. Additionally, calf vein DVTs do not necessarily require anticoagulation unless they migrate proximally.

If the Patient Has a Calf Vein Deep Venous Thrombosis, What Is the Probability that It Will Migrate Proximally?

Several studies have noted that the risk for proximal migration is 25% to 30%.

What Is the Likelihood That a Patient with a Negative Lower Extremity Doppler Test Result Will Have a Calf Vein Deep Venous Thrombosis that Will Migrate Proximally?

As we can see from the last two questions, a patient with a suspected DVT but a negative duplex ultrasonographic result has approximately a 5% chance of having a calf vein DVT. If 30% of calf DVTs migrate, then the probability or absolute risk for having a migratory calf vein DVT is simply $0.05 \times 0.3 = 1.5\%$. To assess the clinical significance of this number, it is helpful to put this data into a more user-friendly form called the number needed to treat, or for our purposes, the number needed to miss (NNM):

$$NNM = 1 \div \text{absolute risk for a migratory calf vein DVT}$$

Using our example, NNM = 1 ÷ 1.5% = 1 ÷ 0.015 = 67.

Therefore, 1 out of every 67 patients with a first negative lower extremity duplex ultrasonographic result will have a calf vein DVT that migrates proximally. That is why follow-up testing is recommended in most instances.

How Often Does a Patient Need to Be Followed Up after a First Negative Lower Extremity Ultrasonographic Result?

Based on older studies, the management of patients with a negative duplex ultrasonographic result required at least two follow-up tests over the course of several weeks. However, recent evidence suggests that only one follow-up ultrasonography test (5–7 days after the first negative test) may be sufficient. In one study the negative predictive value of two negative tests 5 to 7 days apart was 99.4%.

Suggested Reading

Birdwell B, Raskob GE, Whitsett TL. The clinical validity of normal compression ultrasonography in outpatients suspected of having deep venous thromboses. *Ann Intern Med* 1998;128:1–7.

Pini M, Marchini L, Giordano A. Diagnostic strategies in venous thromboembolism. *Haematologica* 1999;84:535–540.

Hirsh J, Hoak H. Management of deep vein thrombosis and pulmonary embolism. AHA Statement for Healthcare Professionals. *Circulation* 1996;93:2212–2245.

Birdwell B. Recent clinical trials in the diagnosis of deep vein thrombosis. *Curr Opin Hematol* 1999;6:275–279.

IX
Infectious Diseases

51

Adult Vaccines: Pneumococcal and Influenza Vaccination

Susan M. Ray

1. What are the indications for pneumococcal and influenza vaccinations and how effective are the vaccines?
2. What are the contraindications for and adverse effects of pneumococcal and influenza vaccinations?
3. What are recent developments in the formulations of pneumococcal and influenza vaccines?

Discussion

What Are the Indications for Pneumococcal and Influenza Vaccinations in Adults and How Effective Are the Vaccines?

Adults at increased risk for invasive pneumococcal disease [*Streptococcus pneumoniae* isolated from a normally sterile site, e.g., blood, cerebrospinal fluid (CSF)] or complications from the disease should be vaccinated. Adults at risk fall into three categories:

1. Older adults ($\geq$65 years)
2. Individuals with immunocompromising conditions that decrease the antibody response to polysaccharide antigens [e.g., congenital immunodeficiency, human immunodeficiency virus (HIV) infection, leukemia, lymphoma, multiple myeloma, Hodgkin disease, generalized malignancy, organ or bone marrow transplantation, therapy with alkylating agents, antimetabolites, or systemic corticosteroids, or chronic renal failure] or increase the rate of loss of protective antibodies [functional or anatomic asplenia (sickle cell disease), nephrotic syndrome]
3. Immunocompetent adults with chronic medical conditions that increase the likelihood of developing invasive pneumococcal disease or complications from invasive pneumococcal disease (chronic cardiovascular disease, chronic lung disease, diabetes, liver disease, alcohol abuse, CSF leak)

In general, pneumococcal vaccine should be given once to adults with indications. Revaccination at 5 years is recommended for adults who are at highest risk of serious disease or those who are likely to have a rapid decline in response or a suboptimal antibody response, including asplenic individuals and the immunocompromised persons listed above. Patients over 65 should receive a second dose of vaccine if they received a first dose of vaccine over 5 years earlier and were under 65 at the time. Over 90% of adults who present with invasive pneumococcal disease have one or more of the vaccine indications outlined above. The 23 serotypes included in the currently available pneumococcal polysaccharide account for over 90% of the serotypes from invasive disease isolates. The efficacy of the vaccine varies depending on the age and underlying immune status of the patient. Data from case-control and indirect cohort studies indicate an overall vaccine efficacy of 50% to 70% in the prevention of invasive pneumococcal disease. Efficacy in prevention of invasive pneumococcal disease by underlying disease status ranges from 75% to 80% in healthy elderly patients to 50% to 60% in immunocompetent adults with chronic medical conditions. Efficacy in immunocompromised adults is significantly less, but vaccination of this group is still recommended because the potential benefits of vaccination far outweigh any risk from the vaccine. A recent study by Nichol et al. demonstrated a 43% reduction in the risk of hospitalization for pneumonia and influenza and a 29% reduction in the risk of death in elderly persons with chronic lung disease who received pneumococcal vaccine. Pneumococcal vaccine is cost saving in the prevention of bacteremia and hospitalization: from $8 to $300 per person vaccinated.

Annual influenza vaccination is strongly recommended for groups of persons who are at increased risk for complications from influenza or have a high prevalence of medical conditions associated with increased risk for influenza complications [age ≥50 years, residents of long-term care facilities, persons with chronic heart or lung disease (including asthma), diabetes, renal failure, hemoglobinopathies, or immunosuppression (including HIV), and women who will be in the second or third trimester of pregnancy during the influenza season] and persons who could transmit influenza to other persons at risk of complications from infection (health-care workers in hospitals, clinics, long-term care facilities and home health and emergency response settings, and household members of persons at high risk). The inactivated influenza vaccine is manufactured annually and is composed of three strains of influenza (2 type A and 1 type B) predicted most likely to resemble the circulating viruses in the United States in the upcoming winter. The effectiveness of the vaccine varies with the age and immunocompetence of the vaccine recipient and the strength of antigenic match between the circulating virus and vaccine strains. When antigenic match is good, the vaccine is 70% to 90% effective in preventing influenza illness in immunocompetent adults under 65 (such as health-care workers). The vaccine may be less immunogenic in the elderly and immunocompromised and thus afford less protection (30%–40%) against upper respiratory tract infection. However, it is 30% to 70% effective in preventing influenza-related hospitalization in the elderly and 80% effective in preventing influenza-related death among elderly nursing home residents. In the Nichol et al. study cited above, the benefits of pneumococcal and influenza vaccinations during the influenza season were additive in elderly patients with chronic lung disease, with a 72% reduction in the incidence of hospitalization and an 82% reduction in the risk of death compared with patients who received neither vaccination.

What Are the Contraindications to and Adverse Effects of Pneumococcal and Influenza Vaccinations?

Contraindications to pneumococcal vaccination are few and include previous hypersensitivity to the vaccine and previous receipt of one or two doses of the vaccine (depending on timing and revaccination recommendation). It is recommended that women of childbearing age be vaccinated before becoming pregnant, because the safety of the pneumococcal vaccine during the first trimester of pregnancy has not been evaluated. Approximately half the patients who receive the pneumococcal vaccine develop mild pain, erythema, and swelling at the injection site lasting less than 48 hours. The incidence of moderate local reactions (redness or swelling >4 inches in diameter) is increased in persons who are revaccinated (11%) compared with those receiving a first vaccine (3%). Fever, myalgias, or severe local induration are rare. Anaphylaxis has only rarely been reported (0 cases out of 7,531 patients vaccinated in nine randomized, controlled trials).

Contraindications to influenza vaccine include hypersensitivity to eggs or any component of the vaccine and acute febrile illness. Minor respiratory illnesses with or without fever do not constitute a contraindication to immunization. The most frequent side effect of influenza vaccination is a sore arm (reported in 10%–64% of patients) lasting 2 days or less. Fever, malaise, and myalgias can occur after vaccination, but in several studies comparing influenza vaccine and placebo, such systemic symptoms are no more common in the vaccine group than the placebo group. Such symptoms following vaccination have been associated with intercurrent upper respiratory tract infection (an infection observed in >50% of patients in the 6 weeks following influenza vaccination). Immediate hypersensitivity reactions can occur; most are likely caused by residual egg protein. Hypersensitivity to thimerosal (a mercury-containing compound used as a preservative in some influenza vaccine formulations) may result in local, delayed-type hypersensitivity reactions following influenza vaccination. In 1976, the swine influenza vaccination program was associated with an increased incidence of Guillain-Barré syndrome (GBS; <10 cases per million persons vaccinated). Epidemiologic investigations have not demonstrated a large increase in GBS associated with subsequent influenza vaccines. If risk does exist, it is quite small (slightly more than 1 additional case per million persons vaccinated), and this risk is substantially less than the risk for severe influenza.

What Are Recent Developments in the Formulations of Pneumococcal and Influenza Vaccines?

Pneumococcal protein conjugate vaccines were developed to address the morbidity and mortality associated with pneumococcal disease in children under 2 years of age, who have the highest rates of invasive pneumococcal disease in childhood (with associated high rates of antimicrobial resistance) and for whom the polysaccharide vaccine was not effective. A large randomized double-blind trial published in 2000 (Black et al. *Pediatr Infect Dis J* 2000;19:187–195) demonstrated that a 7-valent conjugate vaccine (containing serotypes responsible for 85% of pneumococcal disease in infants and children) prevented 94% of invasive disease caused by vaccine serotypes and reduced the number of visits, episodes, recurrent disease, and tube placements due to otitis media. In the same year, the 7-valent conjugate vaccine (Prevnar, Lederle Laboratories, Pearl River, NY/Wyeth-Ayerst Laboratories, Marietta, PA) was licensed by the U.S. Food and Drug Administration for the prevention of invasive disease in infants and toddlers, and the Advisory Committee on Immunization Practices and the American Academy of Pediatrics issued recommendations for routine use of the vaccine in this population. Widespread use of the vaccine is expected to have a large impact on the incidence rates of pneumococcal meningitis and bacteremia in young children. It is possible that a reduction in mucosal carriage rates will be observed; such a reduction could have beneficial effects for adults as well as pediatric contacts of vaccinated children. Possible advantages of the use of conjugate vaccines in adults include the potential for protein conjugate vaccines to induce larger, more functional, and more long-lasting antibody responses in adults who respond poorly to the polysaccharide vaccine (e.g., elderly or HIV infected). It is possible that using one or two doses of conjugate vaccine, followed by booster doses of polysaccharide could provide more effective protection against pneumococcal disease in such populations. Relatively few clinical studies of conjugate vaccines in adults have been reported. Until such studies are conducted, there is no current recommendation for the use of pneumococcal conjugate vaccine in adults.

Intranasally administered, live, attenuated influenza vaccines are currently being used in Russia and are under development in the United States. These vaccines consist of live viruses that induce only mild symptoms and do not replicate well at temperatures found in the lower respiratory tract. Possible advantages of such vaccines include the ability to induce mucosal and systemic antibody responses and the ease and acceptability of an intranasal route of administration. A recent study on the use of the vaccine in healthy adults was associated with a 9% to 24% reduction in febrile respiratory illnesses (all cause) and a 13% to 28% reduction in lost work days. Further studies will be needed to understand how such a formulation might complement or even replace the current injectable inactivated vaccine. Certainly when using a live attenuated influenza vaccine, one could no longer explain that the flu vaccine cannot give you the flu.

Case

A 57-year-old African-American man presents to the medical clinic in October for a routine visit following a recent hospitalization. His medical record indicates that he was hospitalized 2 months previously with unstable angina, new-onset diabetes mellitus, and hypercholesterolemia. Discharge medications included insulin 70/30, metoprolol, nizatidine, and phenytoin. Further review of his chart indicates coronary atherosclerotic heart disease documented by catheterization 2 years previously and alcohol abuse complicated by delirium tremens and alcoholic ketoacidosis in the past. It is noted that he has had eight hospitalizations for chest pain evaluation and seizures over the preceding 4 years. During the same period of time he has been seen in the medical clinic twice and cardiology clinic once. The patient indicates that he has been "really shaken up" by the diagnosis of diabetes because his mother died from complications related to this disease. He reports a new interest in protecting his health and describes his efforts to follow the diabetic diet and insulin regimen and to cut back on his alcohol intake. He wants to know whether he should get the flu shot he has been hearing about on the radio. He thought shots were just for children and he has not had any shots since he was a small boy.

1. Can both influenza and pneumococcal vaccines be given at this clinic visit?
2. What were the missed opportunities for this patient? What are strategies that ensure vaccine is offered and messages that encourage patients to accept the vaccines?
3. What if he reports a history of hives after eating eggs or egg products?

Case Discussion

Can Both Influenza and Pneumococcal Vaccines Be Given at This Clinic Visit?

Yes. This patient should be informed that both pneumococcal and influenza vaccinations are indicated for him because of diabetes and alcohol use. The vaccines can be administered at the same visit in different arms (pneumococcal vaccine 0.5 mL intramuscularly or subcutaneously and influenza vaccine 0.5 mL intramuscularly only) without increasing side effects or decreasing efficacy. He will need a repeat flu vaccine annually until he reaches the age of 65, at which time he should have a second pneumococcal vaccine and continue annual flu vaccines.

What Were the Missed Opportunities for This Patient? What Are Strategies that Ensure Vaccine Is Offered and Messages that Encourage Patients to Accept the Vaccines?

Each hospitalization and clinic visit over the preceding 4 years constituted a missed opportunity for pneumococcal immunization, and any that occurred during flu season were missed opportunities for influenza immunization. This patient is typical of many adults with chronic diseases in that his encounters with the health system were usually prompted by illness and he had few "well" visits to see a health-care provider. Many studies have found that the majority of adults who present with invasive pneumococcal disease have been hospitalized or treated in an outpatient clinic for acute illness in the 5 years preceding their pneumococcal disease. The Advisory Committee on Immunization Practices has recommended that pneumococcal and influenza vaccination programs target hospitalized adults at high risk. In both inpatient and outpatient settings, organizational strategies that result in automatic screening for vaccine indications and prompt providers to give vaccine have proven to be the most effective method for increasing vaccination rates of persons at high risk. It is unusual for high-risk patients to request vaccination as this patient did. Widespread implementation of organizational strategies such as provider reminders or standing orders would make such a request unnecessary. Multiple studies have found that the strongest predictor of a patient receiving influenza or pneumococcal vaccine is physician recommendation. Thus, while a standing order is very useful for ensuring that high-risk patients are offered vaccine appropriately, a clear recommendation from the primary care provider indicating that "I want you to get this shot today" may have additional impact for those reluctant to accept immunization.

What If He Reports a History of Hives after Eating Eggs or Egg Products?

This history indicates that he has an egg allergy, and influenza immunization would be contraindicated. Protocols for safe influenza vaccine immunization in individuals with egg allergy have been published. These studies used specific lots of vaccine known to have a relatively low concentration of egg protein. Commercial preparations of influenza vaccination with higher egg protein concentrations might not be tolerated as well. Chemoprophylaxis with antiviral agents during the influenza season is an alternative for high-risk patients who should not be vaccinated. Both amantadine and rimantadine have been approved for prophylaxis against influenza A and have been studied extensively in nursing home populations as a component of influenza outbreak control. They should not be used as a substitute for vaccination. The newer neuraminidase inhibitors zanamivir (administered by inhalation) and oseltamivir (a tablet) have activity against both influenza A and B and are approved for the treatment of influenza infections. They are not yet approved for prophylaxis, but recent studies show efficacy in preventing influenza illness in healthy adults. There is little experience with use of these agents in patients such as ours with chronic medical conditions.

Suggested Reading

Centers for Disease Control and Prevention. Prevention of pneumococcal disease: recommendations of the Advisory Committee on Immunization Practices (ACIP). *MMWR* 1997;46:1–19.

Centers for Disease Control and Prevention. Prevention and control of influenza: Recommendations of the Advisory Committee on Immunization Practices (ACIP). *MMWR* 2000;49:1–28.

Centers for Disease Control and Prevention. Use of standing orders programs to increase adult vaccination rates. Recommendations of the Advisory Committee on Immunization Practices. *MMWR* 2000;49:15–26.

Jackson L A, Benson P, Sneller V P, et al. Safety of revaccination with pneumococcal polysaccharide vaccine. *JAMA* 1999;281:243–248.

Nichol K L, Baken L, Wuorenma J, et al. The health and economic benefits associated with pneumococcal vaccination of elderly persons with chronic lung disease. *Arch Intern Med* 1999;159:2437–2442.

Nichol K L, Margolis K L, Lind A, et al. Side effects associated with influenza vaccination in healthy working adults. A randomized, placebo-controlled trial. *Arch Intern Med* 1996;156:1546–1550.

52
Pharyngitis
Henry Baffoe-Bonnie

1. What are the various etiologic agents of tonsillopharyngitis?
2. What is the epidemiology of group A β-hemolytic streptococcal pharyngeal infection?
3. How is group A β-hemolytic streptococcal pharyngitis diagnosed?
4. Why is it necessary to treat group A β-hemolytic streptococcal pharyngitis?
5. What treatment options are available?

Discussion
What Are the Various Etiologic Agents of Tonsillopharyngitis?

Pharyngitis and tonsillitis leading to a sore throat are among the most common maladies seen in the outpatient setting. Of the many infectious agents capable of causing tonsillopharyngitis, group A β-hemolytic streptococcus (*Streptococcus pyogenes*), or GAS, stands alone with distinction because of the notorious association with rheumatic fever. In any patient presenting with a sore throat, the physician has the charge of ruling out infection with this pathogen. Other β-hemolytic streptococci (groups C and G) can cause tonsillopharyngitis, especially in teenagers and young adults. Pharyngeal infections with *Neisseria gonorrhoeae* can occur in those who engage in oral sex, especially fellatio. *Arcanobacterium haemolyticum* is a rare cause of bacterial pharyngitis in teenagers and young adults (approximately 3%–5% of cases). There is an associated scarlatiniform rash. Infection with *Mycoplasma pneumoniae* can involve the oropharynx and may be associated with bullous myringitis.

Viral causes include infectious mononucleosis caused by cytomegalovirus or Epstein-Barr virus. Both can have significant pharyngeal involvement. Human herpes simplex virus (HSV) type 1 and 2 infections can both involve the oropharynx even though gingivostomatitis is the main manifestation.

Special mention should be made of the acute retroviral syndrome of human immunodeficiency virus (HIV) infection. Affected patients typically present with fever, lymphadenopathy, myalgias, fatigue, and a nonexudative pharyngitis. A maculopapular rash has been described in 50% to 70% of patients. At the time of presentation, HIV antibodies are typically negative. Diagnosis can be established by detection of the p24 antigen or HIV-1 RNA in serum. Aggressive antiretroviral therapy at the time of diagnosis is advised by most authorities.

Other rare causes of tonsillopharyngitis are discussed in the Suggested Reading list at the end of this discussion.

What Is the Epidemiology of Group A β-Hemolytic Streptococcal (GAS) Pharyngeal Infection?

Group A streptococcus is the most common bacterial cause of tonsillopharyngitis. It is responsible for up to 30% of cases in children and 10% of cases in adults. Of the common bacterial causes of pharyngitis, GAS is the only pathogen for which treatment is mandated. Pharyngitis from GAS most commonly occurs in school-age children who are also more susceptible to develop the dreaded nonsuppurative sequelae of acute rheumatic fever (rare in the Western Hemisphere) and glomerulonephritis. Most infections occur in the cold months. The disease is contagious, with an estimated transmission rate of about 35% to an untreated patient in a family or school environment. Pharyngeal colonization with GAS is common in school-age children; this makes it difficult to delineate whether an acute infection is due to GAS or a concomitant viral infection.

How Is GAS Pharyngitis Diagnosed?

The history and physical examination cannot reliably establish GAS as the causative agent in tonsillopharyngitis. However, the absence of fever and pharyngeal erythema along with the presence of manifestations of the common cold make the diagnosis very unlikely. Throat culture is the gold standard for the diagnosis of GAS pharyngitis. When done properly, the sensitivity is over 90%. The double swab technique is commonly used in most physician offices. Two swabs are obtained: one for the rapid antigen detection test (RADT) and the other for culture if the results of RADT are negative. The specimens should be obtained by vigorous swabbing of both tonsil and the posterior pharynx. This is very important because the sensitivity of culture and the RADT directly correlates with the integrity of the inoculum retrieved. Swabs should be obtained before antibiotics are given. Results from the throat culture usually take 24 to 48 hours. A common dilemma is whether to withhold antibiotics or treat empirically. There is no definite answer. Delaying therapy does not increase the risk of rheumatic fever. If antibiotics are begun empirically, they should be discontinued after a negative culture. The use of RADT is now commonplace. This test has a sensitivity of 80% to 90% and is highly specific for the presence of GAS. A positive result in the office should prompt therapy. In an adult with a negative RADT result, it is reasonable, based on epidemiologic evidence, to withhold treatment and forego obtaining a culture. In a child or adolescent with a negative RADT result, some authorities recommend obtaining a culture, although persuasive arguments are being articulated to the contrary. Whether or not to initiate empiric therapy in this setting will, of course, depend on the clinical presentation.

Why Is It Necessary to Treat GAS Pharyngeal Infections?

Even without antimicrobials, most cases of GAS pharyngitis will resolve with the development of neutralizing antibodies by day 5 to 7 after onset of illness.

The goals of antibiotic therapy are as follows:

- To prevent possible extension of the infection into contiguous structures (e.g., causing retropharyngeal abscess or sinusitis)
- To prevent the nonsuppurative complications of acute rheumatic fever (ARF) and glomerulonephritis. It should be mentioned that in hosts susceptible to ARF (those with a prior history and children, depending on the locale), eradication of GAS from the oropharynx is the goal. The persistence of rheumatogenic strains of GAS in the oropharynx of a predisposed host (after spontaneous or antibiotic-induced resolution of symptoms) can spark an immune response leading to cross-reactivity with cardiac myocytes.
- To shorten the duration of symptoms.
- To decrease infectivity (patients are minimally infectious 24 hours after initiation of appropriate antibiotic therapy)

What Are the Treatment Options for GAS Pharyngeal Infections?

Penicillin is the undisputed drug of choice. It is safe and cheap. GAS has remained exquisitely susceptible to penicillin. Oral penicillin V is preferred over penicillin G because of stability in the acidic gastric environment. A full 10-day course should be taken vigilantly. Even when started a week after onset of illness, penicillin is still effective at preventing attacks of acute rheumatic fever. Recent studies now support the use of twice daily dosing of penicillin to effectively treat GAS pharyngitis. The most used dose is 500 mg twice daily for adults and 250 mg twice daily for children. If compliance is an issue, a single intramuscular injection of benzathine penicillin (600,000 U for children and 1.2 million U for adults) can be given. Some studies have noted a slightly higher recurrence rate with intramuscular penicillin, so whenever possible, the 10-day course should be given. For penicillin-allergic individuals, acceptable alternatives are listed as follows:

- Erythromycin estolate (20–40 mg/kg in two to four divided doses) or the ethyl succinate preparation (40 mg/kg in two to four divided doses) for a full 10 days. Erythromycin base or stearate does not compare with penicillin. GAS resistant to erythromycin is not common in the United States.
- A 5-day course of azithromycin is approved by the U.S. Food and Drug Administration (FDA) as second-line therapy for GAS pharyngitis in patients 16 years and older. The recommended dose is 500 mg the first day and 250 mg for the next 4 days. In one study, clarithromycin demonstrated bacteriologic eradication similar to or superior to penicillin. However, the macrolides are much more expensive than penicillin.
- The FDA-approved cephalosporin oral regimens are cefprodoxine proxetil (10 mg/kg/day in two divided doses for 5 days) and cefuroxime axetil (30 mg/kg/day in two doses for 5 days).
- Clindamycin is an alternative, but its routine use is not advocated because of significant side effects.
- Tetracyclines should never be used because of the prevalence of resistant strains of GAS. Likewise, sulfonamides and bactrim (Septra) should not be used to treat active infections because of their inability to irradicate GAS.

The majority of patients with GAS pharyngitis respond clinically with eradication of GAS organisms from the oropharynx. Posttreatment cultures are not routinely required except in patients who remain symptomatic and those who have had rheumatic fever and have a high risk for recurrence.

Case

A 19-year-old female college student in Boston presented to an emergency room 1 week into the new year complaining of throat pain, fever, headache, and fatigue of 1 day's duration. She was in her usual state of health until 24 hours prior to presentation when she noticed throat discomfort, which progressed to the point of severe pain upon swallowing. Her roommate recorded an oral temp of 102.8°F. She denied a cough, runny nose, earache, or eye irritation. She stated that her two roommates recently got over the "flu." She has never been hospitalized and takes only oral contraceptives.

She stated that because of the unrelenting throat pain she took two pills of "what was left over from a prescription given to her roommate." She could not recall the name of the medication but she stated it was an antibiotic.

A physical examination revealed an ill-appearing female with a blood pressure of 100/60 mm Hg, pulse rate of 112 beats/min, respiratory rate of 24 breaths/min, and an oral temperature of 103.6°F. She had no discernible rash but had bilaterally swollen and erythematous tonsils with a whitish exudate and pharyngeal erythema. Prominent anterior and posterior cervical tender lymphadenopathy was present and she drooled. The rest of the examination was unremarkable.

A white blood cell count was 14,000 with 82% neutrophils. Platelets and hematocrit were normal at 234,000 and 41%, respectively. Basic chemistries and liver enzymes were normal. Results of Monospot and rapid strep tests were both negative.

1. What is the likely diagnosis in this patient?
2. How reliable is the negative rapid strep test?
3. What is your treatment recommendation?

Case Discussion
What Is the Likely Diagnosis in This Patient?

This young college student most likely has GAS pharyngitis. Features of the presentation favoring this diagnosis are as follows: onset in winter, young age, presence of exudates and anterior cervical lymphadenopathy, and absence of upper respiratory symptoms (e.g., runny nose, cough, ear and eye irritation). Infectious mononucleosis is a possibility, but the absence of diffuse adenopathy and a negative monospot make this unlikely. Acute HIV infection is a consideration. However, a maculopapular rash, myalgias and arthralgias are commonly seen in the acute retroviral syndrome. The absence of upper respiratory infection symptoms makes a viral etiology unlikely. *Arcanobacterium haemolyticum* is a rare cause of pharyngitis in her age group, but a scarlatiniform rash is commonly seen.

How Reliable Is the Negative Rapid Strep Test?

The rapid strep test is 80% to 90% sensitive. Prior antibiotic use can be responsible for a negative rapid strep test. In patients like this one who have a high likelihood of streptococcal pharyngotonsillitis, a negative rapid strep test does not effectively rule out the disease, and a throat culture should be sent. It will be appropriate to treat her empirically for GAS pharyngitis pending culture results. Upon receipt of a negative culture, antibiotics should be discontinued.

What Is Your Treatment Recommendation?

The "sharing" of antibiotics should be discouraged. It obfuscates proper diagnosis and most importantly it increases the reservoir of those colonized with virulent strains of GAS. With a positive throat culture, the importance of completing a full course of prescribed antibiotics should be emphasized.

Suggested Reading

Bisno et al. Acute pharyngitis. *N Engl J Med* 2001;334:205–211.

Bisno et al. Diagnosis and management of group A streptococcal pharyngitis: a practice guideline. *Clin Infect Dis* 1997;25;574–583.

Dajani et al. Treatment of acute streptococcal pharyngitis and prevention of rheumatic fever. AHA scientific document 1995.

53
Acute and Chronic Bacterial Sinusitis

Inginia Genao

1. Classify and define sinusitis.
2. What is the pathogenesis and bacteriology of sinusitis?
3. What factors may predispose a patient to sinusitis?
4. What are the clinical features of bacterial sinusitis?
5. What is the diagnostic approach to sinusitis?
6. Review the medical management and referral indications.

Discussion
Classify and Define Sinusitis.

In conjunction with the National Institute of Allergy and Infectious Disease, the American Academy of Allergy, Asthma and Immunology, and the American Academy of Otolaryngology–Head and Neck Surgery Foundation have classified sinusitis as acute, subacute, and chronic.

In acute sinusitis, signs and symptoms suggesting acute inflammation of the sinuses are present for less than 8 weeks. Acute sinusitis is often preceded by an upper respiratory infection (URI); URI symptoms persisting for more than 7 to 10 days suggest the development of acute sinusitis.

Subacute sinusitis involves minimal to moderate signs and symptoms of sinus inflammation. The clinical symptoms persist, sometimes for long periods of time.

In chronic sinusitis, signs and symptoms of inflammation of the sinuses persist for more than 8 to 12 weeks.

What Is the Pathogenesis and Bacteriology of Sinusitis?

The paranasal sinuses are air-filled spaces within the bones of the head. In healthy adults, the air and bone are separated by ciliated epithelium containing goblet cells, nerves, blood and lymphatic vessels, and glandular rich connective tissue. It is important to recognize that the anatomy may vary from person to person or even from side to side on the same person, making it more challenging to define what normal is. The osteomeatal complex is commonly involved in obstruction given the proximity of epithelial cells. Because the maxillary sinuses do not benefit from gravitational drainage, an intact ciliated epithelium is essential. The proximity of the teeth to the maxillary sinus is very important in the pathogenesis of sinusitis.

Streptococcus pneumoniae and *Haemophilus influenzae* have been consistently isolated in cases of acute bacterial sinusitis. However, in chronic sinusitis, no specific pathogen has been isolated on a consistent basis, and multiple organisms have been isolated, ranging from gram-negative organisms to anaerobes to *Staphylococcus aureus*. In patients who are immunocompromised, *Staphylococcus aureus, Moraxella catarrhalis,* and fungi may play a more consistent role.

What Factors May Predispose a Patient to Sinusitis?

- Inflammatory conditions can lead to edematous changes affecting the epithelium and drainage (e.g., URI, allergic rhinitis, rhinitis medicamentosa, sarcoidosis, Wegener granulomatosis).
- Cocaine abuse (snorting) can destroy epithelium.
- Dental infection may spread to the sinuses (maxillary in particular).
- Anatomic abnormalities may lead to obstruction (e.g., nasal polyps, deviated nasal septum).
- Immune disorders [e.g., human immunodeficiency virus (HIV) infection, immunoglobulin A or G deficiencies].
- Genetic disorders associated with ciliary problems (e.g., cystic fibrosis, primary ciliary dyskinesia).
- Sports (e.g., diving, swimming).
- Nasal instrumentation (e.g., nasogastric tube placement).

What Are the Clinical Features of Bacterial Sinusitis?

Signs and symptoms tend to overlap in acute and chronic sinusitis. Sometimes there is not a clear distinction between acute and chronic sinusitis other than chronology of symptoms. In acute sinusitis, patients may present with nasal obstruction, purulent nasal discharge, facial pain, or pressure that is worsened by bending forward or by Valsalva maneuver. Patient also may complain of puffy eyelids, epistaxis, hoarseness, and stuffy eyes. The headache description may correlate with the affected sinus, thereby alerting the physician to possible complications:

- Ethmoidal sinusitis: headache between and behind eyes
- Frontal sinusitis: headache above the eyes, masklike pattern
- Maxillary sinusitis: pain over the teeth, cheeks, ipsilateral temple
- Sphenoidal sinusitis: vertex/occipital headache

Chronic sinusitis is a complication of acute sinusitis. Therefore, patients may experience the above symptoms and also complain of halitosis, hyposmia/anosmia, or a chronic cough arising from postnasal drip.

What Is the Diagnostic Approach to Sinusitis?

Initial diagnosis is usually made on history and physical examination alone. Some investigators have indicated that when the following five clinical entities are present, the predictive probability of bacterial sinusitis is 92%, making other etiologies such as viral, mucosal abnormalities, or hyperreactivity reactions less likely.

- Maxillary toothache
- Poor response to decongestant alone
- Purulent nasal discharge
- Mucopurulence seen on intranasal examination
- Inability to transilluminate sinuses

Keep in mind that transillumination of the sinuses is nonspecific. It is rarely possible to effectively transilluminate the sinuses even in the healthy population. The easiest sinuses to transilluminate are frontal, and they are absent in up to 10% of the population.

Plain sinus film is helpful in excluding sinusitis if negative. A patient with a viral illness or a chronic inflammation would have opacified sinuses with air-fluid levels.

Sinus computed tomography is more sensitive and specific, but it is expensive. It is the modality of choice for providing anatomic information and bone thickening. There are certain guidelines on when to consider ordering a CT scan of the sinuses:

- Recurrent acute sinusitis despite medical therapy
- Chronic sinusitis symptoms despite maximal medical therapy
- Prior to sinus surgery
- Unclear presentation

Nasal endoscopy is relatively invasive and is used for better visualization, biopsy, culture, and even therapy if able to relieve obstruction. There are more consistent data regarding use of nasal endoscopy in obtaining biopsies (e.g., for diagnosis of granulomatous diseases) than use in obtaining cultures.

Sinus aspiration is so far the gold standard, but it is invasive and not routinely done.

What Is the Management Approach and Referral Indication?

Topical and systemic decongestant are vasoconstrictor agents that reduce the thickness of nasal mucosa. Therefore, theoretically, decongestant should improve symptoms, but there are no data available to statistically demonstrate benefits.

Most clinicians agree that mucolytic agents such as guaifenesin should benefit patients with sinusitis, but few data are available to support such treatment.

Mucoevacuants such as saline solution, steam inhalation, heated mist, or dry/hot air are recommended to patients with sinusitis, but no supportive data exist.

The role of corticosteroids in the management of sinusitis is controversial. It is known to decrease mucosal swelling, decrease tissue eosinophilia (histologic hallmark of chronic sinusitis), and shrink nasal polyps, and is therefore thought to help in managing sinusitis. The results of three small studies indicated improvement with topical steroids, but no data from prospective, randomized, controlled studies are available.

Antibiotic use is mostly empiric, and antibiotic resistance has been on the rise. Amoxicillin or trimethoprim/sulfamethoxazole are considered first-line treatment for acute sinusitis. However, we need to be aware of bacteria resistance in the area. When the appropriate antibiotic is instituted, the patient should start to feel better in 3 days or so and the course of antibiotic completed in 10 to 14 days.

In chronic sinusitis, antibiotics should be of broader spectrum, such as amoxicillin/clavulanic acid, and the duration should be for 3 to 4 weeks.

Reasons for referral to an ear, nose, and throat (ENT) specialist include:

- Intracranial complications (meningitis, brain abscess, cavernous sinus thrombosis)
- Extracranial complications (osteomyelitis, orbital cellulitis, decreased visual acuity)
- Nasal polyps
- Treatment failure
- Frequent recurrences
- Nosocomial infections
- Immunocompromised host
- Fungal sinusitis

Case

A 49-year-old man initially seen in an urgent care setting was referred to you for follow-up. He reports getting "pills and stuff for my nose," but with no relief. He reports having a "sinus infection" for 4 months. He cannot breathe through his nose, has decreased perception of taste and smell, and complains of pain in his face and teeth, foul drainage from his nose, and postnasal drip. He requests "a shot to knock it out" since he states he will not take any more pills.

On examination he is afebrile with no facial asymmetry. His eyelids are mildly edematous, conjunctiva are not injected, and ears are within normal limits. There is tenderness over both maxillary sinuses, greatest on the right. None of the sinuses transilluminate. The nasal septum is in the midline. There are no nasal polyps, and the mucosa is erythematous with boggy turbinates and mucopurulent discharge. He has very poor dentition but no evidence of dental abscesses. There is no preauricular or cervical lymphadenopathy, and the rest of the physical examination is within normal limits.

1. What additional information would you like to obtain?
2. What diagnostic tests would you order, if any?
3. How would you treat the patient?

Case Discussion

What Additional Information Would You Like to Obtain?

The signs and symptoms of the initial presentation are important in identifying predisposing conditions such as allergic rhinitis, URI, and poor dentition. A detailed headache description can help identify the sinus involved. A history of recurrent infections can help define the patient's immune status. Information regarding any previous diagnostic workup or previous management (e.g., medications used, the duration of medication use, and his compliance with medications) can be helpful.

What Is Your Diagnosis?

Based on the duration of his symptoms of at least 4 months, tenderness over the maxillary sinuses, pain over the teeth, and purulent nasal discharge, he most likely has chronic maxillary bacterial sinusitis. A further assessment of the patient's immune status would be appropriate, including testing for HIV infection.

How Would You Treat the Patient?

Based on the history, compliance has been an issue and most likely a determining factor in treatment failure. Before any suggestion about medication, you need to determine why he is refusing to take pills. Educating the patient about his illness and treatment is very important. You need to determine if appropriate antibiotic therapy was used and consider antibiotic resistance given the likelihood of noncompliance. A 3- to 4-week course of broad-spectrum antibiotic therapy should be recommended. Decongestants might give symptomatic relief (but may be unacceptable to a patient who does not want to take pills). The patient should be monitored closely for resolution of symptoms and to encourage compliance. With his long-standing symptoms, early referral to an ENT specialist would be indicated.

Suggested Reading

Ahuja G S, et al. What role for antibiotics in otitis media and sinusitis? *Postgrad Med* 1998;104:93–104.
Ferguson B J. Acute and chronic sinusitis. *Postgrad Med* 1995;97:45–57.
Guarderas J C. Rhinitis and sinusitis: office management. *Mayo Clin Proc* 1996;71:882–888.
Reuler J B, et al. Sinusitis: a review for generalists. *West J Med* 1995;163:40–48.

54

Urinary Tract Infections

Linda J. Schultz

1. What is the appropriate evaluation and treatment for uncomplicated urinary tract infections?
2. Which patients should not receive a short course of antibiotic therapy for treatment of an acute urinary tract infection?
3. What is the management of recurrent urinary tract infections?
4. When do you treat and provide prophylaxis for urinary tract infections associated with catheters?
5. When do you screen and treat asymptomatic bacteriuria?

Discussion

What Is the Appropriate Evaluation and Treatment for Uncomplicated Urinary Tract Infections?

Urinary tract infections (UTIs) are significantly more common in women than in men. A UTI is considered "uncomplicated" if it is acute (nonrecurrent) and the patient is a nonpregnant female, under 65 years of age, and without significant comorbidities that could increase the risk of upper tract infection or resistant organisms (e.g., diabetes mellitus, immunosuppression, or structural urologic disease). Although dysuria, frequency, and urgency are the classic symptoms of a UTI, all dysuria is not a UTI. The differential diagnosis in women also includes yeast and *Trichomonas vaginalis* infections, gonorrhea, and chlamydia, as well as atrophic vaginitis in older women. In men, urethritis and prostatitis should be considered. Approximately 80% of uncomplicated UTIs are caused by *Escherichia coli,* with 5% to 15% caused by *Staphylococcus saprophyticus.* Occasionally the etiology is *Klebsiella, Proteus,* or other microorganisms. Risk factors for acute and recurrent UTIs in women include sexual intercourse, delayed postcoital micturition, use of a diaphragm and spermicide, and use of a spermicide alone.

The most common initial test used to make the diagnosis of a UTI is a urine dipstick. Dipstick leukocyte esterase is 75% to 95% sensitive for pyuria. In an uncomplicated UTI, the etiology and antibiotic susceptibility are so predictable that a urine culture is not needed in a classic presentation, and a course of empiric antibiotics is reasonable. If the dipstick test result is negative and the patient has urinary symptoms, urine microscopy and culture should be considered. A positive urine culture has urinary pathogen growth of 100 or more colony-forming units per milliliter. A small study conducted in an emergency department examining the use of urinalysis in patients presenting with possible UTI showed that the addition of urinary microscopy to the initial dipstick results did not alter the course of treatment in 94% of patients.

Several randomized controlled trials published in the late 1980s showed that the optimal antibiotic regimen for young women (nonpregnant) presenting with an acute UTI is a 3-day course of antibiotics. The 3-day regimen has comparable efficacy to the 7-day regimen, but with decreased side effects and decreased cost. The 3-day regimen is also better than the single-dose regimen because the single dose results in lower cure rates and higher recurrence of infection. The low cure rate is due to the drug's rapid excretion. Recommended antibiotics include trimethoprim-sulfamethoxazole, trimethoprim alone, or quinolones. Quinolones are usually only recommended for recurrent or resistant infections due to their cost. The resistance rates are approximately 30% for amoxicillin or sulfamethoxazole alone, 15% to 20% for nitrofurantoin, 5% to 15% for trimethoprim-sulfamethoxazole, and 5% for quinolones (although this may be increasing now).

Which Patients Should Not Receive a Short Course of Antibiotic Therapy for Treatment of an Acute Urinary Tract Infection?

Diabetic patients, pregnant patients, patients over age 65, and patients with recurrent infection should be treated with 7 days of antibiotic therapy. Young men also should be treated for 7 days. Older men usually have an underlying urologic abnormality and should be treated as having a complicated UTI for 14 days with a quinolone. Women with a functional or structural urinary tract abnormality should be treated for 10 to 14 days with a quinolone.

What Is the Management of Recurrent UTIs?

Recurrent UTIs are defined as two or more infections within 6 months or three or more infections in the last year. Risk factors are sexual intercourse, delayed postcoital micturition, diaphragm and spermicide use, spermicide use alone, ABO blood group nonsecretory phenotype, and postmenopausal women with a cystocele, vaginal atrophy, or uterine prolapse. Some women with recurrent urine infections have persistent colonization of the vagina with *E. coli*. This may be due to the absence of hydrogen peroxide–producing lactobacilli in the vagina. Spermicides also cause recurrence of urine infections by altering the normal vaginal flora. Overall the cause of recurrent UTIs is rarely a functional abnormality; therefore, a workup is not recommended. A urine culture should be ordered for women with recurrent infections to look for resistant strains of bacteria.

Several studies performed in the late 1980s support the use of prophylactic antibiotics for recurrent UTIs. Patients experience a statistically significant decrease in recurrent infection while on antibiotics that did not return for 3 to 6 months when off of antibiotics. Two different regimens have been studied. One regimen is a daily antibiotic; the other is a postcoital antibiotic. Both regimens are equally effective. The antibiotics found to be effective are trimethoprim-sulfamethoxazole at one double-strength tablet, nitrofurantoin at 50 mg, and quinolones (ciprofloxacin at

125 or 250 mg). Nitrofurantoin was found to be more effective than trimethoprim alone due to the higher resistance that developed with trimethoprim. Women who took prophylactic antibiotics were found to have a decrease in vaginal *E. coli* and a decrease in *Enterobacter* in the intestine, vagina, and periurethral area. The most recent study on prophylaxis shows that ciprofloxacin is an effective agent for prophylaxis under either regimen with minimal resistance developing. In this and other studies, the postcoital regimen was better tolerated with fewer side effects and a decrease in the total cost of antibiotics. The postcoital regimen should be used especially if the infections are temporally related to sexual intercourse. A third regimen is patient initiated therapy. When patients begin to have symptoms, they can treat themselves with a 3-day course of antibiotics.

When Do You Treat and Provide Prophylaxis for Urinary Tract Infections Associated with Catheters?

If the patient with an indwelling urinary catheter has symptoms suggesting a UTI, treat as a complicated UTI for 10 to 14 days. The infections are usually polymicrobial. Intermittent catheterization results in a lower rate of bacteriuria than long-term indwelling catheters. Patients need to use sterile techniques during intermittent catheterization. If an indwelling catheter has been used long term, the catheter should be changed intermittently because organisms adhere to the catheter and make biofilms to protect themselves. Treating asymptomatic episodes does not reduce complications of bacteriuria in patients with long-term catheters.

Prophylactic regimens are not effective in patients with long-term indwelling catheters. In patients who use intermittent catheterization, oral antibiotic prophylaxis or bladder irrigation with antibiotic solutions can be used.

When Do You Screen and Treat Asymptomatic Bacteriuria?

Asymptomatic bacteriuria is especially common in nursing home residents. Complications are rare in this group of patients and do not justify screening or routine use of prophylactic antibiotics. If a culture is obtained, criteria for infection is generally greater than 10 to the 5th colony forming units per milliliter.

Screening for UTI should only be performed on two occasions: before urologic surgery and during the first trimester of pregnancy. If asymptomatic infection is treated preoperatively, there is a decrease in postoperative complications, including bacteremia. Pregnant patients should be treated to decrease the risk of acute pyelonephritis, premature births, and low-birth-weight babies. Monthly urine cultures need to be obtained following initial culture in pregnant patients.

Case

A 35-year-old woman complains of dysuria. She has associated frequency and urgency but denies hematuria. She denies fever, chills, and vomiting. She has had "bladder infections" with similar symptoms in the past but none in the past 5 years. She is sexually active with one stable partner. She denies vaginal discharge or abdominal pain. For contraception she recently changed from oral contraceptive pills to a diaphragm and spermicide. Her last menstrual period was 7 days ago, and her periods are regular.

Physical examination reveals a blood pressure of 130/70 mm Hg, and she is afebrile. Her abdomen is soft with active bowel sounds. She has mild suprapubic tenderness but no costavertebral angle tenderness. Her urine dipstick is positive for both nitrate and leukocyte esterase.

1. What is the initial management of this patient?
2. The patient returns 2 months later with the same symptoms. A urine culture is performed and she is treated with trimethoprim-sulfamethoxazole double strength twice daily for 7 days. The urine culture grows *E. coli,* sensitive to trimethoprim-sulfamethoxazole. What is the diagnosis and management?
3. She returns again 2 months later with the same symptoms. On her third visit, what changes in management should be discussed?

Case Discussion
What Is the Initial Management of This Patient?

This patient has all of the classic symptoms of an uncomplicated UTI. She has no evidence of pyelonephritis or vaginitis by history or examination. Her urine dipstick test result is positive. Her last UTI by her report was 5 years ago, so she does not meet criteria for recurrent infections at this time. Because the most likely offending organism is *E. coli* and she has not been on antibiotics recently, a urine culture is not needed. She is started on trimethoprim-sulfamethoxazole double-strength twice daily for 3 days.

The Patient Returns 2 Months Later with the Same Symptoms. What Is the Diagnosis and Management?

Because the patient returns 2 months after the initial infection and has had two infections in the past 6 months, she is diagnosed with recurrent UTIs. At this time a urine culture is performed to evaluate susceptibility of the organism. She is treated for 7 days with the trimethoprim-sulfa, because this is no longer an uncomplicated UTI. The patient is also educated on the risk factors of recurrent UTIs, which for her include sexual intercourse and the use of a diaphragm and spermicide. However, she decides to continue to use the same method of birth control.

She Returns Again 2 Months Later with the Same Symptoms. On Her Third Visit, What Changes in Management Should Be Discussed?

She is treated again for 7 days with trimethoprim-sulfamethoxazole because her cultures have been sensitive. At this time prophylactic antibiotics are discussed, including the everyday and post-coital regimens. Because the infections are somewhat temporally related to sexual intercourse, she decides on the postcoital regimen. She is given nitrofurantoin 50 mg to take after sexual intercourse.

Suggested Reading

Gupta K, Stapleton A E, et al. Inverse association of H_2O_2-producing lactobacilli and vaginal *Escherichia coli* colonization in women with recurrent urinary tract infections. *J Infect Dis* 1998;178: 446–450.

Hooton T M, Scholes D, et al. A prospective study of risk factors for symptomatic urinary tract infection in young women. *N Engl J Med* 1996;335:468–474.

Hooton T M, Winter C, et al. Randomized comparative trial and cost analysis of 3-day antimicrobial regimens for treatment of acute cystitis in women. *JAMA* 1995;273:41–45.

Jou W W, Powers R D. Utility of dipstick urinalysis as a guide to management of adults with suspected infection or hematuria. *South Med J* 1998;91:266–269.

Melekos M D, Asbach H W, et al. Post-intercourse versus daily ciprofloxacin prophylaxis for recurrent urinary tract infections in premenopausal women. *J Urol* 1997;157:935–939.

Stamm W E, Hooton T M. Management of urinary tract infections in adults. *N Engl J Med* 1993;1328–1334.

55

Sexually Transmitted Diseases: Cervicitis, Urethritis, and Pelvic Inflammatory Disease

Linda J. Schultz

1. What are the clinical presentations and differential diagnoses for urethritis and cervicitis?
2. How are urethritis and cervicitis diagnosed and treated?
3. What are the clinical characteristics and causes of pelvic inflammatory disease?
4. What is the treatment for pelvic inflammatory disease, and when is hospitalization recommended?
5. What are the current CDC prevention and counseling guidelines for sexually transmitted diseases?

Discussion

What Are the Clinical Presentations and Differential Diagnoses for Urethritis and Cervicitis?

The symptoms of urethritis in a man include mucopurulent or purulent penile discharge and dysuria. Asymptomatic infections are common. *Neisseria gonorrhoeae* is one of the leading causes of urethritis in men. *Chlamydia trachomatis* is the most frequent cause of nongonococcal urethritis (NGU), accounting for approximately 25% to 55% of cases. Other causes of NGU include *Ureaplasma urealyticum, Mycoplasma genitalium, Trichomonas vaginalis,* and herpes simplex virus. Testing for *U. urealyticum* or *M. genitalium* is not recommended. However, testing for *Trichomonas* is recommended when urethritis symptoms persist following empiric treatment for nongonococcal urethritis.

The symptoms of cervicitis are a vaginal discharge or vaginal bleeding. On examination, women are found to have purulent or mucopurulent discharge in the endocervical canal and a friable cervix. However, about 75% of women with cervicitis have few or no symptoms and no findings on examination. Many women who appear to have an uncomplicated cervical infection already have a subclinical upper reproductive tract infection. The differential diagnosis for cervicitis includes *Chlamydia trachomatis* and *Neisseria gonorrhoeae*. *Chlamydia* is the most common bacterial sexually transmitted disease (STD) in the United States, causing approximately 4 million infections each year. An estimated 1 in 10 adolescent girls and 1 in 20 women of reproductive age are infected. Without treatment, 20% to 40% of women with *Chlamydia* develop pelvic inflammatory disease (PID). In women, chlamydia can lead to PID, ectopic pregnancy, and infertility.

How Are Urethritis and Cervicitis Diagnosed and Treated?

For men with urethritis, the diagnosis of NGU is made by evidence of any of the following: a purulent discharge, a Gram stain with five white blood cells (WBCs) per high-power field and no evidence of *Neisseria* gonorrhea, or a positive leukocyte esterase test result on first-void urine. Gonococcal urethritis is diagnosed by a Gram stain result with WBCs containing intracellular gram-negative diplococci. The diagnosis can also be made by urethral culture.

Cervicitis from gonorrhea is diagnosed clinically and with cultures; Gram staining is not recommended. For years, cell culture has been considered the method for diagnosing chlamydia, but the less sensitive enzyme immunoassays (86%–93%) have been widely used in laboratories with a high workload. Ligase chain reactions, a DNA amplification technique, have improved sensitivity and are nearly 100% specific. The sensitivity decreases when first-void urine samples are used instead of genital swabs. The sensitivity for *Chlamydia* in the urine still far exceeds that achieved by culture of the swabs. Due to the asymptomatic nature and the serious sequelae of chlamydial infection, adolescents and women 20 to 24 years of age should be screened if they are sexually active, particularly those who have new or multiple sex partners and do not consistently use barrier contraceptives.

Patients are often coinfected with gonorrhea and chlamydia, which led to the recommendation that empiric treatment should cover both organisms. Empiric treatment is indicated for patients who are high risk or are unlikely to return for follow-up. Common treatment options include coverage of gonorrhea with one intramuscular 125-mg dose of ceftriaxone, one oral 400-mg dose of cefixime, one 500-mg dose of ciprofloxacin, or one 400-mg dose of ofloxacin plus one 1-g dose of azithromycin or 100 mg doxycycline twice daily for 7 days to cover *C. trachomatis*. Ceftriaxone has a better cure rate for gonorrhea (99.1%) compared with cefixime's cure rate (97.1%), but cefixime has the advantage of oral dosing. Cases of *N. gonorrhoeae* resistant to fluoroquinolones have been reported from many areas of the world, and are becoming widespread in parts of Asia. As of 1997, less than 0.05% of isolates from the United States at the Centers for Disease Control and Prevention (CDC) were quinolone resistant. Azithromycin and doxycycline are equally efficacious in the treatment of chlamydia. Azithromycin has the advantage of administration in a single dose and thus can be used for directly observed therapy. Tetracyclines and fluoroquinolones are contraindicated during pregnancy.

What Are the Clinical Characteristics and Causes of Pelvic Inflammatory Disease?

Pelvic inflammatory disease includes a spectrum of inflammatory disorders of the upper female genital tract, including any combination of endometritis, salpingitis, tuboovarian abscess, and pelvic peritonitis. PID is difficult to diagnose because many women have subtle or mild symptoms. Because of the difficulty of diagnosis and the potential for damage to the reproductive organs (even with mild PID), health-care providers should maintain a low threshold for the diagnosis and treatment of PID. Empiric treatment of PID should be given if the patient has lower abdominal tenderness, adnexal tenderness, or cervical motion tenderness, and no other causes can be found. Additional criteria that support a diagnosis of PID include temperature over 101°F, abnormal cervical or vaginal discharge, elevated erythrocyte sedimentation rate, elevated C-reactive protein, and documentation of gonorrhea or *Chlamydia*. The definitive criteria for diagnosis is warranted in only selected cases and is made by evidence of endometritis by endometrial biopsy, thick fluid-filled tubes with or without free pelvic fluid by ultrasonography, or laparoscopic abnormalities.

As stated earlier, the most common organisms are *N. gonorrhoeae* and *C. trachomatis*. However, organisms that can be part of the vaginal flora can contribute to PID (anaerobes, *G. vaginalis, H. influenzae,* enteric gram-negative rods, and *Streptococcus agalactiae*). PID causes chronic pelvic pain and damage to the reproductive organs, leading to ectopic pregnancies and infertility. Permanent damage to the fallopian tubes can result from a single episode of PID but is even more common with each successive episode. Thirty percent of infertility in women may be related to past STDs and PID.

What Is the Treatment for Pelvic Inflammatory Disease and When Is Hospitalization Recommended?

Several treatment regimens have been shown to improve patient outcomes at short-term follow-up, but few investigators have determined the incidence of long-term complications. There are also no current data comparing the efficacy of intravenous and oral therapy or inpatient and outpatient treatment. Outpatient regimens include one intramuscular dose of 250 mg ceftriaxone, one intramuscular dose of 2 g cefoxitin plus 1 g probenecid orally, or most other third-generation cephalosporins plus 100 mg doxycycline twice daily for 14 days. An alternative regimen is 400 mg ofloxacin twice daily for 14 days plus 500 mg metronidazole twice daily for 14 days. The major difference in treatment between cervicitis and PID is the increase in the length of treatment for chlamydia with doxycyclin at 14 days and single g dose. Azithromycin is not effective.

The following are criteria for hospitalization based on observational data:

- A surgical emergency cannot be excluded.
- Pregnancy.
- Nonreponse to oral antibiotics within 72 hours.
- The patient is unable to follow or tolerate an outpatient regimen.
- The patient has nausea/vomiting or high fever, suggesting a severe illness or presence of a tuboovarian abscess.
- The patient is immunodeficient.

If hospitalization is required, the recommended antibiotic regimen is intravenous cephalosporin plus doxycycline or clindamycin and gentamicin together.

What Are the Current CDC Prevention and Counseling Guidelines for Sexually Transmitted Diseases?

1. The health-care provider must take an accurate sexual history. This history should be part of the clinical review of systems.
2. When risk factors have been identified, the provider has an opportunity to deliver prevention messages.
3. The messages should include a description of specific actions that the patient can take to avoid acquiring or transmitting STDs: specifically, the use of condoms and spermicides to prevent infection and abstinence during STD-related symptoms.
4. Once a patient is diagnosed with any STD, the sexual partners should be advised to seek testing and treatment. Patients should be encouraged to notify their partners, but many local health departments can assist in notification of reportable STDs [human immunodeficiency virus (HIV), syphilis, gonorrhea, chlamydia, and hepatitis B].
5. Once a patient is diagnosed with any STD, he or she should be offered testing for other STDs, especially HIV.
6. Patients with STDs should be tested for hepatitis B and offered hepatitis A and B vaccines if appropriate.

Case

A 34-year-old woman presents complaining of vaginal discharge. She has had the discharge for 2 weeks and describes it as yellow and thick. She also has noticed some mild abdominal pain in the lower quadrants over the past 3 days. She reports subjective fevers but no nausea or vomiting. She denies any dysuria or vaginal itching. Her sexual history includes two new partners in the past 2 months. She has not used condoms, because she believes her tubal ligation performed 8 years ago will protect her from pregnancy. Her last menstrual period was 2 weeks ago, and her periods are regular. Her past history includes four vaginal deliveries without complications. She has a history of gonorrhea several years ago.

On physical examination she is afebrile and well appearing. On pelvic examination there is mild inguinal lymphadenopathy. The vulva and vagina are normal. The cervix is friable and there is a copious amount of yellow discharge from the os. The uterus and adnexa are tender, and there is mild cervical motion tenderness.

1. What is her diagnosis?
2. What treatment should be given?
3. What else should be done at the visit?

Case Discussion

What Is Her Diagnosis?

The patient has PID given the discharge from the os and the adnexal and cervical motion tenderness. The patient should be treated empirically for PID because she is tender on pelvic examination, even though she does not have a fever. The most likely cause is chlamydia or *Neisseria* gnorrhea, and tests should be performed for both organisms.

What Treatment Should Be Given?

The patient does not have an indication for hospitalization; therefore, she can be treated as an outpatient with close follow-up. She is treated with a single intramuscular dose of 250 mg ceftriaxone and 100 mg doxycycline twice daily for 14 days. She is scheduled for a follow-up examination in 48 hours to ensure that her infection is not worsening. Pregnancy is highly unlikely in this patient because she has had a tubal ligation. If there is any question of pregnancy, her β human chorionic gonadotropin (βHCG) level should be checked to help determine if the patient should be admitted and to guide the choice of antibiotics.

What Else Should Be Done at the Visit?

Most importantly, the patient should receive counseling on STDs and HIV. She should be educated on barrier contraception and its use to prevent infections. The patient should be offered screening tests for HIV, hepatitis, and syphilis. Finally the patient should tell her partner of her diagnosis and encourage him to be tested. The patient should not have sexual intercourse even with a condom until she and the partner are treated.

Suggested Reading

Carne C. Recent advances: sexually transmitted infections. *BMJ* 1998;317:129–132.

Caul E O, Horner P J, et al. Population-based screening programs for *Chlamydia trachomatis. Lancet* 1997;349:1070–1071.

Centers for Disease Control and Prevention (CDC). *Guidelines for treatment of sexually transmitted disease,* Atlanta. CDC, 1998.

Ho Gloria Y F, Bierman R, et al. Natural history of cervicovaginal papillomavirus infection in young women. *N Engl J Med* 1998;338:423–428.

Mishell D R, Stenchever M A, Droegemueller W, et al., eds. *Comprehensive gynecology,* 3rd ed. St. Louis: CV Mosby, 1997.

56

Sexually Transmitted Diseases: Genital Ulcers and Warts

Linda J. Schultz

1. What is the differential diagnosis for genital ulcers?
2. What are the characteristics and treatment for herpes simplex virus, including the treatment of recurrent episodes?
3. What are the characteristics, diagnosis, and treatment for the stages of syphilis?
4. What are the characteristics, diagnosis, and treatment for chancroid, granuloma inguinale, and lymphogranuloma venereum?
5. What are the characteristics and treatment for warts due to human papillomavirus?

Discussion

What Is the Differential Diagnosis for Genital Ulcers?

The differential diagnosis for genital ulcers includes herpes simplex virus (HSV), syphilis, chancroid, granuloma inguinale, and lymphogranuloma venereum (LGV).

What Are the Characteristics and Treatment for Herpes Simplex Virus, Including the Treatment of Recurrent Episodes?

Genital herpes is caused by either HSV-1 or HSV-2. Only five percent to 30% of first episodes are caused by HSV-1. Clinical recurrences are much less frequent for HSV-1 (55% chance of recurrence within 1 year) than HSV-2 (80% chance of recurrence in 1 year). HSV-2 has been diagnosed in approximately 45 million persons in the United States, and it is believed that many remain undiagnosed.

Herpes lesions begin as erythematous papules followed by grouped vesicles, which may evolve into pustules. Prior to the eruption of vesicles, patients often experience a prodrome of burning or itching. The lesions may turn into large ulcers. Local symptoms of genital herpes include dysuria, pain, pruritis, and tender inguinal lymphadenopathy. In general, the initial outbreak is usually more severe than subsequent outbreaks and can include fever, malaise, and myalgias.

For the first episode, the diagnosis is made by culture of the ulcer. Typing the strain is helpful to predict recurrence rate and for counseling. Management consists of antiviral therapy and counseling. Three antiviral medications have been shown in randomized trials to provide clinical benefit: acyclovir at 400 mg three times daily for 7 to 10 days, famciclovir at 250 mg three times daily for 7 to 10 days, and valacyclovir at 1 g twice daily for 7 to 10 days. Valacyclovir is almost completely converted to acyclovir in the body, and both famciclovir and valacyclovir have good oral bioavailability. Topical acyclovir is substantially less effective than the systemic drugs; therefore, its use is discouraged. Counseling should include information on the natural history of the disease, preventing transmission, the risk of neonatal infection, and the benefits of antiviral treatment. Patients should be aware that viral shedding and risk of transmission can occur even during asymptomatic periods.

Most patients with genital HSV-2 have recurrent episodes of genital lesions. Episodic or suppressive antiviral therapy might shorten the duration of lesions or decrease the number of recurrences. Episodic treatment and should be started during the prodromal phase or within 1 day of the onset of lesions. Antiviral treatment can be given for 5 days. In patients with frequent recurrences (six or more per year), daily suppressive therapy reduces the frequency of recurrences by approximately 75%. For suppressive therapy, antivirals are given twice daily instead of three times a day. Because the frequency of recurrences decreases over time, discontinuation of suppressive therapy should be attempted after 1 year. Suppressive treatment with acyclovir reduces but does not eliminate asymptomatic viral shedding.

What Are the Characteristics, Diagnosis, and Treatment for the Stages of Syphilis?

Syphilis, caused by the spirochete *Treponema pallidum,* is a systemic disease characterized by multiple stages. Syphilis is classified as primary, secondary, latent, or tertiary.

Primary infection is characterized by a painless ulcer, also called a chancre. It is typically round with raised borders and a serous exudate. The ulcer occurs approximately 3 weeks after the primary exposure. Nontender adenopathy also may be present.

Secondary infection appears 2 to 10 weeks after the primary infection. The characteristic skin lesions are round macules and papules on the trunk, hands, and palms. Condylomata lata also occur and are soft, flat-topped, moist, pale papules or plaques that may become confluent. These are generally found in the anogenital region. Patients also can develop patchy alopecia and white-gray mucous membrane patches. Systemic findings include fever, generalized lymphadenopathy, and splenomegaly.

Latent syphilis is the stage where patients are seroreactive but there are no clinical signs or symptoms of the infection. This stage varies in duration from 2 to 20 years. Latent syphilis is divided into early latent, acquired within the preceding year, and late latent syphilis or syphilis of unknown duration. Early latent syphilis can be diagnosed by documented seroconversion within the past year, unequivocal symptoms of primary or secondary syphilis within the past year, or a sex partner who had primary, secondary, or early latent syphilis within the past year.

Tertiary syphilis is now rare and develops in approximately 33% of patients left untreated. Tertiary infection involves cardiac, neurologic, ophthalmic, auditory, or gummatous (cold abscess with necrotic center) lesions. The skin lesions are granulomatous, reddish brown papules and nodules.

The definitive tests for diagnosing early syphilis are dark-field examination and direct fluorescent antibody test of a lesion exudate or tissue. A presumptive diagnosis is made with the two types of serologic tests that become positive 4 to 6 weeks after exposure: nontreponemal and treponemal. Nontreponemal tests include the venereal disease research laboratory (VDRL) and rapid plasma reagent (RPR); treponemal tests include fluorescent treponemal antibody absorbed (FTA-ABS) and microhemagglutination assay for antibody to *T. pallidum* (MHA-TP). Because various medical conditions, including connective tissue diseases, pregnancy, and multiple infectious diseases, can result in a false-positive nontreponemal test result, an adjunctive treponemal test should be used. Nontreponemal test antibody titers usually correlate with disease activity and should be reported by the lab. A fourfold change in titer, equivalent to a change of two dilutions (from 1:16 to 1:4), is usually considered a clinically significant change. Sequential serologic tests should be performed using the same test at the same laboratory; RPR titers are often slightly higher than VDRL titers. The RPR and VDRL tests are equally valid. Most nontreponemal tests will eventually become nonreactive after treatment, but in some patients nontreponemal antibodies can persist at a low titer for a long period or indefinitely. Most patients with reactive treponemal tests will have a reactive test for the rest of their lives regardless of treatment. However, 15% to 25% of patients treated during the primary stage will have a negative treponemal test after 2 to 3 years. Treponemal test antibodies correlate poorly with disease activity and should not be used to assess treatment response.

The treatment of primary, secondary, and early latent syphilis is a single dose of benzathine penicillin G 2.4 million units administered intramuscularly. For patients allergic to penicillin, doxycycline 100 mg twice daily or tetracycline 500 mg four times daily for 2 weeks can be used. Late latent syphilis or latent syphilis of unknown duration should be treated with benzathine penicillin G 2.4 million units intramuscularly once weekly for 3 weeks. Again, doxycycline or tetracycline can be used for penicillin-allergic patients, but should be given for 4 weeks.

Invasion of the central nervous system by *T. pallidum* with resultant cerebrospinal fluid (CSF) abnormalities is common in patients with primary or secondary syphilis, but neurosyphilis develops in only a few patients after treatment. Therefore, unless clinical signs or symptoms of neurologic or ophthalmic involvement are present, lumbar puncture is not recommended for routine evaluation of patients who have primary or secondary syphilis. Patients with symptoms or signs of neurologic or ophthalmic disease (uveitis) should be evaluated for neurosyphilis and syphilitic eye disease. The evaluation should include CSF analysis and an ocular slit-lamp examination.

Patients should be reexamined clinically and serologically at both 6 and 12 months after treatment. If signs and symptoms persist or there is a fourfold increase in nontreponemal test titer, they probably have been reinfected or failed treatment. These patients should be retreated and retested for the human immunodeficiency virus (HIV), and a lumbar puncture should be performed if reinfection is not certain. If there is not a fourfold decrease in titers at 6 months, the patient should be retested for HIV, retreated, and a CSF examination considered. The regimen for retreatment is three weekly intramuscular injections of benzathine penicillin G 2.4 million units.

What Are the Characteristics, Diagnosis, and Treatment for Chancroid, Granuloma Inguinale and Lymphogranuloma Venereum?

Chancroid is caused by *Haemophilus ducreyi,* a gram-negative rod. The symptoms are painful ulcers with an erythematous halo and tender inguinal lymphadenopathy. A painful ulcer with suppurative inguinal adenopathy is typical. The adenopathy may drain spontaneously. A definitive diagnosis requires identification of *H. ducreyi* on a special culture medium that is not widely available. A probable diagnosis of *H. ducreyi* is made if the patient has one or more painful ulcers, there is no evidence of *T. pallidum* by dark-field examination or serology, or the patient has regional lymphadenopathy that is not felt to be secondary to HIV disease. Polymerase chain reaction (PCR) testing may become available for diagnostic use in the near future. Treatment options include oral azithromycin 1 g, ciprofloxacin 500 mg twice daily for 3 days, erythromycin 500 mg four times daily for 7 days, or a single intramuscular injection with ceftriaxone 250 mg.

Patients should be reexamined 3 to 7 days after treatment. The ulcers should improve symptomatically in 3 days and objectively in 7 days after therapy. The fluctuant lymphadenopathy may resolve more slowly than the ulcers and may require drainage.

Granuloma inguinale is rare in the United States, but is endemic in India, New Guinea, central Australia, and southern Africa. It is caused by an intracellular gram-negative bacterium, *Calymmatobacterium granulomatis.* The disease presents as painless, progressive, ulcerative lesions that are beefy red without regional lymphadenopathy. The lesions are highly vascular and bleed easily. Diagnosis requires visualization of dark-staining Donovan bodies on tissue crush preparation or biopsy. Treatment options include 3 weeks of trimethoprim-sulfamethoxazole double strength twice daily, doxycycline 100 mg twice daily, ciprofloxacin 750 mg twice daily, or erythromycin 500 mg four times daily. The addition of an aminoglycoside should be considered if lesions do not respond within the first few days.

Lymphogranuloma venereum is a rare disease in the United States. It is caused by the invasive forms of *Chlamydia trachomatis.* The symptoms begin with a self-limited ulcer at the inoculation site, but most patients present with unilateral inguinal or femoral tender lymphadenopathy that develops 1 to 4 weeks after the ulcer. The lymphadenopathy may drain spontaneously and form sinus tracts. Some patients might have proctocolitis or inflammatory involvement of perirectal or perianal lymphatic tissue. The diagnosis is made serologically and by exclusion of other causes of inguinal lymphadenopathy and genital ulcers. Treatment options include doxycycline 100 mg twice daily or erythromycin 500 mg four times daily for 21 days.

What Are the Characteristics and Treatment for Warts Due to Human Papillomavirus?

There are more than 20 types of human papillomavirus (HPV). Most HPV infections are asymptomatic, subclinical, or unrecognized. Types 6 and 11 usually cause visible genital warts. These two types are rarely associated with invasive squamous cell carcinoma of the external genitalia. HPV types 16, 18, 31, 33, and 35 have been strongly associated with cervical dysplasia. These types also have been associated with external genital squamous intraepithelial neoplasia, vaginal, anal, and cervical intraepithelial dysplasia, and squamous cell carcinoma. All women with genital warts should be followed closely with Papanicolaou (Pap) smears looking for dysplasia.

Although most infections are asymptomatic, genital warts can be painful, friable, or pruritic, depending on their size and location. The diagnosis is made clinically or by biopsy if the clinical diagnosis is uncertain (e.g., the lesions do not respond to therapy, the disease worsens with therapy, the patient is immunocompromised, or the warts are pigmented, indurated, fixed, or ulcerated). There are no data supporting the use of type-specific HPV nucleic acid tests in the routine diagnosis or management of visible genital warts.

The primary goal of treatment is the removal of symptomatic warts. Treatment can induce wart-free periods in most patients. The removal of warts may or may not decrease infectivity. The use of condoms may reduce but does not eliminate the risk of transmission to uninfected partners. If left untreated, visible genital warts may resolve, remain unchanged, or increase in size or number. No evidence indicates that treatment of visible warts affects the development of cervical cancer. Treatment options can be divided into patient-applied therapies and provider-administered therapies. Treatment is guided by location of warts, patient preference, available resources, and experience of health-care provider.

Patients can apply Podofilox or Imiquimod. Health-care providers can apply podophyllin resin or trichloracetic acid (TCA), or perform cryotherapy or surgery to remove the warts. Exophytic cervical warts should be treated by an expert. Vaginal warts can be treated with podophyllin, trichloracetic acid/dichoroacetic acid (TCA/BCA), or cryotherapy. Urethral meatal warts can be treated with podophyllin or cryotherapy. Anal warts can be treated with TCA/BCA, cryotherapy, or surgery.

Case

A 25-year-old woman notices an ulcer on her vulva after having sex with a new partner. She states the ulcer is not painful and noticed it only as she was using the bathroom. She denies any history of genital ulcers or other sexually transmitted diseases (STDs). She denies any vaginal discharge or abdominal pain. She uses oral contraceptive pills for birth control and has regular periods, but does not routinely use condoms.

On pelvic examination she has nontender, mild inguinal lymphadenopathy bilaterally. The vulva has several small fleshy colored papules clustered together on the labia. At the entrance to the vagina, there is a nontender ulcer with raised borders. There is no vaginal discharge and the cervix is pink. The uterus and adnexa are nontender.

1. What is the most likely cause of her ulcer?
2. What tests should be performed to confirm the diagnosis?
3. What treatment should be given now?

Case Discussion

What Is the Most Likely Cause of Her Ulcer?

The most likely diagnosis of the single nontender ulcer is primary syphilis. Chancroid presents as a painful ulcer with prominent adenopathy. Granuloma inguinale causes a painless ulcer also, but no adenopathy. LGV has prominent, tender adenopathy. Granuloma inguinale and LGV are both rare in the United States, and the patient has not traveled recently on further questioning. The fleshy colored papules are genital warts caused by HPV.

What Tests Should Be Performed to Confirm the Diagnosis?

For immediate diagnosis of the ulcer, a dark-field examination is needed. RPR or VDRL with a treponemal test should be ordered. Because the patient is at risk for other STDs, other laboratory studies are indicated, including culture for gonorrhea, a chlamydia assay, HIV test, and hepatitis profile. Given the genital warts observed on examination, a Pap smear is appropriate to look for dysplasia associated with HPV.

The dark-field examination result was positive and the RPR titer was 1:128. The rest of her test results were normal, including the Pap smear.

What Treatment Should Be Given Now?

The patient should be treated for primary syphilis with a single dose of intramuscular benzathine penicillin 2.4 million units. She can also be treated with podophyllin for the genital warts. Most importantly, she should be educated on the transmission of STDs and the risks of HIV infection.

Suggested Reading

Carne C. Recent advances: sexually transmitted infections. *BMJ* 1998;317:129–132.

Caul E O, Horner P J, et al. Population-based screening programs for *Chlamydia trachomatis. Lancet* 1997;349:1070–1071.

Centers for Disease Control and Prevention (CDC). *Guidelines for treatment of sexually transmitted disease,* Atlanta. CDC, 1998.

Ho Gloria Y F, Bierman R, et al. Natural history of cervicovaginal papillomavirus infection in young women. *N Engl J Med* 1998;338:423–428.

Mishell D R, Stenchever M A, Droegemueller W, et al., eds. *Comprehensive gynecology,* 3rd ed. St. Louis: CV Mosby, 1997.

57

Outpatient Management of Human Immunodeficiency Virus Infection

Henry Baffoe-Bonnie
Shanta Zimmer

1. What are the important features of the history in the initial evaluation of the HIV-infected patient?
2. What are the important features of the physical examination in the initial evaluation of the HIV-infected patient?
3. What tests should be obtained in the initial evaluation?
4. What preventive measures should be emphasized?

Discussion

What Are the Important Features of the History in the Initial Evaluation of the HIV-Infected Patient?

The primary care physician encountering a patient newly diagnosed with human immunodeficiency virus (HIV) infection must perform a detailed history and physical examination. For the history, it is important to probe for the presence of constitutional symptoms (e.g., night sweats, fever, weight loss, and fatigue).

The past medical history should include an assessment of existent chronic illnesses, a history of prior opportunistic infections or potential AIDS-defining illnesses, and a history of sexually transmitted diseases (STDs), hepatitis, and varicella-zoster (chicken pox or shingles). It is important to establish whether the patient has been in an environment considered high risk for contracting tuberculosis (e.g., jail/prison, a homeless shelter) or has had close contact with persons known to have active tuberculosis. Results of prior skin testing for tuberculosis should be obtained.

In addition to covering use of tobacco, alcohol, and drugs, the social history should include questions on occupation, hobbies, pets, and travel. Certain infections endemic to specific regions have the proclivity to reactivate in immunocompromised hosts; histoplasmosis is endemic in the Ohio and Mississippi river valleys, and coccidioidomycosis is endemic in the desert southwest. Patients should be questioned on current sexual practices and counseled on high-risk behaviors that could lead to further viral transmission. They should be strongly encouraged to inform prior sexual contacts of their diagnosis and urge them to seek HIV testing.

Despite significant advances in HIV care, a new diagnosis engenders a heavy psychological burden, and depression is not uncommon. Primary care physicians should probe for symptoms of depression and, if found, offer treatment in the form of medication or counseling.

What Are the Important Features of the Physical Examination in the Initial Evaluation of the HIV-Infected Patient?

A thorough baseline physical examination encompassing all organ systems should be performed. Vital signs should include a baseline weight. Common skin ailments (e.g., psoriasis, seborrheic dermatitis and folliculitis) tend to be more pronounced in HIV-infected individuals. It is important to look for the lesions of herpes simplex and condylomata acuminata, especially in the anogenital areas, and treat accordingly. Other less common skin diseases that may be more specific for HIV disease include Kaposi sarcoma (KS) and cryptococcus. It is crucial to look for lesions of KS because early treatment is beneficial. KS lesions are often asymptomatic round to oval patches on the skin or mucosa. They are typically pink to deep purple or dark brown. The soft and hard palates of the oral cavity are common sites of occurrence. These lesions often occur as single lesions or in clusters at the same or distant site and eventually become thickened plaques and nodular tumors. Cryptococcal infection can manifest as diffuse skin disease that may appear as papules or nodules. As a general rule, any suspicious skin finding should prompt referral to a dermatologist.

Ocular problems, particularly infections, occur frequently in HIV disease and can result in visual damage if untreated. For this reason, a dilated retinal examination should be performed on the initial encounter and prompt referral to an ophthalmologist should be made for any suspicious complaint or finding. In patients with very low CD4 cell counts ($<50/\mu L$), cytomegalovirus (CMV) eye disease is prevalent. Patients with CMV infection typically complain of "floaters" or abnormal spots floating in front of their eyes.

The newly infected female should have a Papanicolaou smear that should be repeated yearly. An abnormal Pap smear should be referred for immediate colposcopy. The incidence of cervical dysplasia is higher in HIV-infected women.

As part of a thorough physical examination, a good neurologic and mental status examination should be performed. Special attention should be focused on muscle strength, deep tendon reflexes, and the sensory examination because disorders such as progressive myelopathy can be caused by an opportunistic infection or HIV itself. If impairment in reality testing is detected, the clinician should ascertain from family members and friends whether the mental impairment is acute (e.g., consistent with delirium) or more chronic or progressive (suggesting dementia). The workup of mental status change in the newly infected HIV patient should include a lumbar puncture. The diagnosis of HIV dementia warrants consultation with an infectious disease specialist and therapy with antiretroviral agents.

What Tests Should Be Ordered?

Several laboratory tests should be obtained at the initial encounter, including a baseline complete blood count and chemistries. Although current HIV serology techniques are very specific, false-positive test results can occur. Repeat testing may be indicated, particularly among those tested through an anonymous program or those with high CD4 cell counts, undetectable viral loads, and no symptoms.

A baseline CD4 cell count should be obtained at the initial evaluation. The CD4 cell count is used to stage the disease and remains the benchmark for risk assessment. There is a seasonal and diurnal variation in the values. Some clinicians obtain two values at two different times. It is important for the primary care physician to know that the CD4 cell count is substantially affected by (a) intercurrent illness (e.g., severe upper respiratory infection, pneumonia) and (b) use of corticosteroids. The CD4 cell count should not be obtained in the office under these circumstances. It is best to wait about a week after recovery from an illness or after stopping steroids.

Viral load is used to assess prognosis, determine the need for antiretroviral therapy, and define a baseline value to judge the response to therapy. In the asymptomatic newly infected patient presenting to the primary care provider, it is appropriate to obtain a baseline value. Its measurement should be deferred in patients with intercurrent illness and recent vaccination. These conditions increase the value.

Syphilis testing should be obtained at the initial visit and repeated yearly. A positive rapid plasma reagent test result in an HIV-infected patient raises the specter of latent syphilis involving the central nervous system. A consultation with an infectious disease specialist is warranted in these situations.

The following hepatitis serologies should be obtained: hepatitis B surface antigen (HBsAg), hepatitis B core antibody (anti-HBcAb), and hepatitis C antibody (anti-HCV). Some authorities advise obtaining baseline antibody testing for hepatitis A (anti-HAV). Newly infected patients should be offered the hepatitis A and B vaccines when not contraindicated. Some newly emerging studies have now brought to light the important association of HIV and hepatitis C coinfection. When coinfection is detected by the primary care physician, referral to a gastroenterologist or an infectious disease specialist should be made.

Testing for varicella immunoglobulin G level should be obtained at the initial visit if a prior history of chickenpox cannot be obtained. A baseline test for evidence of exposure to toxoplasma also should be obtained (toxoplasma IgG).

A baseline test for cytomegalovirus (CMV) antibody should be obtained at the initial visit. Those testing positive should be told to report any vision changes that may be due CMV retinitis. It is crucial that those testing negative do not receive CMV-positive blood products in the future.

Cryptococcal antigen testing is not warranted in the asymptomatic patient unless a history of headache, malaise, or prominent constitutional symptoms is obtained. The primary care physician should be aware that cryptococcal disease can present cutaneously and that headache need not be a prominent feature of cryptococcal meningitis.

Glucose-6-phosphate dehydrogenase deficiency, an X-linked enzyme deficiency, is prevalent in African-American patients, and such patients should be tested for it because the use of drugs with oxidizing potential (e.g., dapsone) among affected patients could lead to hemolytic anemia.

All newly HIV-infected patients should be skin tested for tuberculosis. The Centers for Disease Control and Prevention recommends testing using 5 units of purified protein derivative (PPD). It is not necessary to test for anergy. Suppressive therapy is recommended for those with (a) a positive test, defined as 5 mm of induration or greater, (b) close contact with a patient with active tuberculosis, or (c) a history of a prior positive PPD and no treatment. All patients with a positive PPD should be questioned about the presence of constitutional symptoms (e.g., weight loss, night sweats, fevers) and should undergo chest radiography to look for evidence of old or active tuberculosis. Consultation with an infectious disease specialist is appropriate if the PPD is positive.

A baseline chest radiograph should be obtained in all newly infected HIV patients, regardless of PPD status.

What Preventative Measures Should Be Emphasized?

The United States Preventive Health Service and Infectious Disease Society of America (USPHS/IDSA) has provided guidelines for the prophylaxis of opportunistic infections in the HIV-infected patient.

Pneumocystis carinii *Pneumonia*

With the advent of highly active antiretroviral therapy (HAART), the incidence of *Pneumocystis carinii* pneumonia (PCP) has plummeted. For those newly infected patients with CD4 counts of less than 200/μL, trimethoprim-sulfamethoxazole (TMP-SMX) is still the agent of choice (one double-strength tablet daily or one single-strength tablet daily or one double-strength tablet three times weekly). Those intolerant of TMP-SMX can be offered dapsone 50 mg twice daily or 100 mg once daily. Other regimens exist for those intolerant of TMP-SMX and dapsone. Referral to an infectious disease specialist should be made in such cases. It is now established that prophylaxis for PCP can be safely discontinued in those who respond to HAART with an increase in the CD4 cell count above 200/μL. Recent studies suggest that this applies to even those with prior *Pneumocystis* infection (those on chronic maintenance therapy).

Mycobacterium avium *Complex*

Prophylaxis is indicated in persons with a CD4 count of less than 50/μL. Clarithromycin 500 mg twice daily and azithromycin 1,200 mg weekly are the two most used regimens. Rifabutin 300 mg daily is an alternative, but its use should be under the guidance of an infectious disease specialist because the drug has some interactions with other drugs that HIV patients may be taking. Insufficient data exist at present to recommend discontinuing prophylaxis in those who have responded to HAART with an increase in the CD4 cell count to above 50/μL.

Cytomegalovirus

Routine prophylaxis is not recommended by the USPHS/IDSA guidelines. The decision to initiate prophylaxis in selected high-risk patients (CD4 <50/μL and positive anti-CMV IgG) should be made by an infectious disease specialist.

Toxoplasmosis

For those seropositive for *Toxoplasma gondii* (IgG) and with a CD4 cell count of less than 100/μL, TMP-SMX is appropriate prophylaxis. In such patients the dose of one double-strength tablet daily is more effective than the lower doses, which can be given to prevent *Pneumocystis* infection. Dapsone provides some prophylactic activity, but this has to be supplemented by adding pyrimethamine and leucovorin (50 and 25 mg weekly, respectively). Lifelong therapy is required. Existing data are insufficient to assert that a response to HAART allows for discontinuation of prophylaxis. Seronegative patients should be counseled on risky behavior that can lead to acquisition of new *Toxoplasma* infection. They should refrain from eating raw or undercooked meat, especially undercooked pork, lamb, or venison. All meat should be cooked until an internal temperature of 150°F or until no longer pink. They should be advised to wash their hands after contact with soil. Fruits and vegetables should be thoroughly washed before eating. Patients should be counseled not to handle stray cats or feed their cats raw or undercooked meat. Their cats should be kept indoors. Cat litter should be changed daily, preferably by an HIV-negative, nonpregnant person.

Cryptosporidiosis

No drugs are known to be effective in prophylaxis against cryptosporidiosis. The newly diagnosed patient should be educated on the many ways by which new infection can be acquired. They should be advised to wash their hands thoroughly after contact with human feces (diaper changing), handling pets (especially newborn and very young), and exposure to soil (gardening). Anal-oral sex should be avoided. They should never drink water directly from lakes or rivers. Exposure to lambs and calves should be avoided. Raw oysters should be avoided because cryptosporidial oocysts can survive in oysters for over 2 months.

Bartonella *Infection*

Primary prophylaxis is not recommended. HIV-infected patients who are severely immunocompromised are at very high risk of acquiring *Bartonella* infection, which is transmitted from cats. Patients should avoid being scratched by cats. Cat wounds from scratches should be thoroughly washed promptly. Patients should never allow cats to lick their open wounds or cuts. If a new cat is to be bought or adopted, a healthy more than 1 year old should be selected. Although not absolutely necessary, declawing should be considered.

Varicella Zoster Virus

HIV-infected patients with no history of chickenpox or shingles or those who have tested negative for varicella zoster virus (VZV) IgG should avoid exposure to persons with chickenpox or shingles. At present insufficient data exist on the efficacy of the varicella vaccine in HIV-infected patients, but household contacts of HIV-infected patients who have no history of chickenpox or shingles and are HIV and VZV seronegative should be vaccinated to prevent transmission. If an HIV-infected patient comes into close contact with a patient with chickenpox or shingles, varicella immune globulin should be administered as soon as possible (within 96 hours). There are no data to support the use of acyclovir in this setting.

Hepatitis C Virus Infection

All newly HIV-infected patients should be screened for HCV infection by using enzyme immunoassays (EIA) for the detection of HCV antibody (anti-HCV) in blood. The current USPHS/IDSA recommendation is to confirm all positive test results with the polymerase chain reaction (PCR) technique or recombinant immunoblot assay (RIBA). Primary care providers should know that the EIA may be negative in acute hepatitis C infection for up to 12 weeks. Therefore, when the index of suspicion for acute infection is high as suggested by the history, the initial screening should involve PCR testing for HCV RNA. Those not infected but at risk of acquiring hepatitis C should be aggressively counseled. In the United States, injection drug use is the number one risk factor. Referral to a substance abuse treatment program should be made for injection drug users, and those who continue the behavior should be counseled not to share needles and use bleach to sterilize needles. They should use sterile syringes and boil clean water in drug preparation. They should clean the injection site with an alcohol swab before injection. Syringes and needles should be properly discarded after a single use. The mode of transmission of HCV is not clearly understood, so patients should be counseled on safe sexual practices. Barrier precautions should be emphasized. For those infected with HCV, the use of even moderate quantities of alcohol should be strongly discouraged because the risk of cirrhosis may be much higher in these patients.

Case

A 32-year-old male truck driver presented to the emergency department complaining of flulike symptoms for 3 days. He was in his usual state of health until 3 days prior to presentation, when he developed a sore throat, headache, and intense myalgias. He described prominent photophobia. He took acetaminophen with some relief of symptoms. The next day his symptoms recurred, along with a diffuse rash. He admitted to having unprotected intercourse with prostitutes while on trips. His past medical history is unremarkable. He is not on any medications and reported no allergies. He is married with two children 3 and 5. He has been a truck driver for the past 8 years. His childhood and teenage years were spent in rural Ohio. On physical examination he was ill appearing with a blood pressure of 125/76 mm Hg, pulse 110 beats/min, respiratory rate 20 breaths/min, and an oral temperature of 103°F. A fine maculopapular rash was visible on the whole body, sparing the face. The oropharynx was red with no exudate. There was meningismus. Diffuse lymphadenopathy was present. The balance of the examination was within normal limits, and there was no hepatosplenomegaly. Laboratory values obtained revealed a white blood cell count of 11,000, hematocrit of 30.6%, platelet count of 81,000, aspartate aminotransferase of 112, alanine aminotransferase of 87, total bilirubin of 1.3, and alkaline phosphatase of 156. Results of a monospot test were negative, as were those of an HIV enzyme-linked immunosorbent assay (ELISA). Chest radiography revealed no infiltrates. He was admitted to the hospital. HIV RNA by PCR was detected a day later. A CD4 count obtained a week later was 112/μL.

1. What features of this man's presentation suggest acute HIV infection?
2. How is the diagnosis of acute HIV infection made?
3. What further testing would you consider and what treatment would you provide for this patient?

Case Discussion

What Features of This Man's Presentation Suggest Acute HIV Infection?

Several features of his presentation support the diagnosis of acute HIV infection. He admits to high-risk behavior (e.g., contact with prostitutes). On physical examination, the diffuse lymphadenopathy, nonexudative pharyngitis, meningismus, and maculopapular rash suggest an acute viral syndrome. Infectious mononucleosis is a consideration but unlikely given his age, a negative monospot result, and normal spleen size. Acute infection with CMV is a possibility. The thrombocytopenia noted on his complete blood count can be seen in both the acute retroviral syndrome of HIV, infectious mononucleosis, and CMV infection. The differential diagnosis of fever, meningismus, and a rash includes life-threatening ailments such as Rocky Mountain spotted fever and acute meningitis. It would be prudent to refer such a patient to an emergency department for further evaluation and hospital admission.

How Is the Diagnosis of Acute HIV Infection Made?

Because the HIV ELISA can take many weeks to become positive, detection of HIV RNA by PCR or the p24 antigen can establish acute HIV infection. When the index of suspicion is high, it is crucial to establish the diagnosis promptly. Recent studies have shown the importance of early aggressive HAART.

What Further Testing Would You Consider and What Treatment Would You Provide for This Patient?

As part of the initial evaluation of this patient, a lumbar puncture should be performed to look for evidence of meningitis. Empiric antibiotic coverage would be reasonable if the cerebrospinal fluid results cannot be obtained rapidly or are equivocal. Although the transaminase elevation may be a reflection of his acute systemic illness, it should raise the spector of infection with hepatitis B or C virus. Hepatitis B and C serologies should be obtained. The CD4 count obtained during the acute infection will be low because of the acute illness and is likely to increase significantly with time. In the meantime, the patient needs to be started on prophylaxis for PCP because of his T-cell count of 112/μL. In addition to the initial evaluation outlined above, he should receive the polyvalent pneumococcal vaccine. There is a high rate of invasive pneumococcal disease in HIV patients and a rising tide of resistant strains nationwide. Optimal antigenic response occurs in those with a CD4 count of greater than 200/μL. Those with lower counts may obtain some protective benefit. HIV-positive patients should never receive live virus or bacterial vaccines. Vaccination for measles, mumps, and rubella (MMR) is the only exception. The influenza vaccine is considered safe in patients with HIV but can increase the viral burden load by over 10-fold for about a month.

The patient should be encouraged to inform his wife of his diagnosis. The law varies from state to state on patient confidentiality. It may be helpful to consult the local health department in such instances.

Suggested Reading

Bartlett J G. *Medical management of HIV infection.* Baltimore: Johns Hopkins University Press, 1999. 1999 USPHS/IDSA guidelines for the prevention of opportunistic infections in persons infected with human immunodeficiency virus. Can be obtained at www.cdc.gov.

X
Nephrology

58

Initial Treatment of Hypertension

Laura J. Martin

1. How is hypertension defined and classified?
2. How should risk stratification be performed for the initial treatment of hypertension?
3. What life-style modifications should be recommended to hypertensive patients?
4. What are some considerations in choosing an initial class of antihypertensive medication? ·
5. Which antihypertensive is considered to be first-line during pregnancy?
6. What are some recent findings from the Hypertension Optimal Treatment study and the Antihypertensive and Lipid-Lowering Treatment to Prevent Heart Attack Trial?

Discussion

How Is Hypertension Defined and Classified?

Hypertension is usually defined as systolic blood pressure (SBP) of 140 mm Hg or greater and/or diastolic blood pressure (DBP) of 90 mm Hg or greater. Approximately 43 million Americans have hypertension. It is a leading risk factor for cardiovascular disease, including coronary artery disease (CAD) and stroke. Even though treatment of hypertension has increased in the past 25 years, only 55% of Americans with hypertension are being treated according to the National Health and Nutrition Education Survey III. Even so, mortality rates from CAD and stroke have declined 53% and 60% in the past 25 years, which is thought to be in large part secondary to improvement in blood pressure control.

The sixth report of the Joint National Committee (JNC) on Prevention, Detection, Evaluation, and Treatment of High Blood Pressure is a national guideline published in 1997 that is meant to aid physicians in treating patients with hypertension. The committee uses evidence-based medicine to update recommended approaches in obtaining optimal blood pressure control. The committee recognizes that treatment should be individualized according to the physician's judgment and individual patient's needs. The JNC has provided a classification of stages of blood pressure based on degree of elevation from normal (Table 58.1). Suggested follow-up based on an initial blood pressure measurement is also described (Table 58.2).

Table 58.1. Classification of Blood Pressure in Adults

Optimal BP: SBP < 120 mm Hg and DBP < 80 mm Hg
Normal BP: SBP < 130 mm Hg and DBP < 85 mm Hg
High normal BP: SBP 130–139 mm Hg or DBP 85–89 mm Hg
Hypertension[a]
   Stage 1. SBP 140–159 mm Hg or DBP 90–99 mm Hg
   Stage 2. SBP 160–179 mm Hg or DBP 100–109 mm Hg
   Stage 3. SBP ≥ 180 mm Hg or DBP ≥ 110 mm Hg

[a]Based on average of two or more readings taken at two or more visits after initial screening.
BP, blood pressure; SBP, systolic blood pressure; DBP, diastolic blood pressure.
Adapted from The sixth report of the Joint National Committee on Detection, Evaluation, and Diagnosis of High Blood Pressure. Bethesda: National Institutes of Health, National Heart, Lung and Blood Institute, National High Blood Pressure Education Program, 1997. NIH Publication No. 98-4081; with permission.

How Should Risk Stratification Be Performed for Initial Treatment of Hypertension?

Guidelines on the initial treatment of hypertension for an individual patient include risk stratification for cardiovascular disease. This risk stratification is based on the patient's stage of blood pressure, risk factors for cardiovascular disease, and evidence or lack of evidence of target organ damage, including clinical cardiovascular disease (Table 58.3).

The major risk factors for cardiovascular disease include smoking, dyslipidemia, diabetes mellitus, age ≥ 45 years if male, age ≥ 55 years if female, premature menopause without estrogen replacement, and family history of cardiovascular disease.

In hypertensive patients, components of target organ damage or clinical cardiovascular disease include heart disease, left ventricular hypertrophy, angina, prior myocardial infarction, prior coronary revascularization, heart failure, stroke or transient ischemic attack, nephropathy, peripheral arterial disease, and retinopathy.

What Life-Style Modifications Should Be Recommended to Hypertensive Patients?

Advising hypertensive patients on life-style modification issues is an important component of treating hypertension. Weight loss in overweight patients, exercise,

Table 58.2. Recommendations for Follow-up Based on Initial Blood Pressure

Initial SBP (mm Hg)	Initial DBP (mm Hg)	Recommended Follow-up
<130	<85	Recheck in 2 yr[a]
130–139	85–89	Recheck in 1 yr[a]
140–159	90–99	Confirm within 2 mo
160–179	100–109	Evaluate within 1 mo
≥180	≥110	Evaluate immediately or within 1 wk

[a]Advise on life-style modification.
SBP, systolic blood pressure; DBP, diastolic blood pressure.
Adapted from The sixth report of the Joint National Committee on Detection, Evaluation, and Diagnosis of High Blood Pressure. Bethesda: National Institutes of Health, National Heart, Lung, and Blood Institute, National High Blood Pressure Education Program, 1997. NIH Publication No. 98-4081; with permission.

Table 58.3. Risk Stratification and Treatment

Blood pressure stage	Risk Group A (No risk factors; no TOD/CCD)	Risk Group B (≥1 risk factor, not including DM; no TOD/CCD)	Risk Group C (TOD/CCD and/or DM, with or without other risk factors)
High-normal (130–139/85–89 mm Hg)	LM	LM	Drug therapy[a]
Stage 1 (140–159/90–99 mm Hg)	LM up to 1 yr	LM up to 6 mo[b]	Drug therapy
Stage 2 and 3 (≥160/≥100 mm Hg)	Drug therapy	Drug therapy	Drug therapy

[a]For patients with CHF, renal insufficiency, or diabetes mellitus.
[b]For patients with multiple risk factors, consider drug therapy and life-style modification as initial therapy.
TOD, target organ damage; CCD, clinical cardiovascular disease; DM, diabetes mellitus; LM, life-style modification.
Adapted from The sixth report of the Joint National Committee on Detection, Evaluation, and Diagnosis of High Blood Pressure. Bethesda: National Institutes of Health, National Heart, Lung, and Blood Institute, National High Blood Pressure Education Program, 1997. NIH Publication No. 98-4081; with permission.

tobacco cessation, limiting alcohol intake, and low sodium diet have all been shown to be helpful in reducing blood pressure.

Dietary counseling on low-sodium diets (2.4 g/day) is effective in lowering blood pressure in salt-sensitive individuals. Other recommended dietary measures include maintaining adequate intake of calcium, magnesium, and potassium and reducing intake of dietary saturated fat and cholesterol. In general, weight reduction is recommended for all overweight or obese hypertensive patients with a body mass index (BMI) of 27 kg/m^2 or greater. Referral to a dietitian is helpful in tailoring a specific diet for each patient.

Alcohol intake should be limited to no more than 1 ounce of ethanol per day for men and one-half ounce of ethanol per day for women. A specific recommendation for wine intake is no more than 10 ounces per day.

Physical activity, such as 30 to 40 minutes of brisk walking most days of the week, is a simple exercise prescription that most patients can perform.

What Are Some Considerations in Choosing an Initial Class of Antihypertensive Therapy?

The choice of antihypertensive therapy is somewhat empiric. According to JNC VI, if there is not an indication for another class of medication, a diuretic or β blocker should be chosen based on the results of many randomized controlled trials, which showed a decrease in morbidity and mortality with these agents.

If response to an initial drug choice is inadequate after reaching your optimal dose, a second agent from a different class of antihypertensive can be added. Alternatively, if there are significant side effects with the initial medication, switching to a different agent should be considered. If a diuretic is not chosen as the first drug, it is usually indicated as a second agent because of its additive effect in efficacy.

Antihypertensives from various classes should be sequentially added to the regimen to achieve the patient's optimal blood pressure goal. Low-dose combinations of two agents from different classes have been shown to be efficacious while minimizing the likelihood of dose-dependent side effects.

In some specific clinical situations, there are indications for choosing a particular class of antihypertensive medication. Based on results from randomized controlled trials, the JNC VI recommends using specific agents as follows:

- Diabetes mellitus (type 1 and type 2) with proteinuria: angiotensin-converting enzyme (ACE) inhibitors
- Heart failure: ACE inhibitors and diuretics
- Myocardial infarction: β-blockers (without intrinsic sympathomimetic activity)

Other recommendations include:

- Older persons (with isolated systolic hypertension): diuretics are preferred and long-acting dihydropyridine calcium channel blockers may be considered.
- Patients with renal insufficiency with greater than 1 g/day of proteinuria: blood pressure goal is 125/75 mm Hg; those with less proteinuria have a goal of 130/85 mm Hg; ACE inhibitors should be considered to help slow the progression of nephropathy.
- Patients with diabetes (type 1 and 2): blood pressure goal is 130/85 mm Hg.

Which Antihypertensive Is Considered to Be First-Line During Pregnancy?

Methyldopa is recommended in women whose hypertension is initially diagnosed during pregnancy because it has been extensively evaluated and is considered safe to use for both the mother and fetus. ACE inhibitors and angiotensin II receptor blockers should be avoided during pregnancy because they have been associated with teratogenic effects. β-blockers have been associated with growth retardation of the fetus in early pregnancy, but are considered safe in the latter part of pregnancy.

What Are Some Recent Findings from the Hypertension Optimal Treatment Study and the Antihypertensive and Lipid-Lowering Treatment to Prevent Heart Attack Trial?

The Hypertension Optimal Treatment study addressed the question of what diastolic pressure is optimal to reduce cardiovascular events. The study included 18,790 patients 50 to 80 years of age with diastolic blood pressure of 100 to 115 mm Hg. Patients were randomized to target diastolic blood pressures of 90, 85, or 80 mm Hg. Felodipine was given as baseline antihypertensive therapy, with other agents added as needed according to a five-step regimen. In addition, patients were randomized to receive 75 mg of aspirin or placebo daily along with antihypertensive therapy. Results from the trial were presented in 1998.

The lowest incidence of fatal and nonfatal stroke occurred at a mean blood pressure of 138/83 mm Hg. The lowest risk of cardiovascular mortality occurred at a mean blood pressure of 139/86 mm Hg. This difference in cardiovascular event rates is a trend, which did not reach statistical significance.

In the subgroup of diabetic patients, a 51% reduction in cardiovascular events was seen in the 80 mm Hg target group.

In the subgroup of patients who received aspirin as well as antihypertensive therapy, the incidence of myocardial infarction was reduced by 36%. Seven fatal bleeds and 129 nonfatal bleeds occurred in the aspirin group, whereas 8 fatal bleeds and 70 nonfatal bleeds occurred in the placebo group.

The Antihypertensive and Lipid-Lowering Treatment to Prevent Heart Attack Trial was designed to determine if newer antihypertensive medications reduce the incidence of cardiovascular disease. This study, which began in 1994, involves four arms, including four types of antihypertensives: chlorthalidone, doxazosin, amlodipine, and lisinopril. In January 2000, an independent data review committee recommended stopping the doxazosin treatment arm based on comparison of data with chlorthalidone.

A total of 24,335 patients at least 55 years of age with hypertension and at least one cardiovascular risk factor randomly received either doxazosin or chlorthalidone at one of 625 centers in the United States and Canada. Total mortality between the two groups did not differ at four years, but the doxazosin arm had a higher risk of stroke [relative risk (RR) = 1.19; p = 0.04] and combined cardiovascular disease (RR 1.24; p < .001). The risk of congestive heart failure was doubled in the doxazosin group (8.13%) as compared with the chlorthalidone group (4.45%). Based on these findings, doxazosin should not be considered as a first-line antihypertensive.

Case

A 46-year-old man presents to your office for an initial visit. He relates that he has a history of borderline elevated blood pressure and type II diabetes mellitus. He has been following a low-sodium, American Diabetic Association (ADA) diet for the past 6 months. He brings medical records from his previous practitioner, revealing several previous blood pressure readings. Six months prior to this visit his blood pressure was 148/92 mm Hg (right arm) and 142/90 mm Hg (left arm). Three months prior his blood pressure was 144/90 mm Hg (right arm) and 140/92 mm Hg (left arm). He currently is feeling well. His family history is remarkable for hypertension in his brother and father. He takes no medications.

Physical examination reveals seated blood pressures of 146/94 mm Hg (right arm) and 144/90 mm Hg (left arm); standing blood pressures of 140/92 mm Hg (right arm) and 142/94 mm Hg (left arm); pulse of 80 beats/min; weight of 195 pounds; and height of 5 feet 10 inches. The remainder of the examination is unremarkable.

Laboratory results from 3 months prior are remarkable for serum creatinine 1.5 mg/dL, potassium 3.8 mEq/L, glucose 124 mg/dL, urinalysis with 2+ protein, and total cholesterol 264 mg/dL.

1. How should this patient be risk stratified according to JNC VI criteria?
2. Which life-style modifications should be recommended to this patient?
3. What special considerations influence the choice of initial antihypertensive therapy?

Case Discussion
How Should This Patient Be Risk Stratified According to JNC VI Criteria?

This patient has documented elevated blood pressures on at least three separate office visits in the past 6 months. According to the JNC VI classification system, he is categorized as having stage I hypertension (Table 58.1). Because he has diabetes mellitus and evidence of nephropathy, drug therapy should be initiated along with life-style modification (Table 58.3). According to the JNC guidelines, goal blood pressure in patients with diabetes mellitus or proteinuria is less than or equal to 130/85 mm Hg. In those patients with greater than 1g/24 hours proteinuria, goal blood pressure is 125/75 mm Hg.

Which Life-Style Modifications Should Be Recommended to This Patient?

This patient should continue to follow a low-sodium, ADA diet. Using the equation BMI = [weight (pounds)/height (inches)^2] $\times$ 703, his BMI is calculated as 28 kg/m^2. In general, all patients with a BMI greater than or equal to 27 kg/m^2 should be counseled to lose weight. He also should be counseled on the benefits of regular exercise and limiting alcohol intake. In view of his elevated cholesterol, he should be advised to follow a low-fat, low-cholesterol diet. A fasting lipid profile should be obtained to further delineate his high-density lipoprotein, low-density lipoprotein, and triglyceride levels.

What Special Considerations Influence the Choice of Initial Antihypertensive Therapy?

Because this patient has diabetes mellitus and proteinuria, an ACE inhibitor is considered to be first-line therapy to treat his hypertension and slow the progression of his nephropathy. In many patients, ACE inhibitors can reduce the glomerular filtration rate. It is thus recommended that serum creatinine and potassium levels be checked approximately 10 to 14 days after the initiation of ACE inhibitors.

Suggested Reading

Furberg C D, Wright J T, Davis B R, et al. Major cardiovascular events in hypertensive patients randomized to doxazosin vs chlorthalidone: the antihypertensive and lipid-lowering treatment to prevent heart attack trial. *JAMA* 2000;283:1967–1975.

Hansson, L, Zanchetti A, Carruthers S, et al. Effects of intensive blood-pressure lowering and low-dose aspirin in patients with hypertension: principle results of the Hypertension Optimal Treatment (HOT) randomized trial. *Lancet* 1998;351:1755–1762.

National Institutes of Health. *The sixth report of the Joint National Committee on Detection, Evaluation, and Diagnosis of High Blood Pressure.* Bethesda, MD: National Institutes of Health, National Heart, Lung, and Blood Institute, National High Blood Pressure Education Program, 1997. National Institutes of Health Publication No. 98-4081.

Staessen J A, Fagard R, Thisjs L, et al. Randomized double-blind comparison of placebo and active treatment for older patients with isolated systolic hypertension. *Lancet* 1997;350:757.

Systolic Hypertension in Elderly Program Cooperative Research Group. Implications of the Systolic Hypertension in Elderly Program. *Hypertension* 1993;21:335–343.

59

Resistant Hypertension

Laura J. Martin

1. How is resistant hypertension defined?
2. What measures can improve patient compliance to antihypertensive therapy?
3. What are some medication-related causes of resistant hypertension?
4. Ingestion of which medications and substances can increase blood pressure?
5. When should "white coat" hypertension be suspected?
6. When should pseudohypertension be suspected?
7. What are some common secondary causes of hypertension?

Discussion

How Is Resistant Hypertension Defined?

Resistant hypertension can be defined as blood pressure that cannot be reduced to below 140/90 mm Hg in a patient taking three or more antihypertensive medications prescribed at near maximal dose, one being a diuretic. In elderly patients with isolated systolic hypertension, those with persistent systolic blood pressure of greater than 160 mm Hg while on three antihypertensive medications are classified as having resistant hypertension.

There are several etiologies to consider in patients with resistant hypertension. Some common causes include noncompliance with medications, "white coat" hypertension, pseudohypertension, volume overload, and ingestion of medications or substances that increase blood pressure. Secondary hypertension is present in less than 5% of patients with resistant hypertension.

What Measures Can Improve Patient Compliance to Antihypertensive Therapy?

It is thought that noncompliance to antihypertensive therapy may contribute to lack of adequate control of blood pressure in up to two thirds of patients with hypertension. Physicians can help assure adherence to therapy by providing accurate information to patients about their health status and encouraging patients to participate in their care.

The Joint National Committee (JNC) on Prevention, Detection, Evaluation, and Treatment of High Blood Pressure in their sixth report has described guidelines to help improve patient compliance with therapy (Table 59.1).

Table 59.1. Guidelines to Improve Patient Adherence to Antihypertensive Therapy

Be aware of signs of patient nonadherence to antihypertensive therapy.
Establish the goal of therapy: to reduce BP to nonhypertensive levels with minimal or no adverse effects.
Educate patients about the disease, and involve them and their families in its treatment. Have them measure blood pressure at home.
Maintain contact with patients; consider telecommunication.
Keep care inexpensive and simple.
Encourage life-style modifications.
Integrate pill taking into routine activities of daily living.
Prescribe medications according to pharmacologic principles, favoring long-acting formulations.
Be willing to stop unsuccessful therapy and try a different approach.
Anticipate adverse effects, and adjust therapy to prevent, minimize, or ameliorate side effects.
Continue to add effective and tolerated drugs, stepwise, in sufficient doses to achieve the goal of therapy.
Encourage a positive attitude about achieving therapeutic goals.
Consider using nurse case management.

Adapted from The sixth report of the Joint National Committee on Detection, Evaluation, and Diagnosis of High Blood Pressure. Bethesda: National Institutes of Health, National Heart, Lung, and Blood Institute, Blood Pressure Education Program, 1997. NIH Publication No. 98-4081; with permission.

What Are Some Medication-Related Causes of Resistant Hypertension?

Medication-related causes are involved in many cases of resistant hypertension. In some cases, a higher dose of medication may be all that is needed. If compliance is of concern, use of combination pills (two antihypertensives in one pill) may improve adherence.

In choosing an antihypertensive agent, it is important to consider the half-life of the medication. Some agents may have a rapid inactivation and may not provide 24-hour efficacy. Choosing an agent with a longer half-life may improve blood pressure control.

Volume overload may be a factor in many patients. Salt-sensitive patients who consume a high sodium diet may have an increased plasma volume, leading to resistant hypertension. Counseling patients on low-sodium diets is helpful in this situation. In addition, patients with renal insufficiency, as well as some patients with normal renal function, sometimes develop volume overload, leading to increased blood pressure. Thiazides or loop diuretics are recommended in these patients. In patients with normal renal function, thiazide diuretics generally have been found to be more effective in treating hypertension than furosemide because thiazides have a longer half-life.

Ingestion of Which Medications and Substances Can Increase Blood Pressure?

Alcohol, caffeine, and licorice can contribute to resistant hypertension. Other substances noted to increase blood pressure include tobacco, cocaine, and other illicit drugs. Patients should be counseled on dietary measures and life-style changes in order to help them achieve their goal blood pressure. Common medications that can contribute to hypertension include sympathomimetics, nasal decongestants, appetite suppressants, oral contraceptives, steroids, cyclosporine, erythropoietin, venlafaxine, and nonsteroidal antiinflammatory drugs.

When Should "White Coat" Hypertension Be Suspected?

White coat hypertension has been estimated to affect blood pressure readings in approximately 20% of office visits to a physician. This diagnosis should be considered in patients with hypertension who report that their blood pressure readings are consistently normal outside of the physician's office. It also should be suspected in patients who develop symptoms of dizziness or weakness on antihypertensive medications. Patients who describe these symptoms may possibly be experiencing hypotension as a side effect of their medications. When white coat hypertension is suspected, a 24-hour ambulatory blood pressure monitor is helpful in establishing the diagnosis.

When Should Pseudohypertension Be Suspected?

Pseudohypertension can be seen in older patients with calcified arteries. In those with pseudohypertension, systolic blood pressure readings taken with a blood pressure cuff may be higher than the true intraarterial pressure. This is because compression of the calcified brachial artery may require a cuff pressure greater than the true intraarterial pressure. The diastolic pressure also may be higher than true intraarterial pressure because the brachial artery may stop vibrating more quickly, causing earlier resolution of the Korotkoff sounds. Confirmation of this diagnosis requires that the patient have a direct measurement of arterial pressure (e.g., with an arterial line).

What Are Some Common Secondary Causes of Hypertension?

Secondary hypertension should be a consideration in certain patients with resistant hypertension. Renal artery stenosis should be suspected in those with a history of peripheral vascular disease or abdominal bruit. It also should be suspected in older patients with previously well-controlled blood pressure who develop resistant hypertension and in patients who develop acute renal insufficiency after initiating treatment with an angiotensin converting enzyme (ACE) inhibitor.

Evaluation for pheochromocytoma should be considered in patients with palpitations, paroxysmal headaches, and pallor. Patients with a pheochromocytoma may experience an increase in blood pressure on β-blockers.

Workup for primary hyperaldosteronism should be considered in patients with persistent unexplained hypokalemia and resistant hypertension. Other potential secondary causes to consider include Cushing syndrome, coarctation of the aorta, obstructive sleep apnea, and hyperparathyroidism.

Case

A 60-year-old man presents to your office for follow-up of hypertension diagnosed 15 years ago. He currently is feeling well. There are no symptoms of chest pain, shortness of breath, or edema. He reports that his blood pressure checked 1 week ago with an automated cuff at his pharmacy was normal. He finds it difficult to adhere to a low-sodium diet, but reports good compliance with his medication regimen. His current medications include hydrochlorothiazide 50 mg daily, lisinopril 40 mg daily, felodipine 20 mg daily, and ibuprofen.

In reviewing his medical records, you find several blood pressure measurements from previous visits. Six months ago, his blood pressure was 160/100 mm Hg; 3 months ago, it was 150/96 mm Hg.

Physical examination today reveals blood pressures of 150/92 mm Hg (right arm) and 152/96 mm Hg (left arm), pulse of 76 beats/min, weight of 206 pounds, and height of 69 inches. His cardiovascular examination reveals an abdominal bruit as well as a left femoral bruit. The rest of the examination is unremarkable.

Recent laboratory results include sodium 140 mEq/L, potassium 4.0 mEq/L, creatinine 1.8 mg/dL, total cholesterol 296 mg/dL, and calcium 8.6 mEq/L; electrocardiogram shows a normal sinus rhythm with evidence of left ventricular hypertrophy.

1. What life-style modifications and medication changes may be helpful in treating this patient's resistant hypertension?
2. Could this patient have white coat hypertension?
3. Is secondary hypertension a consideration?

Case Discussion

What Life-Style Modifications and Medication Changes May Be Helpful in Treating This Patient's Resistant Hypertension?

Adherence to a low-sodium diet is important, particularly because he has renal insufficiency and possibly an increased plasma volume. Because he has a significantly decreased creatinine clearance, it may be beneficial to switch from a thiazide to a loop diuretic.

Nonsteroidal antiinflammatory drugs (NSAIDs) can decrease the efficacy of many antihypertensive medications. They are known to cause fluid retention. Switching from ibuprofen to acetaminophen may help to improve his blood pressure. In addition, he should be asked about and counseled on use of over-the-counter medications and other substances that can elevate blood pressure.

Obesity is strongly associated with hypertension. The benefits of weight loss in treating his hypertension should be discussed. Based on his current weight and height, his body mass index (BMI) is 30 kg/m^2, indicating that he is obese. In general, hypertensive patients with a BMI greater than or equal to 27 kg/m^2 should be counseled to lose weight.

Obstructive sleep apnea (OSA) is commonly associated with both hypertension and obesity. If he has symptoms consistent with OSA, such as snoring and daytime somnolence, then a sleep study should be considered.

Could This Patient Have White Coat Hypertension?

This patient reports a normal blood pressure reading outside of the practitioner's office 1 week ago. However, the findings of abdominal and femoral bruits, left ventricular hypertrophy, and an elevated creatinine level indicate that he has significant clinical cardiovascular disease and target organ damage likely secondary to hypertension. These findings are not consistent with white coat hypertension.

Is Secondary Hypertension a Consideration?

The findings of an abdominal and a left femoral artery bruit on examination along with the finding of his elevated cholesterol indicate probable peripheral vascular disease. In view of these findings, his age, and resistant hypertension, renal artery stenosis could be a possible secondary cause of his hypertension. Diagnostic workup for renal artery stenosis should be considered.

Suggested Reading

Graves J W. Management of difficult to control hypertension. *Mayo Clin Proc* 2000:278–284.

Kaplan N M, Rose B D. Resistant hypertension. *Up to Date* 1998;8:1.

National Institutes of Health. *The sixth report of the Joint National Committee on Detection, Evaluation, and Diagnosis of High Blood Pressure.* Bethesda, MD: National Institutes of Health, National Heart, Lung, and Blood Institute, Blood Pressure Education Program, 1997. National Institutes of Health Publication No. 98-4081.

Report of the U.S. Preventive Services Task Force. *Guide to clinical preventive services*, 2nd ed. Baltimore: Williams & Wilkins, 1996.

Setaro J F, Black H R. Current concepts: refractory hypertension. *N Engl J Med* 1992;327:543.

60
Secondary Hypertension

Jennifer Kleinbart

1. What are the causes of secondary hypertension?
2. Which clinical features are associated with the different causes of secondary hypertension?
3. What is the diagnostic approach to renovascular hypertension and how should it be managed?
4. What is the diagnostic approach to hyperaldosteronism?
5. How is pheochromocytoma diagnosed?

Discussion

What Are the Causes of Secondary Hypertension?

Secondary causes of hypertension occur in 5% of all hypertensive individuals. After renal parenchymal disease, the most common causes of secondary hypertension are renovascular disease, occurring in 0.5% to 3% of hypertensive patients, and primary hyperaldosteronism (PHA), found in 0.05% to 2% of hypertensive patients. Pheochromocytoma occurs in less than 0.2% of hypertensive patients. Other less common causes include Cushing disease, aortic coarctation, hypothyroidism, hypercalcemia, porphyria, carcinoid syndrome, central nervous system tumors, and autonomic hyperreflexia associated with spinal cord lesions. Sleep apnea may be associated with hypertension as well. Finally, drugs such as anabolic steroids, corticosteroids, caffeine, cocaine, ethanol, nicotine, sympathomimetics (β agonists, phenylpropanolamine, pseudoephedrine), nonsteroidal antiinflammatory agents, tricyclic antidepressants, and oral contraceptives should be considered in the evaluation of hypertension.

Which Clinical Features Are Associated with Secondary Hypertension?

Resistant hypertension can be defined as blood pressure of over 140/90 mm Hg (or over 160/90 mm Hg in patients over 60 years of age) while the patient is being treated with maximal doses of at least three antihypertensive agents for an adequate time to assess their effectiveness. It is associated with a secondary cause of hypertension in less than 5% of cases. Previously well-controlled hypertension that becomes difficult to control should also raise concerns of a secondary cause.

Features associated with renovascular hypertension (RVH) include newly diagnosed hypertension in a patient under 25 years of age, especially with no family history of hypertension, or in a patient over 60 years of age. Renal failure of uncertain etiology, acute renal failure precipitated by angiotensin-converting enzyme (ACE) inhibitor or angiotensin receptor blocker use, and the presence of an abdominal bruit or diffuse atherosclerotic disease should raise the suspicion of RVH.

Moderate to severe hypertension that may be refractory is typical of hyperaldosteronism. Elevated aldosterone leads to hypokalemia, hypernatremia, metabolic alkalosis, and hyperglycemia. The serum potassium is less than 3.6 mEq/L in approximately 80% of cases. Mild hypernatremia results from decreased release of vasopressin secondary to volume expansion or hypokalemia. Increased fasting plasma glucose occurs in 25% of patients due to suppression of insulin secretion and activity by chronic potassium depletion.

Pheochromocytoma is associated with episodic headache, palpitations, and diaphoresis. Orthostatic hypotension also may occur. Proximal muscle weakness and hyperglycemia suggest Cushing syndrome.

What Is the Diagnostic Approach to Renovascular Hypertension and How Should It Be Managed?

Arteriography is the gold standard for diagnosing RVH; however, associated complications of renal failure (1%–2%), contrast reaction, and cholesterol embolization limit its use as a screening test. Arteriography should be used for confirmation and quantification of renal artery stenosis (RAS). Intraarterial digital subtraction angiography, which uses lower doses of contrast, is an alternative to arteriography. When the use of ionic contrast dye is contraindicated, arteriography with gadolinium or CO_2 can be performed. Stenosis of more than 50% is considered significant.

Several noninvasive tests are available to screen for RVH. Magnetic resonance angiography (MRA) is the most accurate if high-quality equipment is used. Nuclear scanning is less sensitive and specific.

Renal scintigraphy measures each kidney's uptake of a nuclear label to estimate renal function. Two types of nuclear labels may be used: technetium 99m–DPTA (diethylenetriamine pentaacetic acid), a marker of glomerular filtration rate, and MAG3 (mercaptoacetyltriglycine), a marker of renal blood flow. MAG3 may provide better imaging than DPTA when renal function is impaired and should be used when the creatinine level is over 2.5 mg/dL. With normal renal function, DPTA provides higher sensitivity.

Nuclear scanning performed after the administration of captopril (captopril renal scan) may improve diagnostic accuracy. Angiotensin II is important for maintaining glomerular filtration when renal perfusion is compromised. Reduction in angiotensin II by ACE inhibition leads to impairment of renal function if the renal artery is stenotic, resulting in decreased uptake on the affected side. The increased asymmetry after captopril increases the test's sensitivity. Test accuracy depends on the cutoff for renal uptake: with a cutoff value of less than 35% uptake by the affected kidney, sensitivity is approximately 70% for unilateral RAS and 60% for bilateral RAS, with a specificity of 90%.

An elevated plasma renin level may raise suspicion for RVH, but the renin level may be normal in up to 50% of patients with RVH and elevated in over 10% of patients with essential hypertension. Therefore, it is an inadequate screening test.

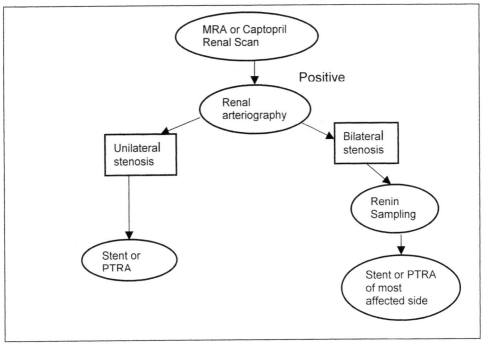

Figure 60.1. Approach to suspected renovascular hypertension.

In summary, if suspected based on clinical features, high-quality MRA is the initial diagnostic procedure of choice to evaluate RVH. If not available, a captopril renal scan should be performed. Given a high clinical index of suspicion, a negative nuclear scan does not rule out the diagnosis of renal artery stenosis, and further testing may still be warranted. Arteriography is used to confirm the diagnosis and guide treatment (Fig. 60.1).

Without intervention, approximately 10% of stenoses greater than 60% occlude within 2 years. Interventional treatment options include percutaneous transluminal renal angioplasty (PTRA) and stent placement. Stenting provides higher initial patency rates (98%–100%), with a restenosis rate of 8% to 12% at 6 months. The rate of reocclusion with PTRA is 25% to 65%.

Clinical benefits of achieving renal artery patency include slowing the rate of progression to renal failure and normalization or improvement of hypertension. Seventy percent of those whose arteries remain patent have improvement or stabilization of renal function. Patients with preserved renal function are more likely to remain normotensive after intervention.

What Is the Diagnostic Approach to Primary Hyperaldosteronism?

Hypertensive patients with spontaneous hypokalemia and a 24-hour urine potassium of greater than 30 mmol during hypokalemia should be evaluated for PHA. The diagnostic approach to PHA involves several steps. First, the biochemical presence of PHA is confirmed, followed by determination of the particular cause of increased aldosterone production. Next, anatomy is defined by imaging. Imaging should not be the initial diagnostic approach to suspected hyperaldosteronism, because many adrenal masses are nonfunctional.

Upright plasma renin activity is suppressed in 97% of patients with PHA, but this also may occur in 30% of patients with essential hypertension. The ratio of the plasma aldosterone level to plasma renin activity (PAC:PRA ratio) is a more useful test. When measured in the morning in the upright position, patients with PHA will have a PAC:PRA ratio of over 20, and in most cases over 30.

Primary hyperaldosteronism is confirmed by the aldosterone (saline) suppression test, which measures aldosterone and renin levels after sodium loading. Normally, aldosterone production is suppressed by volume expansion, but when aldosterone production is autonomous, the usual inhibition is absent and the aldosterone level remains elevated.

The aldosterone (saline) suppression test is conducted by infusing 2 L of 0.9% normal saline over 4 hours in the morning (8:00 A.M. to 12:00 P.M.), while in the supine position, followed by measurement of plasma aldosterone and renin. An aldosterone level of less than 8.5 ng/dL excludes PHA (Fig. 60.2). Alternatively, an oral sodium load may be administered with 2 to 3 g NaCl tablets at each meal for 3 days, followed by a 24-hour urine collection. PHA is diagnosed if the 24-hour urine aldosterone is greater than 14 μg, with a 24-hour urine Na of over 200 mEq (confirming adequate Na repletion). Because sodium loading may exacerbate hypokale-

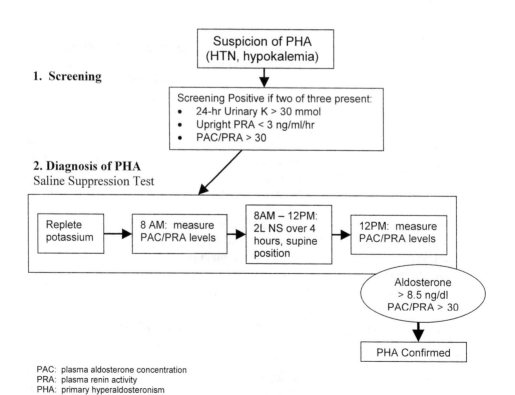

1. Screening

2. Diagnosis of PHA
Saline Suppression Test

PAC: plasma aldosterone concentration
PRA: plasma renin activity
PHA: primary hyperaldosteronism

Figure 60.2. Diagnostic approach to hyperaldosteronism.

mia, potassium should be repleted before testing. Prior to and during testing, antihypertensive agents least likely to affect renin or aldosterone production, such as α_1 blockers, should be used, and diuretics, ACE inhibitors, and β-blockers should be discontinued.

After PHA is confirmed, the cause of hyperaldosteronism must be identified. Possible causes include aldosterone-producing adenoma, accounting for 65% of PHA cases, idiopathic hyperaldosteronism with bilateral adrenal hyperplasia, found in 25% of cases, primary adrenal hyperplasia (may be unilateral or bilateral), glucocorticoid-remediable hyperaldosteronism (where aldosterone production is regulated by adrenocorticotropic hormone), and aldosterone-producing carcinoma, a rare finding.

To distinguish an aldosterone-producing adenoma from idiopathic hyperaldosteronism, measurement of plasma aldosterone level, plasma renin activity, and 18-hydroxycorticosterone is performed after the patient has been sitting upright for 2 to 4 hours. With an aldosterone-producing adenoma, aldosterone production is autonomous and typically does not increase in response to angiotensin II or upright position. If idiopathic hyperaldosteronism is the cause of the PHA, the aldosterone response to angiotensin II is exaggerated and increases after postural testing. Primary adrenal hyperplasia responds similarly to an aldosterone-producing adenoma.

Following biochemical diagnosis, computerized tomography or magnetic resonance imaging is used for adrenal assessment. A unilateral mass larger than 1 cm is consistent with an aldosterone-producing adenoma. A mass larger than 3 cm suggests malignancy.

Adrenalectomy is indicated for an aldosterone-producing adenoma, resulting in improvement or resolution of hypertension in 70% of patients, and resolution of hypokalemia in 100%. Idiopathic hyperaldosteronism should be managed medically with spironolactone up to 400 mg daily or amiloride 5 to 30 mg daily (fewer side effects than spironolactone), which effectively controls blood pressure and hypokalemia.

How Is Pheochromocytoma Diagnosed?

Pheochromocytoma is diagnosed by finding elevated free catecholamines, or the catecholamine metabolites metanephrine and vanillylmandelic acid (VMA) in a 24-hour urine collection. Drugs such as labetalol, propranolol (may interfere with the assay for metanephrines), buspirone, and monoamine oxidase inhibitors should be discontinued before testing.

Case

Your clinic patient is a 50-year-old white man with a 20-year history of hypertension, hyperlipidemia, and tobacco abuse. Despite compliance with dietary measures and medications, his blood pressure has been difficult to control on several agents. He currently takes atenolol 100 mg, nifedipine 90 mg, hydrochlorothiazide 25 mg, as well as aspirin and simvastatin. On physical examination, his blood pressure is 170/98 mm Hg. Cardiac examination is normal, and there are no carotid, femoral, or abdominal bruits. Pedal pulses are 1+. Laboratory testing shows a creatinine level of 1.4 mg/dL and potassium of 3.4 mEq/L.

1. Which clinical features are consistent with secondary hypertension?
2. How would you proceed with your evaluation?

Case Discussion

Which Clinical Features Are Consistent with Secondary Hypertension?

This patient has refractory hypertension, with uncontrolled blood pressure on maximal doses of three antihypertensive agents, increasing the likelihood of a secondary cause of hypertension. With his history of hyperlipidemia, tobacco abuse, and possible peripheral vascular disease (diminished pedal pulses), atherosclerotic renal vascular disease should be suspected. This is further suggested by a slightly elevated creatinine and low potassium.

How Would You Proceed with Your Evaluation?

Evaluation should begin with MRA or a captopril renal scan. A positive test result would be followed by angiography with stenting as the preferred therapy.

Suggested Reading

Renovascular Hypertension

Derkx F, Schalekamp M. Renal artery stenosis and hypertension. *Lancet* 344:237–239.
Harden P N, et al. Effect of renal-artery stenting on progression of renovascular renal failure. *Lancet* 1997;349:1133.
Plouin P, Chatellier G, Darne B, et al. Blood pressure outcome of angioplasty in atherosclerotic renal artery stenosis: a randomized trial. *Hypertension* 1998;31:823.
Van Jaarsveld B C, Krijnen P, Derkx F, et al. The place of renal scintigraphy in the diagnosis of renal artery stenosis: fifteen years of clinical experience. *Arch Intern Med* 1997;157:1226.
Xue F, et al. Outcome and cost comparison of percutaneous transluminal renal angioplasty, renal arterial stent placement, and renal arterial bypass grafting. *Radiology* 1999;212:378.

Hyperaldosteronism

Blevins L S, Wand G S. Primary aldosteronism: an endocrine perspective. *Radiology* 1992;184:599–600.
Ganguly A. Primary aldosteronism. *N Engl J Med* 1998;339:1828–1834.
Stewart P M. Mineralocorticoid hypertension. *Lancet* 1999;353:1341–1347.
Young W, Hogan M J, Klee G G, et al. Primary aldosteronism: diagnosis and treatment. *Mayo Clin Proc* 1990;65:96–110.

61
Acute Renal Failure

Nina S. Garas
Byard F. Edwards

1. Define acute renal failure.
2. How can acute renal failure be categorized, and what are the common causes for each category?
3. What are the common historical and physical findings?
4. Which laboratory studies can be helpful in the diagnosis of acute renal failure?
5. What are the treatment options?
6. What are the indications for dialysis?

Discussion
Define Acute Renal Failure.

Acute renal failure (ARF) is a clinical syndrome characterized by rapid deterioration of renal function that occurs within days (as opposed to weeks or months in subacute renal failure or years in chronic renal failure). The principal feature of ARF is an abrupt decline in glomerular filtration rate (GFR), resulting in the retention of nitrogenous wastes such as urea and creatinine (azotemia).

How Can Acute Renal Failure Be Categorized, and What Are the Common Causes for Each Category?

Acute renal failure can be categorized into three categories:

1. Prerenal failure is a functional, rapidly reversible reduction in GFR, caused by renal hypoperfusion without any parenchymal damage to the kidney (Table 61.1).
2. Intrarenal failure is caused by damage to the renal tubules, interstitium, glomeruli, or vessels (Table 61.2).
3. Postrenal failure occurs when urinary outflow tracts are obstructed (Table 61.3).

Table 61.1. Major Causes of Prerenal Failure

Intravascular volume depletion
Decreased cardiac output
Decreased renal perfusion with normal/high cardiac output
Renovascular obstruction

What Are the Common Historical and Physical Findings?

Frequently, patients with acute renal failure are asymptomatic. However, if the renal failure is severe, weakness, loss of appetite, nausea, and/or symptoms of fluid retention and decreased urine output may be present. Acute renal failure secondary to glomerulonephritis or a renal artery stenosis will frequently be associated with accelerated hypertension. In hospitalized patients, acute renal failure is most commonly diagnosed following an increase in serum creatinine. Careful history taking and a thorough chart review are necessary to confirm the presence of acute versus chronic renal failure and to determine its cause.

Vital signs and an assessment of volume status are critical. Volume contraction and congestive heart failure may result in hypoperfusion of the kidney. Orthostatic hypotension, tachycardia, skin tenting, and dry mucous membranes suggest renal failure secondary to volume contraction. Edema, elevated jugular venous pressure, a third heart sound, and evidence of pulmonary congestion indicate congestive heart failure. An enlarged prostate, palpable bladder, or increased postvoid residual volume raise the possibility of an outlet obstruction. Evaluation of the skin may reveal a rash in allergic interstitial nephritis or vasculitis, purpura in vasculitis, and blue toes in cholesterol emboli.

Which Laboratory Studies Can Be Helpful in the Diagnosis of Acute Renal Failure?

Blood Chemistry

Serum blood urea nitrogen (BUN) and creatinine are elevated. An elevated BUN:creatinine ratio often implies prerenal azotemia. Conditions such as a high-protein diet, gastrointestinal bleeding, and glucocorticoid treatment can increase BUN. Serum creatinine is a more specific indicator of GFR.

Urinalysis

Urinalysis is a crucial part of the diagnostic evaluation of ARF. The spun specimen should be examined within 30 minutes of voiding. The urine dipstick will indicate

Table 61.2. Major Causes of Intrarenal Failure

Acute tubular necrosis
Tubulointerstitial nephritis
Rapidly progressive glomerulonephritis
Vascular causes

Table 61.3. Major Causes of Postrenal Failure

Prostatic hypertrophy
Neoplasm: prostate, bladder, cervix, colorectal
Nephrolithiasis
Neurogenic bladder
Papillary necrosis
Retroperitoneal fibrosis

the urine pH, specific gravity, protein, urobilinogen, leukocytes, and nitrites. A high pH (>7) will be present with urease-splitting organisms (*Proteus, Providencia, Klebsiella, Pseudomonas,* and enterococci) and suggests the possibility of a staghorn calculus. Proteinuria greater than 30 mg/dL is detectable by dipstick. Urobilinogen is elevated in hepatitis. Leukocytes may be present in a urinary tract infection as well as an interstitial nephritis, but the nitrite is positive only if bacteria are present. Yeast does not induce a positive nitrite test.

A normal urine sediment, or one with hyaline casts, may be found before and after renal failure. Multiple coarse granular casts with free epithelial cells are pathognomonic for acute tubular necrosis (ATN). Crystalluria may be indicative of an obstructing stone. The presence of dysmorphic red blood cells (RBCs) with or without RBC casts raises the suspicion of glomerulonephritis, particularly rapidly progressive glomerulonephritis in the presence of ARF.

A spot urine protein:creatinine ratio (mg/dL) may be easily obtained in an outpatient setting and has a high correlation with a quantitative 24-hour urine test that measures total urinary protein. The spot urine ratio of protein creatine can be used to estimate the urinary protein excreted in 24 hours. A protein-creatine ratio of greater that 3.0 or 3.5 mg indicates protein excretion rates of greater thatn 3.0 or 3.5g/24 h. Estimated urinary creatinine excretion (mg/24 h) may be estimated using the following formulas:

- Males: [28 − (0.21 × age)] × lean body weight (LBW, kg)
- Females: [24 − (0.17 × age)] × LBW (kg)
- Male LBW: 106 pounds for first 60 inches in height, then 6 pounds for each additional inch
- Female LBW: 100 pounds for first 60 inches in height, then 5 pounds for each additional inch
- Kilograms = pounds ÷ 2.2

Urine Indices

Urine osmolality, urinary sodium concentration, and fractional excretion of sodium (FE_{Na}) help differentiate between prerenal azotemia and tubular necrosis. In prerenal azotemia, the reabsorptive capacity of the tubular cells and the concentrating ability of the kidney are preserved. Both of these functions are impaired in tubular necrosis. One of the earliest functional defects seen with tubular damage is loss of the ability to concentrate the urine. Of note, the FE_{Na} and the urine sodium concentration are difficult to interpret with concurrent diuretic therapy, because natriuresis raises the FE_{Na} even in patients with prerenal disease. Urine sodium and FE_{Na} must be interpreted in light of sodium intake and clinical volume status (Table 61.4).

$$FE_{Na} = [(U_{Na} \times P_{Cr}) / (P_{Na} \times U_{Cr})] \times 100$$

Table 61.4. Tests to Distinguish Prerenal Azotemia from ATN

Test	Prerenal Azotemia	ATN
BUN/plasma creatinine	>20:1	10–15:1
Urine specific gravity	>1.020	<1.010
Urine osmolality	>500 mOsm/kg	<350
Urine sodium	<20 mEq/L	>40 mEq/L
FE_{Na}	<1%	>1%
Urine sediment	Normal, hyaline casts	Granular casts, tubular cells

ATN, acute tubular necrosis; BUN, blood urea nitrogen; FE_{Na}, fractional excretion of sodium.

Blood Count

Leukocytosis may be present with sepsis. Eosinophilia may be seen in allergic interstitial nephritis, vasculitis, or atheroembolic disease. Patients with microangiopathic hemolytic disease may have thrombocytopenia, anemia, and schistocytes.

Other Laboratory Tests

In some circumstances, further studies are required to establish the diagnosis of ARF. If multiple myeloma is suspected, serum and urine immunoelectrophoresis should be checked. Positive antinuclear antibody and anti-DNA antibodies support the diagnosis of lupus nephritis, whereas a positive antineutrophil cytoplasmic autoantibody (ANCA) indicates vasculitis. Antiglomerular basement membrane antibodies are specific for Goodpasture syndrome. Cryoglobulin studies, hepatitis B and C serologies, C3, C4, and antistreptococcal antibody titers may be useful in evaluating glomerular disease.

Ultrasonography

Renal ultrasonography is indicated if the renal anatomy is unknown and the etiology of the renal failure is in doubt. Organ size and number, cortical thickness, echogenicity, cysts, and obstruction may be readily determined without risk to the patient.

Biopsy

Renal biopsy is not indicated when the etiology of the ARF is known and the patient's renal function favorably responds to therapy. Prerenal azotemia, postrenal failure, cholesterol embolization, and most cases of ATN are diagnosed clinically. However, if a glomerulonephritis of undetermined etiology or severity is suspected, or the ARF is in a transplanted kidney, then a renal biopsy should be performed in a timely manner.

What Is the Management for Acute Renal Failure?

If intravenous contrast must be used in a high-risk patient (diabetics and those with a creatinine clearance (Cr_{Cl}) of <50 mL/min), pre- and postvolume expansion with half normal saline and minimal dosing of iodinated contrast should be performed.

Using nontraditional contrast media such as carbon dioxide and gadolinium prevents contrast-induced renal injury.

Nonsteroidal antiinflammatory drugs (NSAIDs) and angiotensin-converting enzyme (ACE) inhibitors should be avoided in patients with ARF. When aminoglycosides are administered, doses should be adjusted for the estimated GFR and blood levels should be monitored.

$$\text{Estimated } Cr_{Cl} \text{ (mL/min)} = \frac{[(140 - \text{age}) \times \text{lean body wt (kg)}]}{P_{Cr} \times 72 \times 0.85 \text{ for females.}}$$

Immediate Care

- Initiate treatment of life-threatening electrolyte disorders immediately.
- Correct volume contraction and hypotension.
- Look for and treat obstruction (by Foley catheter).
- Obtain diagnostic urinary studies before administering diuretics or intravenous fluids.
- Adjust drug doses to estimated renal function.
- Reassess volume status and electrolytes.

Conservative Medical Management of Acute Renal Failure

Fluid management is essential to prevent volume depletion, which may contribute to ARF by decreasing renal perfusion. In the hospital, monitor daily fluid input and output as well as daily weights. Serum electrolytes, BUN, creatinine, calcium, and phosphate should be measured frequently.

Protein, sodium, potassium, and phosphate intake should be limited.

Hyperkalemia is common and if mild can be treated with dietary restriction and potassium-binding resins. Marked hyperkalemia or hyperkalemia accompanied by electrocardiographic abnormalities requires immediate medical therapy (e.g., calcium gluconate, insulin and glucose, nebulized β-agonists, and if accompanied by a metabolic acidosis, sodium bicarbonate). Hyperkalemia unresponsive to medical therapy is an indication for dialysis.

Metabolic acidosis that is mild (≥ 20 mEq/L) does not require therapy. More marked acidosis should be corrected with oral sodium bicarbonate. Each 650-mg tablet contains 8 mEq of bicarbonate. The daily titratable acid load in mEq equals the lean body weight (LBW) (kg). The bicarbonate required to balance the acid load can be calculated as follows:

$$\text{Required bicarbonate replacement (mEq/day)} = [(24 - \text{serum } HCO_3) \div 24] \times LBW$$

Acidosis that is unresponsive to medical therapy is an indication for dialysis. Drug doses should be adjusted for the level of renal function.

Anemia does not occur in ARF until the GFR is less than 30 mL/min for several weeks. Therefore, secondary causes of the anemia should be sought. Major bleeding sources should be excluded. Erythropoietin (EPO) is expensive and not effective as short-term therapy for anemia. EPO therapy is indicated in chronic renal insufficiency, in which the anemia is attributed primarily to decreased endogenous EPO production.

What Are the Indications for Dialysis?

- Hyperkalemia in a patient with ARF unresponsive to nondialytic management
- Life-threatening volume overload unresponsive to the usual measures (e.g., diuretics)
- Life-threatening intoxications that are dialyzable
- Uremia (encephalopathy, pericarditis, anorexia, platelet dysfunction)

Case

A 62-year-old woman presents with weakness, anorexia, and fatigue of 5 days' duration. One month ago she had symptoms suggestive of a viral infection. At that time her serum creatinine was 1.0 mg/dL and her weight 65 kg. A review of her systems is negative for any shortness of breath, nausea, vomiting, diarrhea, dysuria, or hematuria.

Past medical history includes congestive heart failure, hypertension, and osteoarthritis. Her current medications include lisinopril, furosemide, and naproxen.

Physical examination shows her height to be 5 feet 7 inches, weight 63 kg, sitting blood pressure 128/60 mm Hg with a pulse of 85 beats/min, and standing blood pressure 110/50 mm Hg with a pulse of 100 beats/min. Dry mucous membranes are noted; there is no jugular venous distension; cardiac examination reveals normal S_1 and S_2; lungs are clear to auscultation; there are no abdominal masses or bruits; no rash is present; there is no lower extremity edema; and the skin tents.

Laboratory testing reveals sodium 148 mEq/L, potassium 5.0 mEq/L, chloride 110 mEq/L, bicarbonate 27 mEq/L, BUN 50 mg/dL, and creatinine 2.1 mg/dL. Urinalysis shows specific gravity of 1.025, trace protein on dipstick, and a few hyaline casts.

1. Is this acute or chronic renal failure?
2. What can cause this type of renal failure with a normal urinalysis?
3. How can urine indices help in distinguishing the etiology of renal failure?
4. What can you do to prevent acute renal failure?

Case Discussion

Is This Acute or Chronic Renal Failure?

Although the patient has chronic renal failure with an estimated Cr_{Cl} of 56 mL/min, a serum creatinine of 1.0, and an estimated LBW of 61 kg, she now presents with acute on chronic renal failure with an estimated Cr_{Cl} of 26 mL/min (a reduction in renal function by 50%).

What Can Cause This Type of Renal Failure with a Normal Urinalysis?

This patient likely developed renal failure secondary to diuretic-induced volume contraction, and renal vessel autonomic dysfunction from the NSAID and ACE inhibitor therapies.

How Can Urine Indices Help in Distinguishing the Etiology of Renal Failure?

Urine osmolality, urinary sodium concentration, and fractional excretion of sodium will help differentiate between prerenal azotemia and tubular necrosis in this patient. In prerenal states, the fractional excretion of sodium is usually less than 1%. Intrinsic renal failure with tubular damage results in a FE_{Na} of greater than 1%. (See Tables 61.1 through 61.3 for additional tests to distinguish prerenal azotemia from ATN.)

What Can You Do to Prevent Acute Renal Failure?

The patient is 2 kg below her previous weight. Diuretic therapy should be stopped, and if anorexia prevents adequate volume intake, intravenous fluids of normal saline should be administered until the volume is repleted. The patient should be initiated on a 2-g sodium diet to limit the need for diuretic therapy. Water should be taken ad libitum to replete her deficit of approximately 3 L or given as 5% dextrose in water after repleting her intravascular volume. The NSAID therapy should be stopped to allow afferent vasodilation, increased glomerular filtration pressure, and kaliuresis. Acetaminophen may be tried as an alternate therapy for her arthritic pain. The ACE inhibitor should be held and then cautiously reintroduced following the resolution of her ARF with frequent assessment of the patient's creatinine and potassium.

Suggested Reading

Dinour D. *Rakel: Conn's current therapy,* 51st ed. 1999:714–722.

DuBose T D, Warnock M D, Mehta R L, et al. Acute renal failure in the 21st century: recommendations for management and outcomes assessment. *Am J Kidney Dis* 1997;29:793–799.

Rose B D. *Pathophysiology of renal disease,* 2nd ed. New York: McGraw-Hill, 1987:680–693.

Star R A. Treatment of acute renal failure. *Kidney Int* 1998;54:1817–1831.

Thadhani R, Pascual M, Bonventre J V. Medical progress: acute renal failure. *N Engl J Med* 1996;334:1448–1460.

62

Chronic Renal Failure

Byard F. Edwards

1. How is renal insufficiency defined and measured?
2. What metabolic derangements are anticipated with chronic renal failure?
3. What interventions are required prior to the initiation of replacement therapy?
4. What renal replacement therapy is available and who gets it?
5. When does the primary care physician refer to the nephrologist?

Discussion

How Is Renal Insufficiency Defined and Measured?

Although arbitrarily defined, mild renal insufficiency may be considered when the glomerular filtration rate (GFR) is impaired, but greater than 70 mL/min. Moderate insufficiency ranges from a GFR of 70 to 30 mL/min, whereas severe insufficiency is a GFR below 30 mL/min. End-stage renal disease (ESRD) occurs when the GFR is less than 10 mL/min.

Renal function can be defined in many ways. An estimated or measured creatinine clearance (Cr_{Cl}) commonly defines renal function, but this measurement is only an approximation of the GFR. Creatinine, once filtered, is neither metabolized nor reabsorbed and as such is an inexpensive, readily available index of clearance. However, several caveats exist. Creatinine is secreted by the proximal tubules and is filtered by the glomeruli. In severe renal insufficiency, the secretion of creatinine may account for up to 35% of the total excreted load. To prevent an overestimation of GFR, the secretion of creatinine may be blocked with cimetidine (400 mg orally twice daily) begun 48 hours prior to urine collection and continued during urine collection. If the patient is near ESRD, then the non–cimetidine-treated Cr_{Cl} may be averaged with the urea clearance to obtain a closer approximation of the GFR. Urea clearance is underestimated as a result of increased distal tubule reabsorption to the same degree that Cr_{Cl} is overestimated by proximal tubule secretion.

Estimation of the Cr_{Cl} in mL/min may be calculated from the Cockcroft-Gault equation:

$$\text{Estimated } Cr_{Cl} = \frac{(140 - \text{age}) \times \text{LBW} \times 0.85 \text{ for females}}{72 \times S_{Cr}}$$

where LBW = lean body weight in kilograms and S_{Cr} = serum creatinine in mg/dL.

LBW may be estimated from the following equations:

- Male LBW = 106 pounds for the first 60 inches of height and 6 pounds for each additional inch of height.
- Female LBW = 100 pounds for the first 60 inches of height and 5 pounds for each additional inch of height.
- Kilograms = pounds ÷ 2.2.

Creatinine derives from muscle metabolism; the weight associated with excessive fat must be disregarded if an accurate estimate of the Cr_{Cl} is to be obtained.

An estimated creatinine excretion may be used to judge the adequacy of a patient's 24-hour urine collection and for calculating the estimated Cr_{Cl}:

- For men, estimated 24-hour urine creatinine (mg/day) = [28 − (0.21 × age)] × LBW in kg.
- For women, estimated 24-hour urine creatinine (mg/day) = [24 − (0.17 × age)] × LBW in kg.

The Cr_{Cl} may then be calculated as follows:

$$Cr_{Cl} \text{ (mL/min)} = \frac{\text{Estimated 24-hour urine creatinine (mg/24 h)} \times 100 \text{ ml/dL}}{1{,}440 \text{ min/24 h} \times S_{Cr} \text{ (mg/dL)}}$$

What Metabolic Derangements Are Anticipated with Chronic Renal Failure?

The kidney's myriad functions wane as renal failure progresses. Declining clearance is reflected in an increased S_{Cr} level unless the patient is suffering from a reduced LBW. The cachexia associated with ESRD may obscure a declining GFR.

Volume homeostasis may be lost as the function of glomerular filtration and tubular concentration is lost. Antidiuretic hormone receptor dysfunction and diminished urea concentration gradient limit distal tubular concentration.

Decreased hormonal production of erythropoietin and 1,25 dihydroxycholecalciferol (vitamin D) produces progressive anemia and mineral derangements. Vitamin D increases gut absorption of calcium and phosphorus, promotes bone osteoclastic activity, and inhibits parathyroid activity. Vitamin D production and activity become limited early in renal failure (GFR < 70 mL/min), and the lowered calcium serum level results in hyperparathyroidism, bone demineralization, and hyperphosphatemia. Erythropoietin stimulates bone marrow production of red blood cells. Anemia usually develops with moderate to severe renal impairment unless the patient has polycystic kidney disease or a tumor producing the hormone.

Metabolic acidosis progresses as the tubules lose the ability to generate ammonia and trap hydrogen as an ammonium ion within the tubular lumen. The increased hydrogen ion concentration in the blood places increased demands on the body's largest buffer source, bone, resulting in bone demineralization, hypercalcemia, and hyperphosphatemia. The acidosis also contributes to increased protein catabolism, decreased muscle mass, hyperkalemia, and impaired growth hormone release.

What Interventions Are Required Prior to the Initiation of Replacement Therapy?

Reversible etiologies of the renal failure should be sought and rectified in the hopes of preserving and prolonging native renal function. Hydronephrosis may be visualized through ultrasonography and corrected by ureteral or percutaneous stenting. If the obstruction is for longer than several weeks, the GFR may not improve, but the increased urine production may simplify fluid management. Renal artery stenosis (RAS) is best assessed through carbon dioxide arteriography or magnetic resonance imaging. Correction of the RAS may not improve the GFR as often as it improves the management of the patient's hypertension.

Optimal therapy specifically tailored to the patient and the etiology of the renal failure should be provided. Therefore, the etiology of the renal failure should be diligently sought if successful therapeutic intervention is thought possible. Hypertension should be controlled to 120/70 mm Hg unless significant renal arterial disease is present. Diabetics should maintain the hemoglobin A1C at 7.0% or less. Proteinuria should be minimized to limit progressive renal disease, malnutrition, and dyslipidemia. Hepatitis B and C, human immunodeficiency virus (HIV), connective tissue diseases including systemic lupus erythematosus and vasculitis, and atherosclerosis should be aggressively treated when possible.

A review of nephrotoxic compounds—including those that may contribute to interstitial nephritis (nonsteroidal antiinflammatory drugs and sulfonamides) or decrease GFR [angiotensin-converting enzyme (ACE) inhibitors, angiotensin receptor blockers (ARBs), verapamil, and diltiazem]—should be undertaken. Verapamil and diltiazem preferentially vasodilate the efferent arterioles, thereby decreasing the glomerular filtration pressure, GFR, and proteinuria. Below a GFR of 20 mL/min, the renal reserve to preserve homeostasis is limited, and the risk of hyperkalemia and symptoms of uremia or volume overload may outweigh the protective attributes of the ACE inhibitors and ARBs.

Dose adjustment of medicines excreted through the kidneys should be made repeatedly as renal function declines. Atenolol, which has 40% excretion through the kidneys, should be discontinued in severe renal insufficiency. Digoxin, amoxicillin, famodipine, gabapentin, and alendronate are some of the common pharmaceuticals that must be adjusted for renal impairment. Medicines containing aluminum, magnesium, and phosphorus should be avoided (magnesium aluminum hydroxide, aluminum hydroxide, magnesium citrate, magnesium oxide, and sodium phosphate enemas).

Dietary adjustments are necessary and frequently the most difficult of the changes to implement. Daily caloric intake should equal 35 kcal/kg LBW. Protein should be limited to 0.6 g/kg LBW if diabetic, and 0.8 g/kg LBW if nondiabetic. An additional amount of protein equal to the grams of daily excreted urinary protein is added if the patient is nephrotic. Cooked egg whites are an excellent source of inexpensive protein. Phosphorus is limited to 15 mg/g of dietary protein. Phosphorus-rich foods include dairy products, colas, pastries, beans, and leafy green vegetables. Sodium (Na) and potassium (K) should be limited to 2 g per day unless the patient wastes potassium as a result of diuretic therapy or type I or II renal tubule acidosis (RTA). Sodium-rich foods include salted or cured meats, canned goods, meat sauces, soy sauce, ketchup, and all restaurant foods. Potassium-rich foods include tomatoes, potatoes, bananas, raisins, and most citrus fruits. Apples, pears, grapes and grapefruit are lower in potassium content. Potassium content can be lowered in potatoes by thinly slicing and soaking in water overnight prior to use. Repeated referral to a qualified dietitian will improve the probability of the patient's compliance. Estimations of the patient's compliance can be made through spot urine collections for sodium, potassium, urea, protein, and creatinine.

- Estimated daily urine volume (EDUV) (L/day) = estimated 24-hour urine creatinine (mg/day) ÷ spot urine creatinine (mg/dL) ÷ 10 dL/L
- Estimated daily Na or K intake (mEq/day) = spot urine Na or K (mEq/L) × EDUV (L/day)
- Sodium conversion of mEq to mg = mEq × 23 mg/mEq
- Potassium conversion of mEq to mg = mEq × 39 mg/mEq
- Estimated daily urine urea (EDUU) (mg/day) = spot urine urea (mg/dL) × EDUV (L/day) × 10 dL/L
- Estimated daily urine protein (mg/d) = spot urine protein (mg/dL) ÷ spot urine creatinine (mg/dL) × estimated 24-hour urine creatinine (mg/day)
- Estimated protein intake (mg/day) = 6.25 [EDUU + (30 mg/kg/day × kg LBW)] + estimated daily urine protein (mg/day)

Therapy to replace lost renal function should begin in a timely manner. Bicarbonate should be orally replaced to maintain the acid-base balance. Each day the body produces 1 mEq of titratable acid for every kg of LBW. The quantity of daily supplemental bicarbonate may be calculated as follows:

$$\text{Supplemental HCO}_3 \text{ required (mEq/day)} = [(24 \text{ mEq/L} - \text{serum HCO}_3) \text{ (mEq/L)} \div 24 \text{ mEq/L}] \times \text{LBW in kg}$$

Each 650-mg tablet of sodium bicarbonate contains 8 mEq of HCO_3.

Phosphate binders must be taken with meals to absorb both secreted phosphates used in digestion and phosphates released from food during digestion. Calcium carbonate is the cheapest binder and may be obtained by taking one to five 500- to 650-mg calcium tablets per meal, which should maintain the serum phosphorus at a level less than 5 mEq/L. However, calcium carbonate also gives the highest calcium load to the patient and may promote metastatic calcification of the soft tissues, including the vessels. Calcium carbonate requires an acidic gastric fluid to dissolve, limiting its utility in patients using acid blockade therapy. Alternative binders include calcium acetate (667 mg per tablet) and sevelamer (800 mg per tablet), taken as two to five tablets per meal. Sevelamer has the advantage of containing no calcium and additionally lowers the serum cholesterol. However, it is extremely expensive. Citrate-based medicines should be avoided because their use increases aluminum absorption in the gut and may lead to osteomalacia and encephalopathy.

Vitamin D (1,25 dihydroxycholecalciferol) production declines below a GFR of 70 mL/min. Vitamin D replacement may begin once the serum phosphorus level is controlled. Vitamin D replacement therapy consists of oral 1,25 dihydroxycholecalciferol or vitamin D analogues taken 3 days a week to limit the intact parathyroid hormone (PTH) level to less than 200 pg/mL. Vitamin D analogues have the advantage of limiting phosphorus absorption in the gut, but are more expensive than 1,25 dihydroxycholecalciferol. Serum calcium, phosphorus, albumin, and intact PTH levels should be monitored at least monthly while on vitamin D therapy.

Anemia can be treated with erythropoietin once the iron saturation is increased and maintained above 20%. Intravenous iron sucrose may be required to maintain adequate iron levels; oral iron therapy is poorly tolerated. The patient should be encouraged to eat iron-rich foods and to use cast-iron cookware for meal preparation. Erythropoietin is administered subcutaneously weekly with a starting dose of 100 to 150 U/kg LBW. The dose adjusted every 2 to 4 weeks to achieve a hemoglobin level of 11 to 12 g/dL. Hemoglobin levels should be monitored every 2 to 4 weeks and iron saturation every month.

What Renal Replacement Therapy Is Available and Who Gets It?

Three therapeutic options currently exist to provide chronic renal replacement therapy. Peritoneal dialysis (PD) allows home therapy and mobility for travel. The diet is restricted only for phosphorus and total caloric intake. Those patients with severe cardiomyopathy or coronary artery disease who cannot tolerate intermittent dialysis three times a week, or those who wish to maintain an independent life-style, should consider PD. Contraindications include abdominal adhesions, unrepaired herniations, ascites, severe malnutrition, and an unsuitable home environment.

Hemodialysis (HD) can be provided at home if a willing partner is available and used either intermittently three times a week or daily. The vast majority of replacement therapy in the United States is intermittent HD provided three times a week in an outpatient dialysis facility. Severe water, sodium, potassium, and phosphorus dietary restrictions apply to those using intermittent dialysis.

Transplantation of a living or cadaveric donor kidney will restore renal function, allowing the resumption of a relatively normal life-style. Potential transplantation recipients must be in good health, without cancer for at least 5 years, without active hepatitis B, C, or HIV, and with a suitable psychological profile to optimize medical compliance.

When Does the Primary Care Physician Refer to the Nephrologist?

Referral to a subspecialist should occur when the diagnosis is in doubt, the selection and management of the optimal therapies are uncertain, or a renal replacement therapy is required. Preparation for renal replacement therapy, dialysis, or kidney transplantation should be initiated when the GFR approaches 20 mL/min/1.73 m^2.

Failure to diagnose and properly manage renal failure will rapidly result in ESRD. Mortality on dialysis therapy averages 20% per year, with an average survival time of 7 years. The prevention or delay of ESRD will greatly impact the patient's life expectancy.

Case

Mr. Y, a 57-year-old type II diabetic, presents for an initial examination after changing from a preferred provider organization to a health maintenance organization insurance policy. His medical history is notable for uncontrolled hypertension, a 5-year history of type II diabetes mellitus (DM) that was poorly controlled on oral therapy and later insulin therapy, no known retinopathy or neuropathy, and chronic edema. His social history is notable for a sedentary life-style and a divorce many years ago. He lives with his girlfriend and frequently dines out for his meals.

Current medicines include insulin, lisinopril, and sildenafil.

Physical examination is notable for a sitting blood pressure of 160/92 mm Hg with a pulse of 84, weight of 195 pounds, benign fundi, soft S_4 gallop, protuberant abdomen with the right liver lobe palpated four finger breaths below the costal margin, lower limbs with 1+ pitting edema extending to the mid-calf, skin with a crude tattoo over the right deltoid, small violaceous nodules on the legs, and no neurologic deficits.

Laboratory values are notable for Na =134 mEq/L, K= 5.1 mEq/L, HCO_3 = 21 mEq/L, BUN = 21 mg/dL, creatinine = 1.5 mg/dL, glucose = 184 mg/dL, and hemoglobin A1C = 8%. Urinalysis shows 4+ protein on urine dipstick with no casts present. Spiculated RBCs = 15 per high-power field on microscopic examination.

1. What vital information is lacking?
2. What information can be extracted from the initial laboratory results?
3. What is the differential for the cause of the renal failure?
4. What should be the next laboratory tests?
5. How should this patient be managed?

Case Discussion

What Vital Information Is Lacking?

The patient's height will be necessary to estimate his LBW. Mr. Y is 5 feet 11 inches tall. His estimated LBW is 172 pounds, or 78 kg.

What Information Can Be Extracted from the Initial Laboratory Results?

1. The patient has an estimated Cr_{Cl} of 60 mL/min.
2. The patient probably has type 4 RTA. His estimated daily HCO_3 deficit is 9.7 mEq.
3. The patient probably has a nephrotic syndrome with an associated lipid disorder.
4. The patient has poorly controlled DM with an average blood glucose of 176 mg/dL derived from the equation: average blood glucose = (33 × hemoglobin A1C) − 88.
5. The hyponatremia is associated with a volume overload.

What Is the Differential for the Cause of the Renal Failure?

There is little evidence that DM is the cause of the nephropathy. The duration of the diagnosis for DM in Mr. Y is 5 years; overt diabetic nephropathy generally occurs after 10 years of DM. Diabetic retinopathy usually precedes nephropathy and is absent in this patient. Hypertension may lead to glomerular sclerosis but is seldom associated with nephrotic range proteinuria. Ultrasonography would disclose enlarged kidneys if the nephropathy resulted from diabetes, and smaller, echodense kidneys if due to hypertension. Ultrasonography would also rule out obstruction as a cause of renal failure.

There is no evidence for RAS; bruits are absent and the patient has hyperkalemia. There is no evidence that a cardiomyopathy is contributing to the nephropathy. The mean arterial pressure is 115 mm Hg; there is no hypoperfusion. Spiculated RBCs in the urine suggests the presence of nephritis. Palpable purpura suggests the presence of vasculitis. Multiple myeloma should be ruled out in light of his age and degree of proteinuria. The patient has increased risks for sexually transmitted diseases, including HIV, hepatitis B and C, and syphilis.

What Should Be the Next Laboratory Tests?

- Renal ultrasonography demonstrated bilateral, normal density kidneys that measured 10.9 cm in length without evidence of obstruction.
- Serum calcium = 7.0 mEq/L, phosphorus = 5.0 mg/dL, albumin = 2.0 g/dL, and intact PTH = 70 pg/mL.
- Aspartate aminotransferase = 215 U/L, alanine aminotransferase = 105 U/L, total bilirubin = 1.2 mg/dL.
- Total cholesterol = 265 mg/dL, triglyceride = 300 mg/dL, high-density lipoprotein = 40 mg/dL, low-density lipoprotein = 165 mg/dL.
- Results of HIV enzyme-linked immunosorbent assay, hepatitis B surface antigen, and rapid plasma reagent test were negative. Hepatitis C antibody was positive. Cryoglobulin screen was positive.
- C3 and C4 were decreased.
- Antinuclear antibody and antineutrophil cytoplasmic antibody (ANCA) were normal.
- Serum protein electrophoresis and urine protein electrophoresis were normal.
- Spot urine protein = 300 mg/dL, creatinine = 50 mg/dL, Na = 85 mEq/L, chloride = 80 mEq/L, K = 35 mEq/L, urea = 370 mg/dL, osmolarity = 275.

How Should This Patient Be Managed?

The patient should be referred to a nephrologist to consider a renal biopsy and a gastroenterologist to evaluate the hepatitis C. The patient should be referred to a dietitian to learn restrictions regarding sodium (2 g/day), potassium (2 g/day), phosphorus (1,000 mg), and protein (54 g/day) and to reinforce compliance with an American Diabetes Association, lipid-lowering diet. The patient currently consumes approximately 4.9 g sodium, 3.4 g potassium, and 80 g protein each day.

Diltiazem and a thiazide diuretic should be added to the medicines to lower the blood pressure to the goal of 120/70 mm Hg. Diltiazem improves the proteinuria; a thiazide diuretic improves the volume and hyperkalemia. However, if significant hypercalcemia develops, the thiazide should be discontinued.

Given the patient's type 4 RTA (urinary gap = 40+) and hyperkalemia, the potassium should be lowered with diet and thiazide therapy before a higher dose of ACE inhibitor therapy is tried. Bicarbonate therapy (one 650-mg tablet daily to replace his 9 mEq/day deficit) will also improve the hyperkalemia.

Hyperphosphatemia should be controlled through dietary measures and utilization of phosphate binders prior to treating the mild hyperparathyroidism with vitamin D.

Volume should be reduced through dietary salt restriction and thiazide medications.

Dyslipidemia should be treated by improving the proteinuria and diet, with additional pharmaceutical therapy added as needed.

His diabetes needs improved control through dietary intervention, weight reduction, and exercise.

The patient should be counseled on his sexually transmitted disease.

Suggested Reading

Food and Nutrition Information Center. United States Department of Agriculture. Available at http://www.nal.usda.gov/fnic/

McCarthy J T. A practical approach to the management of patients with chronic renal failure. *Mayo Clin Proc* 1999;74:269–273.

National Institute of Diabetes and Digestive and Kidney Diseases (NIDDK). Available at http://www.niddk.nih.gov/

Nephron Information Center. Available at http://www.nephron.com/

Rahman M, Smith M C. Chronic renal insufficiency: a diagnostic and therapeutic approach. *Arch Intern Med* 1998;158:1743–1752.

Schrier R W, ed. *Atlas of diseases of the kidney.* Available at http://www.kidneyatlas.org/

Tufts Nutrition Navigator. Tufts University. Available at http://www.navigator.tufts.edu/index.html

United States Renal Data System (USRDS). Available at: http://www.usrds.org/

63
Proteinuria

Yacob Ghebremeskel
Byard F. Edwards

1. What is the underlying pathologic process in proteinuria?
2. What is the significance of microalbuminuria in diabetic patients?
3. What are the major types of overt proteinuria?
4. What are the complications of nephrotic syndrome?

Discussion

What Is the Underlying Pathologic Process in Proteinuria?

Glomerular capillaries are highly efficient filters that allow free passage of water and small dissolved solutes while inhibiting the passage of macromolecules, the blood's formed elements, and most proteins. The filters are composed of three successive elements through which the filtrate must pass to enter the tubules: the fenestrated endothelium, the glomerular basement membrane (GBM) fenestrated matrix, and the visceral epithelial cells (i.e., podocytes), with their slit diaphragms. Molecular size and charge are the primary determinants of the filtrate's composition.

The fenestrae have radii that range from 40 to 45 Å in the GBM to 400 Å in the endothelial cells. Negatively charged polyanionic glycoproteins cover the surfaces and influence the filtration of charged macromolecules. At any given radius, anionic molecules are significantly restricted, and cationic molecules are significantly enhanced in their filtration when compared with neutral molecules.

Molecular size is also a barrier to filtration; the glomerular capillary structures function as a size-selective sieve. Small neutral molecules, such as inulin with a radius of 14 Å, pass freely until a radius of 20 Å is reached. Thereafter, size is a progressive barrier with little passage for molecules the size of albumin with a 36 Å radius and none at 42 Å.

Pore size and number can vary with glomerular diseases; abnormal channels may develop in the GBM, resulting in a loss of size selectivity. The loss of negatively charged glycoproteins in the glomerular capillary wall structures results in a loss of charge selectivity: both cationic and anionic macromolecules are filtered to the same degree as the neutral macromolecules. Significant albuminuria and proteinuria can occur. Urine containing more than 30 mg of albumin or 150 mg of protein per 24 hours is abnormal.

What Is the Significance of Microalbuminuria in Diabetic Patients?

Microalbuminuria is defined as persistent urinary albumin excretion of 30 to 300 mg/day. Urinary albumin excretion of more than 300 mg/day is considered overt proteinuria. Microalbuminuria is the earliest clinical finding of diabetic nephropathy and at times precedes the onset of overt type 2 diabetes mellitus. Progression from microalbuminuria to overt proteinuria occurs in 20% to 40% of white patients with type 2 diabetes mellitus within 10 years. Early detection and treatment of microalbuminuria can slow the progression of diabetic renal disease. A number of studies have suggested that microalbuminuria is an independent risk factor for cardiovascular mortality in both type 1 and type 2 diabetic patients.

What Are the Major Types of Proteinuria?

Proteinuria can result from increased glomerular filtration of macromolecules (glomerular), decreased tubular absorption of normally filtered low molecular weight proteins (tubular), or increased excretion of abnormally produced proteins (overflow).

The distinction of nephrotic (>3 g/24 h/1.73 m^2) versus non-nephrotic proteinuria is of clinical significance. Non-nephrotic proteinuria has a more favorable outcome associated with prolonged renal function and less dyslipidemia, edema, malnutrition, infections, and thrombosis.

Glomerular proteinuria results from glomerular disease. Anatomic changes, including glomerular sclerosis (focal segmental or diffuse glomerulosclerosis, diabetes), mesangial proliferation (membranoproliferative), and GBM thickening with subepithelial deposits (membranous), may be present, or there may be no apparent change other than foot process effacement as seen in minimal change nephropathy.

Tubular proteinuria increases when the proximal tubules are injured from intrinsic disease or tubulointerstitial nephritis. These proteins are low molecular weight, normally nearly completely resorbed, and are not detectable by urine dipstick analysis.

Increased production and excretion of immunoglobulin light chains leads to an overflow proteinuria that is not detectable by urine dipstick chemistry. Sulfosalicylic acid precipitates all protein present in the urine and can be used to screen for the presence of a paraprotein. Urine electrophoresis with immunofixation can be used to quantify the paraprotein excretion and discern whether it is a kappa or lambda type.

Seventy percent of nephrotic syndromes in the United States result from a secondary disease (primarily diabetes mellitus). A study of 233 renal biopsies performed in adults with nephrotic syndrome without systemic diseases such as diabetes, hypertension, and systemic lupus erythematosus, found that the most common causes were membranous nephropathy and glomerular sclerosis (33% each), minimal change disease (15%), and amyloidosis (4%). The most common primary glomerular disease that causes nephrotic syndrome in adults in the U.S. is membranous glomerulonephritis. In African-American patients, glomerulosclerosis is the most common primary glomerular disease.

What Are the Complications of Nephrotic Syndrome?

Edema

The major cause of edema in nephrotic syndrome is primary sodium retention. This is due to decreased tubular response to atrial natriuretic peptide, which results in an increase in sodium absorption in the distal tubules and reduced oncotic pressure that limits resorption of the interstitial fluid. These patients require low sodium diets (2 g/day) and high doses of loop diuretics to maintain an optimal fluid status.

Thromboembolism

The hypercoagulable state in nephrotic syndrome is multifactorial. A decrease in antithrombin III, protein C, and protein S, combined with increased procoagulatory factors and thrombocytosis, play important roles. The cumulative incidence of thromboembolic complications in nephrotic patients is nearly 50%. Renal vein thrombosis is frequent in patients with membranous glomerulonephritis. Predictors of thromboembolic complications include a serum albumin of less than 2.5 g/dL, proteinuria greater than 10 g/day, antithrombin III, protein C or protein S level less than 75% of normal level, and hypovolemia. Some experts recommend primary preventive anticoagulation in nephrotic patients with a serum albumin level of less than 2 g/dL. The benefit of anticoagulation is much higher than the risk of bleeding in this group of patients. Nephrotic patients with prior thromboembolic events require prophylactic anticoagulation.

Infection

Patients with nephrotic syndrome are prone to infection by encapsulated bacteria. Due to decreased levels of immunoglobulin G and complement factor B, pneumococcal vaccination is essential.

Hyperlipidemia

Dyslipidemia may occur because of overproduction of apoprotein B and decreased catabolism of apoprotein B, chylomicrons, and very low-density lipoprotein (VLDL). These patients generally require lipid-lowering agents.

Diminished Carrier Proteins

The plasma levels of many protein-bound drugs, hormones, and vitamins are low. Free drug levels of some drugs may be high and can cause drug toxicity.

Case

A 52-year-old man presents to the urgent care center complaining of early morning periorbital facial swelling beginning 3 weeks prior to this visit. The swelling generally goes away a few hours after he gets up and moves around. He also has noticed that his legs get swollen after a few hours of standing. He has had no chest pain or dyspnea. He sleeps on one pillow.

His past medical history is significant for type 2 diabetes mellitus, hypertension, and hypercholesterolemia. His medications include nifedipine, simvastatin, aspirin, and glipizide XL.

Physical examination is significant for a blood pressure of 180/90 mm Hg. Head, eyes, ears, nose, and throat examination reveals periorbital edema. The lungs are clear to auscultation. Heart examination reveals a regular rate and rhythm with a II/VI holosystolic murmur. The abdomen is soft and nontender; there is 2+ lower extremity edema. Laboratory studies show blood urea nitrogen of 24 mg/dL, creatinine 1.7 mg/dL, glucose 200 mg/dL, cholesterol 245 mg/dL, and 24-hour urinary protein 3.9 g. Chest radiograph is clear.

1. What is the most likely diagnosis?
2. How do you evaluate a patient with nephrotic syndrome?
3. Discuss the different treatment modalities.

Case Discussion

What Is the Most Likely Diagnosis?

The most likely diagnosis in this patient is a nephrotic syndrome secondary to diabetic nephropathy. He meets all the criteria for nephrotic syndrome.

How Do You Evaluate a Patient with Proteinuria?

Evaluation of a patient with proteinuria begins with a thorough history and physical examination. This will help to disclose contributing systemic diseases such as diabetes mellitus, hypertension, connective tissue diseases, and hepatitis, as well as benign conditions such as extreme physical exertion that may cause transient proteinuria.

The 24-hour urinary protein is the gold standard test for quantifying proteinuria. However, this test requires the patient's cooperation and completion of a proper urine collection for 24 hours. Therefore, the initial screening for proteinuria is done by urine dipstick. These firm plastic strips contain a paper area impregnated with an indicator sensitive to albumin and other parameters. It does not detect nonalbumin proteinuria, such as light chain proteins. The test becomes positive when the urinary albumin concentration exceeds 10 mg/dL. Therefore, it is concentration dependent. Concentrated urine and excreted iodinated contrast can give false-positive results. Dilute urine may give a false-negative result. The extent of color change is proportional to an albumin concentration of up to 2 g/dL. In a patient with urinary tract infection, the test should be repeated after treatment. If the dipstick is negative, microalbuminuria can be screened by obtaining a spot urine albumin:creatinine ratio.

The mid-morning and mid-afternoon albumin:creatinine ratio correlates well with the 24-hour urine albumin excretion, is inexpensive and readily available during the office visit. A random albumin:creatinine ratio of above 30 μg/mg defines the presence of microalbuminuria. A random protein:creatinine ratio of above 3 mg/mg defines the presence of a nephrotic syndrome. A microscopic examination of the spun urine sediment should be performed to assess for hematuria, pyuria, casts, bacteria, and lipiduria. If the urine sediment is unremarkable, the urinalysis should be repeated on the next visit. If the diagnosis of nephrotic range proteinuria is confirmed either by a spot urine protein:creatinine ratio or 24-hour urine collection, further evaluation is required, including serum electrolytes, total protein, albumin, lipid profile, hepatitis B surface antigen, hepatitis C antibody, serum protein electrophoresis, urine protein electrophoresis, human immunodeficiency virus, rapid plasma reagent, antinuclear antibody, C3, and C4.

If the patient is under 30 years of age, split urinary protein measurement is required to assess for orthostatic proteinuria. Two urine samples are collected. One is the urine voided after arising from bed until returning to bed. The second is the urine voided starting 2 hours after returning to bed until the patient arises from bed. If the proteinuria is present only while standing, then orthostatic proteinuria is present. No further assessment is necessary, and the patient should be assured of the condition's benign prognosis.

If the urine dipstick chemistry is negative, but the spot urine protein:creatinine ratio is greater than 0.3 mg/mg, then a urinary immunoelectrophoresis should be performed to assess for multiple myeloma and paraproteinuria.

Patients with persistent proteinuria should undergo renal ultrasonography to assess the number and size of the kidneys, determine the echogenicity, and assess for cysts, stones, hydronephrosis, and cortical thickness. Reflux uropathy and polycystic kidney disease may induce significant proteinuria. All patients with an uncertain etiology of the proteinuria should be referred to a qualified nephrologist.

Discuss the Different Treatment Modalities.

Treatment of diabetic nephropathy includes excellent blood pressure and diabetic control. Studies have shown that patients with a hemoglobin A1C above 8.5% have a higher rate of albuminuria. Lowering hemoglobin A1C to less than 7% is essential. Aggressive blood pressure control is important in all patients with proteinuria. Target blood pressure in patients with frank proteinuria is less than 125/75 mm Hg. Angiotensin-converting enzyme (ACE) inhibitors have been repeatedly shown to decrease proteinuria in both diabetic and nondiabetic patients. Recent studies confirm a positive effect of angiotensin receptor blockers in reducing proteinuria. Nondihydropyridine calcium channel blockers also have been shown to reduce proteinuria. Recent studies have shown that dihydropyridine calcium channel blockers reduce proteinuria when combined with an ACE inhibitor. Serum chemistries should be monitored frequently for changes in the electrolytes and renal function.

Proteinuria promotes renal failure. A low-protein diet (0.6 g/kg lean body weight for diabetics and 0.8 g/kg lean body weight for nondiabetics) is recommended to avoid malnutrition and hyperfiltration of the protein load. Additional dietary protein supplementation equaling the amount of daily urine protein excretion is required with the nephrotic syndrome.

Nephrotic patients avidly absorb sodium and require a low sodium (2 g/day) diet to avoid anasarca. Atrial natriuretic peptide resistance limits tubular sodium excretion. Higher doses of loop diuretics are required to maintain a diuresis because the loop diuretics have an increased volume of distribution and a decreased intratubular free concentration with the nephrotic syndrome.

Aggressive cholesterol reduction can be achieved with diet and drug therapy. Nephrotic patients generally have high low-density lipoprotein, VLDL, and triglyceride levels.

Pneumococcal vaccination should be given to every nephrotic patient, because immunoglobulins are lost in renal excretion.

The patient should be referred to a qualified nephrologist to assess the need for a renal biopsy and tailor the therapeutic interventions to the biopsy results.

Suggested Reading

Alzaid A A. Microalbuminuria in patients with NIDDM: an overview. *Diabetes Care* 1996;19:79.

Brater D C. Diuretic therapy. *N Engl J Med* 1998;6:387.

Kloke, et al. Antihypertensive treatment of patients with proteinuric renal diseases. *Kidney Int* 1998;53:1559.

Orth S R, Ritz E. The nephrotic syndrome. *N Engl J Med* 1998;338:1202.

Rose B D. Evaluation of isolated proteinuria. *Up to Date* 2000;8:1–6.

Schrier R W, Fassett R G. A critique of the overfill hypothesis of sodium and water retention in nephrotic syndrome. *Kidney Int* 1998;53:1111.

64

Hyponatremia

Todd S. Perlstein

- Discussion   *400*
- Case   *402*
- Case Discussion   *403*

1. What are the common outpatient presentations of hyponatremia?
2. What pathologic state is indicated by hyponatremia?
3. What are the steps in the workup of hyponatremia?
4. What are the therapeutic considerations in the treatment of hyponatremia?

Discussion

What Are the Common Outpatient Presentations of Hyponatremia?

In the ambulatory setting, hyponatremia is often an unexpected finding in an asymptomatic patient. Initial symptoms caused by hyponatremia can often be protean in nature, including malaise, weakness, muscle cramping, abdominal discomfort, and vomiting. More severe symptoms are neurologic, beginning with lethargy, and progressing to seizures and coma.

It is important to appreciate that not only is the absolute sodium concentration important in determining the severity of symptoms, but also the rate at which that sodium concentration was achieved. A patient whose hyponatremia developed slowly might be asymptomatic with a serum sodium of 105 mEq/L, whereas a sodium of 118 mEq/L that developed acutely might lead to coma and death.

What Pathologic State Is Indicated by Hyponatremia?

Hyponatremia indicates that total body water is increased relative to total body solute. It is important to note that although the principal extracellular solute is sodium, the principal intracellular solute is potassium, and total body potassium is an important determinant of the serum sodium. The serum sodium concentration provides no information about total body solute content, only its relative amount compared with water. One exception to this is hypertonic hyponatremia, examples of which are hyperglycemia or hyponatremia following mannitol infusion. Another exception is pseudohyponatremia, an artifact of measuring the serum sodium that can occur in severe hyperlipidemia and hyperproteinemia.

Water can be increased relative to total body solute whether solute content is high, low, or normal. It is best to approach hyponatremia in terms of total body solute content. Clinically, solute content is best measured by estimating volume status; thus, we will discuss hyponatremia in terms of volume status.

Hypervolemic hyponatremia occurs when there is abnormal retention of solute and water, with water retained in excess of solute. Congestive heart failure, cirrhosis, nephrotic syndrome, and pregnancy are clinical states that cause hypervolemic hyponatremia. Activation of the renin–angiotensin–aldosterone system, nonosmotic stimulation of antidiuretic hormone (ADH), and sympathetic nervous system activation are thought to be the underlying pathophysiologic mechanisms by which abnormal solute and water retention occur. In renal insufficiency, decreased ability of the kidneys to excrete free water may contribute to hyponatremia. Pregnancy is associated with a resetting of the osmostat, leading to a reduction in serum sodium of 5 to 6 mEq/L.

Hypovolemic hyponatremia occurs in conditions of solute loss in excess of water loss, or solute loss with ingestion of free water. Thiazide diuretics cause natriuresis and aquaresis, but because their site of action is the distal convoluted tubule and cortical collecting duct, they interfere with the kidney's ability to excrete free water and can cause hyponatremia. Both thiazide and loop diuretics cause significant kaliuresis, and depletion of this intracellular solute can contribute to hyponatremia. Solute loss through the gastrointestinal tract, for example by vomiting or diarrhea, combined with oral intake of free water, also can lead to hyponatremia. In hypovolemic hyponatremia, nonosmotic stimulation of ADH secretion is a key mediator.

Euvolemic hyponatremia most often occurs because of abnormal ADH secretion or action. ADH secretion can be stimulated by a wide variety of causes. Drugs such as opioids, nonsteroidal anti-inflammatory drugs (NSAIDs), antidepressants, and sulfonylureas can cause euvolemic hyponatremia by either enhancing ADH release or potentiating its action on the kidney. Pain, nausea, and anxiety have all been associated with ADH secretion. Multiple central nervous system diseases and pulmonary diseases can stimulate ADH secretion. ADH can be produced ectopically by a tumor.

Hypothyroidism and adrenal insufficiency are endocrinopathies that are associated with a decreased ability of the kidney to excrete free water.

Because there is a limit to the kidney's ability to produce dilute urine, inadequate solute ingestion can lead to hyponatremia. This can occur in alcohol abusers who do not eat sufficiently and is referred to as beer potomania. Pathologic water ingestion can outstrip the kidney's ability to excrete free water, a condition known as psychogenic polydipsia. This most often occurs in patients with schizophrenia, who have been shown to have abnormalities in ADH secretion.

What Is the Approach to the Workup of Hyponatremia?

The workup of hyponatremia begins with a thorough history. Of primary importance is determining whether the hyponatremia is symptomatic, as will be discussed later.

Inciting events, such as excessive solute loss via sweating or via the gastrointestinal tract, or intense pain or emotional stress, should be investigated. The history should be reviewed for predisposing medical or psychiatric conditions. The medication list should be reviewed, with adverse effects referenced when unsure. The social history should include drinking (both alcohol and water) and eating habits. The review of systems should look for clues to cardiac, pulmonary, renal, hepatic, or neurologic disease, as well as evidence of an endocrinopathy.

The physical examination is primarily focused on determination of volume status. Blood pressure and pulse should be checked both lying and standing. Edema must be carefully sought out. A thorough neurologic examination, including mental status and reflexes, should be performed. The examiner should keep in mind the differential diagnosis of hyponatremia, thus looking for signs of heart failure, cirrhosis, hypothyroidism, and pulmonary and neurologic disease.

The laboratory examination begins with electrolytes. Hypertonic hyponatremia and pseudohyponatremia should be ruled out by measuring serum osmolarity, lipids, and total protein. Renal function should be checked, with a comparison of the blood urea nitrogen (BUN) with creatinine for an indication of volume status. The uric acid is generally normal or elevated in hypovolemic and hypervolemic hyponatremia, whereas it is nearly always low in euvolemic hyponatremia. In euvolemic hyponatremia, a low urine osmolality suggests either psychogenic polydipsia or inadequate solute ingestion. A chest radiograph should be checked for an active pulmonary process, and a focal finding on neurologic examination should prompt neuroimaging. Hyponatremia occurs in up to 30% of patients with acquired immunodeficiency syndrome, and testing for human immunodeficiency virus should be considered when no etiology is apparent. Pregnancy should be ruled out.

What Are the Important Considerations in the Management of Hyponatremia?

Primum non nocere has been the mantra of treating hyponatremia. Too rapid correction of hyponatremia can cause an osmolar demyelination syndrome known as central pontine myelinolysis, which causes permanent neurologic injury or even death. It has been common practice to actively correct only severely symptomatic chronic hyponatremia or acute hyponatremia. Recently it has been demonstrated that in chronic symptomatic hyponatremia, water restriction alone is associated with worse neurologic outcomes. This same study confirmed that overly aggressive therapy is also associated with poor neurologic outcomes. In general, increasing the sodium by 6 to 8 mEq/L will correct the symptoms. A reasonable therapeutic strategy would be to actively correct all symptomatic hyponatremia with intravenous saline, with a goal of increasing the serum sodium either to 120 mEq/L or by 10 mEq/L, whichever is less, in the first 24 hours. In patients with severe neurologic symptoms, such as seizures, the goal should be to rapidly increase the sodium by 6 to 8 mEq/L, which should stop the seizure activity, but again not to exceed 120 mEq/L or an increase of 10 mEq/L in the first 24 hours.

Case

A 76-year-old woman was in your office 10 days ago for follow-up of an elevated blood pressure. She is known to have hypertension, as well as hypothyroidism, diabetes mellitus, and depression. Her medications include lisinopril, glipizide, levothyroxine, sertraline, and aspirin. Her blood pressure was 150/90 mm Hg, pulse

70 beats/min, and weight 56 kg. On that day, her serum chemistry was as follows: sodium 140 mEq/L, potassium 4.2 mEq/L, chloride 105 mEq/L, bicarbonate 25 mEq/L, BUN 16 mg/dL, and creatinine 1.0 mg/dL. Blood counts were normal. You began hydrochlorothiazide 25 mg, with follow up scheduled for 2 weeks.

Eight days later, the patient is brought in by her family because of weakness, muscle cramping, and emesis. Her blood pressure is 120/60 mm Hg, pulse 90 beats/min, and weight 54.5 kg. Orthostatic vital signs are not checked because she immediately becomes symptomatic upon standing. On neurologic examination, the patient is notably fatigued but otherwise normal. Today, her sodium is 124 mEq/L, potassium 3.1 mEq/L, chloride 85 mEq/L, bicarbonate 29 mEq/L, BUN 24 mg/dL, and creatinine 1.2 mg/dL.

1. What is the most likely cause of her hyponatremia?
2. How should she be treated?
3. What else might predispose her to hyponatremia?

Case Discussion

What Is the Most Likely Cause of Her Hyponatremia?

The most likely cause is her thiazide diuretic. As stated earlier, thiazides act on the distal convoluted tubule and the cortical collecting duct of the kidney and therefore interfere with its ability to produce dilute urine. The hypokalemia reflects a significant loss of intracellular solute, which further contributes to the hyponatremia.

Elderly patients, especially women, are particularly susceptible to thiazide diuretic-induced hyponatremia. This patient's creatinine is within the normal laboratory range. However, her glomerular filtration rate calculated by the Cockcroft-Gault equation is only 42 mL/min. Her decreased renal function limits her ability to clear free water, and the thiazide diuretic amplifies this.

How Should She Be Treated?

The patient has three problems: volume depletion, hyponatremia, and hypokalemia. Her volume deficit should be corrected with isotonic saline. This will begin to correct her serum sodium as well. Her sodium should be followed closely to ensure that it does not rise too rapidly. Her intravenous fluids also should contain potassium, which will also contribute to the normalization of her serum sodium. In hypovolemic hyponatremia, hypertonic fluids are often not necessary to correct the serum sodium, and are almost never indicated when serum sodium exceeds 120 mEq/L. Of course her thiazide diuretic should be discontinued. Water restriction is not recommended in hypovolemic patients. Once her volume is corrected, her serum sodium should be checked. Her sodium should not be increased to greater than 134 mEq/L in the first 24 hours.

What Else Might Predispose Her to Hyponatremia?

Her major predisposing factor was her renal insufficiency. She is on a selective serotonin reuptake inhibitor antidepressant, which has been associated with hyponatremia, particularly in the elderly. If her levothyroxine dose is inadequate, hypothyroidism might be contributing as well.

Suggested Reading

Ayus J C, Arieff A I. Chronic hyponatremic encephalopathy in postmenopausal women. *JAMA* 1999;281:2299–2304.

Berl T, Robertson GL. *Pathophysiology of water metabolism.* In: Brenner BM, eds. *Brenner & Rector's the kidney*, 6th ed. Philadelphia: WB Saunders, 2000.

Mange K, Matsura D, et al. Language guiding therapy: the case of dehydration versus volume depletion. *Ann Intern Med* 1997;127:848–853.

Rose B D. *Clinical physiology of acid-base and electrolyte disorders*, 4th ed. New York: McGraw-Hill, 1994.

Sterns R H, Spital A, Clark E C. *Disorders of water balance.* In: Kokko JP, Tannen RL, eds. *Fluids and electrolytes*, 3rd ed. Philadelphia: WB Saunders, 1996.

XI
Neurology

65

Dizziness and Vertigo

Yvonne J. Braver

1. What are the basic mechanisms of balance?
2. What is vertigo, and how do we distinguish it from other forms of dizziness?
3. How does the history help in differentiating between peripheral and central vestibular and nonvestibular causes of vertigo?
4. How do the physical examination and laboratory tests help in differentiating between peripheral and central vestibular and nonvestibular causes of vertigo?
5. Describe the clinical picture and treatment for the following common causes of vertigo: benign paroxysmal positional vertigo, vestibular neuronitis (labyrinthitis), and Ménière's disease.

Discussion

What Are the Basic Mechanisms of Balance?

Vestibular, visual, and somatosensory receptors provide information about the position of the head and body in space. Vestibular receptor neurons in the ear consist of ciliated hair cells within the paired anterior, posterior, and horizontal semicircular canals, the utricle, and the saccule. Peripheral vestibular receptors emit impulses when stimulated by motion. These impulses get transmitted through cranial nerve VIII and then through the internal auditory canal. The impulses emerge in the cerebellopontine angle, where they synapse in ipsilateral and contralateral vestibular nuclei. Visual receptors provide a stable retinal image during head movement. Somatosensory receptors provide information about gravity, position, and motion of muscles and joints. Dizziness results from a mismatch or imbalance in any of these receptors.

What Is Vertigo, and How Do We Distinguish It from Other Forms of Dizziness?

Vertigo is the illusion of motion between the patient and outside world when they are in fact not moving. Nausea, vomiting, pallor, and perspiration often accompany vertigo. Objective vertigo is defined by the perception that the world is moving while the patient remains still. In subjective vertigo the perception is of the body moving while the world remains still. Unfortunately the distinction between objective and subjective vertigo does not help to localize the lesion. A peripheral vestibular lesion (semicircular canal, utricle, or peripheral nerve) accounts for 85% of complaints of vertigo. Central lesions (beyond the cerebellopontine angle) account for the other 15%.

Presyncope occurs when patients have the perception they are about to faint, but there is no loss of consciousness. Patients complain of symptoms suggesting decreased cerebral perfusion; they typically describe a woozy feeling with sinking spells, buzzing in the head, rubbery legs, frequent falls, visual field constriction, pallor, perspiration, and nausea. The differential diagnosis for presyncope is the same as that of a true syncopal episode. These patients are at high risk for cardiac disease, arrhythmia, orthostatic hypotension, vasovagal syndromes, and bradycardia.

Dysequilibrium is defined by the sensation of losing balance. There is no illusory movement or sense of loss of consciousness. Dysequilibrium is common in the elderly because of declining sensory inputs from worsening vision and hearing, and declining postural reflexes from arthritis and joint abnormalities. Dysequilibrium can be accentuated in the elderly when they are in unfamiliar environments, in dim light, or on uneven ground. In the young, disequilibrium should prompt a workup for significant neurologic disease.

Lightheadedness and the feelings of being outside one's body are usually of psychogenic origin. Patients may describe a feeling of impending doom, shortness of breath, headache, palpitations, and perioral numbness. Forced hyperventilation can often reproduce the symptoms. Anxiety, major depression, somatization disorders, and panic attacks can often cause these symptoms in the young, but rarely in the elderly.

How Does the History Help in Differentiating Between Peripheral and Central Vestibular and Nonvestibular Causes of Vertigo?

An accurate history and thorough physical examination should produce a diagnosis in a majority of patients with a complaint of dizziness. The physician should differentiate peripheral and central vestibular lesions from nonvestibular illnesses. Peripheral vestibular lesions (e.g., benign paroxysmal positional vertigo) are typically benign and self-limiting. Central vestibular lesions can represent a mass lesion or a neurologic emergency such as a posterior cerebellar stroke. Patients at high risk for heart disease or stroke should have a thorough cardiovascular examination and a search for potentially life-threatening nonvestibular etiologies.

A sensation of vertigo indicates a vestibular disorder either of peripheral or central origin. Important historical clues come from determining the onset and duration of symptoms. In general, vertigo of sudden onset with intermittent symptoms points toward an inner ear problem. Symptoms lasting less than 1 minute are suggestive of benign paroxysmal positional vertigo (BPPV). Symptoms lasting many hours are associated with Ménière's disease, whereas those lasting more than 24 hours point toward viral labyrinthitis or a central lesion. A central nervous system mass lesion tends to have a gradual onset with continuous or progressive symptoms. Transient ischemic attacks or stroke (e.g., posterior circulation) also must be considered when symptoms are acute in onset but last from minutes to hours.

Vertiginous symptoms brought on by a change in position suggest vestibular disease. If a specific movement, such as turning in bed, produces symptoms, suspect BPPV and otolith dysfunction. A tendency to list to one side or a reluctance to bend over can indicate peripheral or central vestibular disease. Some patients develop "top shelf" vertigo or even "drop attacks" when looking up or working overhead. This can be from an acute reduction of cerebral perfusion in the posterior circulation due to cervical osteophytes (degenerative joint disease in the neck) impinging on the vertebral basilar arteries during neck extension. Complaints of hearing loss, fullness or pressure in the ear, tinnitus, and perception of sounds being unusually loud or distorted usually originate peripherally in the cochlea. However, when a patient complains of both tinnitus and hearing loss, consider a brain tumor or acoustic neuroma. Presentations of altered mental status and dizziness require a workup for drug toxicity, metabolic disorders, cerebellar hemorrhage, or infarct. A headache and dizziness raises concern about meningitis, stroke, aneurysm, migraine, and systemic illness. Sudden onset of nausea, vomiting, and dizziness suggest labyrinthitis. Any focal, localizing neurologic symptoms or ataxia suggest a cerebellar or central lesion.

How Do the Physical Examination and Other Tests Help in Differentiating Between Peripheral and Central Vestibular and Nonvestibular Causes of Vertigo?

The physical examination should concentrate on cardiovascular and neurologic findings. Uncontrolled hypertension can cause vasospasm and reduce blood flow to the vestibular labyrinths, resulting in vertigo. Orthostatic hypotension can cause decreased cerebral perfusion.

Nystagmus is the objective finding to the subjective complaint of vertigo. Horizontal or rotary nystagmus can occur with central or peripheral lesions. Vertical nystagmus results from a central lesion. The slow component of nystagmus is caused by vestibular stimulation through a reflex arc from the semicircular canal to the extraocular muscles. The fast component returns the eyes to the resting position and points away from the affected side. The fast component requires a functioning cerebral cortex and is not present in comatose patients or in patients under anesthesia. The direction of the slow and fast component of nystagmus should be noted on physical examination.

The Dix-Hallpike maneuver can be used to provoke nystagmus when BPPV is suspected. This procedure should be used therapeutically, rather than for diagnosis of BPPV. Repeated use of the Dix-Hallpike maneuver in the direction of the lesion can eliminate nystagmus and reduce vertigo.

Peripheral lesions of the cochlea or cochlear division of cranial nerve VIII can cause sensorineural hearing loss. Lesions of the vestibular nuclei or temporal lobe can cause central deafness. Conductive hearing loss is caused by disorders of the external and middle ear. The external auditory canal should be examined for evidence of trauma, foreign body, or infection. Cerumen impaction can be a fairly debilitating and easily cured cause of vertigo. Fluid, infection, and perforation can affect the tympanic membrane. Mastoiditis is associated with erythema, edema, and tenderness.

Any laboratory evaluation should be directed toward suspected conditions, such as hypoglycemia or drug toxicity. If brain imaging is indicated, magnetic resonance imaging with gadolinium is best for detecting brainstem and vestibular structures.

Describe the Clinical Picture and Treatment for the Following Common Causes of Vertigo: Benign Paroxysmal Positional Vertigo, Vestibular Neuronitis (Labyrinthitis), and Ménière's Disease.

Benign paroxysmal positional vertigo is the most common cause of vertigo. Patients develop brief episodes of vertigo (<1 minute) with change in position. Patients describe sudden onset of rotational vertigo when rolling over in bed, bending forward, or reaching up to a high shelf. BPPV is thought to result when free, floating otoliths are disrupted in the labyrinth with head movement. Otolith dysfunction is typically idiopathic, but can be caused by head injury, viral labyrinthitis, or vascular occlusion. Nystagmus occurs with the fast component moving away from the side of the lesion.

Benign paroxysmal positional vertigo is typically self-limited, with recovery in about 3 months. The patient's natural tendency is to avoid movements that provoke symptoms, but desensitization with habituation training can help recovery. Patients should lie safely on their bed or on the floor and roll several times daily in the position that causes symptoms. Additionally, the Eply maneuver, a variation of the Dix-Hallpike maneuver, can be used to move the otolith out of the semicircular canals and relieve BPPV of the ear. Use the Eply maneuver in the direction of the lesion and repeat as many times as necessary until nystagmus disappears.

Vestibular neuritis (labyrinthitis) presents with sudden severe vertigo, nausea, and vomiting that may last several days. Half of patients report a viral upper respiratory infection prior to onset of symptoms. Unsteadiness may persist for several weeks after resolution of vertigo. Treatment is generally supportive, with meclizine for dizziness, or antiemetics for nausea.

Ménière's disease presents with aural fullness, fluctuating sensorineural hearing loss, tinnitus, and vertigo. Attacks of vertigo become severe over a few minutes then slowly subside over several hours. The hearing loss, which can be permanent, localizes the side of the lesion. In Ménière's there is an excessive accumulation of endolymph, expanding and rupturing the labyrinth. This causes hearing loss and vertigo. Treatment is aimed at preventing osmotic shifts in the endolymph with vasodilators and diuretics. Salt, tobacco, and caffeine restriction also may be helpful. Surgery to destroy the labyrinth, and hearing on the affected side, may be necessary in refractory cases of Ménière's disease.

Case

A 72-year-old woman with a past medical history significant for hypertension and hyperlipidemia presents with a 2-week complaint of a dizzy feeling that occurs when she turns over in bed in the morning or arises from a chair. She feels like the room is spinning around her for about 30 seconds. Sometimes she feels a little nauseated and begins to perspire when this happens, but she has not vomited. She also feels a little woozy, like her legs are turning to rubber, when she goes to the bathroom at night. She denies associated chest pain, shortness of breath, palpitations, weakness, fever, cough, or congestion. She denies any recent falls, loss of consciousness, or injuries. She denies slurred speech, change in hearing, or vision. Medications include atenolol, started 4 weeks prior to presentation, hydrochlorothiazide, simvastatin, and daily aspirin.

On physical examination, her blood pressure is 120/72 mm Hg and her pulse rate is 62 beats/min while supine. Upon standing, her blood pressure is 105/60 mm Hg and her pulse rate is 62 beats/min. Results of a thorough examination are normal, except for spontaneous horizontal nystagmus with the fast component toward the left during the right-side head-down position. Nystagmus and symptoms of vertigo occurred after a 5-second latency.

1. What are some special considerations in the differential diagnosis for older patients with dizziness?
2. What are the likely causes of vertigo in this patient, and how should it be treated?
3. What special precautions should this patient take?

Case Discussion

What Are Some Special Considerations in the Differential Diagnosis for Older Patients with Dizziness?

Symptoms of dizziness increase with advanced age often due to disruption of vestibular, visual, and somatosensory receptors. Older patients also have a higher incidence of comorbidities such as coronary artery disease, carotid artery stenosis, and central neurologic lesions. In a recent study (Lawson et al., 1999), 46% of geriatric patients with dizziness had syncope and falls associated with their dizziness. A cardiac diagnosis was found in 28% of patients, and 18% had more than one cause of dizziness. Anxiety disorders are rarely a cause of dizziness in the elderly.

What Are the Likely Causes of Vertigo in This Patient and How Should It Be Treated?

This patient presents with symptoms and physical findings suggesting two different processes: recurrent episodes of acute vertigo and a "woozy feeling" upon standing. Her vertiginous symptoms are highly consistent with BPPV; this disease is benign and generally self-limited. Treatment options include habituation training where the patient practices maneuvers that reproduce symptoms in order to desensitize her from the sense of vertigo. Attempt to remove free-floating debris from the affected posterior semicircular canal through repeated use of the Dix-Hallpike maneuver.

The "woozy" sensation upon getting up to use the bathroom at night suggests presyncope due to orthostatic hypotension, and on examination the patient is orthostatic by blood pressure. Dehydration should be considered because it is common in the elderly, partly due to a decreased sense of thirst. Review of her medications shows that she is on a β-blocker and a diuretic for treatment of hypertension. An adjustment in her medications might relieve her symptoms of orthostatic hypotension.

What Special Precautions Should This Patient Take?

Dizziness and vertigo can place a geriatric patient at high risk for falls and injury. Elderly patients are at a higher risk for hip fractures with associated morbidity and mortality. Patients should be instructed on specific fall precautions, including moving slowly from and laying, to sitting, to standing position to avoid orthostatic hypotension. Patients should remove area rugs from the home that increase the potential for falls. A nightlight should be on at all times. A cane or walker should be used to improve balance. Maintaining adequate hydration, particularly in the summer months, is important to emphasize as well.

Suggested Reading

Balough R W. Dizziness: neurologic emergencies. *Neurol Clin* 1998;16:305.
Furman J M, Cass S P. Primary care: benign positional vertigo. *N Engl J Med* 1999;341:1590.
Hotson J R, Baloh R W. Current concepts: acute vestibular syndrome. *N Engl J Med* 1998;339:680.
Lawson J, Fitzgerald J, Birchall J, Aldren C P, Kenny R A. Diagnosis of geriatric patients with severe dizziness. *J Am Geriatr Soc* 1999;47:12.

66
Migraine Headache

Murtaza Cassoobhoy

1. Distinguish migraine headache from other kinds of headaches, particularly tension, cluster, and analgesic.
2. What is the current understanding of the pathophysiology of migraine headache?
3. What are the nonpharmacologic options for the treatment of migraine headache?
4. What abortive pharmacologic therapies are available currently?
5. What medications are available for prophylaxis and when should they be used?

Discussion

Distinguish Migraine Headache from Other Kinds of Headaches, Particularly Tension, Cluster, and Analgesic.

In order to effectively treat a patient with a headache disorder, it is extremely important to categorize the type of headache (or headaches) a patient is experiencing. The International Headache Society has developed comprehensive diagnostic criteria for the many different types of headaches. The most common ones that can be classified are migraine with aura (previously termed classical), migraine without aura (previously termed common), tension, cluster, and analgesic.

Simplified diagnostic criteria for migraine without aura include:

- Attacks lasting 4 to 72 hours
- At least two of the following four headache characteristics:
  - Unilateral location
  - Pulsating quality
  - Moderate to severe intensity
  - Aggravated by movement
- At least one associated symptom:
  - Nausea or vomiting
  - Photophobia and phonophobia

Simplified diagnostic criteria for migraine with aura include at least three of the following four characteristics:

1. One or more transient focal neurologic aura symptoms
2. Gradual development of aura symptom over more than 4 minutes, or several symptoms in succession

3. Aura symptoms last 4 to 60 minutes
4. Headache following or accompanying aura within 60 minutes

The diagnostic criteria of tension headaches are basically the opposite of migraine without aura:

1. Bilateral
2. Nonpulsating
3. Mild to moderate severity (usually not disabling)
4. Not aggravated by movement
5. None or only mild nausea or photophobia

Cluster headaches are much more common in men (8:1 ratio). The pain is periorbital, excruciating, and deep (not pulsatile). The same side is affected every time and can be associated with nasal congestion, lacrimation, and redness of the eye on the affected side. The headaches tend to occur at the same time every day for many days. There may be long headache-free intervals.

Analgesic headaches are common in patients that chronically use antimigraine or analgesic drugs, especially those that contain caffeine. Patients have a gradual increase in headache frequency with resultant increase in drug use followed by a change in headache characteristics. Daily use of a low-dose analgesic is much riskier for analgesic headaches than occasional use of large doses. The headache initially worsens when the analgesics are discontinued but should improve after a few weeks.

What Is the Current Understanding of the Pathophysiology of Migraine Headache?

Our current understanding of the pathogenesis of migraine headaches is incomplete. Patients with migraine are susceptible to cortical hyperexcitability by having a lower threshold and an increased response to certain triggers. The lower threshold is felt to be determined by genetic factors (possibly involving ion channel function). Specific triggers that can set off the cortical hyperexcitability include hormonal fluctuation, certain foods, altered sleep pattern, emotional or physical stress, and drugs.

The aura associated with migraines is currently thought to be caused by a cortical spreading depression (CSD), a depolarization wave that propagates across the brain cortex, resulting in significant dysfunction of brain ion homeostasis. The human visual cortex, due to a low ratio of glial cells to neuronal cells, may have a reduced local threshold for CSD.

Patients with migraine headaches have low serotonin levels between attacks and increased levels during attacks. The serotonin release during an attack is probably a self-defense mechanism rather than the cause of the migraine as originally thought.

What Are the Nonpharmacologic Options for the Treatment of Migraine Headache?

Nonpharmacologic options for migraine management include patient education and behavioral therapy. Patient education allows patients to take an active role in the management of their headaches. They should understand that although the condition is not curable, effective therapy can lessen the severity, duration, and frequency of their attacks. Behavioral therapy is composed of developing regular, healthful life-style habits and avoiding specific triggers. Healthful life-style habits include a regular schedule of sleep, meals, and physical activity. Triggers such as stress, altered sleep pattern, menses, physical activity, alcohol, excess caffeine use or withdrawal, foods containing monosodium glutamate (Chinese food, canned soups, seasonings), tyramine (cheese, red wines), nitrites (cured meat), or aspartame (diet sodas, artificial sweeteners) can induce migraines. When patients develop a migraine, they should be advised to lie down in a quiet, dark room. Vigorous scalp massage or cold compress to the affected area can help reduce the symptoms.

What Abortive Pharmacologic Therapies Are Currently Available?

Pharmacologic options include analgesics, ergot alkaloids or triptans. Acetaminophen and nonsteroidal antiinflammatory drugs (NSAIDs) are useful in mild to moderate attacks. Oral absorption is impaired in migraine attacks, even in nonnauseated patients, and promethazine or metoclopramide 30 minutes before or with analgesics can help their absorption. A combination of isomethaptene, acetaminophen, and dichloralpherazone, known as midrin, and a combination of caffeine and bultalbital, sold as fiorinal, both have addictive potential and a propensity to induce headaches with long-term use. The U.S. Food and Drug Administration (FDA) lists midrin as only possibly effective for migraine headache, and fiorinal is only approved for tension headache.

Ergot alkaloids were previously the only drugs specifically used for migraine. They have a high affinity for a wide range of receptors, including serotonin, dopamine, and adrenergic. In controlled trials, ergotamine has proved to be effective in about 50% of patients and can be given via the oral, sublingual, rectal, or nasal route. The addition of caffeine to ergotamine enhances its absorption. Dihydroergotamine can be given parenterally and is useful in the emergency room setting to treat the acute migraine attack.

Four triptans are currently available for the treatment of migraine headache: naratriptan, rizatriptan, sumatriptan, and zolmitriptan. They share similar chemical structures and mechanisms of action. They are selective serotonin receptor agonists, particularly for the 1B and 1D receptor subtypes. There are subtle differences between the four. Zolmitriptan and rizatriptan are more lipid soluble and may have a more rapid onset of action than oral sumatriptan. Naratriptan has a longer half-life but a slower onset of action. There is no clear therapeutic advantage of one over the other. If one triptan does not work on at least two occasions, a different triptan can be tried. One triptan may be better tolerated than another in terms of side effects. The formulation of the triptan (administered nasally, orally, or subcutaneously) may influence the choice as well, such as when a patient has severe nausea and is unable to tolerate oral medications.

Sumatriptan was the first triptan available and so we have the most clinical experience with it. It is available in subcutaneous injection, nasal spray, or oral tablet formulation. The injection and nasal spray act within 15 minutes, and the tablets take about 1 hour to work. It is recommended that patients receiving injectable sumatriptan for the first time should be observed for 30 to 45 minutes after the dose in case of adverse reactions.

Both triptans and ergotamines are vasoconstricters and so contraindicated in patients with coronary atherosclerotic heart disease and uncontrolled hypertension. Also patients with basilar or hemiplegic migraine should not receive triptans. They can cause neck or chest discomfort (especially injectable sumatriptan), and patients should be advised of this side effect. Usually they are well tolerated.

What Medications Are Available for Prophylaxis and When Should They Be Used?

Prophylactic treatment should be considered in patients with more than two or three attacks a month that are severe enough to limit activity. They also should be considered in patients in whom abortive agents have been ineffective, poorly tolerated, or contraindicated. Menstrual-induced or other predictable migraine attacks may sometimes be prevented by a brief course of ergotamine or NSAIDs taken for several days before and during the first few days of menstruation.

Only four drugs are currently approved by the FDA for migraine prophylaxis, but many more are commonly used and are listed in Table 66.1. The choice of a prophylactic agent should be based on the patient's comorbid conditions. For example, if a patient is also suffering from depression, an antidepressant can be tried, or if a pa-

Table 66.1. Drugs Commonly Used for Migraine Prophylaxis

Drug	Side Effects	Contraindications
Beta blockers Nadolol Propranolol[a] Atenolol Timolol[a] Metoprolol	Hypotension, weight gain, depression, insomnia, impotence, nightmares, decreased tolerance to exercise, bradycardia	Uncontrolled asthma, chronic obstructive pulmonary disease, heart block, sick sinus syndrome
Anticonvulsant Divalproex sodium[a]	Lethargy, anorexia, indigestion, diarrhea, skin rash, alopecia, hepatoxicity	Impaired liver function
Antidepressants Amitriptyline Nortriptyline Imipramine Desipramine Doxepin Trazadone Fluoxetine	Dry mouth, sedation, decreased libido, orthostatic hypotension, arrhythmia	Impaired liver function, angle closure glaucoma, hyperthyroidism, thyroid medication use
Calcium channel blockers Verapamil Nifedipine Diltiazem Nimodipine	Constipation, dizziness, hypotension	Heart block, sick sinus syndrome, congestive heart failure
Serotonin antagonist Methylsergide[a]	Nausea, muscle cramps, abdominal pain, weight gain, peripheral artery spasm, retroperitoneal, pulmonary or endocardial fibrosis	Impaired liver function, coadministration of phenytoin, carbamazepine or phenobarbital

[a]Approved by the Food and Drug Administration for migraine prophylaxis.
Adapted from Migraine Prophylaxis. *Hosp Med*, 34(10):13–14, 19–21, 25, October 1998.

tient has hypertension, a β-blocker or calcium channel blocker may be more appropriate. The drug should be used for at least 2 to 3 months before deeming it a failure. If it is successful, it should be continued for at least 6 months and then tapering considered.

Case

A 19-year-old college student presents to the student health center for evaluation of recurrent headaches. She has suffered from headaches for the past 3 years, described as diffuse, and usually precipitated by hunger or fatigue. They are of mild intensity, have no associated symptoms, and are easily relieved by acetaminophen.

In the past month since starting college she has had two severe, disabling headaches that have required her to take multiple acetaminophen and ibuprofen tablets without significant relief. She turns off all the lights in her room and has to ask her roommate to leave the room. The headache is preceded by zig-zag lines in her peripheral vision and tingling in her fingers that lasts for a few minutes. The headache is always one sided and can last for 3 to 4 hours. She feels drained after the headache. She recalls her father having such severe headaches when she was a child. She has been taking oral contraceptive pills for the past 3 months. She is very concerned she may have a brain tumor.

Results of the physical examination, including a detailed neurologic examination, are completely normal.

1. What different types of headaches does she have?
2. Does she need any radiologic imaging studies?
3. What may have triggered these attacks?
4. What initial therapy can be suggested?

Case Discussion
What Different Types of Headaches Does She Have?

By history it appears that she has two different types of headache. The first headache is most likely a tension-type headache given that it is bilateral, mild, and has no associated symptoms. The more recent headache fulfills the diagnostic criteria for migraine headache with aura. Aura symptoms are most commonly visual (scintillating scotomas, zig-zag patterns, blind spots) but also can be sensory (paresthesia) or aphasia. The headache is also disabling, unilateral, and associated with photophobia.

Does She Need Any Radiologic Imaging Studies?

No. Given the clear history of migraine headaches, a probable family history, and a completely normal neurologic examination, no further tests are needed at this time. The patient must be educated extensively about her diagnosis. Indications for considering a neuroimaging study (such as computerized tomography or magnetic resonance imaging) include the following:

- A history suggestive of subarachnoid hemorrhage (e.g., patients presenting with the "worst headache of their life," accompanied by neck stiffness or photophobia)
- An abnormal neurologic examination, raising the suspicion of an intracranial mass
- A persistent headache that is worsening or changing over time, does not fit the tension type pattern, and has not responded to medication
- A history of aura symptoms or loss of consciousness, suggestive of a seizure rather than migraine
- A personality change associated with the headache that is noticed by the family or the patient

What May Have Triggered These Attacks?

The oral contraceptive pills that she has recently started using may have triggered these attacks. Oral contraceptive pills that contain estrogen and progesterone (combination pills) are associated with migraine headaches. Progestin-only pills rarely cause migraines. She has made significant life changes (starting college) recently, and these may have lowered her threshold for the migraine headaches.

What Initial Therapy Can Be Suggested?

She should be advised to stop using the oral contraceptives, and other birth control methods should be discussed. If she is taking a combination oral contraceptive, she could be switched to a progestin-only pill. She must receive extensive education about migraine headaches, particularly how to recognize the symptoms and the nonpharmacological therapies discussed earlier. She should be reassured that it is a treatable condition and not life threatening. Given the severity of the headaches and that analgesics have been ineffective, it would be reasonable to try a triptan at the onset of the headache. The choice of the triptan depends on the formulation that the patient is most comfortable using, either oral, injection, or nasal spray.

For the tension headaches she can continue using acetaminophen or ibuprofen.

Suggested Reading

Bartleson J. Treatment of migraine headaches. *Mayo Clin Proc* 1999;74:702–708.
Ferrari M. Migraine. *Lancet* 1998;351:1043–1051.
Smith T. Migraine prevention need no longer be a headache. *Hosp Med* 34(10):13–14, 19–21, 25.

67
Carotid Stenosis

Murtaza Cassoobhoy

1. What is the clinical significance of a carotid bruit?
2. What is the risk for stroke in asymptomatic carotid stenosis/symptomatic carotid stenosis?
3. What is the standard medical treatment for carotid stenosis?
4. What three major questions must be addressed when deciding whether or not to perform a carotid endarterectomy? In whom should carotid endarterectomy be considered?

Discussion

What Is the Clinical Significance of a Carotid Bruit?

Listening to the carotid arteries should be part of every complete physical examination. Carotid bruits may be heard in states of increased vascular flow such as thyrotoxicosis and anemia, or in patients with arteriovenous fistulas used for hemodialysis. Most commonly, however, carotid bruits are caused by atherosclerosis and are considered markers for more widespread vascular disease. Systolic murmurs radiating to the neck can be differentiated from carotid bruits in that they are normally loudest over the precordium; venous hums are more prominent in diastole and can be stopped by compression of the internal jugular vein.

Upon finding a carotid bruit, it is essential to find out if the patient has had transient ischemic attack (TIA) symptoms or a history of stroke in the distribution of the carotid artery. This distinguishes asymptomatic carotid stenosis from the symptomatic type and is crucial in evaluating and treating a patient with carotid stenosis.

Asymptomatic carotid bruits are relatively common, and their prevalence increases with age. About 2% of the population 45 to 54 years have bruits; this increases to about 8% in the age group of 75 years or older. In asymptomatic patients under 75 years of age, the presence of a carotid bruit increases the chance of having a stroke by threefold (0.5% vs. 1.5%) or of dying from ischemic heart disease. Interestingly, in people over 75 with an asymptomatic bruit, there is no apparent increased risk for stroke. Further workup of an asymptomatic carotid bruit depends on the clinical situation. A workup for the bruit is indicated if the patient is without comorbid conditions that would significantly increase surgical morbidity/mortality, is willing to undergo further (possibly invasive) evaluation and surgery [carotid endarterectomy (CEA)], and has a life expectancy of at least 5 years. If the patient is not a surgical candidate, the patient should be medically treated for presumed steno-sis and educated about the symptoms of a TIA. Further workup is not necessary.

Anyone who has had a TIA or stroke in the carotid distribution should undergo further imaging of the carotid artery as part of the workup regardless of the pres-ence or absence of a carotid bruit. In a symptomatic patient, the presence of a ca-rotid bruit does not reliably predict high-grade stenosis (>70%). On the other hand the absence of a bruit cannot be used to rule out carotid stenosis as a cause of the symptoms.

What Is the Risk for Stroke in Asymptomatic Carotid Stenosis and Symptomatic Carotid Stenosis?

Two recently published clinical trials have provided useful information regarding stroke risk among patients with carotid stenosis. The European Carotid Surgery Trial assessed the 3-year risk for stroke in asymptomatic patients based on the de-gree of carotid stenosis (e.g., mild, moderate, and severe):

- Mild (0–29%): 1.8% 3-year risk (0.6%/yr)
- Moderate (30%–69%): 2.1% 3-year risk (0.7%/yr)
- Severe (70%–99%): 5.7% 3-year risk (1.9%/yr)

The North American Symptomatic Carotid Endarterectomy Trial (NASCET) was able to provide data on stroke risk in patients with symptomatic carotid stenosis based on degree of stenosis (mild, moderate, moderately severe, and severe):

- Mild (0–29%) 0.6% 3-year risk
- Moderate (30%–49%) 18.7% 5-year risk
- Moderately severe (50%–69%) 22.2% 5-year risk
- Severe (70%–99%) 26% 2-year risk

In summary, in asymptomatic patients, carotid stenosis (<70%) presents a rela-tively low risk for stroke; whereas severe stenosis (≥70%) presents a higher risk. Symptomatic patients (e.g., TIA or prior stroke) have a significantly increased risk for stroke. This risk increases as the degree of stenosis worsens.

What Is the Standard Medical Treatment for Carotid Stenosis?

Aggressive risk factor modification and medical therapy with antiplatelet agents is extremely important and significantly lowers a patient's risk for stroke.

Hypertension is the most powerful and treatable risk factor for stroke. A meta-analysis of randomized trials found that an average reduction in diastolic blood pressure of 6 mm Hg results in a 42% reduction in stroke incidence. The Systolic Hypertension in the Elderly study, in patients over 60 years of age showed that treatment of isolated systolic hypertension reduced stroke incidence by 36%.

Smoking substantially increases the risk for stroke, with the relative risk value 1.5 to 2.2. The degree of risk is proportional to the number of cigarettes smoked. Smoking cessation begins to reduce the risk immediately.

There is increasing evidence that lowering cholesterol and low-density lipoprotein (LDL) levels decreases the risk for stroke, and the National Cholesterol Education Panel guidelines should be followed closely.

In patients with diabetes mellitus, intensive treatment of hyperglycemia has been shown to reduce the risk for microvascular complications and may help reduce macrovascular complications, including stroke.

Antiplatelet Therapy

Aspirin has been conclusively shown to reduce the risk for TIA, stroke, and death in patients at risk for stroke. The optimum dose is controversial, and the acceptable range is 50 to 1,300 mg a day. The American Heart Association (AHA) recommends 325 mg/day because of fewer side effects and better compliance.

Ticlopidine (ticlid) and clopidogrel (plavix) inhibit adenosine diphosphate–induced platelet aggregation and are slightly better than aspirin at reducing the risk for stroke. These drugs are second line due to side effects (particularly with ticlopidine, which may induce diarrhea, rash, and neutropenia) and cost, and are recommended for patients who are unable to tolerate aspirin or have failed aspirin therapy.

A combination of dipyridamole (200 mg extended release) and aspirin (25 mg, Aggrenox, Boehringer Ingelheim) has been approved by the U.S. Food and Drug Administration for use in stroke prevention. The combination was better at reducing stroke risk when compared with low-dose aspirin (25 mg twice a day). The side effect profile is similar to that for aspirin but does involve a higher incidence of headache.

Currently, aspirin is the preferred antiplatelet agent in the prevention of stroke because of long-term experience, favorable side effect profile, and low cost. The other agents should be used in patients who are unable to tolerate aspirin because of side effects or have symptoms of TIA or stroke on aspirin.

What Three Major Questions Must Be Addressed When Deciding Whether or Not to Perform a Carotid Endarterectomy? In Whom Should Carotid Endarterectomy Be Considered?

Prior to deciding whether or not to perform a CEA, the following questions must be addressed:

1. Is the patient symptomatic or asymptomatic?
2. What is the degree of stenosis?
3. What is the risk of surgical morbidity/mortality? (including patient risk due to comorbid conditions and surgeon's experience)

Carotid endarterectomy should only be considered in the following three groups of patients:

1. Symptomatic patients with greater than 70% stenosis
2. Symptomatic patients with 50% to 70% stenosis
3. Asymptomatic patients with greater than 60% stenosis

In symptomatic patients with greater than 70% stenosis, CEA is clearly proven to benefit the patient as long as the surgical risk is less than 6%.

In symptomatic patients with 50% to 70% stenosis, CEA may be beneficial for patients with certain risk profiles and whose surgical risk is less than 2%. Men, patients who have had a recent stroke (rather than TIAs), and those who have sustained hemispheric (rather than retinal) TIAs benefit the most.

In asymptomatic patients with greater than 60% stenosis, CEA may be beneficial for patients with a life expectancy of at least 5 years whose surgical risk is less than 3%.

When considering CEA in any patient, it is important to explain the risks and potential benefits of the procedure to the patient so they can become an active part of the decision-making process. They have to understand that surgery puts them at an initial increased risk for stoke or death but that there may be a long-term benefit in preventing stroke. If they are asymptomatic and decide against surgery, it is essential to educate them on the warning signs of TIAs so they can seek immediate medical attention and reconsider CEA.

Case

A 60-year-old man is seen for the first time to establish a relationship with a primary care physician. He has no complaints at this time, and his past medical history is significant for hypertension. He has been taking hydrochlorathiazide for 2 years and tolerating it without problems. Both his parents died in their eighties, his father from an apparent heart attack and his mother from breast cancer. He has a 40-pack/year smoking history and currently smokes one pack a day. He has been walking about 2 miles three times a week for the past 3 years. A cardiac and pulmonary review of systems is normal.

On physical examination his weight is 174 pounds, height 6 feet, blood pressure 156/94 mm Hg, and pulse 84 beats/min. He has a left carotid bruit heard best in systole. No abdominal or femoral bruits are heard, and the peripheral pulses in his feet are easily palpable. No cardiac murmurs or gallops are audible. The rest of the examination is unremarkable.

Laboratory studies show normal chemistries and total cholesterol of 220 mg/dL with a LDL level of 150 mg/dL and high-density lipoprotein level of 40 mg/dL.

1. What information is crucial at this point and why?
2. What do you tell him, and would you proceed with a workup?
3. What diagnostic options are available?
4. What treatment must you start at this point? What other treatment should you consider?
5. What would you recommend now?

Case Discussion

What Information Is Crucial at This Point and Why?

There is a significant difference in the risk for stroke and treatment of carotid stenosis depending on whether a patient is symptomatic (TIA or previous stroke in the distribution of the stenotic carotid artery) or asymptomatic from the stenosis, so this information is very important. He should be specifically asked about one-sided weakness or paresthesia, dysarthria, aphasia, and amaurosis fugax (transient loss of vision in one eye, usually described as "a shade that comes down," due to platelets or cholesterol embolization to the ophthalmic artery commonly from a carotid artery plaque). Vague symptoms such as dizziness, vertigo, syncope, and blurred vision should not be characterized as a TIA.

The patient denies any of these symptoms he is asked about and is obviously very concerned about the sound you heard in his neck. He asks you, "Doc, am I going to have a stroke?"

What Do You Tell Him, and Would You Proceed with a Workup?

The presence of a carotid bruit in the patient increases his risk of having a stroke compared with someone who does not, but only from 0.5% to 1.5% a year. It is important to discuss his other risk factors for stroke, which are hypertension and cigarette smoking. Hypertension is the most prevalent and modifiable risk factor for stroke, and its treatment will substantially reduce his chances of having a stroke. Cigarette smoking is an independent determinant of carotid artery plaque thickness, and by smoking he is 1.5 times more likely to have a stroke than compared with a nonsmoker.

It is important to quantify the degree of stenosis of a carotid bruit in this patient because it could influence his treatment options. He may be a candidate for CEA if the stenosis is greater than 60%.

What Diagnostic Options Are Available?

The best initial test is carotid Doppler ultrasonography because of safety, cost, and accuracy for severe stenosis. Its limitations are that it cannot always distinguish occlusion from very severe stenosis (>95%), and its accuracy is operator dependent.

Magnetic resonance angiography is a promising but expensive test. It is safe and has the advantage of looking at carotid, vertebral, and intracranial arteries.

Angiography remains the goal standard because it is very accurate and can distinguish 99% stenosis from complete occlusion. Its limitation is that it is invasive and carries a 0.5% to 1% risk for severe complications, even with experienced radiologists. Some centers that have found their Doppler results to correlate extremely well with angiography have been using Doppler alone before CEA. Also, combining Doppler, MRA (to increase accuracy), and bypass angiography is being studied. Currently many surgeons require angiography before performing CEA.

Carotid duplex ultrasonography shows 70% stenosis on the left and mild, non–flow-limiting stenosis on the right.

What Treatment Must You Start at This Point? What Other Treatment Should You Consider?

His blood pressure must be treated aggressively to a goal of less than 130/85 mm Hg. He should be strongly encouraged to stop smoking, and nicotine replacement therapy can be discussed as an aid to help him quit. Given that he has more than two cardiac risk factors (male, >55 years of age, hypertension, tobacco use, and peripheral vascular disease), his minimum goal LDL is less than 130 mg/dL according to the National Cholesterol Education Program guidelines. Because he is likely to have subclinical atherosclerotic heart disease, many clinicians would be even more aggressive with his LDL cholesterol, using less than 100 as their target. He should be started on a low-fat, low-cholesterol diet, and medication to lower his cholesterol should be considered. Aspirin therapy at 325 mg a day must be started as well.

The role of CEA should be discussed with the patient. He should be informed of the up-front risk of surgery, with a possible benefit of stroke risk reduction over the long term. Presuming he has no evidence of coronary atherosclerosis, his risk of undergoing the procedure is very low. However, the surgeon's experience with the procedure also should be factored in. Only if his surgical risk is felt to be less than 3% should CEA be considered. He also should be educated on the signs and symptoms of TIAs so that he can recognize them and seek immediate medical attention.

The patient is very anxious about surgical intervention at this time and chooses medical therapy. Two years later he presents after a sudden loss of vision in his left eye that resolved within a few minutes. He remembers you warning him of such symptoms. After a thorough evaluation you conclude that he likely had an episode of amaurosis fugax secondary to the left carotid stenosis.

What Would You Recommend Now?

Because he is now having symptoms from the carotid stenosis, his chances of having a stroke are significantly increased. If his surgical risk is estimated to be less than 6%, CEA should be strongly recommended. An angiogram would likely be needed before the procedure. Medical therapy should be continued, and clopidogrel or dipyridamole and aspirin combination could be considered instead of aspirin alone.

Suggested Reading

Albers G, Hart R, Lutsep H, et al. Supplement to the guidelines for the management of transient ischemic attacks. *Stroke* 1999;30:2502–2511.

Biller J, Feinberg W, Castaldo J, et al. AHA: guidelines for CEA. *Stroke* 1998;29:554–562.

European Carotid Surgery Trialists' Collaborative Group. Randomized trial of endarterectomy for recently symptomatic carotid stenosis: final results of the MRC European Carotid surgery trial. *Lancet* 1998;351:1379–1389.

NASCET Collaborators. Beneficial effect of CEA in symptomatic patients with high grade stenosis. *N Engl J Med* 1991;325:445–453.

68

Carpal Tunnel Syndrome

Laura J. Martin

1. How is carpal tunnel syndrome classified?
2. What is the typical clinical picture of carpal tunnel syndrome?
3. What is the pathophysiology of carpal tunnel syndrome?
4. How is carpal tunnel syndrome diagnosed?
5. What treatment options are recommended?

Discussion

How Is Carpal Tunnel Syndrome Classified?

Carpal tunnel syndrome can be classified into acute and chronic forms. Acute carpal tunnel syndrome is usually seen when there is a rapid accumulation of fluid or increase of edema within the carpal canal. This can occur following trauma to the distal upper extremity, most commonly a distal radius fracture. It also has been seen in hemophiliacs and patients on anticoagulants who experience bleeding into the carpal tunnel. In this scenario, acute compression of the median nerve occurs, leading to ischemia of the nerve. Emergent surgical decompression may be indicated to decompress the carpal tunnel. In cases of prolonged ischemia of 8 or more hours, the patient may develop permanent damage to the affected median nerve.

Chronic carpal tunnel syndrome is sometimes classified as early, intermediate, or advanced. Patients with early carpal tunnel syndrome have usually experienced mild, intermittent symptoms for less than 1 year. Symptoms mainly occur at night or with activity. Patients with intermediate carpal tunnel syndrome usually demonstrate constant numbness and paresthesias in the median nerve distribution. At physical examination, patients with the advanced form usually demonstrate sensory loss in the distribution of the median nerve as well as thenar atrophy.

What Is the Typical Clinical Picture of Carpal Tunnel Syndrome?

Carpal tunnel syndrome is the most common entrapment neuropathy of the upper extremity. It has been estimated that about 1 million American adults seek treatment for carpal tunnel syndrome each year. It is considered to be the most prevalent repetitive motion disorder in the United States.

Carpal tunnel syndrome usually occurs in middle-aged people and is three times more prevalent in women than in men. Typical findings include pain and paresthesias in the hand in the median nerve distribution (thumb, index, long, and the radial aspect of the ring fingers). In some cases there may be associated pain in the forearm or upper arm. These symptoms usually worsen at night and with specific activities. Symptoms may be provoked by sleep, sustained hand positions, and repetitive motion of the hand or wrist. Changing the hand position or shaking the hand can sometimes bring about improvement of symptoms. Some patients also may experience weakness or clumsiness of the hand.

There are many predisposing factors for carpal tunnel syndrome. Some common factors include obesity, hypothyroidism, diabetes mellitus, pregnancy, rheumatoid arthritis, and gout. Several occupations have been associated with increased risk for carpal tunnel syndrome as a repetitive motion disorder. These include chicken processing, meat packing, grocery checking, and data processing, among others.

What Is the Pathophysiology of Carpal Tunnel Syndrome?

The transverse carpal ligament is a semi-rigid structure that functions as the roof of the carpal tunnel. It is confluent with the antebrachial fascia of the distal forearm. Structures passing through the carpal tunnel include the median nerve and three ligaments: the flexor pollicis longus, flexor digitorum superficialis, and flexor digitorum profundus.

After passing directly beneath the transverse carpal ligament, the median nerve divides into sensory and motor branches. The sensory branches supply the thumb, index, long, and radial aspect of the ring fingers, whereas the motor branches supply the superficial head of the flexor pollicis brevis, abductor pollicis brevis, opponens pollicis, and lumbricals of the index and long fingers.

Carpal tunnel syndrome occurs when there is an increase in the interstitial pressure of the carpal tunnel canal, leading to median nerve compression. With compression, the median nerve can develop ischemia. Impaired conduction may occur, leading to symptoms of pain and paresthesias. Chronic ischemia may lead to endoneural edema, intraneural fibrosis, and nerve fiber degeneration, which in some cases may be irreversible.

How Is Carpal Tunnel Syndrome Diagnosed?

Standard screening tests for carpal tunnel syndrome include the Tinel sign test, Phalen sign test, and sensory testing. A positive Tinel sign test result is defined as paresthesias in the median nerve distribution upon percussion of the median nerve at the carpal creases of the wrist. In some cases paresthesias may be limited to the long finger. Phalen's testing is performed by having the patient hold the wrist in a maximally flexed position for 30 to 60 seconds. Wrist flexion leads to narrowing of the carpal tunnel with resulting compression of the median nerve. As in Tinel's test, a positive test comprises paresthesias in the median nerve distribution. Sensory testing may reveal decreased sensation in the thumb, index, long, or radial aspect of the ring fingers.

Another useful screening test looks at thumb abduction strength. This test evaluates the strength of the abductor pollicis brevis that is innervated by the median nerve. It can be performed by having the patient raise the thumb perpendicular to the palm. The practitioner then applies downward pressure on the thumb and compares the strength to the thumb of the opposite hand. In severe cases, both thenar muscle weakness and wasting may be noted on physical examination. Dry skin on the thumb, index, and long fingers also may be seen.

Standard diagnostic testing to help confirm the diagnosis includes nerve conduction and in some cases electomyographic studies. Nerve conduction studies have been shown to have a sensitivity of about 90%. Thus, there are some patients with classic findings for carpal tunnel syndrome who have normal nerve conduction results. It has been shown that these patients usually respond very well to standard treatment.

The differential diagnosis for carpal tunnel syndrome includes cervical radiculopathy, peripheral neuropathy, brachial plexopathy, and thoracic outlet syndrome. Nerve conduction and electromyographic studies are useful to exclude or confirm alternate diagnoses. Imaging of the wrist can be helpful to evaluate for bone or joint deformity. Cervical spine films may be performed to evaluate for possible cervical radiculopathy. A chest film is useful if brachial plexopathy or thoracic outlet syndrome is suspected.

It is important to determine if the patient with carpal tunnel syndrome may have an associated underlying systemic disorder. Tests for hypothyroidism, diabetes mellitus, gout, and rheumatoid arthritis may be ordered if there is sufficient clinical suspicion. Pregnancy should be a consideration in young women of childbearing age.

What Treatment Options Are Recommended?

Nonsurgical therapy is considered to be first line unless there is evidence of a progressive motor or sensory deficit on physical examination or electrodiagnostic testing. Initial therapy may include the following:

- Avoidance or modification of activities that exacerbate symptoms
- Wrist splints (wrist should be in neutral position without flexion or extension)
- Non steroidal antiinflammatory drugs
- Diuretics in patients with arm edema

Steroid injection into the carpal tunnel may be helpful if initial therapy is ineffective. Repeat injections can be performed up to three times at 3- to 6-week intervals. Potential complications include infection, tendon rupture, median nerve damage, and reflex sympathetic dystrophy.

Surgical therapy is a consideration in patients with progressive motor or sensory deficits or persistent symptoms after nonsurgical treatment. The main goal of carpal tunnel surgery is decompression of the median nerve by transecting the transverse carpal ligament. The two most commonly performed surgical techniques are open carpal tunnel release and endoscopic carpal tunnel release.

Case

A 55-year-old woman with a history of type II diabetes mellitus presents to your office complaining of bilateral pain and paresthesias in her hands over the past 3 months. She relates that this pain began about 6 weeks after beginning a new job as a medical transcriptionist. The paresthesias occur in the thumb, index, long, and radial aspect of the ring fingers bilaterally. She noticed that the pain is worse in the evening after typing on her computer keyboard for several hours. She relates no symptoms of extremity weakness and no problems with hand grasp. Her only current medication is metformin.

Physical examination shows a blood pressure of 130/82 mm Hg, weight 190 pounds, and height 65 inches. On examination of the extremities, there is no edema and no thenar muscle atrophy. There is diminished thumb abduction strength bilaterally with a positive Tinel sign and positive Phalen sign. There are no sensory or motor deficits.

Laboratory results include glucose 156 mg/dL, creatinine 1.0 mg/dL, hemoglobin A1C 7.5%, and thyroid-stimulating hormone 14 µIU/mL.

1. What findings in this patient's history and physical examination contribute to a possible diagnosis of carpal tunnel syndrome?
2. What further testing may be helpful?
3. What therapy would you initiate for this patient?

Case Discussion

What Findings in This Patient's History and Physical Examination Contribute to a Possible Diagnosis of Carpal Tunnel Syndrome?

She has some of the classic findings of carpal tunnel syndrome, including pain and paresthesias in her hands. Physical examination findings pointing toward the diagnosis include positive Tinel and Phalen signs and decreased thumb abduction bilaterally. She has evidence of several systemic disorders that are associated with carpal tunnel syndrome. These include obesity, type II diabetes mellitus, and hypothyroidism. She also is employed as a medical transcriptionist, which requires repetitive motion that may exacerbate her symptoms.

What Further Testing May Be Helpful?

Clinically there is a high index of suspicion for a diagnosis of carpal tunnel syndrome. If further confirmation is desired, then nerve conduction studies and possibly electromyographic studies can be considered. Standard electrodiagnostic testing includes sensory conduction studies across the wrist of the median nerve and one other sensory nerve in the symptomatic limb. Motor conduction studies of the median nerve recording from the thenar muscle and one other nerve in the symptomatic limb also can be helpful in selected cases.

What Therapy Would You Initiate for This Patient?

In patients with carpal tunnel syndrome, any underlying associated systemic disorders should be treated. In this patient, optimizing the treatment of her type II diabetes mellitus and initiating treatment for hypothyroidism will be helpful. Treatment of her obesity is indicated as well.

Noninvasive treatment of carpal tunnel syndrome is considered to be first line for most patients as long as there is no evidence of progressive or severe motor or sensory deficits. Initial treatment for this patient may include wrist splints applied in the neutral position and nonsteroidal antiinflammatory drugs. Modifying her work station in her medical transcriptionist job to optimize ergonomic design may be beneficial. In mild cases of carpal tunnel syndrome, some improvement may be expected in 2 weeks, with duration of care lasting up to 6 months.

Suggested Reading

American Academy of Neurology. Practice parameter: carpal tunnel syndrome. *Neurology* 1993;43: 2406.

American Academy of Neurology, American Association of Electrodiagnostic Medicine, American Academy of Physical Medicine and Rehabilitation. Practice parameter for electrodiagnostic studies in carpal tunnel syndrome. *Neurology* 1993;43:2404.

Atcheson S G, Ward J R, Lowe W. Concurrent medical disease in work-related carpal tunnel syndrome. *Arch Intern Med* 1998;158:1506.

D'Arcy C A, McGee S. Does this patient have carpal tunnel syndrome? *JAMA* 2000:283:3110.

Kerwin G, Williams C S, Seiler J G. The pathophysiology of carpal tunnel syndrome. *Hand Clin* 1996;12:243.

Kulick R G. Carpal tunnel syndrome. *Orthop Clin North Am* 1996;27:345.

69
Tremor

Jonathan M. Flacker

- Discussion   *429*
- Case   *434*
- Case Discussion   *434*

1. What is tremor?
2. How is tremor classified?
3. What medications are used to treat tremors?
4. What are the nonpharmacologic treatments for tremor?

Discussion
What Is Tremor?

Tremor is an involuntary, rhythmic muscle contraction characterized by back-and-forth oscillations of a body part. Specifically this involves reciprocally innervated, antagonistic muscle groups, resulting in movement of a body part around a fixed plane in space. This differentiates tremor from other disorders of involuntary movements such as dystonias (slow, sustained muscle contractions), chorea (arrythmic, rapid muscle jerks), athetosis (slow, writhing movements), and tics. Tremor can affect any part of the body, with the hands being the most common area afflicted. Tremors may be fine (barely noticeable), medium (somewhat noticeable), or coarse (large, obvious movement). The frequency of oscillation may be slow (3–5 Hertz, or cycles per second), intermediate (5–8 Hertz), or rapid (9–12 Hertz). Tremors are responsible for substantial functional impairment as well as social isolation due to embarrassment.

How Is Tremor Classified?

Tremors may be classified according to the position and context in which they occur, or the pathophysiologic condition responsible for the tremor. For the purposes of this discussion, the basic contextual classification of tremors will be outlined, and some specific etiologies of tremor will then be discussed.

Contextual Classification of Tremors

Resting Tremor

Resting tremors are also often called repose or static tremors. These tremors occur while the muscle (not patient) is at rest (i.e., no voluntary muscle activity). The tremor tends to abate with voluntary movement, and thus has less functional consequences than other forms of tremor. For example, a tremor occurring while the hands are at rest on the patient's lap, but not when reaching for a cup, would likely be a resting tremor. This is a common tremor in those with Parkinson disease. Multisystems atrophy and progressive supranuclear palsy may have a rest tremor similar to Parkinson disease, but it is usually unilateral and of lower amplitude that the parkinsonian tremor.

Action Tremors

These tremors occur during voluntary muscle movement and are subdivided into several general categories. Kinetic tremor is also often called intention tremor. Although some use these terms synonymously, it is best to reserve the term *intention tremor* only for those tremors that increase at the end of a visually guided task. The term *kinetic tremor* is more general and designates any tremor that occurs during goal-directed action. Common kinetic tremors include physiologic tremor and essential tremor (ET). Less common variants include dystonic tremor (occurring in muscles affected by dystonia), isometric tremor (occurring when the muscle contraction is opposed by a fixed object), and isolated voice tremor.

Goal-directed tremors, also called task-specific tremors, are sometimes categorized with kinetic tremors. These occur during specific, skilled tasks. Several variants have been described, including tremors occurring during speaking (vocal tremor), handwriting (writing tremor), or standing (orthostatic tremor). The primary writing tremor may be familial.

Postural tremors occur during antigravity posture, such as holding the hands out. Chronic neuroleptic use may result in a postural tremor. Some patients with parkinsonism may have a postural tremor in addition to the typical resting tremor.

Psychogenic Tremor

Psychogenic tremor is also called hysterical tremor. This tremor may manifest as either a resting tremor, kinetic tremor, or both. Psychogenic tremor may be due to a primary psychiatric disorder. It usually does not involve the fingers.

Classification by Common Etiologies of Tremor

Parkinsonian Tremor

The tremor of parkinsonism typically occurs at rest, diminishes with action, and manifests as a slow (4–6 Hertz), "pill-rolling" motion. In Parkinson disease the tremor often begins unilaterally and affects the hands. It also may involve the head, trunk, or jaws.

Essential Tremor

Essential tremor is a kinetic tremor, and may be the most common movement disorder, occurring in up to 1.7% of people. This tremor is postural, with a wide range of frequency (4–11 Hz) depending on the involved body part. Distal involvement manifests as a higher frequency tremor than proximal involvement. ET usually begins in the young adult years (second to sixth decades), and prevalence increases with age. The hands are commonly involved, but the tremor also may manifest in the arms, legs, head, jaw, and tongue.

There is often a family history of tremor. ET may occur sporadically or may be inherited as an autosomal-dominant trait. Gene penetrance is nearly complete by the age of 65 to 70 years. Some patients may self-medicate with alcohol because they notice that this often improves the tremor.

Some persons with ET-like tremor also have other neurologic findings that make it difficult to definitively make a diagnosis of ET. Such patients are often designated as having an "indeterminate tremor syndrome." ET-like tremors also have been described in association with neuropathic diseases such as demyelinating syndromes, Guillain-Barré, and dysgammaglobulinemic neuropathy.

Physiologic Tremor

All humans have a physiologic tremor, although it may be more pronounced in some persons. Such tremors tend to have a rapid frequency in younger individuals, and slow to an intermediate frequency with increasing age. Stress, anxiety, hyperthyroidism, alcohol intoxication, drug withdrawal, and certain medications (β-agonists, methylxanthines) may enhance this tremor. Beta blockers tend to ameliorate the tremor.

Alcohol Withdrawal Tremor

Alcohol withdrawal tremor superficially appears similar to ET, but is usually a bit more rapid. Usually there is no family history of tremor, and this tremor is typically not as debilitating as ET. Alcohol withdrawal tremor affects only the hands, and likely results from the overactivity in the central nervous system that results from alcohol withdrawal.

Cerebellar Tremor

Cerebellar tremors may manifest differently depending on the site of involvement. The most common cerebellar tremor results from damage to a hemisphere or nuclei that produce a unilateral intention or goal-directed tremor. If the lesion is midline, then the tremor may be present bilaterally and involve the trunk and head as well as the arms.

Rubral tremor refers to the "wing-beating" tremor produced by damage to the red nucleus, which may be present at both rest and posture.

Cerebellar postural tremor is commonly slow (2.5–4 Hertz) when severe and occurs with action and posture. It is generally a proximal (trunk) tremor that fluctuates, but generally worsens with prolonged posture. It is faster (10 Hertz) when mild and manifests distally in the extremities. This tremor is commonly seen with multiple sclerosis, although cerebellar degeneration and stroke may result in this phenomenology.

Cerebellar tremors manifest with an increase in amplitude as the patient's extremity approaches the target (with goal-directed movement). Other signs of cerebellar damage are often evident on physical examination. Tremors arising from the cerebellum, brainstem, or thalamus are now commonly categorized together as Holmes tremor.

Orthostatic Tremor

Orthostatic tremor is a postural tremor that involves the legs, and usually occurs in older adults. It is worse on standing and is alleviated by sitting or walking. This tremor generally manifests as a feeling of weakness, imbalance, or trembling in the legs. It is a rapid tremor (13–18 Hertz) whose etiology is unknown, and may or may not be associated with orthostasis. Although some investigators have suggested that a repetitive thumping over the hamstrings during standing is diagnostic for this tremor, electromyography is generally used to demonstrate orthostatic tremor.

Psychogenic Tremor

This tremor may occur in any setting, including rest, action, or antigravity posture. Usually this tremor begins abruptly, does not progress, is difficult to classify, and spontaneously remits.

What Medications Are Used to Treat Tremors?

Certainly the treatment of tremor depends on the underlying cause. Thus, the first step in determining the treatment of tremor is to identify a specific etiology. In addition, before embarking on a course of pharmacologic treatment, the functional and aesthetic impact of the tremor must be assessed in order to determine if the benefits of treatment outweigh the potential burdens and side effects.

Resting Tremor

This form of tremor is most commonly seen in Parkinson disease and is usually managed with antiparkinsonian therapy. This may include medication or surgery. Levodopa/carbidopa combinations are often used, but anticholinergics such as amatidine can be considered if tremor is the only target symptom. Beta blockers also may be tried. Clozapine may be of use, although the rare side effect of agranulocytosis should give one pause before recommending this drug.

Essential Tremor

Two medications are commonly used for the treatment of ET. The first are β-blockers, of which propranolol is the best studied. The typical dose ranges from 80 to 320 mg/day. Other β-blockers such as metoprolol and nadolol also may be tried. Equally effective in the treatment of ET is primidone, an anticonvulsant that is typically used in doses of 25 to 750 mg/day. This agent may cause confusion and lethargy in older individuals, especially at higher doses. Primidone has the advantage of not affecting blood pressure, pulse, or exercise tolerance. Alcohol also may relieve ET, but is not recommended because of the risk of abuse.

Second-line drug therapies for the treatment of ET include nadolol (which may be effective treatment for individuals who were previously responsive to propranolol), methazolamide, gabapentin, and clozapine. Interestingly, theophylline also has been reported to reduce ET. Benzodiazepines may have some limited utility for ET. Some patients with ET who do not respond to drug therapy may be considered for local injections of botulinum toxin.

Alcohol Withdrawal Tremor

The tremor of alcohol withdrawal is usually treated in conjunction with treatment of the hyperadrenergic withdrawal state. If additional treatment is required, then propranolol in doses of 40 to 80 mg twice daily may be tried.

Cerebellar Tremor

Treatment of cerebellar tremor may be difficult and frustrating. No specific treatment has been clearly established. If there is a significant resting component, levodopa/carbidopa, clozapine, or anticholinergics may be tried. Clonazepam and odansatron have been reported to be of some benefit. Isoniazid has been used with some success in patients with multiple sclerosis and cerebellar tremor.

Goal-Directed Tremor

Treatment often depends on the specific area and body part involved. Primidone is often tried.

Postural Tremor

Postural tremor is often treated with levodopa/carbidopa or primidone, although the efficacy of this approach is unclear. Small trials suggest that clonazepam, chlordiazepoxide, gabapentin, pramipexole, and valproate may have some utility for postural tremor. Propranolol does not seem to be effective.

Psychogenic Tremor

The treatment of psychogenic tremor is directed at the underlying psychiatric condition. Most typically these tremors resolve over time, with or without treatment.

What Are the Nonpharmacologic Treatments for Tremor?

For some tremors such as ET, caffeine (e.g., in soda, coffee, tea, chocolate, etc.) and other stimulants should be eliminated from the diet. Occupational therapy consultation is often helpful to allow the patient to adapt to the functional consequences of their tremor. Exercises with 1- to 2-pound weights strapped to the wrist may help to promote hand stability, and weighted utensils may improve self-feeding ability. In certain individuals, a small quantity of alcohol may decrease tremors; however, this approach to treating ET is controversial and not generally recommended. Although consumption of small amounts of alcohol may pose no risk to some people, it may lead to alcohol dependence in other susceptible individuals. In addition, there may be a rebound worsening of ET symptoms the day after alcohol consumption. Thalamotomy or deep brain stimulation may be considered, especially in refractory cases.

Case

Ms. James, a 68-year-old retired former schoolteacher, comes to see you because she is having problems with "the shakes." She first noticed the shaking about 5 years ago, but it has steadily gotten worse. Now she sometimes spills drinks if the cup is too full, and she can no longer quilt.

Her past medical history is remarkable for mild hypertension for which she takes hydrochlorothiazide. On examination she has a rapid, bilateral kinetic tremor of the hands. She has no other focal neurologic findings.

1. What is the likely diagnosis and what are the important aspects of the history gleaned from this patient?
2. What treatment would you recommend now?

Case Discussion

What Is the Likely Diagnosis and What Are the Important Aspects of the History Gleaned from This Patient?

You suspect she has an ET. It is therefore important to inquire about other family members who may have tremor. Because she may simply have an enhanced physiologic tremor, you should ask about stress, anxiety, and caffeine and nicotine use. It is useful to note whether alcohol abates the tremor. Signs of hyperthyroidism also should be sought.

What Treatment Would You Recommend Now?

Once any of the above-mentioned contributing factors have been removed, one must determine if the impairment from tremor is impacting on function or quality of life. If so, then the next step may be to add a medication. If blood pressure control is inadequate, then adding a β-blocker may treat both the tremor and hypertension. Even if blood pressure is at an acceptable level, exchanging hydrochlorothiazide for a β-blocker could be considered. Alternatively, primidone also would be reasonable in this setting. Referral to an occupational therapist should also be considered.

Suggested Reading

Deuschl G, Wenzelburger R, Raethjen J. Tremor. *Curr Opin Neurol* 2000;13:437–443.
Habib-ur-Rehman. Diagnosis and management of tremor. *Arch Intern Med* 2000;160:2438–2444.
Louis E D. Essential tremor. *Arch Neurol* 2000;57:1522–1524.
www.essentialtremor.org: The official website of the International Tremor Foundation.

70
Parkinson Disease
Jonathan M. Flacker

1. What is the epidemiology of Parkinson disease?
2. What are the parkinsonism syndromes?
3. What medications are used to treat Parkinson disease?
4. What are the surgical options for treating Parkinson disease?
5. What other nonpharmacologic interventions may be helpful in Parkinson disease?

Discussion
What Is the Epidemiology of Parkinson Disease?

Parkinson disease (PD) is a disorder of the central nervous system first described in the early 1800s. It is estimated that PD affects 1 to 1.5 million people in the United States, most over the age of 50, with peak occurrence at about 75 years of age. PD occurs in all ethnic groups throughout the world, and affects males somewhat more commonly than females. Nearly one third of all PD cases are familial, and a small subset appears to be autosomal dominant; however, the majority exhibit no clear inheritance pattern. Because PD leads to substantial functional impairment, it is a common contributor to institutionalization, and the prevalence in U.S. nursing homes is estimated to be about 7%. Data from Europe suggest that up to 20% of older patients with PD will eventually be institutionalized.

What Are the Parkinsonism Syndromes?

Parkinsonism is a syndrome, or a constellation of symptoms. Idiopathic Parkinson disease (IPD) is just one cause of parkinsonism. The parkinsonism syndrome consists of rigidity, tremor, bradykinesia, and postural instability.

Rigidity, an increased tone or stiffness in the muscles, is present at all times and often increases with movement. Manifestations include a "masked" facial expression and smooth resistance with superimposed "cogwheeling" (ratchetlike resistance) during passive range of motion.

The tremor is typically a "pill-rolling" tremor of the fingers that is present in repose, and suppressed with movement. It may be unilateral.

Bradykinesia, or slowness of movement, is characterized by a delay in initiating movements. Bradykinesia is especially evident during feeding, writing, and walking.

Postural instability consists of retropulsion (a tendency to fall backward) during standing, propulsion (a tendency to fall forward during gait), decreased or nonexistent arm swing, festination (shuffling steps), and sudden freezing spells.

The parkinsonism syndrome may have several causes.

Idiopathic Parkinson Disease

This cause of parkinsonism results from idiopathic loss of dopaminergic neurons in the substantia nigra and basal ganglia. Pathologic examination of the brain shows intracellular inclusions known as Lewy bodies. People with IPD may have many other associated symptoms. These include depression, sleep disturbances, dizziness, stooped posture, constipation, dementia, and problems with speech, breathing, swallowing, and sexual function. It is important to note that different patients experience different symptoms. Rates of progression also may vary substantially, with some patients reaching a completely dependent state in 3 to 5 years and others enjoying many years of functionality. There are no specific tests for IPD, and diagnosis is based on a history and physical examination that evaluates the patient's symptoms and their severity. Clinically diagnosed IPD shows classic pathologic signs at autopsy in about 75% of cases. Neuroimaging is generally not necessary unless the presentation is atypical.

Secondary Parkinsonism

In these conditions the phenomenology of parkinsonism results from a known cause other than IPD. For example, many people experienced secondary parkinsonism following the influenza epidemic in the Unites States from 1915 to 1926. Medications have been implicated in this syndrome, including most neuroleptics (including olanzapine), selective serotonin reuptake inhibitors, metoclopramide, reserpine, and methyldopa. Toxins such as carbon monoxide, manganese, and MPTP (1-methyl-4-phenyl-1,2,3,6-tetrahydropyridine, injected by some intravenous drug users) should be considered if the history suggests an exposure. Hypoparathyroidism (with basal ganglia calcification), lacunar infarcts, brain tumors, anoxia, and head trauma each may precipitate parkinsonism.

Parkinson-Plus Syndromes

These conditions result from dopaminergic neuronal loss in the basal ganglia, as well as dysfunction of other brain systems. They include progressive supranuclear palsy, primary autonomic failure, olivopontocerebellar atrophy, and corticobasilar atrophy. These problems may bear some phenomenologic similarities to PD. Unfortunately, the Parkinson-plus syndromes do not generally respond to dopamine replacement.

Dementia with Lewy Bodies

This condition consists of cognitive impairment in the presence of signs of parkinsonism. Typically, vivid hallucinations and delusions are present, and the patients may experience severe adverse effects from neuroleptics. Pathology consists of Lewy bodies in the frontal lobe regions of the brain. These patients often do not respond well to carbidopa/levodopa, but may get some improvement from cholinesterase inhibitors such as donepazil.

What Medications Are Used to Treat Parkinson Disease?

If symptoms are serious enough, a trial of anti-Parkinson drugs may be indicated. Drug therapy for IPD typically provides relief for about 10 to 15 years or more. It is reasonable to delay pharmacologic treatment of IPD until symptoms cause functional impairment because of the side effects associated with these medications, the lack of any clear disease-modifying agents, and concern over long-term neurotoxicity of dopamine agonists. Potential side effects include hypotension, dry mouth, nausea, dizziness, confusion, hallucinations, drowsiness, increased abnormal movements, and insomnia. Medications commonly used to treat IPD are listed in Table 70.1 and described below.

Levodopa is a precursor of dopamine. If used by itself, high doses of levodopa are required and often lead to debilitating side effects such as severe nausea and vomiting. When combined with the peripheral tissue dopa-decarboxylase inhibitor, carbidopa, much lower doses of levodopa are required. Carbidopa/levodopa is commonly used to treat IPD. If there is no symptomatic improvement at a daily dose of 600 mg of carbidopa/levodopa, then the patient likely has a levodopa-unresponsive cause of parkinsonism, and the medication should be stopped.

Table 70.1. Medications Commonly Used to Treat Parkinson Disease

Medication	Starting Dose	Typical Dose	Maximum Dose	Typical Indication
Carbidopa/ levodopa	12.5/50–25/100 mg b.i.d. to t.i.d.	25/100 mg q.i.d.	Total daily levodopa dose of 2,000 mg	Initial dopamine replacement
Controlled release carbidopa/ levodopa	25/200 mg b.i.d.	50/200 mg t.i.d.	Total daily levodopa dose of 2,400 mg	Replacement for short-acting carbidopa/levodopa to treat peak dose dyskinesias and wearing off of dose
Amantadine	100 mg daily	100 mg b.i.d.	100 mg b.i.d.	Early mild tremor; add-on therapy to carbidopa/levodopa
Trihexyphenidyl	1 mg b.i.d.	2.5 mg b.i.d.	5 mg b.i.d.	Early mild tremor; add-on therapy to carbidopa/levodopa
Selegiline	5 mg daily	5 mg daily	5 mg b.i.d.	Early Parkinson disease; add-on therapy to carbidopa/levodopa; slows progression?
Pergolide	0.05 mg daily	0.25 mg q.i.d.	1.25 mg q.i.d.	Add-on therapy to carbidopa/levodopa
Tolcapone	100 mg b.i.d.	200 mg t.i.d.	200 mg t.i.d.	Second-line add-on therapy for frequent on-off episodes

b.i.d., twice daily; t.i.d., three times daily; q.i.d., four times daily

Side effects such as large uncontrollable movements called "dyskinesias" especially at peak dose times, and end-dose "off" episodes may be treated with long-acting preparations. Long-acting preparations require 20% higher doses because they are less bioavailable. Cognitive impairment also may develop after many years. Some researchers also believe that levodopa in the brain may result in damage to neurons over time from too much stimulation (excitoxicity).

Carbidopa/levodopa should be taken on an empty stomach, about 15 minutes prior to eating, with 4 to 5 ounces of nondairy fluid. If the medication causes nausea, a small cracker or bite of fruit can be taken with any doses required between meals, and ginger also may be useful. Few patients with IPD need to alter the amount or timing of protein intake to avoid interfering with carbidopa/levodopa absorption. Most commonly such patients experience significant on/off motor fluctuations, and typically need to take carbidopa/levodopa six or more times per day.

Amantadine hydrochloride is an antiinfluenza medication that is both mildly anticholinergic, and an indirect-acting dopamine agonist. It is thought to work in IPD by either blocking the reuptake of dopamine or by increasing the release of dopamine by neurons, thereby increasing the supply of dopamine in the synapses. Amantadine is widely used as an early monotherapy, particularly for tremors. When its benefits seem to lessen, stopping the drug for a short period and then reintroducing it may result in efficacy again for a time. Amantadine also may have significant adverse cognitive effects.

Anticholinergics (e.g., trihexyphenidyl, benztropine mesylate, and procyclidine) decrease the activity of the neurotransmitter acetylcholine, which works in balance with dopamine in the brain. They do not act directly on the dopaminergic system. They are most effective in the control of mild tremor, especially early in the course of IPD. These drugs are contraindicated in those with glaucoma, prostatic hyperplasia, and dementia. They are also problematic in older patients because they tend to cause sedation, confusion, hallucinations, urinary retention, dry mouth, and blurred vision.

Selegiline works by inhibition of monoamine oxidase B, thus inhibiting the metabolism of dopamine. It is often used early in IPD to provide symptomatic relief. Selegiline also has been promoted as slowing the progression of PD, but this claim is not well substantiated. Selegiline may delay the need for carbidopa/levodopa when prescribed in the earliest stage of PD, and may boost the effects of carbidopa/levodopa in later stage PD.

Dopamine agonists are drugs that activate the dopamine receptor directly and can be taken alone or in combination with carbidopa/levodopa. Agonists available in the United States include bromocriptine, pergolide, pramipexole, and ropinirole.

Catechol-o-methyltransferase (COMT) inhibitors such as tolcapone and entacapone represent a new class of Parkinson medications. These drugs must be taken with levodopa. They prolong the duration of symptom relief by blocking the action of an enzyme that breaks down levodopa before it reaches the brain. They may be especially efficacious for reducing the number and severity of "off" spells (periods of significant increased tone and freezing). These are second-line agents whose use has been limited by severe hepatotoxicity.

What Are the Surgical Options for Treating Parkinson Disease?

Four surgical options are available to individuals for whom more conventional drug therapies have proven inadequate. To ensure the best results, surgical candidates must fit certain criteria before surgery can be considered. Candidates must have the specific symptoms treatable by the procedure, and they should be otherwise healthy and usually relatively young (e.g., under age 65 or 70). All procedures carry some risk, so careful selection of patients is required.

Pallidotomy

This procedure fell out of favor with the advent of levodopa. In recent times magnetic resonance imaging has allowed pallidotomy to be performed with great precision. Pallidotomy may be indicated for patients who have developed dyskinetic movements in reaction to their medications, and may help correct problems with slow movement, tremor, and imbalance. It is performed with the patient conscious. Pallidotomy targets the globus pallidus, and uses an electrode to destroy the cells in this area. The most serious risk is the possibility of stroke. Other risks include partial loss of vision, speech and swallowing difficulties, and confusion.

Thalamotomy

Thalamotomy surgically destroys cells in the brain's thalamus to correct a disabling tremor in the hands or arms for persons with few other symptoms. Risks are considered low. Immediate improvement is seen in 80% to 90% of patients after the operation; full recuperation generally takes 6 weeks.

Deep Brain Stimulation

This technique is especially helpful for uncontrollable movements. It is based on the technology of cardiac pacemakers. Electrodes are implanted in the thalamus or globus pallidus and connected to a pacemaker-like device, which the patient can switch on or off in response to symptoms.

Brain Tissue Transplants

Although they have produced encouraging results, transplantation surgeries are still experimental. Most recently, scientists are working with genetically engineered cells and a variety of animal cells that can be made to produce dopamine, rather than human fetal tissue.

What Other Nonpharmacologic Interventions May Be Helpful in Parkinson Disease?

Physical and Speech Therapy

Physical, occupational or speech therapy may be helpful for some patients. Physical therapy and muscle strengthening exercises can be important in the management of parkinsonism. A physical therapist can help develop and monitor a home exercise program that includes strengthening and flexing all limbs, stretching legs and feet, walking, and breathing exercises. An occupational therapist can help maintain maximum function in everyday activities. A speech therapist can help the person with PD improve voice volume, quality, and articulation. Therapeutic exercises such as verbalizations and tongue movements may be helpful. Being unable to articulate can be very frustrating, and reassurance and support should be provided.

Nutrition

Idiopathic PD slows gastric motility, so small amounts of food eaten frequently may be tolerated better than three larger meals per day. Liquid supplements can be useful for maintaining weight. Such supplements are not necessary if the patient consumes an adequate amount of a variety of foods. Many providers also recommend daily vitamin and mineral supplementation. It is believed that excess free radicals in the brain can damage brain cells, so antioxidants are also often recommended. Because the natural sense of thirst diminishes with age, it is also important to recommend drinking water on a schedule. This will enhance the absorption of nutrients and medications, and also reduce the risk of dehydration.

Mood/Cognitive Disorders

Depression and anxiety are common in patients with IPD. A careful evaluation is warranted because the facial expression and slowness can make the patients appear depressed even when no mood disorder is present. If depression is present it should be treated. Whether IPD itself is a cause of dementia is controversial, but certainly dementia may coexist with IPD.

Because IPD is a progressive condition, attempts to identify a health-care proxy and clarify advance directives regarding such issues as resuscitation and tube feeding should be made early in the course of the disease.

Case

A 69-year-old man who was formerly employed in a battery manufacturing plant comes to see you at the urging of his wife. She has noticed that her husband takes longer to get ready in the morning. She says he seems to have more trouble walking and is afraid he might fall and get hurt. Always a soft-spoken man, his voice is now hard to understand much of the time. He has developed a slight tremor in the left hand and she worries he might have had a stroke. The patient says he feels fine, and recalls for you stories about his amateur boxing career as a young man. He only complains that he tires more easily than he used to. He says his wife is a "worrier" and his problems are just part of "being old."

The patient's past medical history is remarkable for mild depression treated with paroxetine, hypertension treated with hydrochlorothiazide, and gastroesophageal reflux treated with omeperazole and metoclopramide. He has not had surgery. He denies hallucinations or delusions and his wife agrees these are not present. On examination, his blood pressure is 168/84 mm Hg and pulse is 72 beats/min. He has decreased facial expression and slowness in movement. He has reduced arm sway when he walks, short, shuffling steps, and difficulty turning, and tends to lean backward when standing still. The tone is increased in both arms, but more on the left. He has a slight tremor in the left hand, which abates when he reaches for objects. A Mini-mental status examination score is 26/30. The rest of the history, physical, and laboratory findings are unremarkable.

1. Does the patient have IPD?
2. What treatment is in order now?

Case Discussion
Does the Patient Have IPD?

The patient has the cardinal signs of parkinsonism (rigidity, tremor, bradykinesia, and postural instability), but the diagnosis of IPD is by no means certain. He is on multiple medicines that could cause parkinsonism such as paroxetine and metoclopramide. Furthermore, given his elevated blood pressure, a lacunar infarct leading to parkinsonism is possible. As a former worker in a battery manufacturing plant, he may have been exposed to manganese. Head trauma from his years as a boxer might also be contributing to his parkinsonism. His presentation is not consistent with a Parkinson-plus syndrome, and his intact cognition and lack of hallucinations makes dementia with Lewy bodies less likely.

What Treatment Is in Order Now?

Attempts at discontinuing paroxetine and metoclopramide should be made prior to the initiation of any pharmacotherapy directed at IPD. If you conclude that his functional impairment is significant, a trial of carbidopa/levodopa would be in order. If he failed to respond to this trial, then another cause of parkinsonism would be presumed to be present. Speech therapy consultation may be in order to improve the intelligibility of his speech.

Suggested Reading

Gorell J M, Rybicki B A, Cole Johnson C, Peterson E. Occupational metal exposures and the risk of Parkinson disease. *Neuroepidemiology* 1999;18:303–308.

http://www.apdaparkinson.com/; The American Parkinson Disease Association. A good starting point for information about Parkinson disease.

http://pdweb.mgh.harvard.edu/; The Parkinson's Web, a joint effort by Massachusetts General Hospital and Harvard University. This site has good information for families, patients, and physicians.

http://www.parkinsons-foundation.org/. Parkinson's Disease Foundation, Inc. A good starting point for information about Parkinson disease.

Lang A E, Lozano A M. Parkinson's disease: first of two parts. *N Engl J Med* 1998;339:1044–1053.

Lang A E, Lozano A M. Parkinson's disease: second of two parts. *N Engl J Med* 1998;339:1130–1143.

Mitchell S L, Kiely D K, Kiel D P, Lipsitz L A. The epidemiology, clinical characteristics, and natural history of older nursing home residents with a diagnosis of parkinson's disease. *J Am Geriatr Soc* 1996;44:394–399.

Parkinson J. *An essay on the shaking palsy.* London: Sherwood, Neely, & Jones, 1871.

Payami H; Zareparsi S. Genetic epidemiology of Parkinson's disease. *J Geriatr Psychiatry Neurol* 1998; 11:98–106.

71
Dementia

Inginia Genao

1. What is dementia and which associated risk factors have been identified?
2. Review briefly the different dementia syndromes.
3. What is your approach in diagnosing dementia?
4. Review the nonpharmacologic and pharmacologic management of dementia.

Discussion

What Is Dementia and Which Associated Risk Factors Have Been Identified?

Dementia is characterized by an acquired and persistent loss of cognitive and intellectual abilities, severe enough to interfere with daily functioning and quality of life without impairment of consciousness. Alzheimer disease (AD) is the most common form of dementia in the elderly, accounting for 60% to 80% of all cases and currently affecting 4 million Americans and 15 million people worldwide. The incidence increases steadily from 0.5% at the age of 65 years to 47% by the age of 85 years. Dementia has a tremendous negative impact on the quality of life of patients and caretakers at emotional, physical, and financial levels. The cost of caring for one person with dementia at home or in a nursing home is more than $47,000 per year. This figure contributes to a total estimated cost of more than $100 billion per year in the United States. Risk factors associated with AD are listed in Table 71.1.

Review Briefly the Different Dementia Syndromes.

Alzheimer Disease

- Most common of dementia syndromes
- Primary degenerative disease of the brain
- Progressive decline, sometimes with mild plateaus, affecting multiple cognitive domains:
  - Progressive memory impairment, especially short-term memory
  - Initially, mild impairment of attention and recall of remote events that worsens with time
  - Progressive disorientation with respect to time and place

Table 71.1. Risk Factors Associated with Alzheimer Disease (AD)

Major	Minor

Age (strongest risk factor, particularly in AD)
Family history
    Autosomal-dominant forms of AD are
        associated with early onset
    Apolipoprotein E epsilon 4 allele is associated
        with late-onset AD
    Chromosomal gene mutations in chromosome 1,
        14, 21
    Patients with a first-degree relative with
        dementia have a 10%–30% increase risk of
        developing the disorder
Down syndrome
	Head trauma
	History of depression
	Low education level
	Organic solvent exposure
	Gender: approximately 16% of women surviving
	    to an average life expectancy will develop AD
	    compared with 6% of men

- Language: difficulties finding words and naming parts of objects; decreased verbal comprehension with intact ability to repeat phrases
- Visual and spatial abilities: difficulties in recognizing faces; misperceptions (e.g., mistaking shrubs in the yard for people)
- Activities of daily living: apraxia (e.g., inability to dress or use silverware properly); acalculia; inability to perform complex tasks such as meal preparation; inability to maintain personal hygiene
- Personality changes: increase in passivity or hostility, stubbornness, decreased emotional expression, paranoid delusions (e.g., accusations of theft, marital infidelity, persecution)
- Hallucinations: visual (e.g., deceased parents/siblings, unknown intruders, and animals are frequently seen)
- Depression/anxiety
- Neurologic functions usually normal early in the disease process; motor deficits present later on
- Average survival after the time of diagnosis is 8 to 10 years, but range is variable

Vascular Dementia

- Second most common form of dementia
- Decline depends on severity of underlying cerebrovascular disease. Common associated cerebrovascular diseases include systemic lupus erythematosus, neurosyphilis, Lyme disease, endocarditis, hypertension, stroke, and subarachnoid hemorrhage
- Historical/physical examination findings that favor diagnosis:
  - Fluctuating course
  - Focal neurologic signs and symptoms in the setting of cognitive deficits
  - Relative preservation of personality
  - Abrupt onset with stepwise deterioration
  - Infarct on brain imaging
  - Triad: gait disturbance, urinary incontinence, cognitive decline

Dementia of the Frontal Lobe

- Rare cause of dementia

- Impairment of executive function such as initiation, goal setting, and planning
- Disinhibited behavior with normal or mildly abnormal cognitive testing
- Most patients deny that they have a problem
- Subtype: Pick disease—presents with logorrhea (abundant unfocused speech), echolalia (spontaneous repetition of words or phrases), palilalia (compulsive repetition of phrases)

Dementia with Parkinsonism

- About 30% of patients with Parkinson disease develop dementia
- Difficult to diagnose because rigidity and postural instability is present in about 30% of patients with AD
- Frequently progresses more rapidly than AD
- Presents with psychomotor slowing
- Delusions and hallucinations early in the course of the disease are common and might be exacerbated by treatment of parkinsonism
- Lewy body dementia: most common dementia associated with Parkinson disease that presents with marked hallucinations, delusions and fluctuating mental status

Normal Pressure Hydrocephalus

- Poorly understood cause of dementia
- Characterized by the triad of gait disorder, urinary incontinence, cognitive decline (triad is not specific; can be present in patients with vascular dementia)
- Diagnosis confirmed by Miller-Fisher test (objective gait assessment before and after the removal of 30 mL of cerebrospinal fluid). This test also predicts the likelihood of successful treatment with ventriculoperitoneal shunting

What Is Your Approach in Diagnosing Dementia?

The approach to the diagnosis of dementia starts with a very detailed history because dementia is a clinical diagnosis (i.e., there are no tests that confirm the diagnosis). The gold standard is brain biopsy/autopsy.

History

- Mode of onset: abrupt versus gradual
- Progression: stepwise versus continuous decline versus fluctuating course
- Duration of symptoms
- Detailed history of chief complaint—any problems with activities listed below:
  - Learning and retaining new information (trouble remembering recent conversations, events, appointments; frequently misplacing objects)
  - Handling complex tasks (inability to balance a checkbook or to cook a meal)
  - Reasoning ability (inability to reply to questions with a reasonable plan; e.g., difficulty in answering the questions "What should you do if you find a stamped envelope in the street?" or "How is an apple like a banana?")
  - Spatial ability and orientation (inability to navigate around familiar places)
  - Language (difficulty finding words or following conversations)

- Behavior (noticeably more passive or less responsive; irritable; suspicious; misinterprets visual or auditory stimuli)
- Detailed medication list including over-the-counter and herbal medicines
- Past medical history, social history and family history
- Review of systems, including psychiatric and neurologic symptoms, history of head trauma, and environmental toxin exposure

Physical Examination

- A full neurologic examination is warranted in all patients with suspected AD.
- Assess cognitive function with the Mini-Mental Status Examination.
- Order tests as tailored by the history and physical examination. The American Academy of Neurology recommends obtaining the following: complete blood count (CBC), chemistry panel, calcium, phosphate, liver profile, thyroid-stimulating hormone (TSH), erythrocyte sedimentation rate, serum vitamin B_{12}, and syphilis serology [the rapid plasma reagent test may be nonreactive in neurosyphilis; therefore, a fluorescent treponemal antibody absorption (FTA-ABS) test also should be ordered].
- The cost effectiveness of including all of these laboratory tests in a routine workup has been questioned due to the low likelihood (<10%) of identifying a reversible dementia. Therefore, test ordering can be tailored to patients with a compatible history or physical findings.

Neuroimaging Studies

- Most patients do not require computed tomography (CT) or magnetic resonance imaging (MRI) for a diagnosis of AD.
- Imaging studies do not seem to improve the diagnostic accuracy in patients without focal neurologic deficits or atypical features.
- Demented patients with atherosclerotic disease or its associated risk factors may have silent cerebrovascular disease. Abnormal findings on neuroimaging may lead to more aggressive management of risk factors, such as diabetes mellitus, hypertension, hyperlipidemia, and tobacco use.
- Head CT is important for patients with acute onset of cognitive decline and rapid neurologic deterioration.
- Neuroimaging is also indicated when there are historical features and physical examination findings suggestive of a central nervous system bleed, or embolic/thrombotic stroke.

Review the Nonpharmacologic and Pharmacologic Management of Dementia.

Nonpharmacologic Management

Educate patients, family members, and caregivers on dementia and its complications, disease progression, and prognosis. Discuss medication side effects and expected therapeutic response. For instance, it is helpful to explain that some of the

Table 71.2. Therapeutic Response to Medication in Alzheimer

Usually Responsive	Sometimes Responsive	Usually Refractory
Depression	Apathy	Wandering
Hallucinations	Anxiety	Repetitive questions
Delusions	Episodic outbursts	Repetitive behaviors
Insomnia	Aggressive behaviors	Mirror talking

common symptoms and behaviors associated with AD are more likely to improve with medication than others (Table 71.2).

Address behavior and social environment:

- Safety issues
- Legal/financial planning
- Caregiver health
- Structured activity availability and support systems

Pharmacologic Management

There are several cognitive and functional enhancers that can be used in the treatment of AD.

Acetylcholinesterase Inhibitors

- These agents increase acetylcholine at the synaptic cleft by inhibiting acetylcholinesterase. Donepezil and tacrine are the only drugs approved for AD treatment in the United States. Donepezil is discussed here because it is widely used, best tolerated, and easier to administer than tacrine.
- Donepezil is an reversible, selective anticholinesterase inhibitor with minimal peripheral action and a longer half-life than tacrine.
- Dosing is once per day.
- The most frequent side effects are nausea, diarrhea, and vomiting.
- A small improvement in cognitive function has been shown in a few studies in patients with mild to moderate disease. One study showed that cognitive function returned to its initial pretreatment state after donepezil was discontinued. There are no controlled studies available to provide information on long-term benefits and safety.

Antioxidants

- Alpha-tocopherol (vitamin E), selegiline, and *Ginkgo biloba* extracts are thought to have antioxidant properties.
- Selegiline is a monoamine oxidase inhibitor with antioxidant properties that increase brain catecholamines.
- A 2-year controlled study using 2,000 IU of vitamin E and 10 mg of selegiline together and individually showed no difference in cognitive function. Vitamin E decreased the late complications of AD (nursing home placement, severe dementia, and death) by 5 to 7 months compared with placebo. No added benefit was observed from combining it with selegiline

- It is recommended to administer vitamin E, given its safe profile, and avoid selegiline given its potential for other medication interactions and unclear benefits.
- *Ginkgo biloba* is thought to have antiinflammatory as well as antioxidant properties. It is also thought to improve cerebral circulation in elderly patients.
- Small studies have shown that *Ginkgo biloba* increases cognitive function slightly.

Antiinflammatory Medication

- Findings from a small study suggested that patients who received the nonsteroidal antiinflammatory drug (NSAID) indomethacin were more clinically stable compared with placebo.
- NSAIDs are not recommended for routine use given their potential side effects, especially in the elderly.

Hormone Replacement Therapy

- Hormone replacement therapy (HRT) is thought to decrease vascular disease, decrease trophic effects on the brain, and have antiinflammatory/antioxidant effects.
- Limited data have suggested a decrease relative risk for AD in postmenopausal women treated with HRT.
- Limited data exist regarding the treatment of patients who already have AD.
- HRT is not recommended solely for the prevention or treatment of AD.

Case

Mr. CR is an 80-year-old man with a high school education who comes to you for the first time accompanied by his daughter. You were the primary care provider to his wife who died a year ago. You recall her telling you that "he has been driving me crazy for years." Mr. CR appears distant and disengaged as you listen to his daughter's story:

> Doctor, my father has changed! He is irritable and argumentative. He forgets things all the time; he is always misplacing his glasses. I moved in with him because he has not been taking care of himself or paying the bills. One thing that I have noticed is that he gets lost in the neighborhood. Maybe he is just getting old.

Mr. CR has not made any comments and does not appear concerned. There is no history of medication allergy and he is not on any medications, including over-the-counter or herbal medicines. Past medical history is remarkable for osteoarthritis. Family history is not known. Social history reveals that he is a retired church minister. He smoked cigarettes in the remote past and he has no history of alcohol or recreational drug use.

On physical examination he appears physically healthy, younger than his stated age. His blood pressure is 140/80 mm Hg; pulse is regular at 80 beats/min and respiratory rate is 18 breaths/min. He is afebrile. A thorough physical examination, including neurologic examination, is unremarkable. His Folstein Mini-Mental Status Examination score is 18/30 (normal, >23). Laboratory data reveal a normal CBC, renal function, electrolytes, TSH, liver profile, vitamin B_{12}, folate, and treponemal test.

1. What is your response to the daughter's statement, "Maybe he is just getting old"?
2. Would you order an imaging study in this patient?
3. What reversible causes of dementia do you need to consider in this patient?

Case Discussion

What Is Your Response to the Daughter's Statement, "Maybe He Is Just Getting Old"?

It is common for family members and even health-care providers to attribute signs of dementia to the normal aging process. This patient's cognitive decline has been progressive, and his daily function has been quite affected, indicating a possible diagnosis of dementia.

Would You Order an Imaging Study in This Patient?

This patient has no neurologic physical findings to indicate a brain neuroimaging study. Without physical findings, CT or MRI imaging studies are nonspecific in identifying findings that correlate with dementia. One exception is vascular dementia, where white matter disease has been reported in patients with normal cognitive function.

Cerebral atrophy on neuroimaging studies tends to correlate more with aging than with dementia. A neuroimaging study would not change the management in this patient and is therefore not thought to be necessary at this time.

What Reversible Causes of Dementia Do You Need to Consider in This Patient?

This patient does not have clinical signs of any systemic illnesses such as congestive heart failure, pulmonary insufficiency, or liver disease. However, findings consistent with thyroid disease, hyponatremia, or hypocalcemia can be nonspecific, particularly in the elderly, and might need to be ruled out. Depression is also difficult to discern from dementia in some cases and tends to coexist with dementia. Some physicians might consider "empirically" treating for depression, especially in this patient whose wife died a year ago. As discussed above, laboratory tests ordered should be guided by clinical suspicion. Syphilis serology (FTA-ABS) should be ordered in case syphilis has gone untreated.

Suggested Reading

Geldmacher D S, et al. Evaluation of dementia. *N Engl J Med* 1996;335:330–336.

Quinn J, Kaye J. *Treatment of Alzheimer's disease.* Bayer Corporation, Pharmaceutical Division, 1999.

Shadlen M F. Approach to the diagnosis of dementia. *Up To Date* 1999;7.

Small G W, et al. Diagnosis and treatment of dementia in the aged. *West J Med* 1981;135:469–481.

Winograd C H, et al. Physician management of the demented patient. *J Am Geriatr Soc* 1986;34:295–308.

XII
Psychiatry

72

Alcohol Use Disorders

Anuradha Paranjape

1. How are alcohol use disorders classified?
2. What is the rationale behind the definitions of safe or moderate drinking levels?
3. Should one screen routinely for alcohol use disorders? Why?
4. What approach should one take toward identification of an alcohol use disorder?
5. What initial steps can be taken as a clinician to help a patient with an alcohol use disorder?

Discussion

How Are Alcohol Use Disorders Classified?

One standard drink is defined as 12 g of alcohol, which is the amount of alcohol in 180 mL (6 ounces) of wine, 360 mL (12 ounces) of beer, or 45 mL (1.5 ounces) of 90-proof spirit. An abstainer is a someone who does not drink alcohol. At one end of the spectrum of alcohol use is regular use in moderation without adverse consequences to the drinkers themselves or to those around them. At the other end are drinkers who suffer adverse physiologic, psychological, and economic consequences as a result of their drinking. Between the two ends lies a continuum of drinkers with varying alcohol consumption patterns. The *Diagnostic and Statistical Manual of Mental Disorders,* 3rd revised edition (DSM-III-R), of the American Psychiatric Association has outlined guidelines for the diagnosis of substance abuse disorders. The DSM-III-R recognizes two categories: alcohol abuse and alcohol dependence. Table 72.1 outlines these definitions. It also defines the concept of moderate and at-risk drinking as defined by the National Institute of Alcohol Abuse and Alcoholism, which distinguishes levels of alcohol consumption based on health risks.

What Is the Rationale Behind the Definitions of Safe or Moderate Drinking Levels?

The rationale behind the "safe" levels of two drinks per day in men and one drink per day in women comes from large population studies. Multiple prospective studies have defined the risk of all-cause mortality and alcohol consumption. In general, a U or J shaped association between alcohol consumption and mortality has been described for both sexes. In two prospective studies, with 300,000 men, increased mortality was found among men consuming more than two to three drinks per day.

Table 72.1. Spectrum of Alcohol Abuse

Alcohol dependence: *maladaptive pattern over 12-mo period with three or more items present* (DSM-III-R criteria)	Substance often taken in larger amounts or over a longer period than the person intended (loss of control)
	Persistent desire or one or more unsuccessful attempts to cut down or control substance use
	Great deal of time spent in activities necessary for getting, taking, or recovering from use
	Withdrawal symptoms
	Use to prevent or relieve withdrawal symptoms
	Recurrent use when substance is physically hazardous *or* frequent intoxication or withdrawal symptoms when expected to perform major role obligations at work, school, or home
	Important social occupational or recreational activities given up or reduced
	Continued substance use despite knowledge of having social, psychological, or physical problems caused or exacerbated by use
Alcohol abuse: *maladaptive pattern with one or more of following items present over a 12-mo period* (DSM III R criteria	Continued use despite persistent social, psychological, occupation or physical problems caused or exacerbated by use; recurrent use in hazardous situations
At-risk drinking (NIAAA definition)	Men: >14 drinks/wk; >4 drinks/occasion
	Women: >7 drinks/wk; >3 drinks/occasion
Moderate drinking (NIAAA definition)	Men: ≤2 drinks/day
	Women: ≤1 drink/day

Adapted from O'Connor P G, Schottenfield R S. Patients with alcohol problems. *N Engl J Med* 1998;338:592–601; with permission.

Women drinking more than approximately 2.5 drinks per day had increased mortality. The difference in mortality has a physiologic basis; women have both a lower volume of alcohol distribution and decreased activity of gastric alcohol dehydrogenase. This difference results in higher alcohol levels in women per ounce of alcohol consumed. The reason that binge drinking is considered to be an at-risk drinking pattern is also based on population survey data. The National Health and Nutrition Education Survey follow-up study has demonstrated that episodic (binge) consumption of more than four drinks per day is associated with increased odds of death from injury of 1.9, whereas episodic consumption of more than eight drinks per day increases these odds to 3.3.

Should One Screen Routinely for Alcohol Use Disorders? If so, Why?

A decision to screen for a disease depends on a few factors: the burden of disease, availability of screening measures, and availability of interventions once a disease is detected. Generally one will screen for a disorder that is prevalent, when screening measures are available and where intervention upon screening has been found to be effective. Alcohol dependence, abuse, and at-risk drinking are very common. They are more common among patients seen by physicians than among the general population. The lifetime prevalence of alcohol abuse or dependence is higher than in the general population and ranges from 16% to 36% among current drinkers. The prevalence of at-risk or problem drinking is also high (4% to 33%), with higher rates reported in men.

Alcohol use disorders result in a myriad of health problems at multiple levels, including medical, behavioral, and psychosocial problems. The medical consequences of alcohol use are well known to the clinician: liver cirrhosis, alcoholic hepatitis, alcohol withdrawal seizures, and pancreatitis are but a few of the many complications of prolonged and heavy alcohol use. As seen above, at-risk drinking and binge drinking are also associated with increased morbidity and mortality. Alcohol has been linked to violent crime, fires, burns, suicides, and fatal and nonfatal traffic accidents. The costs to society from alcoholism are also great, ranging in the billions of dollars. As will be discussed below, a number of screening tools are available for the early detection of alcohol dependence and problem drinking. It has also been shown that, once detected, five minutes of physician advice is effective to get patients to stop drinking. Routine universal screening is recommended by several professional organizations, including the American Medical Association, and prevention guidelines have been issued by the U.S. Preventive Services Task Force. Clinicians should incorporate brief counseling into routine patient care and consider referral for alcohol dependent-patients into rehabilitation programs.

What Approach Should One Take toward Identification of an Alcohol Use Disorder?

It is important to bear in mind that the diagnosis of an alcohol use disorder is rarely accomplished in one visit, unlike other medical problems. O'Connor and Schottenfield have described a simple four-step clinical approach that can be incorporated into daily practice. The first step is to ask all patients about current and previous alcohol use. A good way of initiating a discussion about drinking is to ask a question such as, "Do you drink alcohol, including beer, wine or distilled spirits?" as part of the patient's routine health history along with other questions about smoking, drug use, seatbelt use, and safe sexual practices. Prefacing the social history with a statement like, "These are questions that I ask everyone I see" will facilitate disclosure, because it has been presented as a routine matter and the alcohol-dependent patient does not feel singled out. Because genetic predisposition and family environment are risk factors for alcohol problems, the family history should also include questions on alcohol use.

The second step is to obtain detailed information about quantity used and frequency of use:

- "On a typical day, how much do you drink?"
- "On average, how many days a week do you drink?"
- "What is the maximum number of drinks that you have had on one occasion?"

These questions will help the clinician to differentiate moderate drinking from at-risk drinking and binge drinking. Step 3 is the administration of a screening instrument to detect alcohol problems. The most commonly used questionnaire is the CAGE (Fig. 72.1). The CAGE was developed in 1968 by Ewing et al. and since then has been extensively studied and validated in several populations.

The sensitivity of the CAGE questionnaire to detect lifetime alcohol use problems ranges from 60% to 95% for a positive result (answering yes to two or more of the four CAGE questions). Buschbaum et al. have estimated the sensitivity and specificity of a positive CAGE result to be 75% and 91%, respectively. Using these numbers, if 10% of patients are expected to have an alcohol use disorder, any pa-

- Have you ever felt you ought to **C**ut down on your drinking?

- Have people **A**nnoyed you by criticizing your drinking?

- Have you ever felt bad or **G**uilty about your drinking?

- Have you ever had a drink the first thing in the morning to steady your nerves or get rid of a hangover? (**E**ye-opener)

Figure 72.1. The CAGE questionnaire. (Ewing JA. Detecting alcoholism, the CAGE questionnaire. JAMA 1984;252:1905–1907.

tient who answers yes to two or more of the four CAGE questions will have a 47% chance being one of those 10% patients. The utility of the CAGE increases if one takes into account the number of positive responses that the patient gives. Using this method and assuming that 10% of all patients are expected to have an alcohol use disorder, the chance that your patient is one of those 10% if he or she answers yes to zero, one, two, three, or all four CAGE questions is 2%, 14%, 33%, 59%, and 92%, respectively. Thus, a negative CAGE result should rule out alcohol dependency, whereas four positive responses most certainly "rules in" alcohol dependency in this patient population. The drawback to using CAGE is that it was designed to detect alcohol dependency, not at-risk drinking. The sensitivity is less when used to screen women and elderly patients because of a lower prevalence. Yet another screening instrument, the Alcohol Use Disorders Identification Test (AUDIT) was developed under the aegis of the World Health Organization to overcome some of these shortcomings. AUDIT incorporates quantity and frequency items, is able to detect at-risk drinking, and is a sensitive screen for different racial, gender, and ethnic groups. However, the instrument consists of 10 questions and is too long to be incorporated into a routine office visit. Thus, what most experts recommend is to use a brief screening instrument, such as the CAGE, and to supplement it with questions regarding duration, quantity, and frequency of use.

Step 4 is the final step, and is based on the results of screening. Here one should ask targeted questions to look for signs of problem drinking and dependence, including interpersonal, work-related, and legal problems, to separate abuse and dependency from at-risk drinking. The medical history should be reviewed to identify problems such as hypertension, depression, injuries, sexual dysfunction, and sleep disorders. Laboratory tests should be reviewed or checked for evidence of liver or red blood cell abnormalities, the so-called red flags of alcohol dependence. One should also ask about other forms of substance abuse because the rate of polysubstance use is high.

What Initial Steps Can Be Taken as a Clinician to Help a Patient with an Alcohol Use Disorder?

As mentioned above, alcohol use disorders fall outside the usual biomedical model of disease. Social factors influence these disorders more than others, and the diagnosis of the problem is difficult. Unlike other medical diseases, the solution to the problem has to be patient centered for it to succeed. Abstinence from alcohol is heavily dependent on the patient's readiness to change his or her behavior. Prochaska and DiClemente's stages of change model has now been adapted for substance abuse, which includes alcohol use. The patient's stage of change—precontemplation, contemplation, determination, action, maintenance, or relapse—can be identified during the patient interview once an alcohol problem has been detected. To do so, one must explore the patient's perception of his or her alcohol problem. This can be done by simply asking in a nonjudgmental fashion if he or she perceives drinking to be a problem. Identifying a specific alcohol-related problem and asking the patient how much he or she perceives this problem to be a result of alcohol is another strategy. Once the clinician has determined how ready the patient seems to stop drinking, (i.e., change behavior), the patient can be counseled appropriately. In short, patient-centered counseling sessions (called brief interventions) designed to enhance the patient's motivation to change behavior (in this case drinking habits), have been shown to be effective at promoting and maintaining abstinence. In randomized trials, increased referrals to treatment programs, reduced self-reported drinking rates, and improved self-reported work performance have all been shown to result from such interventions. A detailed discussion of motivational interviewing is beyond the scope of this chapter, but Table 72.2 briefly illustrates the various interview approaches described by Samet et al. that the clinician can adapt.

Table 72.2. Counseling Approach Based on Stages of Change Model

Stages of Readiness to Change	Interview Approach
Precontemplation: *patient does not recognize that alcohol use could be a problem*	Express concern about patient. State nonjudgmentally that alcohol is a problem. Agree to disagree about severity of problem. Consider abstinence trial to clarify issue. Suggest bringing family member to an appointment. Explore patient's perception of the problem. Emphasize the importance of seeing the patient again.
Contemplation: *patient is aware that alcohol use is a problem but unsure how negative the consequences may be*	Elicit positive and negative aspects of alcohol use. Ask about positive and negative aspects of past periods of abstinence. Summarize patient's comments on use and abstinence and make explicit discrepancies between values and actions. Consider a trial of abstinence.
Determination: *patient has made a decision to seek help for alcohol problem*	Acknowledge self-sufficiency of decision to seek treatment. Support self-efficacy. Affirm patient's ability to successfully seek treatment. Help patient decide an appropriate achievable action. Caution that the road ahead is tough, but important. Explain that relapse will not affect your patient–physician relationship.
Action: *patient has sought help, may be on medications to ameliorate symptoms* Maintenance: *patient has successfully completed a treatment program*	Be a source of encouragement and support. Acknowledge the discomforting aspects of withdrawal. Reinforce the importance of remaining abstinent. Anticipate difficulties as a means of preventing relapse. Recognize the patient's struggle. Support the patient's resolve. Reiterate that relapse should not disrupt your relationship with the program.
Relapse: *distinct part of the process of change and is not failure to change*	Explore what can be learned from the relapse. Express concern, disappointment. Emphasize positive aspects of effort to seek care. Support patient's self-efficacy, so that recovery seems attainable.

Adapted from Samet JH, Rollnick S, Barnes H. Beyond CAGE, a brief clinical approach after decision of substance abuse. Arch Intern Med 1996;156:2287–2293; with permission.

Anyone with a pattern of drinking that is not safe should be counseled. Patients with at-risk drinking patterns sometimes are more challenging because they are less likely to see their drinking to be a problem. The importance of empathy, support, and the efficacy of physician intervention are worth mentioning again. It is also important to remember that change will only happen when the patient is ready to change, hence the stress on an approach tailored to the patient's readiness to change. Advising someone with an alcohol use problem who is in the precontemplative stage to "go and join Alcoholics Anonymous" and leaving it at that is not only ineffective, but will possibly undermine the physician–patient relationship as well.

Case

N.B. is a taciturn veteran patient seen by you for the past 2 years for primary care. He is hypertensive, and often presents with a heart rate in the high 90s and tremors. Physical examination so far has been unremarkable and you have not noticed any clinical signs of liver dysfunction. On a few occasions over the past 2 years, you have noticed a definite whiff of alcohol on his breath. The previous provider had noted "occasional" alcohol use in his chart notes. Recent laboratory tests obtained for other reasons have revealed a macrocytic anemia, and an aspartate aminotransferase (AST) level of 80 U/L.

1. Do you think this patient has an alcohol use problem?
2. You are certain that he is alcohol dependent and that he would benefit from referral for further evaluation and counseling. How would you approach this with him?
3. What would you recommend to the patient regarding his alcohol use?

Case Discussion

Do You Think This Patient Has an Alcohol Use Problem?

Despite the chart notes about occasional alcohol use, there are a few concerning signs on physical examination and laboratory values that hint at a problem. Apart from subjective observations of the whiff of alcohol on his breath and tremors, he is hypertensive, and has changes on his blood smear (macrocytic anemia) and an elevated AST that are consistent with alcohol use. He has several red flags mentioned in step 4 of the clinical approach, and is a current drinker. Further assessment depends the CAGE score and an assessment of quantity and frequency of use and information on whether the drinking has caused interpersonal, work-related, and legal issues. It also depends on whether or not there is evidence of loss of control, of tolerance, and a history of withdrawal symptoms.

The patient says he drinks a couple of beers a day, up to a six-pack on the weekend. He says, however, that he is not "like one of those drunks or winos who drinks all the time." However, he also tells you that the amount he needs to feel any sort of effect from alcohol has increased over the past few years. On further questioning, you discover that he has had his driver's license revoked for driving under the influence in the past 6 months, and that he has kept to himself since he lost his job a few months ago. He tells you that he had started sneaking a beer now and then on the job in the few months before getting fired. He scores 3 out of 4 on the CAGE.

You Are Certain that He Is Alcohol Dependent and that He Would Benefit from Referral for Further Evaluation and Counseling. How Would You Approach This with Him?

As described above, the next step is to solicit the patient's opinion about his drinking to see if he views it as a problem. One way of doing this would be to ask if his recent personal difficulties could have resulted from alcohol.

The patient says that he is aware that his drinking has escalated recently, and that this may have led to his being fired. He then reiterates that he is not drunk all the time and does not think that the alcohol has contributed to any health problems.

What Would You Recommend to the Patient Regarding His Alcohol Use?

The patient recognizes some of the problems that result from his drinking, but not all of them. He is in the contemplative stage and would best be helped by a few minutes of discussion concerning the positive and negative aspects of drinking as elicited from the patient. His opinion should be followed by your own opinion about the negative aspects of drinking, to reinforce his views and add to them. Next, one should suggest a trial of abstinence. Because abstinence is hard to achieve and takes time, a follow-up appointment should be scheduled. At future visits, once the patient demonstrates the willingness to abstain, he or she should be referred to a local rehabilitation program, just as one would refer a patient to a subspecialist for subspecialty care.

Suggested Reading

Kitchens J M. Does this patient have an alcohol problem? *JAMA* 1994;272:1782–1787.

National Institute of Alcohol Abuse and Alcoholism. The physician's guide to helping patients with alcohol problems. Washington, DC: U.S. Government Printing Office, 1995. National Institutes of Health Publication No. 95-3769.

O'Connor P G, Schottenfield R S. Patients with alcohol problems. *N Engl J Med* 1998;338:592–601.

Samet J H, Rollnick S, Barnes H. Beyond CAGE. A brief clinical approach after detection of substance abuse. *Arch Intern Med* 1996;156:2287–2293.

73
Anxiety

Michael T. Compton
Andrew C. Furman

1. How prevalent are anxiety disorders, and other disorders associated with anxiety, in the general U.S. population?
2. What is the differential diagnosis of anxiety in the ambulatory medicine setting?
3. What are the treatments of choice for anxiety disorders?
4. When is referral to a psychiatrist indicated for patients presenting with anxiety?

Discussion

How Prevalent Are Anxiety Disorders, and Other Disorders Associated with Anxiety, in the General U.S. Population?

Patients with anxiety often present to primary care settings, frequently for somatic complaints and symptoms associated with their anxiety. Anxiety disorders and other illnesses causing clinically significant anxiety can cause devastating socioeconomic consequences and can seriously adversely impact quality of life. The National Comorbidity Survey assessed the prevalence of psychiatric disorders in the United States by administering a research diagnostic interview to over 8,000 individuals. This study revealed that the lifetime prevalence of any anxiety disorder is 19.2% in men and 30.5% in women. Mood disorders and substance use disorders are also highly prevalent, with lifetime prevalence rates of approximately 19% and 27%, respectively. The rates of cooccurrence of an anxiety disorder with a depressive disorder, a substance use disorder (abuse or dependence), or both, are also high.

What Is the Differential Diagnosis of Anxiety in the Ambulatory Medicine Setting?

Anxiety is a distressing emotion often accompanied by physiologic symptoms that may be a transient affective state, a chronic dysfunctional mood, or a discretely defined psychiatric syndrome. In the ambulatory care setting, anxiety often presents as somatic complaints, such as dizziness, dysphagia, dyspnea, flushing, muscle tension, nausea, palpitations, paresthesias, tremulousness, or sweating. Emotional and cognitive symptoms include fatigue, fear, hypervigilance, insomnia, irritability, nervousness, poor concentration, restlessness, and worry. The differential diagnosis of the common complaint of anxiety is quite extensive. In fact, one could argue that many medical and most psychiatric diagnoses are associated with various symptoms of anxiety.

Current psychiatric diagnosis is based on a system that is purely descriptive, as outlined in the fourth edition of the *Diagnostic and Statistical Manual of Mental Disorders* (DSM-IV). Therein, when the primary expression of the illness is in the form of symptoms of anxiety, the illness is termed an *anxiety disorder.* The DSM-IV provides criteria for 11 specific anxiety disorders, which are briefly described below.

Panic disorder without agoraphobia consists of recurrent unexpected panic attacks. A panic attack is characterized as a discrete period of intense fear or discomfort during which four or more symptoms develop abruptly and peak within 10 minutes. Symptoms include palpitations, sweating, trembling, shortness of breath, sensation of choking, nausea, dizziness, derealization or depersonalization, fear of losing control, fear of dying, paresthesias, and chills or hot flushes. In panic disorder, the patient has a persistent concern about having additional attacks, worries about the consequences of the attack, or has a change in behavior due to the attack. In *panic disorder with agoraphobia,* the patient also demonstrates symptoms of agoraphobia, which is anxiety about being in places or situations from which escape might be difficult; and such situations are avoided or endured with marked distress. *Agoraphobia* without history of panic disorder describes patients who have agoraphobia related to fear of developing panic-like symptoms, but criteria have never been met for panic disorder.

Specific phobia represents a marked and persistent fear that is excessive or unreasonable, related to a specific object or situation (such as flying, heights, animals, seeing blood). Exposure to the phobic stimulus almost invariably provokes an immediate anxiety response, the person recognizes the fear as excessive, the stimulus is avoided, and the anxiety interferes significantly with functioning. *Social phobia* (frequently referred to as social anxiety disorder) consists of a marked and persistent fear of social or performance situations. The individual fears embarrassment, and the feared social situations provoke anxiety responses. The fear is recognized as excessive, but social situations are avoided or endured with intense anxiety or distress. Fear of negative evaluation is the critical cognitive feature of social phobia.

Obsessive-compulsive disorder consists of either obsessions (recurrent intrusive thoughts) or compulsions (repetitive behaviors that the person feels driven to perform in response to an obsession). Generalized anxiety disorder involves excessive anxiety and worry occurring more days than not for at least 6 months, about a number of events and activities. The individual finds it difficult to control the worry, and the worry is associated with three or more symptoms, including restlessness, being easily fatigued, difficulty concentrating, irritability, muscle tension, and difficulty sleeping. *Generalized anxiety disorder* commonly occurs comorbidly with depression or other anxiety disorders.

Acute stress disorder and *posttraumatic stress disorder* occur in individuals exposed to a traumatic event that evokes intense fear, helplessness, or horror. The traumatic experience is persistently reexperienced (in the form of flashbacks, dreams, intrusive memories, or psychological or physiologic reactivity to cues that symbolize the traumatic event), and the individual avoids stimuli that arouse recollections. These disorders cause marked symptoms of anxiety or increased arousal. In acute stress disorder, the symptoms persist for less than 1 month, and the trauma causes dissociative symptoms, including a sense of numbing or detachment, reduced awareness of surroundings, derealization, depersonalization, or amnesia.

The DSM-IV also provides diagnoses for *anxiety disorder due to a general medical condition* and *substance-induced anxiety disorder.* Some medical conditions that can be physiologically associated with significant anxiety include angina, arrhythmias, carcinoid syndrome, chronic obstructive pulmonary disease, endocrine disturbances (pituitary, adrenal, parathyroid, and thyroid dysfunction), heavy metal poisoning, hypoglycemia, hypoxia, inflammatory disorders such as lupus erythematosus, many neurologic disorders, pheochromocytoma, systemic malignancies, uremia, and vitamin deficiency states. Substance-induced anxiety disorders may be physiologically related to medications (such as corticosteroids, sympathomimetic and vasopressor agents, and theophylline), substance intoxication (amphetamines, caffeine, cocaine, hallucinogens, phencyclidine), or substance withdrawal (alcohol, cocaine, hypnotics/anxiolytics, opioids).

In addition to these anxiety disorders, many other psychiatric disorders can be associated with anxiety symptoms, and must be considered in the differential diagnosis. These include delirium, dementia, schizophrenia and other psychotic disorders, mood disorders, somatoform disorders, sleep disorders, and personality disorders. Clinicians evaluating anxious patients must be especially vigilant for the presence of major depressive disorder, because of the very high degree of comorbidity among depressive disorders and anxiety symptoms or anxiety disorders. Furthermore, anxiety associated with depression increases the risk of suicide, and should be considered a risk factor for suicide among depressed patients.

What Are the Treatments of Choice for Anxiety Disorders?

The psychopharmacologic treatment of anxiety disorders has advanced dramatically over the past 10 years. At present, it is increasingly recognized that agents acting on central serotonergic systems, such as the selective serotonin reuptake inhibitors (SSRIs), have a broad spectrum of anxiolytic action across disorders, even though they were originally developed as antidepressant agents. The treatment of anxiety symptoms and anxiety disorders can be subdivided into two broad categories: psychopharmacologic agents and psychotherapy.

The short-term, acute treatment of anxiety disorders focuses on symptom relief with medications and initiation of psychoeducational and psychological therapies. Antidepressants are the first-line treatments. In panic disorder, although the tricyclic antidepressant (TCA) imipramine has been studied most extensively, SSRIs are currently favored based on their effectiveness and more favorable side effect profile. To avoid or minimize a reaction characterized by increased anxiety in patients with panic disorder, a lower dose of SSRI is usually initiated. Several SSRIs currently have U.S. Food and Drug Administration (FDA) approval for the treatment of panic disorder, and it is assumed that all agents in this category are efficacious. The extended-release form of venlafaxine, a dual serotonin and norepinephrine reuptake inhibitor (SNRI) has been FDA approved for generalized anxiety disorder, in addition to its indication for depression. It is likely that other serotonergically active agents are effective. SSRIs are also efficacious in the treatment of so-cial phobia and posttraumatic stress disorder. Similarly, the serotonergically active TCA clomipramine has been the gold standard treatment for obsessive-compulsive disorder, although SSRIs are currently preferred as first-line agents due to their more favorable side effect profile. Drugs that are less potent blockers of serotonin reuptake than clomipramine (e.g., the TCAs nortriptyline and desipramine) are gen-erally ineffective for obsessive-compulsive disorder. Higher doses of SSRIs may be required in this disorder.

For many anxiety disorders, low doses of benzodiazepines also can be used. They are most useful in the treatment of transient anxiety. The choice of benzodi-azepine depends on potency, half-life, and the patient's hepatic status. Benzodi-azepines should be used cautiously in the elderly, due to increased risk of falls and fractures, and daytime sedation. After being used for a few weeks (while the sero-tonergic agent is beginning to gradually take effect), a careful plan of discontinua-tion is needed, with a slow tapering schedule to avoid potentially dangerous with-drawal phenomena. The risk of physiologic and psychological dependence should be strongly considered in any patient receiving benzodiazepines. These drugs are commonly abused by individuals with diatheses for addiction.

Another anxiolytic agent that should be considered in anxiety disorders is the nonbenzodiazepine serotonin 1A partial agonist, buspirone. Although benzodi-azepines have been the mainstay of treatment for generalized anxiety disorder, bus-pirone has been shown to be as effective as benzodiazepines, although it has a slow onset. Buspirone also has a potential role in the treatment of many other anxiety disorders. Beta blockers have been shown to be effective for performance anxiety, or the specific form of social phobia. There also may be a role for β-blockers for persistent symptoms of autonomic arousal in posttraumatic stress disorder.

Occasionally, other pharmacologic interventions are necessary. For example, monoamine oxidase inhibitors (MAOIs) have established efficacy in the treatment of social phobia. However, the use of these agents is complicated by toxicity or lethality in overdose and the possibility of a hypertensive crisis when taken with certain medications or foods (a special tyramine-restricted diet is required). TCAs are also greatly limited by their unfavorable side effect profile and high toxicity in overdose. MAOIs and TCAs should be prescribed only by clinicians with experi-ence with these agents.

Although current clinical practice generally involves a trial of 3 to 6 months of an effective medication, a longer duration of treatment is often required. It may be good practice to routinely taper and discontinue the medication after 6 to 12 months, allowing at least a month after discontinuation before deciding if restarting is necessary. Relapse after discontinuation of medications is not uncommon, and chronic maintenance therapy is sometimes indicated. Occasionally, combinations of medications are required (e.g., a TCA and an SSRI, or buspirone and an SSRI) for refractory cases.

Psychoeducation should be used in conjunction with medications, especially be-cause anxiety symptoms and anxiety disorders are not widely understood by the general public. Other psychotherapeutic approaches may enhance the outcome of treatment with psychotropic agents. The most extensively studied psychotherapy modality for several anxiety disorders is cognitive-behavioral therapy (CBT). This short-term (12–16 sessions), highly structured psychotherapy examines the pa-tient's thought patterns, cognitive distortions, and maladaptive behavior. For gener-alized anxiety disorder, a combination of relaxation techniques aimed at decreasing arousal, CBT, coping skills training, and alteration of life-style factors are often beneficial. Traditional psychodynamic psychotherapies are often effective in alleviating symptoms of chronic anxiety. Psychotherapy should be conducted by clinicians with experience and expertise in this area.

When Is Referral to a Psychiatrist Indicated for Patients Presenting with Anxiety?

Clinicians evaluating and treating patients with anxiety in the ambulatory care setting must be able to recognize when referral for psychiatric consultation is indicated. In conjunction with the patient, careful consideration should be given to referral for psychotherapy prior to the initiation of pharmacologic agents. When there is any evidence of suicidal thoughts, the patient should be urgently referred for psychiatric evaluation, as well as when there is evidence of psychosis. When conservative or standard pharmacologic approaches do not relieve anxiety, the clinician should refer for further psychiatric intervention. If chronic use of benzodiazepines has been necessary for the treatment of anxiety, psychiatric consultation should be obtained. Anxiety caused by alcohol, benzodiazepine, or opioid withdrawal requires urgent attention, and hospitalization should be considered. When the etiology of anxiety remains unclear, primary care physicians should feel comfortable referring patients for psychiatric consultation.

Case

A 65-year-old woman comes to your office as a new patient, after moving from a neighboring state following the death of her husband several months ago. She has moved in with her daughter's family and will soon run out of her medications. Her past medical history is remarkable for hypothyroidism, diet-controlled hypertension, and mild asthma. Her current medications include levothyroxine and an albuterol inhaler. She denies current physical complaints. Near the end of the history, she mentions that she had started participating in a women's outreach group at the church across the street from your clinic, but had dropped out after about a month because she felt "too jittery to concentrate" on the group's activities. Further questioning reveals that she has been feeling tired, having difficulty falling asleep at night, and prefers to stay at home because of her jitteriness.

Physical examination reveals a healthy-appearing elderly woman with a concerned look on her face. Her blood pressure is 145/90 mm Hg and heart rate is 90 beats/min. Findings from the examination are unremarkable except for a mild fine tremor in her hands bilaterally. Neurologic examination is otherwise within normal limits. When her daughter is invited into the consulting room after the physical examination, she reports that her mother has seemed a little sad, nervous, slow, preoccupied, and forgetful since moving into her home, but she has attributed this to the recent death of her father, and she states, "it's been hard for everybody—I guess it's normal for mother to be having a hard time."

1. What is the differential diagnosis for this patient's symptoms of anxiety?
2. What evaluation and conservative treatments could be initiated?
3. Would referral to a psychiatrist or psychotherapist be useful?

Case Discussion

What Is the Differential Diagnosis for This Patient's Complaint of Anxiety?

When evaluating a patient with anxiety, the clinician must first distinguish between normal and pathologic types of anxiety. Anxiety can be a normal accompaniment of growth, change, new experiences, and finding one's own identity and meaning in life. Pathologic anxiety is an inappropriate response to a given stimulus by virtue of either its intensity or duration. The clinician must be aware of the differential diagnosis for pathologic anxiety, and also must be aware that anxiety can be a component of many medical conditions and other psychiatric disorders, especially depressive disorders.

In formulating a differential diagnosis for this patient's complaints, three categories should be considered: anxiety due to a general medical condition, anxiety due to substances (medications or substances of abuse), and anxiety due to a primary psychiatric condition. A thorough history and physical examination directs the investigation of potential medical illnesses that can cause anxiety. Two obvious conditions that must be considered in this patient are her history of thyroid disease and her postmenopausal status. The signs and symptoms of these conditions should be thoroughly reviewed. Other possible etiologies that must be considered are various medications and substances of abuse. The levothyroxine could clearly cause anxiety if administered in supraphysiologic doses. Further history should clarify the frequency of albuterol use, and its potential temporal relationship to anxiety symptoms. The patient should be questioned about any recent corticosteroid use for asthma or other conditions. Although the history reveals no evidence of substance abuse, all patients should be routinely asked about their use of caffeine, nicotine, alcohol, controlled prescription drugs, and illicit substances.

Several primary psychiatric illnesses should be considered in this patient. Major depressive disorder or subthreshold forms of depression must be considered due to the patient's recent significant psychosocial stressors (death of husband and move from former home) and several depressive symptoms, including anxiety, difficulty concentrating, social withdrawal and isolation, fatigue, and difficulty sleeping. Collateral history provided evidence of sad mood, psychomotor retardation, and forgetfulness. Primary anxiety disorders that should be considered include generalized anxiety disorder and social phobia. Further history should inquire about symptoms of panic attacks and obsessions. Other psychiatric disorders that should be considered include early dementia (and/or pseudodementia) and adjustment disorder with mixed anxiety and depressed mood.

What Evaluation and Conservative Treatments Could Be Initiated?

A thorough history should be gathered, including past psychiatric history. In the review of systems, the clinician should inquire about possible peripheral manifestations of anxiety associated with activation of the autonomic nervous system, including dizziness, elevated pulse, gastrointestinal complaints (such as diarrhea or upset stomach), hyperhidrosis, paresthesias, restlessness, syncope, tachypnea, and tremors. Psychological and cognitive symptoms also should be assessed, including feeling nervous or frightened, and experiencing distortions in perception, concentration, or memory. Suicidality should be thoroughly evaluated, and risk factors for suicide should be assessed.

A thorough physical examination should be performed. Laboratory tests should include thyroid function tests, a calcium level, and other screening as indicated by age and health status. Other commonly ordered tests in the evaluation of depression and anxiety include a complete blood count, screening syphilis serology such as the rapid plasma reagent test, and levels of vitamin B_{12} and folate.

Once a diagnosis of depression or generalized anxiety disorder is established, treatment should be initiated with an SSRI or SNRI. The medication dosage should be titrated upward to a standard dose, and treatment should continue for at least a month before its effectiveness is decided. The short-term use of a low dose of benzodiazepine may be considered, as can a trial of buspirone.

Would Referral to a Psychiatrist or Psychotherapist Be Useful?

Referral for individual psychotherapy may enhance the treatment outcome and provide additional relief of this patient's symptoms. An evaluation for psychotherapy should be conducted by an experienced psychotherapist. If the patient's illness is refractory to standard treatment with a first-line agent, referral to a psychiatrist should be considered. Also, if any evidence of psychosis or suicidality is discovered, referral should be made urgently.

Suggested Reading

American Psychiatric Association. *Diagnostic and statistical manual of mental disorders,* 4th ed revised. Washington, DC: American Psychiatric Association, 2000.

American Psychiatric Association. *Practice guideline for the treatment of patients with major depressive disorder,* revised ed. Washington, DC: American Psychiatric Association, 2000.

Kaplan H I, Sadock B J, eds. *Comprehensive textbook of psychiatry,* 7th ed. Baltimore: Williams & Wilkins, 2000.

Kessler R C, McGonagle K A, Zhao S, et al. Lifetime and 12-month prevalence of DSM-III-R psychiatric disorders in the United States: results from the National Comorbidity Survey. *Arch Gen Psychiatry* 1994;51:8–19.

Schatzberg A F, Nemeroff C B, eds. *The American Psychiatric Press textbook of psychopharmacology,* 2nd ed. Washington, DC: American Psychiatric Press, 1998.

74
Depression

Michael T. Compton
Andrew C. Furman

1. What are the elements of the clinical syndrome of depression?
2. How prevalent is depression in the general U.S. population?
3. What are the treatments of choice for depressive disorders?
4. When is referral to a psychiatrist indicated for patients presenting with depression?

Discussion

What Are the Elements of the Clinical Syndrome of Depression?

According to the *Diagnostic and Statistical Manual of Mental Disorders,* 4th Edition (DSM-IV), the diagnosis of a major depressive disorder depends on the presence of a major depressive episode, namely, at least a 2-week period of five or more symptoms that represent a change from previous functioning. At least one of these symptoms must be either depressed mood (a subjective or observed sense of feeling sad or depressed) or anhedonia (loss of interest or pleasure in activities previously experienced as pleasurable). Other potential symptoms include significant weight loss or weight gain (or decrease or increase in appetite), insomnia or hypersomnia, psychomotor agitation or retardation, fatigue or loss of energy, feelings of worthlessness or excessive/inappropriate guilt, diminished ability to think/concentrate or indecisiveness, and recurrent thoughts of death or suicide. The current diagnostic system is purely descriptive, although the pathophysiology of mood disorders is an area of intense research interest.

Major depressive disorder, single episode refers to the presence of a single major depressive episode whereas *major depressive disorder, recurrent* is used to describe a history of two or more episodes. Such distinctions are useful prognostically due to the increasing likelihood of future recurrence with each successive episode. *Dysthymic disorder* refers to a more chronic but milder form of depression, during which depressed mood exists for at least 2 years and two or more of the aforementioned depressive symptoms persist during this period of time. *Mood disorder due to a general medical condition* and s*ubstance-induced mood disorder* (with depressive features) occur when the depressive episode is the direct physiologic consequence of a general medical condition (such as hypothyroidism, Cushing disease, cerebrovascular accident, or neurosyphilis), a substance of abuse (e.g., cocaine withdrawal) of or as a side effect of a medication (such as older antihypertensives or corticosteroids). In addition to these diagnoses, a number of specifiers can be used to further describe the depressive episode, including those noting the presence of psychotic, catatonic, melancholic, and atypical features, an onset during the post-partum period, or episodes with a seasonal pattern. Depressive conditions also can be disguised by a multitude of somatic complaints or by a predominance of anxiety symptoms.

How Prevalent Is Depression in the General U.S. Population?

Affective disorders are highly prevalent illnesses that significantly impair function-ing, interpersonal relationships, and quality of life. The National Comorbidity Sur-vey interviewed over 8,000 individuals in the United States and found lifetime prevalence rates to be 17.1% for major depressive episode and 6.4% for dysthymia. These disorders underlie 50% to 70% of all cases of suicide, and individuals with serious depression (i.e., requiring hospitalization) have a 15% suicide rate. Epi-demiologic studies reveal that mood disorders are more prevalent among individu-als under the age of 45 (the average age of onset is 20–40 years). Nonetheless, de-pression in older adults is often unrecognized and undertreated. Women suffer from depressive episodes about twice as often as men—a sex difference that begins in early adolescence and persists into midlife. The prevalence of affective disorders does not vary significantly by race or ethnicity. Major depressive disorder appears to be more prevalent in urban residents, among single, divorced, or widowed peo-ple, among unemployed people, in those with a history of negative early childhood experiences, and in those with perceived social stresses. Affective disorders in gen-eral are also more prevalent in individuals with a family history of affective disor-ders, suicide, or alcoholism.

Abundant evidence reveals that many individuals with depression remain undi-agnosed and therefore untreated or inadequately treated. Clearly, due to the sig-nificant psychosocial impairment, disability, increased health-care utilization, and increased morbidity and mortality associated with depression, primary care physi-cians should be proficient in the evaluation and treatment of these disorders.

What Are the Treatments of Choice for Depressive Disorders?

Currently, the first-line treatment for depressive disorders consists of the use of se-lective serotonin reuptake inhibitors (SSRIs) and other newer antidepressants. Compared with the older antidepressant medications, including the monoamine ox-idase inhibitors and tricyclic antidepressants, the newer agents provide comparable efficacy at alleviating depressive symptoms, without the risk of lethality in over-dose and with a more favorable side effect profile. Although the SSRIs (fluoxetine, paroxetine, sertraline, fluvoxamine, and citalopram) and other newer antidepres-sants (venlafaxine XR, bupropion SR, nefazodone, and mirtazapine) are not devoid of side effects, they are easier to dose, provide equal efficacy compared with older agents, and are generally safe in overdose.

Adjunctive medications may be required when the depressive episode is complicated by the presence of psychotic symptoms or anxiety. Antipsychotic medications can usually be discontinued upon resolution of the associated delusions or hallucinations and once the depression is treated adequately to remission. Anxiolytics and hypnotic agents also should be prescribed only on a limited basis, and can usually be tapered and discontinued upon adequate treatment of the depression. When the depressive disorder is the result of a general medical condition or the use of a substance, the underlying disorder must be treated, although the use of antidepressant medications also may be indicated.

Psychotherapy should be considered in all cases of depression, and may be appropriate as monotherapy for cases of mild depression. Electroconvulsive therapy is a highly efficacious treatment for depression, although it is often reserved for depressive illnesses that are refractory to other treatments, are accompanied by psychotic features, are marked by serious suicidality, or are complicated by medical problems that preclude other treatments. Phototherapy may be useful, especially for depressions with a seasonal pattern. Other nonpharmacologic somatic therapies that are being studied include rapid transcranial magnetic stimulation and vagus nerve stimulation.

When Is Referral to a Psychiatrist Indicated for Patients Presenting with Depression?

Several factors warrant referral for psychiatric consultation during the treatment of patients with major depressive disorder. When the depressive episode is accompanied by psychotic features, psychiatric referral is indicated for consultation regarding the possible need for hospitalization and the use of additional medications. When the depressive episode is associated with suicidal thoughts, intent, plans, or attempts, urgent psychiatric evaluation should be obtained. In patients whose depressive episodes are refractory to standard first-line treatment, psychiatric consultation can be useful for assisting with pharmacologic augmentation strategies, for trials of older, more complicated antidepressant medications, for a potential trial of nonpharmacologic somatic treatments, as well as for the addition of psychotherapy. Referral is also indicated in complex cases in which comorbid substance use disorders, medical disorders, or other psychiatric disorders complicate the clinical picture.

Case

A 48-year-old woman has been seen in your office repeatedly over the past 2 months due to numerous vague complaints, including "aches and pains all over" and feeling too tired to accomplish her routine daily activities. Prior to your office visit with her today, she confides in the nurse that she feels like "a nervous wreck," that she cannot sleep at night, and that she no longer feels interested in sex with her husband. Open-ended questioning during your review of her complaints reveals that she has experienced significant anxiety, insomnia, and poor appetite over the past 6 months. She relates her feelings of sadness to an elective hysterectomy 8 months ago, which occurred just a week before her only daughter left home to go to college.

Further history reveals that she has never experienced similar episodes of sadness, and has never used significant alcohol or any other drugs. She does describe that her maternal grandmother had suffered from a "nervous breakdown" in her mid-fifties, and that a sister has a history of several psychiatric hospitalizations for manic-depressive disorder. Her medical history is noncontributory except for the recent hysterectomy for uterine fibroids. She does not take medications, although she has recently tried several nonprescribed herbal remedies for anxiety and insomnia. Her physical examination is normal, although she is noted to have a worried look on her face and to have frequent hand-wringing movements. Her speech is somewhat slow, and she has an increased latency of response, sometimes asking, "I'm sorry, what was your question again?" A thorough laboratory evaluation over the past 2 months has not revealed significant abnormalities.

1. What is the differential diagnosis for this patient's depressive symptoms?
2. What evaluation and conservative treatments could be initiated?
3. What is the relationship between anxiety and depression in this patient?

Case Discussion
What Is the Differential Diagnosis for This Patient's Depressive Symptoms?

The diagnosis of depression relies on the subjective report of the patient's symptoms along with the clinician's objective assessment of history and mental status examination. Several other potential diagnoses should be excluded before initiating treatment. First, any general medical conditions that could be causing the patient's complaints should be ruled-out. Such conditions include endocrinopathies (hypothyroidism, hyperthyroidism, parathyroid disorders, Cushing's syndrome, and surgically-induced menopause), neurological disorders (cerebrovascular accidents, central nervous system lesions, neurosyphilis, multiple sclerosis, neurosarcoidosis, and vasculitis), and other miscellaneous disorders (vitamin deficiencies, anemia, hypoxia, end-stage renal disease, systemic lupus erythematosus and other connective tissue diseases, occult malignancy such as pancreatic cancer, and HIV-associated central nervous system pathology). Most of these disorders can be easily excluded based on the history and physical examination alone. Entities such as menopause and thyroid disorders may need further evaluation. A second category within the differential diagnoses would be depressive disorders due to substances, either prescribed or substances of abuse. A careful medication and substance use history can usually exclude these possibilities.

Once these categories of depressive illnesses are excluded, a third category, that of primary psychiatric disorders, can be considered. Due to the depressive symptoms elicited by the interview, the most likely diagnosis is major depressive disorder, single episode. The family history of bipolar disorder and "nervous breakdown" (possibly major depression) also supports the likelihood of the patient developing a major depressive episode. The clinician should carefully rule out primary anxiety disorders (acute stress disorder, generalized anxiety disorder, obsessive-compulsive disorder, panic disorder, posttraumatic stress disorder, social phobia). In obtaining the history, the patient should be questioned about any past symptoms consistent with hypomania or mania. In doing so, the possibility of a bipolar depression (a major depressive episode in a patient with a history of hypomania or mania) can be excluded. The first-line treatment of bipolar depression (a mood stabilizer such as lithium) is different from the usual treatment of unipolar depression.

What Evaluation and Conservative Treatments Could Be Initiated?

The most important aspects of the evaluation of this depressive episode are a thorough history, mental status examination, and physical examination. Collateral history from a source close to the patient can also be useful in exploring the patient's current depressive symptoms and any past history of psychiatric syndromes. Important findings on the mental status examination might include diminished eye contact, stooped posture, hand-wringing, psychomotor slowing or agitation, increased response latency, decreased rate and rhythm of speech, depressed or anxious mood, tearful or blunted affect, slow thought processes, as well as thought content that is remarkable for excessive guilt, feelings of worthlessness, helplessness or hopelessness, mood-congruent psychotic features, and suicidal ideation. General cognition also might be slow, with impairment in attention, concentration, and memory. As part of the evaluation of depression, a thorough history of past and recent suicidal thoughts, intent, plans, and actions should be obtained. Routine screening laboratory studies to exclude potential medical causes of the depression include complete blood count, basic chemistries, urinalysis, urine drug screen, thyroid stimulating hormone, syphilis serology, levels of vitamin B_{12} and folate, and HIV testing. Other tests should be ordered as indicated, including other laboratory studies or imaging studies of the brain.

The possibility of hormone replacement therapy should be discussed with the patient. Although some of the complaints presented could be due to her possible surgically-induced menopausal status, this is unlikely to account physiologically for the full depressive syndrome. Once the diagnosis of major depressive disorder is confirmed, treatment should be initiated with an SSRI or other newer antidepressant medication. The goal of treatment is full remission of the depressive symptoms. If a partial remission is attained after an adequate trial (4–6 weeks), the dose of the antidepressant should be optimized. If further response is attained, but with less than a full remission, an augmentation strategy can be considered. If the antidepressant does not provide even a partial response, another agent from a different class should be tried. Further refractoriness should prompt psychiatric consultation. Once full remission is achieved, the patient should be continued on the dose of antidepressant used in the acute phase for 16 to 20 weeks (the continuation phase of treatment) to prevent relapse. After this point the antidepressant can be gradually tapered and eventually discontinued, although patients with a history of several episodes or a past severe episode should be continued with maintenance therapy to prevent recurrence of future episodes.

The patient also should be informed about the potential utility of psychotherapy as a monotherapy for a mild depression or as adjunctive therapy for moderate to severe depression. This patient might find psychotherapy beneficial, especially to explore issues related to loss (the recent hysterectomy and the departure of her daughter for college), impairment in role performance and social functioning, and her significant depressive and anxiety symptoms.

What Is the Relationship Between Anxiety and Depression in This Patient?

Depression and anxiety often coexist. A full exploration of both sets of symptoms should be conducted in order to establish the temporal relationship between the syndromes and to rule out any formal comorbidity (e.g., major depressive disorder and panic disorder). An anxiolytic medication is often useful (such as a low dose of clonazapam, a long-acting benzodiazepine), especially around the initiation of treatment with an antidepressant. Once the effects of the antidepressant become noticeable, the anxiety symptoms will often abate as the depression improves. The anxiolytic should then be tapered and discontinued. SSRIs and other newer antidepressants are efficacious in the treatment of many primary anxiety disorders (generalized anxiety disorder, obsessive-compulsive disorder, panic disorder, posttraumatic stress disorder, social phobia) as well as depression. Of special importance is the fact that anxiety associated with the depression is a recognized risk factor for suicide in the depressed individual. This provides further support for the recommendation to monitor and treat the associated anxiety.

Suggested Reading

American Psychiatric Association. *Diagnostic and statistical manual of mental disorders,* 4th ed, text revision. Washington, DC: American Psychiatric Association, 2000.

American Psychiatric Association. *Practice guideline for the treatment of patients with major depressive disorder,* revised ed. Washington, DC: American Psychiatric Association, 2000.

Kaplan H I, Sadock B J, eds. *Comprehensive textbook of psychiatry,* 7th ed. Baltimore: Williams & Wilkins, 2000.

Kessler R C, McGonagle K A, Zhao S, et al. Lifetime and 12-month prevalence of DSM-III-R psychiatric disorders in the United States: results from the National Comorbidity Survey. *Arch Gen Psychiatry* 1994;51:8–19.

Schatzberg A F, Nemeroff C B, eds. *The American Psychiatric Press textbook of psychopharmacology,* 2nd ed. Washington, DC: American Psychiatric Press, 1998.

75
Psychosis

Michael T. Compton
Andrew C. Furman

- Discussion   *470*
- Case   *474*
- Case Discussion   *474*

1. What is psychosis?
2. What is the differential diagnosis for psychosis in the ambulatory medicine setting?
3. What are the current treatments for psychotic disorders?
4. What is the course and prognosis for psychotic disorders?

Discussion
What Is Psychosis?

Psychosis is a syndrome characterized by a gross impairment in reality testing. Such impairment means that individuals incorrectly evaluate the accuracy of their perceptions and thoughts, and make incorrect inferences about external reality, even in the face of contrary evidence. Psychosis is marked by the presence of delusions, hallucinations, or paranoia without insight into their pathological nature. Grossly disorganized speech or disorganized or catatonic behavior is also suggestive of psychosis. Psychosis should not be considered a specific diagnosis. Rather, the syndrome of psychosis can be associated with several psychiatric, medical, and substance-induced disorders.

What Is the Differential Diagnosis for Psychosis in the Ambulatory Medicine Setting?

Currently, psychiatric diagnosis is informed by the fourth edition of the *Diagnostic and Statistical Manual of Mental Disorders* (DSM-IV). Therein, the primary psychotic disorders are classified under the section "schizophrenia and other psychotic disorders." The various diagnoses in this category will be briefly reviewed. Psychosis also can be a secondary phenomenon, due to other disorders. The DSM-IV also provides diagnoses for these cases of secondary psychosis.

Schizophrenia is the prototypical primary psychotic disorder. According to current descriptive nosology, it is characterized by the presence of two or more psychotic symptoms such as delusions, hallucinations, disorganized speech (derailment, loose associations, or tangentiality), grossly disorganized or catatonic behavior, and negative symptoms (such as affective flattening, poverty of speech, and avolition). If certain psychotic symptoms are present (bizarre delusions, hallucinations of running commentary on the person's behavior, or two or more voices conversing with one another), only one of such symptoms is required, because these are considered to be particularly characteristic of schizophrenia. Continuous signs of a disturbance must persist for at least 6 months, and one or more areas of functioning must be markedly below the level achieved prior to the onset. Schizophrenia is further classified into paranoid, disorganized, catatonic, undifferentiated, and residual subtypes, depending on the specific constellation of symptoms present. The psychotic disorder is called *schizophreniform disorder* when the episode lasts at least a month, but less than 6 months. Although a decline in functioning is not a required criterion, patients diagnosed with schizophreniform disorder often progress to schizophrenia.

In *schizoaffective disorder,* a mood episode (major depressive episode, manic episode, or mixed episode) and the active-phase symptoms of schizophrenia occur together and are preceded or followed by at least 2 weeks of delusions or hallucinations without prominent mood symptoms. *Delusional disorder* is characterized by at least 1 month of nonbizarre delusions without other active-phase symptoms of schizophrenia. Unlike in schizophrenia, apart from the impact of the delusions, functioning is not markedly impaired and behavior is not obviously odd or bizarre. *Brief psychotic disorder* consists of psychotic symptoms that last at least 1 day but less than 1 month, with eventual full return to baseline functioning. The disorder may be related to severe stressors (brief reactive psychosis) and may have postpartum onset. *Shared psychotic disorder* is characterized by the presence of a delusion in an individual who is influenced by someone else who has a longer standing delusion with similar content.

Psychotic disorder due to a general medical condition indicates that the psychosis is physiologically related to a medical disturbance, and the primary treatment is therefore directed toward the underlying medical disorder. Many medical conditions can be associated with psychosis, including acquired immune deficiency syndrome, acute intermittent porphyria, carbon monoxide poisoning, central nervous system lesions (neoplasm, stroke, trauma), dementia, heavy metal poisoning, herpes encephalitis, homocystinuria, Huntington's disease, neurosarcoidosis, neurosyphilis, seizures (especially temporal lobe epilepsy), systemic lupus erythematosus, vitamin deficiencies, and Wilson's disease.

Substance-induced psychotic disorder describes psychosis that is a direct physiologic consequence of a drug of abuse, a medication, or toxin exposure. Intoxication or withdrawal from substances such as alcohol, amphetamines, barbiturates and benzodiazepines, cocaine, hallucinogens, and phencyclidine or ketamine can be the cause of psychosis. In some individuals, corticosteroids can cause psychotic and affective symptoms, as can medications associated with delirium (such as anticholinergics and opioids).

Several other psychiatric diagnoses must be included in the differential diagnosis of psychosis. These include delirium, dementia, pervasive developmental disorders of childhood such as autistic disorder, mood disorders accompanied by psychotic features, factitious disorders, dissociative disorders, culture-bound syndromes, and certain personality disorders. The distinction between primary psychotic disorders such as schizophrenia and primary mood disorders such as major depressive disorder or bipolar disorder accompanied by psychotic features is especially important, due to differences in treatment strategies and in prognosis between these two classes of disorders.

What Are the Current Treatments for Psychotic Disorders?

The treatment of psychosis currently involves several modalities. The mainstay of treatment consists of antipsychotic medications. The traditional agents are called conventional antipsychotics, which were previously termed neuroleptics due to their ability to induce neurologic side effects. These are commonly referred to as extrapyramidal side effects and include akathisia (an inner sense of restlessness), acute dystonia such as torticollis and oculogyric crisis, and parkinsonian features, including rigidity, tremor, bradykinesia, masked facies, and shuffling gait. Serious adverse events include irreversible tardive dyskinesia and the potentially lethal neuroleptic malignant syndrome. These medications act by antagonism of dopamine D_2 receptors, which is presumably related to their antipsychotic effect.

Newer medications used to treat psychosis are called atypical antipsychotics, and include four currently available agents approved by the U.S. Food and Drug Administration: clozapine, risperidone, olanzapine, and quetiapine. Clozapine is indicated only for treatment-refractory psychosis due to the 1% to 2% risk of agranulocytosis, therefore necessitating weekly monitoring of blood counts. Atypical agents have significant antagonist activity at the serotonin 5-HT_2 receptor as well as at the D_2 receptor, they are more efficacious for treating the negative symptoms of psychosis, and they are associated with less incidence of extrapyramidal side effects and tardive dyskinesia, and less elevation in prolactin concentrations (though this is not true for risperidone) at standard doses, compared with conventional agents.

The atypical antipsychotics risperidone, olanzapine, and quetiapine are currently the first-line treatment for psychosis. Conventional agents should only be used in cases of intolerance to atypical agents, better demonstrated response to conventional than atypical agents, or strong patient preference, and only when the patient understands the risks (especially the cumulative risk of tardive dyskinesia), benefits, and alternatives. Other agents may be used adjunctively, such as mood stabilizers, antidepressants, and benzodiazepines.

Certain psychosocial interventions, including community, supportive, and rehabilitative services, should also be incorporated into the treatment of psychosis. These treatment modalities have been studied mostly in the context of the schizophrenia spectrum disorders. Psychoeducation of the patient, family, and friends is an important aspect of treatment. Other important forms of psychosocial interventions include case management, social skills training, stress reduction and coping strategies training, family therapy, individual psychotherapy, assertive community treatment, day treatment programs, vocational rehabilitation, supportive housing, and referral to organizations supporting and advocating for family, friends, and patients affected by mental illness, such as the National Alliance for the Mentally Ill (NAMI).

Treatment planning must be tailored around the unique individual, family, social, and psychological profile of each patient with a psychotic disorder. Such treatment planning is best performed through the cooperation of an interdisciplinary team, including psychiatrists, psychologists, social workers, recreation therapists, and vocational rehabilitation therapists, along with involvement from family members. Treatment plans may vary depending on the phase (acute, stabilization, stable phases) and severity of illness.

Hospitalization is sometimes necessary for stabilization on medications, to provide safety from suicidal or homicidal impulses, when grossly disorganized behavior impairs the ability to adequately care for one's basic needs, or for diagnostic purposes. Involuntary hospitalization may be indicated if patients refuse voluntary admission and if the requirements of the local jurisdiction are met. During hospitalization, patients must be appropriately connected with outpatient services in an effort to prevent noncompliance and loss to follow-up after discharge.

What Is the Course and Prognosis for Psychotic Disorders?

In the United States, the lifetime prevalence of schizophrenia is approximately 1%. The peak ages of onset are 15 to 25 for men and 25 to 35 for women. Premorbid symptoms (such as quiet, passive, and introverted personalities, mild negative symptoms, and eccentricities of thought) characteristically begin in adolescence, followed by the development of prodromal symptoms in the months preceding the first episode of frank psychosis. Prodromal symptoms include social withdrawal, loss of interests, deterioration of hygiene and grooming, peculiar behavior, abnormal affects, outbursts of anger, unusual speech, bizarre ideas, and strange perceptual experiences. The onset of psychotic symptoms may be preceded by a social or environmental stressor such as moving away to college or family turmoil.

After a first episode of psychosis, a gradual recovery may be followed by a period of relatively normal functioning. However, the usual course of schizophrenia is one of exacerbations and remissions of psychotic symptoms, without a return to premorbid functioning after relapses. The severity of negative symptoms often increases over time, and subtle cognitive impairments may accumulate, both of which contribute to the frequent occurrence of downward social drift, such as unemployment and homelessness. The negative symptoms of schizophrenia account for a significant portion of the psychosocial morbidity associated with the disorder. Many patients with schizophrenia have increased morbidity and mortality due to medical conditions compared with the general population, in part due to poor health behaviors and the difficulty engaging these patients in traditional medical settings. Suicide is a significant risk and is a common cause of death among patients with schizophrenia—approximately 10% die by suicide, and 20% to 40% attempt suicide at least once during their illness.

Schizophrenia usually carries a worse prognosis than mood disorders, which have more episodic courses with return to baseline functioning between episodes. Many patients with schizophrenia remain significantly impaired by the disorder for their entire lives, requiring comprehensive and continuous care. Good prognostic features include female gender, rapid onset of symptoms, confusion or perplexity at the height of the psychotic episode, good premorbid social and occupational functioning, higher IQ, absence of blunted or flat affect, later age of onset, obvious precipitating factors, depressive symptoms or family history of mood disorders, being married or having good support systems, and predominance of positive symptoms.

The prognosis for psychotic individuals is often much better when the psychosis is associated with other disorders, such as delirium, major depressive disorder, medical conditions, or substance intoxication. In these instances, once the psychosis clears or is adequately treated, return to baseline functioning should be attainable by fully treating the underlying disorder.

Case

A 28-year-old man comes to your office as a new patient, due to the complaint of headaches. He has a history of lymphoma at the age of 18, for which he was treated with chemotherapy. His disease has been in full remission since then. He has no other significant past medical history. Over the past six months, he has noticed dull headaches and difficulty sleeping at night. On further questioning about the details of the headaches, he appears increasingly suspicious and whispers, "I think they're messing with me." When you ask for clarification, he indicates that his co-workers at the warehouse where he works are planning to try to get him fired, and he seems to relate the headaches to this belief. He denies any other physical complaints and refuses to talk further about his beliefs and fears, because he suspects that people might use his medical record to support the plot to get him fired. He denies taking any medications. When asked about drug use, he states that he has been smoking increasing amounts of marijuana in an effort to calm his mind.

Physical examination reveals an unshaven young man with poor hygiene, and with very poor eye contact during the interview. His vital signs are normal, and his physical examination is unremarkable. Neurologic examination is nonfocal, but he seems to have some difficulty cooperating with rapid alternating movement and peripheral visual field testing. He is unwilling to keep his eyes closed for the Romberg test. When his aunt, with whom he lives, is contacted by telephone for collateral history, she reports that the patient actually lost his job 2 months ago. For about the past 4 months, he has tended to stay in his room, and she has heard him talking to himself at night, while he is unable to sleep. She reports that he has never been married, and has lived with her since his mother had a nervous breakdown when the patient was 10 years old. She is unsure about his recent drug use.

1. What is the differential diagnosis for this patient's psychotic symptoms?
2. What other symptoms should be reviewed when gathering history from this patient and his family?
3. What evaluation and treatment should be initiated?

Case Discussion

What Is the Differential Diagnosis for This Patient's Psychotic Symptoms?

When evaluating this patient's new onset of psychosis, three general categories of disorders should be considered. First, the clinician must rule out any underlying general medical conditions that could be causing the psychosis. Given his past history of lymphoma, a central nervous system recurrence of this disease should be seriously considered, especially due to the chief complaint of headaches. Other conditions, such as neurosyphilis, seizure disorder, and endocrinopathy should also be considered. Second, this patient's psychosis could be caused or exacerbated by substance use. Although he endorses the use of marijuana, which may be associated with paranoia in some individuals, one should consider the use of other substances in this presentation. Third, primary psychiatric disorders associated with psychosis should be considered. These include schizophreniform disorder, major depressive disorder with psychotic features, and bipolar disorder with psychotic features. His poor eye contact, withdrawal, and social isolation are signs that could represent depressive symptoms or negative symptoms of a primary psychotic disorder.

What Other Symptoms Should Be Reviewed When Gathering History from This Patient and His Family?

A thorough longitudinal history should be gathered, especially regarding the course of the patient's headaches, suspiciousness and paranoia, delusions, sleep difficulty, social withdrawal, poor hygiene, and talking to himself (which likely represents responding to internal stimuli, or the experience of auditory hallucinations). Such history should be obtained from both the patient and from at least one other collateral source. Social history should include a thorough developmental history, substance use history, legal history, and history of peer relationships and academic, social, and occupational functioning. The details of his mother's psychiatric illness should be obtained, as well as any other family medical and psychiatric history. A thorough review of systems, mental status examination, and Mini-mental status examination should be performed.

A psychiatric review of systems will help to define further the differential diagnosis. The patient and a collateral source should be questioned about depressive symptoms, symptoms of anxiety, and other psychotic symptoms (hallucinations, other delusions, ideas of reference, disorganized or bizarre thoughts or behaviors, and negative symptoms). The occurrence of any recent social stressors also should be reviewed.

What Evaluation and Treatment Should Be Initiated?

The clinician should try to establish and maintain a supportive therapeutic alliance. The patient should also be referred for psychiatric consultation for an evaluation of first-episode psychosis. Indicated laboratory tests include blood counts, chemistries, urinalysis, screening syphilis serology, thyroid function tests, urine drug screen, and levels of vitamins including B_{12} and folate. Other laboratory tests may need to be obtained depending on the full history and physical. An imaging study of the brain, such as computed tomography or magnetic resonance imaging, should be obtained. An electroencephalogram should be considered, especially if further history reveals an episodic nature to the psychosis or the association of motor symptoms. A full psychiatric assessment is indicated, and a battery of psychological testing may be warranted.

In addition to the psychiatric assessment, the patient should begin treatment with an antipsychotic medication. First-line treatment would consist of an atypical antipsychotic: risperidone, olanzapine, or quetiapine. The minimum length of an antipsychotic trial is 4 to 6 weeks at an adequate dosage. If unsuccessful, a trial with another antipsychotic can be tried. The patient should then be maintained on the lowest possible effective dosage. Psychoeducation and the importance of compliance must be provided. Long-acting depot forms of conventional antipsychotics are sometimes necessary (haloperidol or fluphenazine decanoate), especially when noncompliance is an ongoing problem. The psychiatrist should initiate appropriate psychosocial treatment strategies, including psychoeducation, supportive psychotherapy, and connecting the patient with social services and rehabilitative services, especially if the patient is diagnosed with a primary psychotic disorder.

Suggested Reading

American Psychiatric Association. *Diagnostic and statistical manual of mental disorders,* 4th ed, revised. Washington, DC: American Psychiatric Association, 2000.

American Psychiatric Association. *Practice guideline for the treatment of patients with schizophrenia.* Washington, DC: American Psychiatric Association, 1997.

Kaplan H I, Sadock B J, eds. *Comprehensive textbook of psychiatry,* 7th ed. Baltimore: Williams & Wilkins, 2000.

McEvoy J P, Scheifler P L, Frances A. The expert consensus guideline series: treatment of schizophrenia 1999. *J Clin Psychiatry* 1999;60(suppl 11):1–80.

Schatzberg A F, Nemeroff C B, eds. *The American Psychiatric Press textbook of psychopharmacology,* 2nd ed. Washington, DC: American Psychiatric Press, 1998.

XIII
Pulmonology

76

Chronic Obstructive Pulmonary Disease

Gerald W. Staton
Adam N. Strozier

1. How do you define chronic obstructive pulmonary disease?
2. What is the role of chest radiography and pulmonary function studies in the evaluation of chronic obstructive pulmonary disease?
3. What are the benefits of smoking cessation?
4. What drugs are available for the treatment of chronic obstructive pulmonary disease? How and when are they used?
5. Is home oxygen beneficial in chronic obstructive pulmonary disease? What are the criteria for prescribing home oxygen and how is it prescribed?
6. What other treatment modalities are available?

Discussion

How Do You Define Chronic Obstructive Pulmonary Disease?

Chronic obstructive pulmonary disease (COPD) comprises two distinct types of smoking-related lung pathophysiology, each defined in different terms. Chronic bronchitis is defined by the presence of cough for 3 months at a time in each of 2 consecutive years. It is characterized by hypersecretion of mucus and airway inflammation with foci of squamous metaplasia of the respiratory epithelium. Emphysema, on the other hand, is a pathologic diagnosis, characterized by the destruction of the alveolar attachments to blood vessels and bronchioles, with resultant dilation of the alveoli and compression of airways. Although both processes likely occur together in the majority of patients, some will present with signs and symptoms of emphysema alone, such as slowly progressive dyspnea on exertion without productive cough or cyanosis.

What Is the Role of Chest Radiography and Pulmonary Function Studies in the Evaluation of Chronic Obstructive Pulmonary Disease?

Although hyperinflated lungs and bullous changes suggesting emphysema may be present on chest radiography, this modality is not sensitive for diagnosing COPD. Because right heart failure is a complication of end-stage COPD, radiographs can be used to look for right ventricular enlargement and distended hila suggestive of pulmonary hypertension in patients with elevated neck veins, an S_3, or lower extremity edema. The most important role of the chest radiograph lies in helping to exclude other cardiopulmonary diseases that may be contributing to the patient's symptoms.

Pulmonary function tests (PFTs) can assist in determining the severity of airflow obstruction and assessing bronchodilator response. There are three parts to PFTs: spirometry measures the speed with which air escapes the lungs during expiration, lung volumes measure the amount of trapped air after expiration, and the lung's diffusing capacity for carbon monoxide (DLCO) approximates oxygen transfer from the alveolus to the blood. Obstruction is signified by a decrease in the amount of air flowing out through the tracheobronchial tree in the first second of forced expiration, also known as the FEV_1. Air trapping, or hyperinflation, manifests itself as a high residual volume, the amount of air in the lungs after complete, forced expiration. Loss of alveoli from the destructive inflammatory processes in patients with emphysema results in a low DLCO.

Although not essential to the diagnosis of COPD, PFTs provide a baseline against which to compare future measurements, allowing the clinician to gauge the effectiveness of pharmacotherapy and smoking cessation on lung function. They are also helpful in diagnosing otherwise occult causes of cough and dyspnea, such as interstitial lung disease. In addition, patients with an FEV_1 that is less than 35% of the predicted value should have arterial oxygenation assessed, because they may derive a significant mortality benefit from oxygen therapy if their oxygenation is low. Oxygenation can be measured directly by pulse oximetry in the office, or arterial blood gas measurements can be performed with PFTs.

What Are the Benefits of Smoking Cessation?

It is paramount to impress on patients that no intervention is likely to be as effective as smoking cessation in the treatment of COPD. Unfortunately, this remains one of the most daunting tasks of the primary care provider. COPD is progressive in patients who continue to smoke. The rate of decline in lung function returns to normal in patients who quit smoking. Smoking cessation rates roughly double with the use of nicotine replacement or the antidepressant bupropion.

What Drugs Are Available for Treatment of Chronic Obstructive Pulmonary Disease? How and When Are They Used?

It is a matter of some debate as to how much of the airflow obstruction in COPD is reversible. There is undoubtedly only a minimal improvement as measured by spirometry with use of either anticholinergic or β_2-agonist bronchodilators. However, improvement in symptoms of dyspnea and reduction in hyperinflation commonly occur with use of these agents. Starting an anticholinergic inhaler (ipratropium bromide) at two to four puffs three or four times daily may give symptomatic relief. The anticholinergic agents act as bronchodilators, presumably because patients with COPD can have increased vagal tone. Patients, and even some clinicians, view ipratropium as an "as needed" medication, similar to the role of albuterol in asthma. On the contrary, it has a relatively long onset of action as well as half-life, and thus should be prescribed at regular dosing intervals for best effect. A once-daily inhalational anticholinergic, tiotropium, is currently being studied. Studies have shown that adding a β-agonist to the anticholinergic provides additional bronchodilation compared with either drug alone. As is well known, β_2-agonists such as albuterol are quick in onset of action and may be prescribed for use as needed. Long-acting β_2-agonists, such as salmeterol, have the obvious advantage of less frequent dosing intervals.

With the advent of inhalational corticosteroids, there was initial hope that these agents would be as useful in COPD as in asthma. This enthusiasm has not been borne out by trials. Although airway inflammation plays a role in both disease entities, that in COPD is largely macrophage and neutrophil mediated, with few eosinophils, in contrast to asthma. Inhaled steroids have demonstrated no effect on the decline in lung function in COPD, even at high doses. There is some evidence that systemic steroids may provide modest benefit in acute exacerbations of COPD, although with greater risk for toxicity.

Sustained-release oral preparations of the phosphodiesterase inhibitor theophylline have bronchodilator properties, and have been shown to improve respiratory muscle function in COPD patients, and hence exercise tolerance. Unfortunately, theophylline has a narrow therapeutic window, and toxic levels can cause nausea, vomiting, lethal ventricular arrhythmias, and exacerbation of apparent or occult epilepsy. Patients with persistent symptoms on maximal anticholinergic and β_2-agonist therapy may nevertheless benefit from theophylline at a dose of 200 to 400 mg twice daily. Heart failure and cardiac arrhythmias often accompany advanced COPD, and theophylline levels must therefore be followed closely. Intercurrent respiratory infections, hepatic congestion, hepatitis, and a number of antibiotics can raise theophylline levels above the therapeutic range of 8 to 12 mg/mL, and may necessitate dose reductions.

Antiobiotics aimed at common respiratory pathogens such as *Haemophilus influenzae*, *Streptococcus pneumoniae*, and *Mycoplasma pneumoniae* should be considered in patients who present with exacerbations of their symptoms, especially in the presence of fever, leukocytosis, or change in sputum character. All patients with COPD should be offered the Pneumovax (Merck & Co.; Whitehouse Station, NJ) as well as the flu shot in the fall.

Is Home Oxygen Beneficial in Chronic Obstructive Pulmonary Disease? What Are the Criteria for Prescribing Home Oxygen and How Is It Prescribed?

Patients who have an arterial oxygen concentration of less than 55 mm Hg, corresponding to a pulse oximetry reading of less than 88%, should receive oxygen therapy, because it has been proven to reduce mortality and improve quality of life in these patients. Oxygen therapy is expensive, so insurance coverage is very impoortant. The Medicare criteria for home O_2 are: a PaO_2 of less than or equal to 55 mm Hg, corresponding to a saturation of less than 88%, or PaO_2 of 55 to 60 mm Hg (corresponding to a saturation of 88%–90%) with evidence of right heart failure. Patients with hypoxemia at night or during exercise also may benefit from home oxygen. Patients should be strongly cautioned against changing their oxygen flow rates without direct supervision of the prescribing provider, because this may induce carbon dioxide–induced narcosis and hypopnea.

What Other Treatment Modalities Are Available?

It has recently become clear that the inflammatory derangements that occur in COPD are not confined to the lung, and that inflammatory mediators such as tumor necrosis factor-α circulate in these patients, resulting in constitutional symptoms, usually the most marked of which is weight loss. Patients also suffer with weakness over and above their dyspnea, attributable to skeletal muscle wasting. Often overlooked therapeutic avenues in COPD are dietary counseling and exercise training. Exercise improves oxygen extraction, and thus reduces the mechanical burden on the heart and respiratory muscles for any given workload. Referral should be made to an exercise physiologist or physical therapist with experience in the field. Serial weight measurements and nutrition referral (when warranted by resistant weight loss) should be instituted in all patients.

A recently published trial has demonstrated improvement in FEV_1 with lung volume reduction surgery in patients with severe emphysema. Resection of diseased apical segments is thought to allow the relatively normal, remaining lung tissue to expand, thus improving airflow. Patients with end-stage COPD and age under 65, or with a family history of early-onset COPD, should be considered for lung transplantation. Despite the risks of surgery and immunosuppression, overall survival in these patients is improved.

Case

A 58-year-old female nurse presents for a checkup. She reports being healthy and takes no medicines, but on review of systems, she admits to a daily productive cough for the past few years. She also reports missing work three times last year for acute bronchitis, treated with antibiotics. A chest radiograph during her last bout of bronchitis 4 months ago was interpreted as normal. She has noted decreased exercise tolerance over the past year or two but has had no other decline in functional status. She denies hemoptysis, chest pain, orthopnea, paroxysmal nocturnal dyspnea, or lower extremity claudication. Her weight has been stable at 110 pounds. She denies nasal discharge or congestion, or heartburn. She has smoked about 1½ packs of cigarettes daily for 35 to 40 years but does not use alcohol or drugs. She works full time as a nurse in a private office. Her family history is significant for hypertension in her mother. She reports no allergies and medication use. On physical examination, she is a slim female seated comfortably with no use of accessory respiratory muscles. Her blood pressure is 134/78 mm Hg, pulse is 74 beats/min and regular, respiratory rate is 14 breaths/min, and she is afebrile. Her nasal mucosa are normal, as is her oropharynx. She has no lymphadenopathy, thyromegaly, or carotid bruits. On cardiovascular examination, her apical impulse is palpable and nondisplaced; no murmurs, rubs, or gallops are audible. A lung examination demonstrates diffuse mild inspiratory and expiratory wheezes, with slight prolongation of the expiratory phase. Her abdominal examination is unremarkable, and her extremities showed good pulses, and no cyanosis, clubbing, or edema.

1. Does this patient have chronic obstructive pulmonary disease?
2. Would you order a chest radiograph, pulmonary function tests, or other tests?
3. What treatment would you recommend?

Case Discussion

Does This Patient Have Chronic Obstructive Pulmonary Disease?

With a greater than 50 pack per year smoking history, chronic cough, and clinical symptoms, it is likely this patient has developed COPD with chronic bronchitis. Other common etiologies for chronic cough seem less likely. For example, the absence of symptoms of heartburn that is worse with recumbency makes gastroesophageal reflux disease less likely. Absence of coryza and normal-appearing nasal mucosa excludes active rhinitis. She has no symptoms suggestive of postnasal drip or sinusitis. Asthma is usually diagnosed in childhood or early adulthood, making a reactive component to COPD the more likely etiology of the wheezing found on examination. Congestive heart failure is unlikely in our patient given the absence of orthopnea or paroxysmal nocturnal dyspnea by history and lack of elevated jugular venous pressure, a third heart sound, or peripheral edema on physical examination. The lack of chest pain associated with physical activity significantly reduces but does not eliminate the possibility of underlying atherosclerotic heart disease as a contributor to reduced exercise tolerance.

Would You Order a Chest Radiograph, Pulmonary Function Tests, or Other Tests?

A good quality chest radiograph would be warranted to evaluate her cough and decreased exercise tolerance if she has not had one recently. PFTs would be helpful to assess the degree of obstruction, and office pulse oximetry would be useful for an oxygenation assessment. Other tests that should be considered are a hemoglobin level to look for anemia as a cause of decreased exercise tolerance or erythrocytosis as a sign of severe hypoxemia. A cardiovascular risk assessment, including a detailed family history and a fasting lipid profile, is reasonable because of her age and because smoking is a strong risk factor for atherosclerosis. An osteoporosis assessment is also reasonable because she is slim and postmenopausal, and because tobacco accelerates bone loss.

What Treatment Would You Recommend?

Smoking cessation is the most important intervention you can offer her and may require both behavioral counseling and pharmacotherapy. Exercise training and nutritional counseling would be useful life-style interventions. Performing an exercise stress test prior to initiating an exercise program should be considered. Starting an anticholinergic inhaler, ipratropium bromide, at two to four puffs three or four times daily is reasonable for symptomatic relief. Yearly vaccination against influenza and administration of the pneumococcal vaccination is also warranted.

Suggested Reading

Barnes P J. Medical progress: chronic obstructive pulmonary disease. *N Engl J Med* 2000;343:4.

Celli B R et al. American thoracic society standards for the diagnosis and care of patients with chronic obstructive pulmonary disease. *J Respir Crit Care Med* 1995;152(suppl):S77–S120.

Crapo R O. Current concepts: pulmonary-function testing. *N Engl J Med* 1994;331:4.

Ferguson G T, Cherniak R M. Current concepts: management of chronic obstructive pulmonary disease. *N Engl J Med* 1993;328:14.

77

Acute Bronchitis and Acute Exacerbations of Chronic Obstructive Pulmonary Disease

Daniel D. Dressler

1. What are the clinical characteristics of acute bronchitis and acute exacerbations of chronic obstructive pulmonary disease?
2. What are the causes and what alternative diagnoses should be considered?
3. What evidence is available for the use of antibiotics in either situation?
4. What other therapeutic modalities should be used when treating acute bronchitis in an otherwise healthy patient versus an acute exacerbation of chronic obstructive pulmonary disease?

Discussion

What Are the Clinical Characteristics of Acute Bronchitis and Acute Exacerbations of Chronic Obstructive Pulmonary Disease?

Acute bronchitis is the tenth most common diagnosis seen by physicians in the United States, and accounts for 2% to 3% of all visits to internists, family physicians, and general practitioners. It is defined by a symptom complex, and is often distinguished from systemic infection and pneumonia by lack of fever and lack of chest radiograph findings (no infiltrate by definition). The clinical findings in patients with acute bronchitis differ from those in patients with acute exacerbations of chronic bronchitis.

Chronic bronchitis is defined by baseline chronic productive cough; therefore, exacerbations are defined by changes in prior symptoms. Chronic obstructive pulmonary disease (COPD) constitutes a spectrum of disease that includes chronic bronchitis (clinical definition) and emphysema (anatomic definition). Its clinical and economic significance is immense. COPD is the fourth leading cause of death in the United States, and the only one of the top four whose mortality rate is increasing. It is responsible for 13% of hospital admissions. Most of the literature describing and studying acute exacerbations of COPD does not differentiate between exacerbations of chronic bronchitis versus exacerbations of emphysema; therefore, in this summary, exacerbations of chronic bronchitis and exacerbations of COPD will be considered synonymous.

Acute Bronchitis

- Cough with or without sputum production (clear or colored)
- Inflammation of the tracheobronchial tree
- Rhinitis
- Pharyngitis
- Laryngitis
- Normal lung examination (occasionally with wheezes)
- Normal chest radiograph

Acute Exacerbations of Chronic Obstructive Pulmonary Disease

- Increased frequency and/or severity of cough
- Increased sputum volume
- Change in sputum color and consistency
- Increased dyspnea
- Fatigue
- Elevated respiratory rate
- Lung examination variable (may be normal or have diminished breath sounds, rhonchi, or wheezes)
- Chest radiograph unchanged (no infiltrate), by definition

Increased sputum volume, change in sputum color and consistency, and increased dyspnea are clinical characteristics that should be used to determine a patient's need for antibiotics.

What Are the Etiologies of Acute Bronchitis, and What Alternative Diagnoses Should Be Considered?

Although an infectious etiology can be found in only a minority (15%–30%) of patients studied with acute bronchitis, the most frequent identifiable causes of acute bronchitis are viral, including adenovirus, coronavirus, coxsackievirus, influenza, parainfluenza, respiratory syncytial virus, and rhinovirus. Influenza can now be diagnosed with rapid assays, which have sensitivities of 70%–90%. These tests should be considered when clinical suspicion is high (fever, cough, myalgia during flu season).

Although typical bacteria have been recovered from oropharyngeal collections of patients with acute bronchitis, the significance of these findings is unclear, especially considering the high prevalence of these bacteria in normal oropharyngeal flora. Sputum cultures are therefore not helpful in the diagnosis. Atypical bacteria, including *Mycoplasma pneumoniae* and *Chlamydia pneumoniae,* may be associated with 5% to 25% of cases of acute bronchitis. *Bordetella pertussis* may be another significant etiologic agent in adults with acute bronchitis. Infection can occur in adequately vaccinated individuals, especially if 12 or more years has elapsed since the last pertussis vaccination. Pertussis (whooping cough in children) does not have the characteristic "whoop" in adults, but should be considered in patients with recent contact with a person known to have pertussis.

Certain noninfectious conditions should be considered in a patient presenting with symptoms consistent with acute bronchitis, especially in nonsmokers with chronic cough lasting more than a few weeks. These include postnasal drip/rhinitis, gastroesophageal reflux, and asthma. History and therapeutic trials may help clarify diagnoses. Patients who need to frequently clear their throat and those who become symptomatic with occupational, environmental (e.g., cigarette smoke), or medication [e.g., angiotensin-converting enzyme (ACE) inhibitor] exposures may require further evaluation or therapeutic trial for rhinitis. Wheezes on examination may be suggestive of asthma, but be aware that spirometry and methacholine challenges can yield false-positive results in the setting of an acute bronchitis episode. Pneumonia should be considered, especially when symptoms include fever, shortness of breath, and findings on lung examination consistent with consolidation. Chest radiography should be ordered when clinically appropriate.

In a Patient Presenting with an Acute Exacerbation of Chronic Bronchitis, What Are the Possible Causes and What Alternative Diagnoses Should Be Considered?

In patients with chronic bronchitis, bacteria are known to colonize the oropharynx, most commonly *Streptococcus pneumoniae, Haemophilus influenzae,* and *Moraxella catarrhalis.* Recent studies have reported isolation of other gram-negative bacteria, including *Klebsiella pneumoniae* and *Pseudomonas aeruginosa,* especially in patients with severe exacerbations. Some studies have further shown that during infectious exacerbations, compared with stable chronic bronchitis or allergic exacerbations, significantly increased quantities of bacteria can be cultured from the oropharynx, lending support that overgrowth of these organisms may lead to COPD exacerbation.

Other studies have shown some association between acute viral infections and COPD exacerbations (recent large studies revealing only a 20%–30% association, smaller than previously believed). Atypical bacteria such as *Mycoplasma pneumoniae* and *Chlamydia pneumoniae* likely play an even smaller role, affecting up to 10% of cases of COPD exacerbation. However, detection methods often make it difficult to determine the exact relationship of these organisms to infectious exacerbations.

The differential diagnosis of an acute exacerbation of chronic bronchitis is similar to the differential described in acute bronchitis. Particular attention should be directed to environmental exposures and allergens that could be the etiology of an exacerbation. Nonadherence to a stable COPD medical regimen also can lead to acute exacerbations and should be specifically investigated prior to selection of therapeutic intervention.

What Evidence Is Available for the Use of Antibiotics in Either Situation?

Antibiotics are used frequently by physicians to treat acute bronchitis. Survey studies have revealed that two thirds to three fourths of outpatients with acute bronchitis and without underlying lung disease receive antibiotic therapy. Two recent meta-analyses have evaluated the effectiveness of antibiotics in acute bronchitis. They were able to abstract only 10 randomized placebo-controlled trials (ultimately limited to eight and nine articles, respectively, based on inclusion and exclusion criteria). Each trial found a small statistically significant benefit from the use of antibiotics (erythromycin, doxycycline, or trimethoprim-sulfamethoxazole) in acute bronchitis. However, these outcome measures translated into approximately a half day reduction of cough and sputum production. Significantly, 85% of patients in the placebo groups improved. There was no statistical significance in days lost from work, and no trial showed additional antibiotic benefit in smokers or patients with purulent sputum production. The authors of each meta-analysis concluded that the small benefit associated with antibiotics did not outweigh their associated risk of adverse effects or the potential increase in antibiotic resistance. They do not recommend routine antibiotic use in these otherwise well patients presenting with acute bronchitis. They nevertheless submit that further studies will need to evaluate subgroups (e.g., older age, more ill appearing) who may benefit from such therapy.

Antibiotic prescribing similarly pervades medicine with respect to acute bronchitis with underlying COPD. Yet, randomized placebo-controlled trials evaluating antibiotics in this area have been equally as sparse, with fewer than 10 adequate quality trials from which to derive evidence. The largest and best designed of these studies by Anthonisen reported a statistically significant improvement in symptom resolution [Number Needed to Treat (NNT) = 7.6, $p < 0.01$] as well as a significant reduction in treatment failures with deterioration (NNT = 11.1, $p < 0.05$) in antibiotic-treated outpatients compared with placebo. The study further identified three symptoms (of nine evaluated)—increased dyspnea, increased sputum volume, and increased sputum purulence—which if present on patient presentation may be predictive of successful antibiotic response. When all three symptoms were present, the value of antibiotic therapy appeared greatest. Antibiotics were still somewhat beneficial when only two of three symptoms were present, but appeared to confer no benefit when one or none of the three symptoms were present (trial not powered to evaluate statistical significance within each of these subgroups).

More recently a meta-analysis provided a summary estimate of effectiveness of antibiotics in COPD exacerbation using the available randomized, placebo-controlled trials in the literature. It demonstrated a small significant improvement in antibiotic-treated patients compared with placebo, based on pooled outcomes. There was also a statistically significant improvement in peak flow rate (11 L/min) in the antibiotic treated group compared with the placebo group. Although this difference is small, it may represent a substantial effect in these patients with marginal functional reserve. Subanalysis in hospitalized patients revealed even greater effect of antibiotics.

Antibiotic choice should be based on likely organisms (*H. influenzae, S. pneumoniae,* and *M. catarrhalis*) and their local resistance patterns. *M. catarrhalis* and *H. influenzae* have 95% and 30% resistance to amoxicillin, respectively, whereas *H. influenzae* has greater than 40% resistance to erythromycin. Consideration to cover atypical bacteria or potentially highly resistant organisms (e.g., *Pseudomonas*) should be based on severity of illness and clinical judgment. Effective, low-cost antibiotics in COPD exacerbation include doxycycline and trimethoprim-sulfamethoxazole. Alternatives include amoxicillin-clavulanic acid, cephalosporins, newer-generation macrolides (e.g., azithromycin), and newer generation quinolones (e.g., levofloxacin).

What Other Therapeutic Modalities Should Be Used When Treating Acute Bronchitis in an Otherwise Healthy Patient Versus an Acute Exacerbation of Chronic Obstructive Pulmonary Disease?

Symptomatic therapy in acute bronchitis should be emphasized in most patients, including nasal decongestants or ipratropium nasal inhaler for rhinitis symptoms (for allergic rhinitis, an antihistamine or inhaled steroids may be added). Acetaminophen or nonsteroidal antiinflammatory drugs (NSAIDs) may be helpful as well. Two small (n ≤ 46 in each study) randomized controlled trials by Hueston showed that albuterol therapy was associated with statistically significant reduction in the number of patients with persistent cough at 7 days, compared with antibiotics or placebo (61% vs. 91%, NNT = 3–4). Percentage of patients returning to work by day 4 was also statistically significant in one trial (NNT = 4). Thus, inhaled or oral albuterol, a practical intervention with few side effects, may be useful in some patients, but larger studies will need to confirm these effects.

If influenza is diagnosed (rapid assay or high clinical suspicion), therapies that may reduce symptom duration, only if initiated within the first 48 hours of symptoms, include rimantadine or amantadine (for influenza A only) or the newer, more expensive agents anamivir or oseltamivir (for influenza A and B).

In acute exacerbations of COPD, discussion regarding medication adherence and current smoking status and other exposures should be undertaken with all patients. Some of the most important interventions include smoking cessation, frequent bronchodilation therapy (inhaled albuterol and ipratropium), oxygen, mucolytics, and systemic corticosteroids. Consideration of antibiotic therapy should be based on the criteria above. Physicians should have lower threshold for antibiotic therapy when COPD exacerbation requires hospital admission, because this cohort of patients has worse outcomes off therapy.

Case

A 62-year-old man presents to your clinic with a 7-day history of nasal and chest congestion, cough productive of yellow sputum, and raspy voice. He admits to some sore throat but says it is chronic and worse in the mornings. He denies any hemoptysis, chest pain, fever, or chills. He does not feel short of breath and denies any significant dyspnea on exertion. He is a busy businessman and is concerned about being out of work. He wants to know what he can take to get better as rapidly as possible. His past medical history is significant only for moderate obesity and mild hypertension. His only regular medication is lisinopril 10 mg, once each morning. He has been taking over-the-counter Robitussin for the past 2 days without much relief. He has no allergies. He has smoked half a pack of cigarettes per day for 20 years and does not drink alcohol or use drugs. His family history is significant for hypertension.

On physical examination he is moderately obese with occasional paroxysms of productive cough, but is in no respiratory distress. His blood pressure is 144/92 mm Hg, pulse 86 beats/min, respiratory rate 18 breaths/min, and temperature 99.0°F. The oropharynx has moderate erythema and no exudates. There is shoddy cervical lymphadenopathy, good inspiratory effort, occasional rhonchi, no sinus tenderness, no jugular venous distention, and no prolonged expiration.

He has a normal apical impulse, regular rate, normal S_1 and S_2, and no murmurs, rubs, or gallops.

His abdomen is soft, with normal bowel sounds, and the extremities show no clubbing, cyanosis, or edema bilaterally. A posteroanterior and lateral chest radiograph performed in the office demonstrated clear lung fields and normal heart size and diaphragms.

1. What is this patient's diagnosis and what are the likely etiologic agents?
2. What therapies should he receive?
3. Does this patient's smoking status alter your decision of whether or not to give him an antibiotic?

Case Discussion

What Is This Patient's Diagnosis and What Are the Likely Etiologic Agents?

This patient has acute bronchitis, and the likely cause is viral in a patient with no other known disease. Influenza is less likely without fever. Another possibility is *Bordetella pertussis,* especially because more than 12 years has elapsed since his last immunization; exposure history should be obtained. Other possibilities include atypical bacteria.

With his history of chronic sore throat, worse in the morning, the possibility of gastroesophageal reflux disease should be entertained. If further history were to confirm chronic nasal congestion, cough, or postnasal drip, a diagnosis related to chronic rhinitis (allergic, smoking-related, or ACE inhibitor related) should be considered in this patient.

What Therapies Should He Receive?

Because this patient has no underlying lung disease, and no history, physical examination, or chest radiograph findings to suggest baseline COPD (no chronic cough; normal lung examination including normal expiratory phase; and normal chest radiograph, no flattening of diaphragms or chronic interstitial changes), he has no indication for antibiotic therapy. Trials of antibiotics to cover atypical bacteria have not shown improvement in clinical outcomes.

Effective interventions include smoking cessation and symptomatic therapy, which may include decongestants and continuation of mucolytics. If his cough is unbearable, adding agents such as dextromethorphan or codeine to his guafenasin (Robitussin) may have symptomatic benefit. Analgesia with acetaminophen or

NSAIDs may be helpful as well. Many over-the-counter cold preparations often combine analgesics, decongestants, and mucolytics. Although only small studies have shown effectiveness of albuterol in acute bronchitis, the effect was rather significant; it may therefore be a more benign (and effective) choice for patients who want to leave the office with a prescription medication.

If pertussis is suspected by history of recent contact, a trial of erythromycin may be reasonable, although no known studies have evaluated effectiveness in adults.

Does This Patient's Smoking Status Alter Your Decision of Whether or Not to Give Him an Antibiotic?

No. Studies to date have not shown improvement in outcomes in smokers without underlying COPD or other lung disease.

Suggested Reading

Anthonisen N R, Manfreda J, Warren C P W, et al. Antibiotic therapy in exacerbations of chronic obstructive pulmonary disease. *Ann Intern Med* 1987;106:196–204.

Bartlett J G. Acute bronchitis. *Up to Date* 2000;7:1–6.

MacKay D N. Treatment of acute bronchitis in adults without underlying lung disease. *J Gen Intern Med* 1996;11:557–562.

Saint S, Bent S, Vittinghoff E, et al. Antibiotics in chronic obstructive pulmonary disease exacerbations: a meta-analysis. *JAMA* 1995;273:957–960.

Smucny J J, Becker L A, Glazier R H, et al. Are antibiotics effective treatment for acute bronchitis? A meta-analysis. *J Family Pract* 1998;47:453–460.

78
Obstructive Sleep Apnea

Stacy M. Higgins

- Discussion   *491*
- Case   *495*
- Case Discussion   *496*

1. What is the definition and pathophysiology of obstructive sleep apnea?
2. What are some of the clinical manifestations of sleep apnea?
3. How is obstructive sleep apnea diagnosed?
4. What are the complications of untreated obstructive sleep apnea?
5. What treatment options are available?

Discussion

What Is the Definition and Pathophysiology of Obstructive Sleep Apnea?

Sleep apnea is defined as airflow cessation (apnea) and/or reduction (hypopnea) during sleep for 10 seconds or more despite continued ventilatory efforts. The prevalence of sleep apnea is 2% to 4% in the middle-aged population of the United States, with men being affected approximately twice as often as women. It is a significant public health problem, with apneic patients being at significantly increased risk for accidents at home, work, and in traffic.

The most significant risk factor for obstructive sleep apnea (OSA) is obesity, particularly upper body obesity. The incidence of OSA among morbidly obese patients is 12- to 30-fold higher than in the general population. There is also a strong familial component, although this may be because of the familial nature of obesity and inheritance of craniofacial structures.

Although the pathophysiology is not completely understood, most evidence indicates that the pharynx is abnormal in size or collapsibility in patients with OSA. Upper airway size is determined by soft tissue and skeletal factors (e.g., adipose tissue, tonsillar hypertrophy, or craniofacial skeletal abnormalities). During the rapid eye movement (REM) phase of sleep, there is decreased tone of the upper airway muscles, as well as diminished reflexes that protect the pharynx from collapse. An abnormal pharynx is kept open in wakefulness by an appropriate compensatory increase in dilator muscle activity, but during sleep this compensation fails and the airway collapses. Arousal from sleep is required for the return of sufficient pharyngeal dilator muscle activity and adequate airflow. This leads to sleep fragmentation.

What Are Some of the Clinical Manifestations of Sleep Apnea?

The difficulty in diagnosing sleep apnea comes from the fact that many patients present with vague, nonspecific complaints. Snoring, one of the cardinal manifestations of sleep apnea, by itself is a poor predictor of OSA. Daytime sleepiness and fatigue are common, but are nearly universal in our society. Daytime fatigue also may be underreported because of its slow development over time such that patients learn to compensate with naps, sleeping late on days off, and using caffeine. Use of the Epworth Sleepiness Scale (Table 78.1) helps to objectively measure the degree of daytime somnolence. Although controversy exists about the upper limit of normal on the Epworth scale, scores above 10 warrant investigation. Other symptoms include morning headaches, cognitive impairment, depression, nocturnal esophogeal reflux, physically restless sleep, and impotence. Collateral history from the bed partner is helpful because the patient may be unaware of many of these symptoms.

Clinical clues on the physical examination include a crowded upper airway, enlarged soft palate, nasal obstruction, tonsillar hypertrophy, elevated blood pressure, and an increased body mass index (BMI) to greater than 28. Neck circumference ($>$16 inches in men and $>$15 inches in women) has been shown to be a more useful clinical predictor of OSA than the presence of obesity. In a man of average height, a neck circumference of 17 had a sensitivity of 87% and specificity of 79% for OSA.

In order to help the clinician refine which patients need to be referred for further testing, a predictive model using four easily confirmed clinical variables has been developed: presence or absence of hypertension, neck circumference, history of habitual snoring, and observed reports of nocturnal choking or gasping. Using a linear model, combined points give a sleep apnea clinical score (Table 78.2). A score of $<$10 confers a probability of 17% for having sleep apnea (defined as an apnea index

Table 78.1. Epworth Sleepiness Score

How likely are you to doze off or to fall asleep in the following situations, in contrast to just feeling tired? This refers to your usual way of life in recent times.
Use the following scale to choose the most appropriate number for each situation:
   0: would **never** doze
   1: **slight** chance of dozing
   2: **moderate** chance of dozing
   3: **high** chance of dozing

Activity	Chance of Dozing
Sitting and reading	_____
Watching TV	_____
Sitting inactive in a public place	_____
As a passenger in a car for an hour without a break	_____
Lying down to rest in the afternoon when circumstances permit	_____
Sitting and talking to someone	_____
Sitting quietly after a lunch without alcohol	_____
In a car while stopped for a few minutes in traffic	_____
Total /24	

Table 78.2. Sleep Apnea Clinical Score

	Not Hypertensive Historical Features[a]			Hypertensive Historical Features[a]		
	None	One	Both	None	One	Both
Neck circumference (cm)						
28	0	0	1	0	1	2
30	0	0	1	1	2	4
32	0	1	2	1	3	5
34	1	2	3	2	4	8
36	1	3	5	4	6	11
38	2	4	7	5	9	16
40	3	6	10	8	13	22
42	5	8	14	11	18	30
44	7	12	20	15	25	42
46	10	16	18	21	35	58
48	14	23	38	29	48	80
50	19	32	53	40	66	110

[a]Historical features are habitual snoring and partner reports of nocturnal choking or gasping.

>10). A score of >15 confers a probability of 81% for having sleep apnea and requires further testing.

How Is Obstructive Sleep Apnea Diagnosed?

The gold standard for diagnosis is a full night of polysomnography, conducted by a technologist in a sleep laboratory. A full sleep study measures sleep stages and continuity (via electroencephalography and eye movements), respiratory effort, airflow, oxygen saturation, body position, muscle tone, and heart rate (via continuous electrocardiographic monitoring). An apnea index (AI), defined as the number of apneic episodes in 1 hour, is recorded. The presence of five or more episodes of apnea per hour (AI $\geq$ 5) or 30 episodes of apnea over an average night of sleep is considered abnormal. Because there is night-to-night variability in AI, a negative overnight sleep study with high clinical suspicion should prompt a repeat study.

A full sleep study is time consuming, labor intensive, and costly. Because of the large number of patients suspected of having the disease and referred for testing, there are typically long waiting lists. To try and reduce costs and increase the number of patients that can be evaluated, alternative diagnostic strategies that rely on clinical predictors and simplified home (portable) monitoring have gained recent increasing recognition. Whether or not home monitoring is adequate to successfully diagnose OSA is still controversial, and the only approved testing for now is an overnight sleep study.

Because a second study for therapeutic continuous positive airway pressure (CPAP) titration can be an extremely long wait, there has been a trend for split night studies. The first half of the night establishes the diagnosis of sleep apnea, and optimal CPAP dosing is determined during the second half. This method is extremely effective in patients with severe OSA (AI $>$ 20), but not as accurate in optimal dosing for mild OSA.

What Are the Complications of Untreated Obstructive Sleep Apnea?

Hypertension

Approximately 60% of patients with OSA have essential hypertension, yet the contribution of OSA to hypertension remains a controversial subject. There are several confounding variables found in both OSA and hypertension, such as age, sex, obesity, smoking, and alcohol. In 1994, convincing evidence that OSA was an independent risk factor for elevating blood pressure came from the Wisconsin Sleep Cohort Study. In this prospective study, state workers with and without sleep disordered breathing had 24-hour blood pressure monitoring. The results found that subjects with an AI of 5 or more had significantly higher blood pressures than did subjects with snoring but without apnea or subjects with neither snoring nor apnea. The increase in blood pressure was present during both wakefulness and sleep. After controlling for obesity, age, and sex, sleep apnea was still significantly associated with hypertension in a dose-response fashion. In addition, a number of studies that have monitored blood pressure in OSA patients (both hypertensive and normotensive) have found a significant decrease in systemic pressure once therapy has been initiated (CPAP or tracheostomy).

Pulmonary Hypertension and Cor Pulmonale

It seems rational that chronic nocturnal hypoxia leads to hypoxic pulmonary vasoconstriction, eventually leading to sustained pulmonary hypertension. However, whether the hypoxemia associated with repetitive sleep apneas is enough to lead to permanent elevations in pulmonary artery pressure and cor pulmonale is controversial. Most studies have stressed that daytime hypoxia and hypercarbia, perhaps as a consequence of obstructive lung disease or obesity, lead to the development of pulmonary hypertension in sleep apnea patients. Patients with normal lung function and OSA tend to have mild pulmonary hypertension.

Arrhythmias

The most common rhythm disturbances seen in OSA are extreme bradycardia and ventricular asystole lasting longer than 10 seconds. These arrhythmias result from an increase in the vagal tone secondary to hypoventilation, hypoxemia, and respiratory acidosis. Therapy with CPAP eliminates episodic arrhythmias in most patients.

What Treatment Options Are Available?

Behavioral

Weight loss is recommended as a first-line treatment for all obese patients with sleep apnea, and when successful, may significantly lessen the severity of apnea. However, it is usually inadequate alone, and some investigators have found the therapeutic benefit to be inconsistent, and others have reported recurrence of the disease with time despite successful weight loss. Generally, other forms of treatment are necessary.

Alcohol and sedatives should be avoided in all patients with sleep apnea even during daytime hours. They have been shown to cause pharyngeal muscle relaxation, resulting in worsened apnea, and most sedatives potentiate the length of apneas.

Positional therapy is helpful in patients who have more apneic episodes in the supine compared with the lateral position. A tennis ball sewn into the back of pajamas to make sleeping on the back uncomfortable is one suggested method in these patients. The long-term effects of this approach are unclear.

Medical

Continuous positive airway pressure (CPAP) is the treatment of choice for clinically significant sleep apnea, and has been shown to improve cognitive function, daytime sleepiness, mood, and systemic blood pressure. Most importantly, CPAP has been shown to improve survival. Patients must have their CPAPs individually titrated during sleep to the necessary pressure. This is usually done during a second sleep study or in the second half of a split study if apnea is clearly present during the first half. The goal is to find the lowest pressure that eliminates snoring and obstructive breathing events with improvements in sleep continuity.

The main problem with CPAP therapy has been patient compliance. Studies have shown CPAP being used by only 46% of patients as directed (at least 4 hours of sleep for 70% or more of nights).

Oral appliances alter the configuration or compliance of the upper airway by holding the lower jaw forward or holding the tongue forward. A variety of appliances are available, based on the anatomic defect, and they are worn only during sleep and are generally well tolerated. Patients with mild sleep apnea who do not tolerate CPAP are good candidates for an oral appliance trial. Patients with more severe apnea should be encouraged and reinforced on the use of CPAP. If they fail CPAP, oral appliances are used as second-line therapy.

Medication use has had only limited success, the exception being thyroxine in patients who are hypothyroid.

Surgical

Tracheostomy has fallen out of favor with the acceptance of CPAP therapy. It remains an option in a small subgroup of patients with severe apnea who cannot tolerate CPAP, and for whom other interventions are ineffective or unacceptable.

Palatal surgery modifies a site of upper airway closure, but is curative in less than 50% of patients, and preoperative imaging has not improved this success. Laser-assisted uvulopalatoplasty is a new modality in the treatment of OSA. It excises the uvula and portions of the soft palate. Although it improves snoring, there is little supportive evidence in the treatment of moderate to severe OSA.

Case

A 55-year-old man presents to your clinic for follow-up of his hypertension. The patient reports compliance with his diet and hydrochlorothiazide/triamterene 50/75 mg (half a tablet daily) clonidine patch 0.2 mg/day (applied weekly), and labetalol 200 mg twice daily. He is concerned about the morning headaches he has been having, and asks if they are related to his elevated blood pressure. Near the end of the interview, his wife asks if there is anything you can do about his snoring because it is so loud and disruptive, it has been keeping her awake at night. She is also concerned because at times he stops breathing and then gasps for air. On physical examination, his weight is 235 pounds and height 5 feet 10 inches. Blood pressure is 160/85 mm Hg, with a pulse of 62 beats/min. Examination of his oropharynx reveals no tonsillar hypertrophy. His neck circumference is 18 inches. The rest of his examination is unremarkable.

1. What clinical cues suggest these symptoms are due to sleep apnea?
2. What are the options to definitively diagnose obstructive sleep apnea?
3. What are the treatment options?

Case Discussion

What Clinical Cues Suggest These Symptoms Are Due to Sleep Apnea?

Based on the patient's history of hypertension, his wife's report of snoring and gasping, as well as the patient's physical examination, there is a high clinical suspicion for sleep apnea. The Epworth scale can be administered for objective measurement of sleep deprivation and daytime somnolence. A score of 15 or above on the sleep apnea clinical scale will help determine the need for a sleep study.

What Are the Options to Definitively Diagnose Obstructive Sleep Apnea?

The patient can have either a full sleep study or a split-night study. The advantage to a split-night study is that both diagnosis and treatment can be done at the same time. Based on the patient's hourly apnea index, the recommended CPAP titration comes back with the report. However the gold standard remains a full night sleep study.

What Are the Treatment Options?

Given the patient's obesity, weight loss is the first line of treatment to be recommended. In addition, he should be warned to avoid alcohol and over-the-counter sedatives because this may worsen his condition. Based on the severity of apnea defined on the sleep study, and the degree of his clinical symptoms, CPAP would be the treatment of choice.

Suggested Reading

Bahammam A, Kryger M. Decision making in obstructive sleep-disordered breathing. *Clin Chest Med* 1998;19:87–97.

Chaudhary B A, Bliwise D L. Therapy for sleep apnea: who should be treated with CPAP? *J Med Assoc Georgia* 1997;86:230–232.

Flemons W W, Whitelaw W A, et al. Likelihood ratios for a sleep apnea clinical prediction rule. *Am J Respir Crit Care Med* 1994;150:1279–1285.

George C F P. Diagnostic techniques in obstructive sleep apnea. *Prog Cardiovasc Dis* 1999;41:355–366.
Henderson J H, Strollo P J. Medical management of obstructive sleep apnea. *Prog Cardiovasc Dis* 1999;41:377–386.
Hla K M, Young T B, et al. Sleep apnea and hypertension. *Ann Intern Med* 1994;120:382–388.
Johns M W. A new method of measuring sleepiness: the Epworth Sleepiness Scale. *Sleep* 1991;14:540–545.
Skomro R P, Kryger M H. Clinical presentations of obstructive sleep apnea syndrome. *Prog Cardiovasc Dis* 1999;41:331–340.

79
Solitary Pulmonary Nodule
Clyde Watkins, Jr.

1. What characteristics of a solitary pulmonary nodule suggest that it is either benign or malignant?
2. What is the role of imaging radiography in the workup of a solitary pulmonary nodule?
3. How do you determine the probability that a solitary pulmonary nodule is malignant?
4. What is the role of fine-needle aspiration in the evaluation of a solitary pulmonary nodule?

Discussion
What Characteristics of a Solitary Pulmonary Nodule Suggest that It Is Either Benign or Malignant?

The finding of a solitary pulmonary nodule (SPN) on a chest radiograph is a common clinical encounter for primary care physicians. An SPN is defined as having a diameter of 3 cm or less. Currently 1 of every 500 chest radiographs reveals a nodule. Current estimates are that an SPN will prove to be a malignant tumor in 40% of cases.

A clinician should approach an SPN as malignant until proven otherwise. Investigation of an SPN should initially focus on an assessment of the physical characteristics of the nodule as well as an assessment of its stability.

Physical Characteristics of a Solitary Pulmonary Nodule

Rate of Growth

In general, malignant nodules grow at a consistent exponential rate that is expressed as doubling time. A nodule is considered to have doubled in size when its diameter has increased 28% in size. The doubling time of malignant lesions ranges from 25 to 450 days. Most benign tumors show either no or very slow growth (doubling times of >500 days). If an SPN is stable over a 2- to 3-year period (doubling time of >750 days), then it is almost certainly benign.

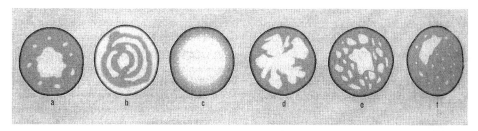

Figure 79.1. Patterns of calcification in solitary pulmonary nodules. **A:** Central. **B:** Laminated. **C:** Diffuse. **D:** Popcorn. **E:** Speckled. **F:** Eccentric.

Calcification

The radiographic detection of calcification is a strong indicator of benign disease. This is particularly true of calcification appearing in either a central, laminated, diffuse, or popcorn pattern. Calcifications appearing in a speckled or eccentric pattern carry a greater likelihood of malignancy and are considered clinically indeterminate (Fig. 79.1).

Margins

The likelihood of cancer is strongly correlated with the appearance of a nodule's edge (Fig. 79.2).

Stability

In the initial evaluation of stability, prior chest films should be reviewed and compared with the current chest films. This is especially important because nodules may be detected in earlier films reported as normal when compared side by side with the current films. If the nodule appears stable over a 2- to 3-year period, then the likelihood of malignancy is small. However, it is still recommended that patients be followed semiannually with chest films or by CT for 2 to 3 years.

What Is the Role of Imaging Radiography in the Workup of a Solitary Pulmonary Nodule?

Computed tomography (CT) is the preferred imaging study in the evaluation and surveillance of an SPN. Although most nodules are seen on plain chest films, CT is clearly superior in the detection of small nodules. High-resolution CT is the most sensitive and specific method for assessing the size and shape, the presence and pattern of calcification, and the margins of an SPN. High-resolution CT also can be used to detect certain benign lesions (hamartomas, arteriovenous malformations) early in the evaluative process. CT also detects the presence of mediastinal adenopathy that can influence surgical plans.

The ability of magnetic resonance imaging (MRI) to detect pulmonary nodules is less than that of CT. Gadolinium-enhanced MRI is equivalent to CT in the characterization of calcific patterns.

Positron emission testing (PET) scans are highly sensitive (95%) for identifying malignancy. Their specificity for malignancy is around 85%. False positive results

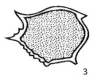

Figure 79.2. Patterns

Type	Appearance	Cancer Probability
1	Regular, smooth	20%
2	Irregular, smooth	33%
3	Spiculated	83%
4	Fuzzy, multispiculated, corona radiata	93%

may occur in lesions that contain active inflammatory tissue. Despite the expense, when PET scanning is available, it is a preferred study to examine the physical characteristics of a solitary pulmonary nodule.

How Do You Determine the Probability that a Solitary Pulmonary Nodule is Malignant?

The initial evaluation of an SPN begins with a thorough history and physical examination. Prior chest films should be sought and compared with the current films, and a CT scan should be obtained.

Once all information is attained, an assessment of the probability of cancer should be made (Table 79.1). The probability assessment is the foundation by which all treatment decisions are based. For example, if a CT scan shows an AVM or hamartoma, both non-neoplastic lesions, then the workup can be terminated. If the evaluation reveals a nonsmoker with a benign pattern of calcification, nodule stability, or very slow growth on prior chest films (doubling time >500 days), then a wait and watch approach may be advocated. If the doubling time of a nodule is

Table 79.1. Variables Predicting Whether a Solitary Pulmonary Nodule is Benign or Malignant

Favoring Benignity	Favoring Malignancy
Age <48 yr	Age >48 yr
Age <30 yr[a] (LR = 0.11)	Age >65 yr[a] (LR = 3.2)
Nodule diameter <1.5 cm	Nodule diameter >1.5 cm
Never smoked[a] (LR = 0.15)	Ever smoked (LR = 1.5)
Currently smokes <10–20 cigarettes per day	Currently smokes >10–20 cigarettes per day
Quit smoking >4 yr ago	Quit smoking <4 yr ago
Nodule edge type 1 (LR = 0.5)	Nodule edge type (LR = 14)[a]
Doubling time >500 days[a]	Doubling time 30–400 days[a]
Calcification in benign pattern[a]	Calcification in indeterminate pattern or none found
Needle biopsy findings	
Specific benign disease[a]	Malignant disease[a]
Nonspecific benign cells	Suspicious cells

[a]Strong indicator.
LR, likelihood ratio for malignancy

less than 400 days in a patient with a history of smoking, then thoracotomy should be pursued. In the case of an uncalcified nodule, or a nodule of unknown stability, the probability assessment is critical. If the patient is judged to have an intermediate level of probability, then needle biopsy may be used to aid diagnosis or a wait and watch approach, using serial CT scan images, with the purpose of prospectively determining nodule stability may be advocated.

What Is the Role of Fine-Needle Aspiration in the Evaluation of a Solitary Pulmonary Nodule?

Fine-needle aspiration (FNA) should be considered as part of a multimodal approach to the management of an SPN. FNA may be most helpful in instances when the probability of malignancy is indeterminate. Otherwise the overall value of FNA in the routine evaluation of an SPN is limited.

Despite the advances in CT technology and FNA needle design, certain technical limitations persist and must be well thought out when considering FNA. First, the diagnostic success of FNA is low in lesions less than 1 cm in diameter. Second, false-negative results of biopsies may be reported in up to 22% of cases, and inadequate samples of diagnostic material may be obtained in up to 18% of cases. Therefore, the absence of malignant cells on sampling does not prove benignity. Third, FNA carries a significant risk of pneumothorax.

Factors that Confer Increased Risk for Pneumothorax from Fine-Needle Aspiration

- Increased lesion depth from the pleura
- Small lesion size
- Lesions surrounded by bullae
- The FNA needle must cross a lung fissure in order to reach a lesion

Case

E.S. is a 68-year-old woman recently seen at a local emergency department for treatment of an exacerbation of chronic obstructive pulmonary disease (COPD). A chest radiograph performed during that evaluation revealed a 1-cm solitary pulmonary nodule located in the right upper lobe. She is referred to you for follow-up evaluation. She has a past medical history of COPD, hypertension, and osteoarthritis. She has a 60-pack/year tobacco history and currently smokes half a pack of cigarettes per day. Her medications include albuterol, ipatropium bromide, lisinopril, and acetaminophen. Her physical examination is significant only for decreased breath sounds. Examination of her most recent chest radiograph reveals a 1-cm nodule located posteriorly in the right upper lobe. The nodule is smooth with rounded edges and is calcified in a laminated pattern. Her lungs are hyperaerated with a small bulla in the apex of the right upper lobe. Her most recent chest radiograph available for comparison was taken 4 years ago and does not show a lung nodule. CT shows the same calcified nodule and no evidence of mediastinal adenopathy.

1. What factors favor benign versus malignant disease?
2. Should this patient be referred for fine-needle aspiration?
3. What are this patient's diagnostic and therapeutic options?

Case Discussion

What Factors Favor Benign Versus Malignant Disease?

Factors favoring benignity include small nodule size (1 cm), pattern of calcification (laminated), and appearance of the nodule's margins (smooth). Factors favoring malignancy include heavy tobacco use (60 packs/year cigarettes) and age. The fact that the nodule was not present on the chest radiograph taken 4 years ago is important, but is not helpful in determining the status of this nodule. Because of the 4-year time frame, the nodule could be actively growing or stable.

Should This Patient Be Referred for Fine-Needle Aspiration?

The nodule's central location, its location close to a bulla, and the patient's history of COPD place her at increased risk for pneumothorax induced by FNA. FNA also has a high rate of false-negative results and nondiagnostic results. A positive FNA result can expedite a referral for thoracotomy. However, a negative FNA result does not rule out malignant disease. The decision to proceed with FNA should be made in concert with the patient's wishes and in consultation with the radiologist.

What Are This Patient's Diagnostic and Therapeutic Options?

The nodule's margins and pattern of calcification are two strong factors suggesting benign disease. The patient's age and strong tobacco history are suggestive of malignant disease. The stability (growth) of the nodule cannot be determined with the available information. FNA is an option to facilitate diagnosis, but the patient has a high risk for pneumothorax. A wait and watch strategy may be the most prudent diagnostic option. After the initial CT scan, serial scans should be obtained at 4 weeks, 6 weeks, and 3 months, and then every 4 to 6 months over a 3-year interval. Any nodule growth should then prompt an evaluation for thoracotomy. The clinician should use this opportunity to counsel the patient on smoking cessation, strongly encourage her to quit, and prescribe pharmacologic agents to assist with quitting if she is interested because they have been shown to double quit rates.

Suggested Reading

Lillington G A. Management of solitary pulmonary nodules. *Postgrad Med* 1997:101:145–150.
Reilly J J, Preparing for pulmonary resection. *Chest* 1997:112(suppl):206–208.
Shaffer K. Role of radiology for imaging and biopsy of solitary pulmonary nodules. *Chest* 1999;116 (suppl):519–522.

XIV
Orthopedics

80

Acute Ankle Injuries

Donald Brady

1. What is the most common type of ankle injury?
2. What physical examination tests can be used to assess for ankle stability?
3. When should a physician order radiographs for ankle injuries?
4. What are the proper steps to take in treating an ankle sprain?

Discussion

What Is the Most Common Type of Ankle Injury?

Ankles are the most commonly injured part of the body. The majority of ankle injuries (88%) are sprain-related. In the United States, over 25,000 people per year sustain ankle sprains; 10% of emergency room visits are related to ankle sprains. Ankle sprains account for 25% of all time lost due to injury in football, basketball, and cross-country running. Up to 40% of ankle sprains may progress to chronic ankle problems.

Given these statistics, it is important to understand the mechanisms of ankle injury and know how to properly treat such injuries. One must never forget the potential impact of ankle injuries on quality of life, loss of work time, and use of healthcare resources.

Ankle sprains are classified into three grades. A grade I (mild) sprain is characterized by some torn ligamentous fibers with minimal hemorrhage, resulting in no ankle laxity or residual instability. Full function and strength are maintained. Grade II (moderate) sprains are incomplete tears of the ligament with mild laxity and instability, a small reduction in function, and possibly some decrease in strength and proprioception. Grade III (severe) sprains are classified by a complete disruption of the ligament, gross instability and laxity, and potentially a complete loss of function, strength, and proprioception (particularly if rehabilitation is deficient or inadequate).

The most common type of ankle sprain involves the lateral ligament complex. This accounts for 85% of all grade III ankle sprains. The lateral ligament complex is composed primarily of three ligaments: the anterior talofibular ligament (ATFL), the calcaneofibular ligament (CFL), and the posterior talofibular ligament (PTFL) (Fig. 80.1). Eighty-five percent of all lateral ligament complex sprains involve the ATFL and CFL.

Lateral sprains most commonly occur from supination and inversion of the foot with external rotation of the tibia on the fixed foot. A sequence of ligamentous in-

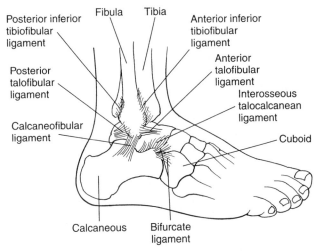

Figure 80.1. Ligaments of the ankle.

juries takes place with an inversion injury. Although it has the greatest strain-to-tear ratio, the ATFL also has the lowest maximal load-to-tear ratio. When a person lands from a jump or is running, the foot is commonly in plantar flexion, which causes the ATFL to be taut or at maximal strain. When inversion occurs in this position, the weight of the person stresses the ATFL to the point of tearing. Subsequently, the CFL, although larger and stronger than the ATFL, begins to tear. Both of these ligaments are integral to talofibular stability.

The PTFL is the strongest of the three ligaments and is rarely injured. Given its attachment posteriorly to the lateral tubercle on the posterior aspect of the talus and anteriorly to the digital fossa of the fibula, it is taut only in severe dorsiflexion. Isolated transection of the PTFL does not lead to ankle instability.

What Physical Examination Tests Can Be Used to Assess for Ankle Stability?

The examiner can use the anterior drawer test to assess the stability of the ATFL. With the knee bent to promote gastrocsoleus relaxation, one should grasp the heel in one hand while holding the lower leg still and then try to translate the foot anteriorly. Movement of a mere 4 mm is considered a positive test result and indicates ATFL instability. A significant amount of muscle guarding can occur and can interfere with test reliability.

The talar tilt test is the best way to evaluate CFL stability. The test is simple: while grasping the lower leg with one hand, use the other to hold the calcaneus and invert and evert the foot. If there is a significant difference between the medial and lateral opening of the ankle mortise of more than 25%, the test result is considered positive for CFL instability. The caveats to this test are that it can be extremely painful, may worsen the existing injury, and may be difficult to perform and evaluate in a person with significant swelling. If the test result is positive and the CFL is torn, the ATFL is also assumed to be torn, thus indicating multiple complete ligamentous ruptures.

The PTFL alone is impossible to assess for instability but can be evaluated in combination with the other distal tibiofibular syndesmosis ligaments (ATFL, inferior transverse ligament, and interosseous ligament) for syndesmotic sprain by performing the squeeze test. This type of injury is rare and usually occurs only with significant force. It most commonly occurs in collision-type injuries like those seen in football, soccer, and ice hockey games. The examiner performs the squeeze test by compressing the tibia and fibula firmly at the mid-shaft region and assessing for pain in the anterolateral region of the ankle or the distal fibula. Pain in either place should be considered positive for syndesmotic injury and probable injury to the PTFL.

When Should a Physician Order Radiographs for Ankle Injuries?

In the past, physicians ordered plain radiographs as part of the evaluation for almost all ankle injuries. However, to many clinicians, this practice seemed excessive and cost ineffective. In the early 1990s, a group of physicians established the Ottawa Ankle Rules, which have proven to be 100% sensitive for fracture and may reduce the need for radiographs by more than 30%. The guidelines are simple. An ankle x-ray series is warranted only under the following circumstances:

- The patient is unable to bear weight on the affected foot/ankle immediately and for four steps in the treatment center, or
- There is bone tenderness at the posterior edge or tip of the lateral or medial malleolus, or
- There is pain at the base of the fifth metatarsal or the navicular bone.

These guidelines should be used only if the patient presents in the first 10 days after injury. The need for radiographs in patients presenting beyond 10 days should be handled on an individual basis, and the input of an orthopedist in any questionable case at any presentation time is advisable.

Computed tomography (CT) and magnetic resonance imaging (MRI) can be used to evaluate ankle injuries but are much more costly. MRI is most useful in evaluating chronic ankle sprains to look for capsular thickening, indicating probable ligamentous injury. Its use, however, is controversial. At least one study found that clinical examination had a greater sensitivity (94%) and specificity (95%) for predicting impingement about the ATFL than did MRI (sensitivity and specificity, 39% and 50%, respectively). CT scans can be useful in patients who fail conservative therapy, have chronic pain, or demonstrate ligamentous instability. CT more accurately measures displacement of lateral complex injuries than plain radiographs, which tend to overestimate displacement.

What Are the Proper Steps to Take in Treating an Ankle Sprain?

Conservative treatment of a lateral ankle sprain should always begin with PRICE: protection, rest, ice, compression, and elevation.

Protection

The goal of protection is to prevent further injury to already damaged structures. Modifying activity—whether home, work, or recreational—reduces exposure to potentially injurious situations. Protective immobilization, including partial or no weight bearing and use of crutches, canes, or walkers, also reduces risk. Bracing the ankle through the use of an elastic bandage, air cast, lace-up stabilizer, splint, or hard cast adds direct protection as well as compression. The choice of modality depends on the patient's willingness and ability to limit use of the ankle while it heals. Without protection, the patient risks not only further injury, but also increased pain and swelling and chronic disability.

Rest

Rest, through partial or no weight bearing, encourages tissue healing and avoids further stressing damaged tissues.

Ice

Ice and other cold compresses have multiple effects in promoting injury healing. The effects of local inflammatory modulators are decreased, the amount of extracellular fluid to be reabsorbed is minimized, and the release of endogenous opioid substances is promoted. The patient must remember to protect the skin to prevent cold burns. A general recommendation is to apply ice or a cold compress for 20 minutes each waking hour for the first 12 to 24 hours post-injury. Studies have shown that cryotherapy, when applied within the first 36 hours post-injury, is better than heat for complete and rapid recovery (average of 13.2 days to full activity for those using cryotherapy in the first 36 hours, 30.4 days when cryotherapy was initiated after the first 36 hours, and 33.3 days for those using heat).

Compression

Compression limits the amount of effusion by physically constraining the extracellular space. When applying compression, whether through an elastic bandage, air cast, or other device, it is important to dorsiflex the foot maximally to constrict the joint space and decrease effusion. This position also limits the strain on the lateral ligament complex, thus approximating torn ends in grade III sprains and lessening the strain on the partially torn ligaments in grade I and II injuries. Some grade III injuries may require either casting or a walking orthosis (with a fixed or hinged ankle). This decision is left to the practitioner, but orthopedic referral should strongly be considered in any questionable cases. Although immobilization may allow more patient mobility, it also may prolong the rehabilitation period and length of time to full recovery.

Elevation

Elevation promotes healing by decompressing the vasculature of the swollen tissues and decreasing dependent edema. While elevating the ankle, the patient needs to support the entire leg to prevent hyperextension of the knee.

Other treatment modalities include the use of nonsteroidal antiinflammatory drugs (NSAIDs) for pain, alternative forms of pain management (acupuncture, biofeedback, etc.), and electrical stimulation to limit effusion (little data on humans to support this).

On average, grade I sprains require 11.7 days before full resumption of athletic activities, grade II sprains 2 to 6 weeks, and grade III sprains typically over 6 weeks. Some reports say grade III sprains require up to 6 months, and only 25% to 60% of grade III patients are asymptomatic at 1 to 4 years postinjury. Negative prognostic indicators for patients with ankle sprains include functional instability, loss of normal ankle kinematics (e.g., talar displacement), recurrent injuries, and younger age.

Case

D.B. is a 30-year-old man who presents to the Urgent Care Clinic after "turning his left ankle" during a basketball game earlier in the afternoon. He says he was driving in for a lay-up and landed on his defender's foot, rolled onto his outer left ankle, and fell to the ground. He thought he heard a "pop" during this episode. He says he has always had good balance and has had no previous ankle injuries. He came to the clinic because the pain was persistent and was not allowing him to rest.

On physical examination, you notice his left ankle is swollen laterally, slightly warm, and tender over the lateral malleolus. There is significant limitation in range of motion, to the point of no active range of motion. He is unable to bear full weight on the ankle, and he cannot take any steps secondary to pain. There is no other point tenderness and no malalignment is noted on examination.

1. Should you obtain radiographs to rule out a fracture? If so, what radiographs should you order?
2. If the injury is merely a sprain, what are the most likely ligaments injured and what tests can you perform to assess their stability?
3. You obtain the ankle radiographs, which are negative. What is your acute treatment plan?
4. D.B. is an avid basketball player and wants to know when he can expect to return to the game. Can you give him an estimated return date and a prognosis for recurrent injury to that ankle?

Case Discussion

Should You Obtain Radiographs to Rule Out a Fracture? If So, What Radiographs Should You Order?

In this case, given that there is point tenderness on the lateral malleolus, plain radiographs are warranted according to the Ottawa Ankle Rules. The clinician should order anteroposterior (AP), lateral, and mortise views (a three-view ankle series).

The AP radiographs are particularly useful to rule out a fifth metatarsal avulsion fracture or an anterior calcaneal injury. Only 14% of ankle ligament tears involve an avulsion injury (usually a fifth metatarsal or a distal fibular fracture); 86% occur within the ligament itself.

If the Injury is Merely a Sprain, What Are the Most Likely Ligaments Injured and What Tests Can You Perform to Assess Their Stability?

Eighty-five percent of all ankle injuries involve the lateral ligamentous complex, comprising the ATFL, CFL, and PTFL. Given that D.B. was landing from a jump, he likely landed with his foot in plantar flexion. With the ankle in plantar flexion, the ATFL is taut, and although it has the highest strain-to-failure ratio in the lateral ligamentous complex, it also has the lowest maximal load-to-failure ratio. Therefore, he most likely sprained the ATFL. You can use the anterior drawer test to test D.B.'s ATFL for stability. The talar tilt test might help to assess CFL stability but, given the limited range of motion, likely will not be useful. The squeeze test will help assess syndesmotic injury and can be performed easily because it does not involve manipulation of the ankle directly.

You Obtain the Films and They Are Negative. What Should Be Your Acute Treatment Plan?

Your treatment plan should involve five major areas: protection, rest, ice, compression, and elevation. He probably should avoid weight bearing for 24 hours, followed by limited weight bearing. An elastic bandage for compression and protection is warranted and should be applied with the foot dorsiflexed as much as possible. Given that he has presented within 4 to 6 hours of injury, ice should be applied 20 minutes of every hour while he is awake to decrease swelling and to relieve pain. He should keep his foot elevated above the level of his heart as much as possible with support behind his knee to avoid hyperextension injury. NSAIDs may help with pain management and to some degree inflammation control.

If you are suspicious of a complete tear of the ligaments or there is some physical evidence of ankle instability (a grade III injury), referral to an orthopedist for evaluation is warranted. Referral also is warranted if there is evidence of locking of the joint, persistent pain, evidence of compartment syndrome, or development of complex regional pain syndrome (formerly called reflex sympathetic dystrophy). Compartment syndrome should be suspected in the setting of pain unrelieved by narcotics, profoundly swollen tissues with taut skin around the ankle, and dysesthesias. Signs of complex regional pain syndrome include intractable pain, trophic changes (swollen, taut skin), excessive growth of nails, and neurosensory changes.

D.B. Is an Avid Basketball Player and Wants to Know When He Can Expect to Return to the Game. Can You Give Him an Estimated Return Date and a Prognosis for Recurrent Injury to That Ankle?

Patients with grade I injuries commonly can return to full activity in 10 days to 2 weeks, with grade II injuries in 2 to 6 weeks, and with grade III injuries return is highly variable, ranging from 6 weeks to 6 months. You should remind him that there is a fair amount of individual variability, especially for grade II and III injuries, and prognosis must be compared with individual response to rehabilitation.

Suggested Reading

Childs S. Acute ankle injury. In: *Lippincott's primary care practice*. Vol. 3, No. 4. Philadelphia: Lippincott Williams & Wilkins, 1999:428–437.

Lentell G, Bass B, Lopez D, et al. The contributions of proprioceptive deficits, muscle function, and anatomic laxity to functional instability of the ankle. *J Orthop Sports Phys Ther* 1995;21:206–215.

Safran M R, Benedetti R S, Bartolozzi A R III, et al. Lateral ankle sprains: a comprehensive review. Part 1: etiology, pathoanatomy, histopathogenesis, and diagnosis. *Med Sci Sports Exerc* 1999;31(suppl): 429–437.

Safran M R, Zachazewski J E, Benedetti R S, et al. Lateral ankle sprains: a comprehensive review. Part 2: treatment and rehabilitation with an emphasis on the athlete. *Med Sci Sports Exerc* 1999;31(suppl): 438–447.

Stiell I G, McKnight R D, Greenberg G H, et al. Implementation of the Ottawa ankle rules. *JAMA* 1994;271:827–832.

81

Acute Knee Pain

Joyce P. Doyle

1. What is the basic anatomy of the knee?
2. What key questions should be asked as part of the history in a patient with acute knee pain?
3. How do you examine the knee for the presence of an effusion?
4. How do you assess the range of motion of the knee?
5. How do you assess the stability of the medial and lateral collateral ligaments of the knee?
6. How do you perform the McMurray and Lachman tests? What knee abnormalities do positive test results suggest?

Discussion

What Is the Basic Anatomy of the Knee?

The knee is the largest and most complex joint in the body. It is the most common site of osteoarthritis and infection, and is particularly vulnerable to injury. The bony structures of the knee joint include the distal femoral condyles, proximal tibial plateau, and patella. The patella is the largest sesamoid bone in the body and it forms within the quadriceps tendon and increases the mechanical advantage of the quadriceps. The intraarticular structures include the medial and lateral menisci (fibrocartilaginous structures that rim and cushion the tibiofemoral articulation), and the anterior and posterior cruciate ligaments, which provide stability for the knee joint. The collateral ligaments stabilize the medial and lateral aspects of the knee.

What Key Questions Should Be Asked as Part of the History in a Patient with Acute Knee Pain?

When a patient presents complaining of acute knee pain, it is important to gather as much information as possible surrounding the onset of pain. Several key questions should be answered:

- Was it truly acute or more insidious?
- Was there an associated fall? If so, describe the details of the fall.
- Was there an associated twisting event or audible pop?

- Did the pain begin immediately?
- Was the patient able to ambulate more than a few steps after the event?
- If swelling is present, did the knee swell up rapidly or after a delay of several hours or on the next day?
- Are there any systemic symptoms suggesting a contributing medical disorder?
- Is there a prior history of injury, pain, or surgery in that knee?

With the patient standing (in a gown), look for a varus or valgus deformity. Observe the patient's ability to walk toward and away from the examination table. With the patient supine on the examining table with knees extended, look for evidence of asymmetric muscle wasting (suggesting a more chronic process). Do not forget the possibility of referred pain from the hip.

How Do You Examine the Knee for the Presence of an Effusion?

The evaluation for a knee effusion is best performed with the patient supine and knees extended and relaxed. First visually inspect the knees. In patients of average build, a hollow is normally present on both sides of the patella. Suspect an effusion if this has filled in.

A visible fluid wave suggests a small to moderate effusion. Using the thumb on one side and the index finger on the other, the examiner simultaneously compresses the hollows of the knee, both medial and lateral to the patella, forcing any fluid into the suprapatellar pouch. The examiner then lifts the hand and presses the suprapatellar pouch while looking at the hollows. The presence of a fluid wave and filling in of the hollows suggests a small to moderate effusion.

A palpable fluid wave suggests a large effusion. In the presence of larger effusions, fluid may return to the hollows too quickly for the examiner to see a fluid wave. The examination technique is initially the same as above: simultaneously compress the hollows of the knee both medial and lateral to the patella using one hand, forcing any fluid into the suprapatellar pouch. Then, without removing the pressure on the hollows from the first hand, compress the suprapatellar pouch. The examiner should feel returning fluid pushing the first hand outward. This technique can be useful in obese patients in whom visualizing a fluid wave will be difficult.

When the knee is very swollen, you must try to distinguish between soft tissue swelling (due to edema or hematoma) and intraarticular fluid. The palpable fluid wave is useful. Large effusions tend to extend into the suprapatella pouch, creating a bulge under the distal quadriceps. Hematomas may be more localized to the site of trauma.

A ballotable patella (moderate effusion) may be present on examination with the knee in full extension, because in this position large effusions may lift the patella. To ballot the patella, the examiner uses two or three fingers to quickly push the patella posteriorly. The patella will descend and strike the femur with a distinct impact. If the effusion is large and tense, however, the effusion may prevent the impact from being felt.

How Do You Assess the Range of Motion of the Knee?

Generally the assessment of range of motion of the knee joint is limited to measurement of extension and flexion. Suspicion of ligamentous injuries, however, requires a more extensive evaluation of range of motion in other planes.

Normally the knees should fully extend to 180 degrees. Knee hyperextension is common, but except in some loose-jointed individuals, hyperextension is generally limited to an additional 10 degrees or less.

Passive extension can be assessed with the patient supine. The examiner raises both of the patient's feet in the air, keeping the medial malleoli together. The degree of extension is noted, with attention to symmetry. Another method of assessing passive extension is the "prone hanging test," where the patient lies prone on the examining table with knees and legs hanging off of the table. Any difference in heel height is noted.

The patient's ability to actively extend the knee is measured with the patient seated on the examining table with legs dangling. The examiner asks the patient to fully extend the knee. If active extension is not full, the examiner should attempt full passive extension. When active extension is less than passive extension, consider problems with the quadriceps tendon or muscle strength or patellofemoral pain. Complete inability to actively extend suggests rupture of the quadriceps or patellar tendons or patellar fracture.

A normal knee can be flexed to 130 to 150 degrees, although people can generally climb stairs and function relatively well with flexion in the range of 110 degrees. Most patients can get each heel to the ipsilateral buttock. In fact, the heel-to-buttock distance can be used to assess small amounts of flexion loss. Loss of flexion is common in effusions, arthritic changes, or patellofemoral pain. Assessment of passive flexion may be painful and not add clinical significance, unless pain is localized to a joint line (e.g., in the case of a meniscus injury).

How Do You Assess the Stability of the Medial and Lateral Collateral Ligaments of the Knee?

The two stability tests for the medial collateral ligament (MCL) and lateral collateral ligament (LCL) are the valgus and varus stress tests. For valgus stress testing, a force directed toward the midline is applied to the knee while an opposing force is applied at the ankle or foot. For varus stress testing, the opposite forces occur; a force directed away from the midline is applied to the knee while an opposing force is applied at the ankle or foot.

Medial collateral ligament injuries most often involve valgus force and usually occur at the ligament's proximal insertion site over the distal femur. The physical examination may show an effusion, along with localized tenderness medially, soft tissue swelling, and ecchymosis extending to the medial joint line.

To perform the valgus stress test, the patient must be supine with the knee in full extension. The examiner lifts the lower limb by grasping it at the ankle. The knee must be fully relaxed so that it falls into full extension. The limb should feel like a dead weight. The examiner then applies a gentle inward force at the knee with an outward force at the ankle, followed by relaxation of these forces. The examiner looks and feels for separation of the femur and tibia medially during the application of the force and a clunk when the femur and tibia move back together after the force is removed. Normally there is no separation with the knee in full extension. The valgus stress test is then applied to the unaffected limb for comparison.

If the test is normal (no laxity found), the examiner should flex the knee 10 to 15 degrees (no more) and repeat the test. Slight flexion removes the contributions of secondary resistance to valgus forces (primarily that of the posteromedial capsule) and focuses the forces on the MCL. A normal valgus stress test result in full extension and an abnormal result with 10 to 15 degrees of flexion suggests isolated MCL damage.

Lateral collateral ligament injuries involving varus forces suggest an LCL injury. Similar to an MCL injury, the physical examination may show an effusion, with localized tenderness laterally, soft tissue swelling, and ecchymosis extending posteriorly across the lateral joint line toward the fibular head.

Varus stress testing is the counterpart to valgus stress testing. Varus forces are applied first with full extension, then with 10 to 15 degrees of knee flexion. The examiner looks and feels for abnormal separation of the femur and tibia laterally. Normally there is no separation with the knee in full extension, but most patients have some natural laxity of the lateral ligaments at 10 to 15 degrees of flexion (generally about 3–5 mm). Thus, it is very important to compare the degree of laxity between the two limbs. As in the case of valgus stress testing, abnormal laxity noted during full extension suggests more extensive damage to the knee.

How Do You Perform the McMurray and Lachman Tests? What Knee Abnormalities Do Positive Test Results Suggest?

The McMurray test is a test for a meniscus injury. The supine patient is asked to flex the involved knee as far as possible. The examiner grasps the patient's hindfoot and externally rotates the foot while placing a varus stress at the knee to compress the medial meniscus. The knee is then passively extended while the examiner palpates the medial joint line with the index finger of the other hand, looking for a click.

The test for a lateral meniscus injury is the converse. The examiner applies an internal rotation valgus force to the flexed knee. The knee is then passively extended, causing pain localized to the lateral joint line.

A positive test result is defined as a complaint of pain localized to the respective joint line and a palpable click felt at this site by the examiner. However, in some cases of medial meniscus injury, the click may not be felt. A click is rarely palpated in a lateral meniscus injury. The presence of localized joint line pain upon passive knee extension is still suggestive of a meniscal injury. False positive results may occur with osteoarthritis.

The Lachman test is a test for anterior knee laxity as seen in ACL injury. It is performed with the knee in 20 to 30 degrees of flexion and the patient supine. The examiner stands next to the examining table on the side to be examined. The examiner grasps the patient's thigh right above the patella with one hand and uses the other hand to grasp below the knee, placing the thumb over the tibial tubercle and the rest of the fingers around the calf. The patient must be fully relaxed, and the limb should feel like dead weight. The examiner pulls forward on the tibia with one hand while pushing backward on the thigh. Because the majority of normal individuals have either no anterior movement or 1 to 2 mm of anterior movement with a very firm end point, anything more than this is considered abnormal. In the presence of an ACL tear, forward translation of the tibia is increased and the end point indefinite.

The Lachman test has replaced the more well known anterior drawer test in the assessment of anterior laxity for several reasons. First, the anterior drawer test requires knee flexion to 90 degrees (rather than 20–30 degrees in the Lachman test). Patients with acute knee injuries often have difficulty flexing to 90 degrees. Second, many patients have considerable anterior laxity at 90 degrees, making laxity interpretation more difficult. Lastly, when flexed to 90 degrees, the hamstring muscles can mask abnormal translation, particularly in patients who are not fully relaxed.

Case 1

A healthy 50-year-old man presents to your office complaining of knee swelling and pain for the past 2 days. Two days ago while swinging a golf club he felt a pop in his left knee and had acute, severe pain. He was able to finish the game, limping and relying heavily on the golf cart, but had to modify his swing to prevent twisting. Over the past 2 days he noted increased swelling, pain with weight bearing, and difficulty flexing his knee. On physical examination he has difficulty weight bearing due to pain, but is able to walk across the room with a limp.

The examination demonstrates a ballotable patella, tenderness at the medial joint line, decreased range of motion (flexion to 90 degrees and unable to fully extend), and a positive McMurray test result.

What Is the Most Likely Diagnosis and Appropriate Approach to This Patient?

The popping sensation and acute pain after twisting is typical of a meniscus tear. Because the meniscus is relatively avascular, bleeding into the joint is slower than in a cruciate ligament tear, and swelling generally occurs more gradually. Joint stability is present on physical examination, but the McMurray test result is positive. Many partial tears will heal with time, and generally a conservative approach is taken at first. Orthopedic referral is recommended but is not emergent. Ordering magnetic resonance imaging (or arthroscopy) should be the orthopedic consultant's decision.

Case 2

A 35-year-old man was playing touch football at a family reunion. He remembers twisting his left knee and falling on the grass while hearing a "pop." He developed severe pain in his left knee and had to be carried off the field due to inability to take a step. His cousin, who had experienced several knee injuries, wrapped his knee in an elastic bandage and lent him crutches and pain pills. The knee became swollen within the hour. Not wanting to go to the emergency department, he made an appointment with you for the next morning. On physical examination, he is unable to bear weight or take a step. He has a swollen left knee with evidence of a moderate sized effusion. There is tenderness with flexion or extension, but no joint laxity with application of medial or lateral stress. The Lachman test result is positive.

What Is the Most Likely Diagnosis and Appropriate Approach to This Patient?

This scenario is typical of an ACL tear. These are serious injuries that may be produced by hyperextension of the knee or a valgus force applied to an externally rotated femur. Patients with suspected ACL tears should be referred to an orthopedist quickly because ligamentous repairs (if indicated) might be performed within the first few days of the injury. The diagnosis generally can be made by history and physical examination, but may be missed, particularly in the case of a partial tear. Plain radiographs are insensitive, but may have one or more of three suggestive findings: (a) avulsion of the intercondylar tubercle, (b) the radiographic drawer sign (anterior displacement of the tibia with respect to the femur), and (c) a Segond fracture (avulsion of a sliver of bone from the proximal lateral tibia). Arthroscopy is the gold standard. MRI has a reported accuracy of 90% when compared with arthroscopy, and ultrasonography has been shown to be useful in the setting of a traumatic hemarthrosis.

Case 3

A healthy 50-year-old man presents to your office with right knee swelling. He has been helping his son with carpentry work over the past 2 weeks and is now unable to kneel due to pain and swelling. He denies knee trauma. On physical examination he is ambulating with minimal difficulty. An egg-like swelling of the right knee anterior to the patella is present with no overlying skin lesions, warmth, or redness. He has decreased knee flexion to 90 degrees.

What Is the Most Likely Diagnosis and Appropriate Approach to This Patient?

This patient's presentation is typical of prepatellar bursitis. Prepatellar bursitis is common in wrestlers, roofers, and carpet layers. These patients may have thickening of the overlying skin. Warmth, erythema, or an overlying skin lesion may suggest infection. A typical size of a prepatellar effusion is 5 cm, although they can be larger. Most patients respond well to conservative treatment with antiinflammatory medicines, compressive wrappings, and avoidance of further trauma. Aspiration with cell count, Gram stain, and culture should be performed if there is suspicion of infection. Corticosteroid injections are not recommended due to the proximity of the patellar and quadriceps tendons.

Suggested Reading

Jacobson K E, Flandry F C. Diagnosis of anterior knee pain. *Clin Sports Med* 1989;8:179–195.

Kalb R L. Evaluation and treatment of acute knee pain. *Hosp Practice* 1997;1:61–63.

Klippel J H, Dieppe P A, Ferri F F. *Primary care rheumatology.* St Louis: CV Mosby, 1999.

McCune W J, Matteson E L, MacGuire A. Evaluation of knee pain. *Primary Care* 1998;15:795–808.

Mercier L R. *Practical orthopedics,* 3rd ed. St. Louis: CV Mosby, 1991.

Reider B. *The orthopaedic physical examination.* Philadelphia: WB Saunders, 1999.

Skinner H B, Scherger J E. Identifying structural hip and knee problems. *Postgrad Med* 1999;106:51–68.

Tandeter H B, Schvartzman P, Stevens M A. Acute knee injuries: use of decision rules for selective radiograph ordering. *Am Fam Physician.* 1999;60:2599–2608.

82
Low Back Pain

Yacob Ghebremeskel

- Discussion   *517*
- Case   *519*
- Case Discussion   *520*

1. What is the pathophysiology of low back pain?
2. What features on history and physical examination suggest the need for further imaging studies?
3. Discuss the different treatment options.

Discussion
What Is the Pathophysiology of Low Back Pain?

The spine consists of the vertebrae joined together by discs anteriorly and facets posterolaterally. These structures are held together by ligaments and muscles attached to the tendons. The spinal cord is located inside the spinal column. Nerve roots pass through the foramina to innervate appropriate dermatomes and muscles.

Functional or organic damage to back structures can cause low back pain. In addition, low back pain can be referred pain originating from intraabdominal structures. Low back pain can be classified into acute (<3 months) and chronic low back pain (>3 months). Depending on the character of the pain, it can be either radicular or nonradicular low back pain.

Radicular pain is characterized as brief, sharp, shooting pain that starts in the middle of the back and radiates to the buttock, posterior thigh, or calf area. The intensity of this pain generally increases with cough, straining (increased intraabdominal pressure), or bending (nerve root stretching). Impingement or irritation of the lumbar nerve roots is responsible for the pain. Major causes of radicular low back pain are listed as follows:

- Intraspinal causes: neurofibroma, ependyloma, meningioma, herniated disc, spinal stenosis, synovial cyst of the facet joint, arteriovenous malformation, and spinal arteriovenous fistulas
- Extraspinal causes: vascular, gynecologic, sacroiliac joint, retroperitoneal neoplasm, lumbosacral plexitis, mononeuropathy, polyneuropathy, herpes zoster, and trauma

Nonradicular pain is characterized as nonspecific low back pain. It is usually localized over the low-back area or at times radiates to the buttock area. Nonradicular pain can be due to muscle sprain, fracture, degenerative joint disease, infection, and psychogenic causes.

What Features on History and Physical Examination Suggest the Need for Further Imaging Studies?

Low back pain is extremely common. Annually, 50% of the working adult population suffers from low back pain; 15% to 20% of these seek medical care. Of all office visits for low back pain, 56% are to family physicians and internists. It is extremely important that primary care providers know the appropriate use of imaging studies in evaluating patients with low back pain.

A thorough history and physical examination can identify patients with potentially dangerous underlying conditions or red flags. The following historical features increase the likelihood of a more serious condition:

1. Preceding major trauma
2. Recent infection
3. Immune suppression
4. Cancer
5. Younger or older age (<20 years or >50 years)
6. Significant weight loss
7. History of intravenous drug abuse
8. Prior evaluation and treatment for low back pain
9. Pain that worsens when supine
10. Bowel or bladder dysfunction

In addition, the characteristics of the pain, location, duration, progression, and alleviating and exacerbating factors should be noted. During the physical examination, it is important to observe the patient's overall appearance. Look at how the patient walks, undresses, and sits on and arises from the chair or examination table. This will give you important information about the severity of the pain and functionality of the patient, and may help you detect discrepancies between the pain and functionality. On physical examination, muscle atrophy or weakness, absence of deep tendon reflexes, laxity of the anal sphincter, and loss of perineal sensation should be noted. In the absence of the aforementioned red flags, there is no need for ordering imaging studies in the acute setting, because 90% of patients recover within 4 weeks.

Discuss the Treatment Options.

Treatment of acute low back pain depends on the etiology of the pain. After excluding red flags, most patients will recover within 4 weeks of conservative therapy. Pain should preferably be treated with acetaminophen, nonsteroid antiinflammatory drugs (NSAIDs), or muscle relaxants. A meta-analysis of 150 trials showed that acetaminophen and NSAIDs are equally effective in the treatment of acute back pain and better than placebo. All NSAIDs are equally effective. Muscle relaxants are superior to placebo, and all are equally effective. Taking the higher rate of side effects of NSAIDs and muscle relaxants into consideration, it is advisable to start with acetaminophen and add NSAIDs as needed. For patients with a higher risk of developing gastrointestinal bleed, consider the newer cyclooxygenase-2 inhibitors. Try to avoid narcotics if possible.

Treatment of chronic low-back pain also may include the use of tricyclic antidepressants and lumbar epidural steroid injection. In one study, patients with chronic low back pain were treated with one, two, or three epidural injections of 80 mg of DepoMedrol. Approximately 60% of patients had varying degree of relief immediately after the injection, but only 24% were asymptomatic at follow-up examination. There was no correlation between the number of injections given and relief of pain. Another study showed no significant difference in low-back pain 6 weeks after epidural steroid injection between patients who were treated with steroid versus saline injection. A meta-analysis of six studies showed that transcutaneous nerve stimulation and acupuncture-like transcutaneous nerve stimulation (ALTENS) reduced pain, and ALTENS improved range of movement in patients with chronic low back pain.

In addition to medical treatment, life-style modification is essential. Patients should stay active after initial treatment of acute pain. Studies have shown that patients who stay active get better sooner. The role of back exercise in the management of low back pain is still unclear. There is insufficient evidence to advise for or against exercise to prevent low back pain. There is also insufficient evidence to advise for or against the routine use of educational intervention, mechanical supports, or risk factor modification to prevent low back pain. However, the standard approach to back pain management generally includes patient education on proper lifting techniques and on signs and symptoms suggesting serious back problems. Patients should be encouraged to stop smoking and drinking alcohol, reduce weight, and participate in regular stretching exercises.

Patients with severe spinal stenosis and herniated disc who do not respond to medical treatment for at least 6 months, have significant neurologic deficit, or have cauda equina syndrome may be considered for low back surgery. Patient selection is extremely important. It is interesting to note that back surgery is performed six times more often in the United States than in the United Kingdom. A meta-analysis of 74 studies showed that 64% of the patients who were treated surgically for lumbar spinal stenosis had good to excellent outcomes. In a retrospective study of 88 patients who underwent laminectomy, 52% were pain free, 17% underwent a second operation, and 30% had severe pain in 3 to 5 years of follow-up. Seven to ten years later the reoperation rate increased to 30%.

Case

A 50-year-old man presents with new-onset lower back pain after lifting a heavy item at work 3 days prior to this visit. The pain is sharp (7/10 in severity) and localized over the lumbar area with no radiation. The pain generally worsens with bending. There is no numbness, muscle weakness, urinary, or bowel incontinence. The patient requests a radiograph.

The physical examination was significant for absence of fever and paraspinal tenderness. The results of a straight leg raise test are negative. He has 5/5 muscle strength, 2+ deep tendon reflexes, intact light touch sensation, and normal rectal tone.

1. What imaging study would you order?
2. What is the sensitivity and specificity of straight leg raising?
3. Discuss the different radiologic examinations used in evaluating low back pain?
4. How do you treat this patient?

Case Discussion

What Imaging Study Would You Order?

Even though the patient has a history of heavy lifting, there is no red flag in the history or physical examination. There is no benefit to ordering any imaging modality in this patient at this point. The patient is rightly concerned about his back, but it is up to the provider to explain to the patient that according to the history and physical examination, he most likely has muscle strain and his prognosis is excellent.

What Is the Sensitivity and Specificity of Straight Leg Raising?

Results of a straight leg raise test are positive when leg elevation at 30 to 70 degrees provokes radicular pain due to nerve root stretching at the L5 and S1 levels. Pain at less than 30 degrees elevation is not radicular. At that level you cannot stretch the nerve roots enough to cause pain. The sensitivity and specificity of the test are 80% and 20%, respectively. Crossed straight leg raising is more specific when the patient complains of radicular pain on contralateral leg elevation. The sensitivity and specificity of this test are 25% and 90%, respectively. Other tests include knee jerk (L3, L4), ankle jerk (S1), toe walking (S1), heel walking (L5), rectal tone, and cremaster reflex.

Discuss the Different Radiologic Examinations Used in Evaluating Low Back Pain.

Diagnostic imaging studies should be used to confirm the information gathered from the history and physical examination. Routine radiography is not recommended during the first month of back problems except when a red flag is noted. Anteroposterior, lateral, and spot L5–S1 spinal radiography is the initial test for evaluating low back pain. Its sensitivity for metastatic bone lesions is 60% to 70%. In one study of patients with metastatic bone disease, 40% of the patients had normal radiographs. In another study of patients with low back pain and an abnormal bone scan, only 67% had abnormal radiographs. Bone scan is extremely sensitive for bone turnover, but it does not yield specific diagnoses. It helps in determining the necessity of additional tests.

Computed tomography (CT) is superior to magnetic resonance imaging (MRI) for bony changes. In one study the sensitivity and specificity of CT for detecting disc herniation were 72% and 77%, respectively. CT with myelography is the gold standard test for the diagnosis of herniated disc. Because myelography is invasive, MRI is commonly used. CT does not allow a multiplanar view of the spine below L3.

Magnetic resonance imaging does not change the management of patients with acute low back pain in the absence of red flags. In one study, 25% of asymptomatic adults under 60 years of age had herniated discs. In another similar study, 25% of asymptomatic adults over 60 years of age had spinal stenosis. In degenerative disc disease there is a decrease in signal intensity within the nucleus pulposis on T2-weighted image. It is important to note that the findings in the MRI may or may not correlate with the clinical picture. As a general rule, it is advisable to refer patients to a spine surgeon if your clinical suspicion is high enough that patients will need back surgery, because an MRI ordered during an initial evaluation may be outdated by the time the patient is evaluated for surgery.

How Do You Treat This Patient?

Patients with acute low back pain with no red flags are treated with conservative therapy, including acetaminophen or NSAIDs. Life-style modification and proper lifting techniques need to be stressed. It is important to reexamine the patient in 4 weeks to see if his low back pain is improved. If not, reevaluate the patient for the presence or absence of any red flag that was not detected at the initial visit and treat accordingly.

Suggested Reading

Lehrich J R, Sheon R P. Treatment of low-back pain unresponsive to conservative management. *Up to Date* 1999.

NSAID and muscle relaxants reduce acute low back pain; manipulation, back schools, and exercise reduce chronic low-back pain. *ACP Journal Club* 1998;128:65.

Rose-Innes A P, Engstrom J W. Low back pain: an algorithmic approach to diagnosis and management. *Geriatrics* 1998;53:26.

Steinberg G G, Akins C M, Baran D T. Orthopedics in primary care. In: Bayley JC, ed. *Thoracic and lumbar spine,* 3rd ed. Philadelphia: Lippincott Williams & Wilkins, 1999:139.

U.S. Department of Health and Human Services. *Acute low back problems in adults: assessment and treatment.* U.S. Department of Health and Human Services, 1994:95-0643.

Walddell G, Feder G, Lewis M. Systemic reviews of bed rest and advice to stay active for low back pain. *Br J Gen Practice* 1997;47:647.

83
Shoulder Pain
Rebecca Babcock Bair

- Discussion   *522*
- Case   *525*
- Case Discussion   *526*

1. What historical information is important in the evaluation of shoulder pain?
2. What are the components of a complete physical examination of the shoulder?
3. Compare and contrast the key historical and physical examination findings of the following common causes of shoulder pain: glenohumeral dislocation, acromioclavicular joint sprain and separation, rotator cuff tear, impingement syndrome, and adhesive capsulitis.
4. How are the above shoulder problems managed?

Discussion
What Historical Information Is Important in the Evaluation of Shoulder Pain?

Key historical points include the patient's age, dominant hand, and work history. Patients also should be asked about sports activities, recent trauma, hobbies, and prior shoulder pain or injuries. In addition, it is helpful to ask about prior physical therapy or joint injections. Finally, one should inquire about the exact location of pain, aggravating activities, stiffness, and limitation in range of motion and arm weakness.

What Are the Components of a Complete Physical Examination of the Shoulder?

A complete shoulder examination begins with visual inspection for any discoloration, abrasions, muscle atrophy, or gross deformity. Gross deformity of the shoulder may indicate glenohumeral dislocation, acromioclavicular strain or separation, or clavicle fracture. One should then palpate the acromioclavicular articulation. Motion of the shoulder girdle causes the acromioclavicular joint to move and makes it easier to identify. The acromioclavicular joint may be tender secondary to osteoarthritis or acromioclavicular joint sprain or separation.

The rotator cuff has clinical importance because degeneration and subsequent tearing of its tendon of insertion is a common condition, which results in weakness and restriction of shoulder movement, particularly in abduction. The rotator cuff can be palpated slightly inferior to the border of the acromion. Any tenderness elicited during palpation may be due to muscle strain, defects, or tears. Of the muscles of the rotator cuff, the supraspinatus is the most commonly ruptured.

Subacromial bursitis is a frequent pathologic finding, which can cause much tenderness and restriction of shoulder motion. Portions of the bursa are palpable just below the acromion. From the lateral edge of the acromion, the bursa extends under the deltoid muscle, separating it from the rotator cuff and allowing each to move freely. The subacromial bursa should be palpated very carefully, because the area can be very tender if bursitis is present.

The quickest way to evaluate a patient's active range of motion is the Apley "scratch" test. First, to test abduction and external rotation, ask the patient to reach behind his or her head and touch the superior medial angle of the opposite scapula. Next, to determine the range of internal rotation and adduction, instruct the patient to reach in front of his or her head and touch the opposite acromion. Finally, to further test internal rotation and adduction, have the patient reach behind his or her back to touch the inferior angle of the opposite scapula. Observe the patient's movement during all phases of testing for any limitation of motion or for any break of normal rhythm or symmetry.

If the patient is unable to perform any of the above motions, passive range of motion testing should be conducted. Passive range of motion is tested by moving the joint through its entire range of motion and noting any limitations.

If a rotator cuff tear is suspected, one can perform the drop arm test. The patient should be instructed to fully abduct his or her arm. The patient should then slowly lower his or her arm to the side. If there are any tears in the rotator cuff, the arm will drop to the side from a position of 90 degrees abduction.

The supraspinatus strength test also can be performed if there is a suspicion of rotator cuff tear. The patient should place both arms in a position of 90 degrees abduction and 30 degrees forward flexion with the thumbs pointing down. The examiner should push down on both arms as the patient resists this pressure. Lack of resistance and presence of pain suggests a rotator cuff tear.

The Hawkins impingement sign is often positive in impingement syndrome or shoulder bursitis. With the patient's arm in a throwing position and flexed forward about 30 degrees, the examiner forcibly internally rotates the humerus. Pain at a reproducible point is a positive test result that indicates impingement of the supraspinatus tendon against the coracoacromial ligament and the acromion.

Glenohumeral Dislocation

Most shoulder dislocations are anterior. Patients with anterior shoulder dislocation commonly hold the affected arm in external rotation and abduction. There is usually an obvious deformity beneath the acromion. Glenohumeral dislocations occur in patients under 30 years of age who have had multiple transient dislocations (subluxations). One should obtain both anteroposterior and axillary radiographs demonstrating the dislocation. Most acute shoulder dislocations can be reduced in the emergency department. There are several methods for reduction of anterior shoulder dislocation. The shoulder joint should then be immobilized for 7 to 10 days to permit capsular healing. The patient should begin early strengthening and range of motion exercises at 2 to 3 weeks. Recurrence rates of anterior shoulder dislocations, particularly in young athletes, are as high as 95%. Educating the patient to avoid voluntarily dislocating the shoulder and to avoid positions of known instability should be a part of the treatment plan.

Recurrent dislocations (two or more) despite a 3-month trial of shoulder rehabilitation exercises should warrant further evaluation by an orthopedic surgeon. Adverse outcomes of anterior shoulder dislocation include pain and weakness of the shoulder joint, persistent instability, and intermittent paresthesias in the arm. Posterior shoulder dislocations are rare, and they occur in the setting of seizures and electrical shocks. Posterior dislocations can easily be missed with routine shoulder radiographs. This type of dislocation is best seen with axillary view radiographs.

Acromioclavicular Joint Sprain and Separation

The acromioclavicular joint and its supporting ligaments are susceptible to injury by overuse and trauma. The ligaments binding the acromion, clavicle, and coracoid process together can be strained, partially torn, or completely disrupted. Acromioclavicular injuries commonly result from a fall onto the tip of the shoulder (acromion). The current classification series recognizes six types of acromioclavicular separations. These injuries are classified on the basis of the degree of separation of the end of the clavicle relative to the acromion. Patients report pain over the acromioclavicular joint, and lifting the arm is painful. Gentle pressure over the acromioclavicular joint elicits pain and the patient will complain of pain when lifting the affected arm. There may be deformity of the acromioclavicular joint. An anteroposterior radiograph of the shoulder may be normal or may show elevation of the distal clavicle.

Nonsurgical treatment is appropriate for mild injuries. This includes wearing a sling for a few days until the pain subsides and applying ice to the area. Nonsteroidal agents are helpful for pain relief. Treatment of more severe injuries is controversial and may include surgery. These patients should be referred to an orthopedic surgeon. Adverse outcomes of acromioclavicular strain and separation include weakness of the shoulder joint and acromioclavicular joint arthritis.

Rotator Cuff Tear

Rotator cuff tears occur primarily in the supraspinatus tendon, which is weakened as a result of many factors, including injury, age, poor blood supply to the tendon, and subacromial impingement. This injury rarely affects people under 40 years of age. Tears are usually due to trauma such as falling onto an outstretched arm or hand; however, sometimes there is no recognized injury. Patients complain of pain over the shoulder radiating to the deltoid region, which often causes difficulty sleeping on the affected side. There also may be weakness of the supraspinatus muscle, catching, and grating, especially when lifting the arm overhead. The examination reveals atrophy of the supraspinatus and infraspinatus muscles, limited range of motion, and tenderness over the tear. Tears occur just proximal to the greater tuberosity of the humerus. Results of a drop arm test will be positive. Patients with suspected rotator cuff tears should be referred to an orthopedist for further evaluation, which may include imaging studies. Treatment consists of nonsteroidal antiinflammatory medications, physical therapy with strengthening exercises, and avoiding overhead activities. Lack of improvement with physical therapy, pain, and significant loss of function necessitate surgical intervention, particularly in younger patients.

The Impingement Syndrome

The impingement syndrome is due to impingement of the tendons of the rotator cuff between the bony structures of the coracoacromial arch (acromion, coracoacromial ligament, acromioclavicular joint, and coracoid process) and the humerus. This generally occurs with abduction of the arm. Impingement syndrome can result in inflammation of the tendons of the rotator cuff, bursa, and biceps tendon; commonly all are affected. A potential complication of impingement syndrome is a rotator cuff tear. Patients complain of anterior and lateral shoulder pain. Patients also complain of night pain and difficulty sleeping on the affected side. Symptoms are usually chronic. Examination reveals atrophy of the supraspinatus and infraspinatus muscles, crepitus when the patient actively lifts the arm, positive Hawkins impingement sign, and tenderness over the inflamed rotator cuff. Shoulder radiographs are usually normal. Treatment consists of nonsteroidal agents, rest, range-of-motion exercises, and subacromial injection of a corticosteroid. If pain persists, referral to an orthopedic surgeon is warranted for possible subacromial decompression.

Adhesive Capsuletis

Adhesive capsulitis is a specific condition with marked decreased active and passive range of motion of the shoulder. The shoulder pain of "frozen shoulder" is classically slow in onset and results from thickening and contraction of the capsule around the glenohumeral joint. Frozen shoulder occurs as a result of immobility following a shoulder injury. Patients often complain of shoulder discomfort, inability to sleep on the affected side, and restricted shoulder movement. The examination reveals significant reduction in both active and passive range of motion of the shoulder joint when compared with the opposite shoulder. Motion of the shoulder joint is painful, and there is tenderness over the rotator cuff. This process is typically slow to improve, often taking more than 2 years to resolve completely. Treatment consists of nonsteroidal agents and physical therapy with a home exercise program. Patients who fail to regain motion after 3 months of conservative treatment need further evaluation by an orthopedist.

Case

A 60-year-old right hand–dominant woman presents with the complaint of gradual onset of right shoulder pain over the past several months. She denies any history of trauma or prior shoulder injuries or surgeries. She reports that the pain is worse at night and she has difficulty sleeping on the affected side. In addition she has weakness and "catching" in the affected shoulder, especially when lifting the arm overhead. The patient is a retired teacher.

Examination of the right shoulder reveals tenderness over the anterior and lateral shoulder. The top and the back of the shoulder appear sunken. Passive range of motion is normal, but active range of motion is limited. She has weakness with abduction, forward elevation, and external rotation.

1. What is the differential diagnosis for the patient's shoulder pain?
2. What tests or physical examination findings will help you make the correct diagnosis?
3. How should you manage this patient's shoulder pain?

Case Discussion

What Is the Differential Diagnosis for the Patient's Shoulder Pain?

The differential diagnosis in this patient includes "frozen shoulder" or adhesive capsulitis (severe loss of both passive and active range of motion), glenohumeral arthritis (pain with any motion and usually evident on plain radiographs), herniated cervical disc (associated neck stiffness and deltoid weakness with absent biceps reflex), impingement syndrome, and rotator cuff tear (weakness of supraspinatus).

What Tests or Physical Examination Findings Will Help You Make the Correct Diagnosis?

A complete examination revealed that the top and the back of the shoulder were sunken, indicating atrophy of the supraspinatus and infraspinatus muscles. In addition, there was pain and crepitation when the patient actively lifted her arm from 60 to 100 degrees (the painful arc of motion). The Neer impingement sign was positive. This test is performed by raising the patient's arm overhead while the scapula is stabilized. If this maneuver elicits pain, the test (Neer impingement sign) is positive for impingement. The Hawkins impingement sign also was positive. This test is performed by placing the patient's arm in a throwing position and flexed forward about 30 degrees. The examiner then forcibly internally rotates the humerus. Pain at a reproducible point is a positive test result, which indicates impingement of the supraspinatus tendon between the coracoacromial arch and the humerus.

One should then perform the supraspinatus strength test. With the patient seated, place both arms in a position of 90 degrees abduction and 30 degrees forward flexion with the thumbs pointing down. Push down on both arms as the patient resists this pressure. Lack of resistance suggests a rotator cuff tear. Passive range of motion in a rotator cuff tear is normal, but active range of motion is limited. Conversely, patients with adhesive capsulitis have limited passive and active range of motion.

Plain radiographs of the shoulder are usually normal with impingement syndrome. This patient was referred to an orthopedic surgeon, who ordered magnetic resonance imaging (MRI) of her right shoulder, confirming the diagnosis of a rotator cuff tear.

How Should You Manage This Patient's Shoulder Pain?

This patient likely has shoulder pain caused by impingement of the acromion, coracoacromial ligament, acromioclavicular joint, and coracoid process on the underlying bursa, biceps tendon, and rotator cuff. This syndrome may be caused by inflammation of any of these structures, and commonly all are affected. One potential outcome is a rotator cuff tear, which the patient appears to have based on physical examination findings. Conservative treatment includes nonsteroidal antiinflammatory medications, physical therapy with strengthening and stretching exercises, and avoiding overhead activities. Corticosteroid injections are controversial and may further weaken the tendon. Complete rotator cuff tears can be repaired surgically. However, not all patients have symptoms severe enough to warrant surgical intervention.

This patient was instructed to take ibuprofen 800 mg orally with meals every 8 hours for 3 weeks. In addition, she was referred to physical therapy for a strengthening and stretching exercise program and instructed to avoid overhead activities for several weeks. She was referred to an orthopedic surgeon who ordered an MRI of the right shoulder. MRI revealed a rotator cuff tear in the supraspinatus tendon, which was probably weakened by subacromial impingement. The orthopedic surgeon recommended continued conservative therapy.

Suggested Reading

Hoppenfield S. *Physical examination of the spine and extremities.* Norwalk, CT: Appleton-Century-Crofts, 1976.

Rockwood, Matsen. *The shoulder.* Philadelphia: WB Saunders, 1998.

Snider R K. *Essentials of musculoskeletal care.* Rosemont, Illinois: American Academy of Orthopedic Surgeons, 1997:70–123.

XV
Rheumatology

84
Osteoarthritis

Allen R. Watson, Jr.
Clyde Watkins, Jr.

1. Review the risk factors for the development of osteoarthritis.
2. Describe the physiology of a normal joint and the mechanisms believed to be involved in the development of osteoarthritis.
3. Review the clinical features and diagnostic criteria for osteoarthritis.
4. Elaborate on the treatment options for osteoarthritis.
5. Review the difference between conventional nonsteroidal antiinflammatory drugs and cyclooxygenase-2 inhibitors.

Discussion

Review the Risk Factors for the Development of Osteoarthritis.

Osteoarthritis (OA) occurs in all races and locations. When it occurs in the setting of predisposing factors, it is classified as secondary OA, whereas when it occurs in the absence of known risk factors, it is classified as primary or idiopathic. Currently recognized risk factors include age, gender (men tend to have higher rates of OA than women until the age of 50 years), obesity, mutations in the type II collagen gene, acquired bone/joint disease (e.g., rheumatoid arthritis, gout, Paget disease), race/ethnicity (e.g., Native Americans have the highest prevalence of OA), prior joint trauma/surgery (e.g., meniscal tear or meniscectomy), and occupations requiring repetitive usage (e.g., cotton mill workers). Of these, age is the strongest risk factor.

Describe the Physiology of a Normal Joint and the Mechanisms Believed to Be Involved in the Development of Osteoarthritis.

See Figs. 84.1 and 84.2. The articular cartilage and the subchondral bone are the primary targets for the destructive processes involved in OA. In the normal joint, cartilage is composed of collagen (predominantly type 2) and proteoglycans, both of which are synthesized by chondrocytes. Proteoglycans are high-molecular-weight molecules that permit the cartilage to retain water and form a highly viscous

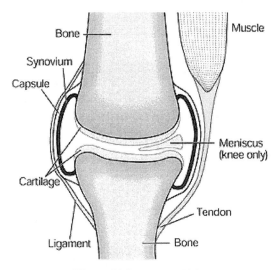

Figure 84.1. A normal joint.

synovial fluid. These properties of cartilage allow it to absorb stress and provide low friction movement of the joint. In the osteoarthritic joint, degradation of the articular cartilage and stiffening of the subchondral bone lead to a joint that is less resilient and mobile. The initiating event in the development of OA is unknown; however, many theories have been proposed to explain the underlying mechanisms that may be involved. Of these, the one that appears the most favored proposes that OA develops when the balance of the synthetic and degradative processes involved in cartilage turnover shifts in favor of cartilage degradation. This theory is supported by the discovery of matrix metalloproteinases (MMPs). They are enzymes that catalyze cartilage degradation, leading to a decrease in the rheologic (viscosity and

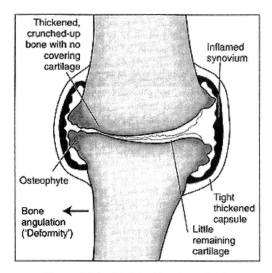

Figure 84.2. A joint with osteoarthritis.

flow) properties of synovial fluid and a breakdown in the joint architecture. In experimental models, MMPs are found in higher concentrations in joints affected by OA. There is also evidence that inflammation plays a role in the development of OA: proinflammatory cytokines, such as tumor necrosis factor-α and interleukin-1, have been found in higher concentrations in OA cartilage and appear to activate MMPs.

Review the Clinical Features and Diagnostic Criteria for Osteoarthritis.

The most common symptom is joint pain that typically affects weight-bearing joints, but can also affect other joints that have been predisposed by trauma, inflammation, or overuse. The pain is usually mild to moderate in severity and worsened by movement of the affected joint. Patients also may have joint stiffness of short duration (5–30 minutes) that improves as the joints are moved. Physical examination may show bony enlargement, decreased range of motion, crepitation, and effusions around affected joints. Radiographs may reveal osteophytes, narrowed joint spaces, sclerotic bone, subchondral cysts, and debris. The American College of Rheumatology has developed criteria that help to identify patients that may have OA of the hand, hip, or knee. With regard to OA of the knee, a combination of clinical and radiographic features gives the highest diagnostic yield. For example, the presence of knee pain and radiographic osteophytes, plus age greater than 50 years, stiffness less than 30 minutes, or crepitus, yields a sensitivity of 91% and a specificity of 86%. The classification criteria developed for the hand and hip differ somewhat but have comparable diagnostic accuracy, with a sensitivity and specificity of 94% and 87% for the hand, and 89% and 91% for the hip.

Elaborate on the Treatment Options for Osteoarthritis.

Treatment options for OA may be divided into nonpharmacologic, pharmacologic, and surgical.

Nonpharmacologic

Options include patient education, monthly telephone contact, weight loss (if overweight), and physical therapy. Patient education and telephone contact increase patients' awareness of ways to manage their illness and lead to decreased pain and physician visits. Weight loss diminishes pain by reducing stress on weight-bearing joints. It also reduces the risk of developing symptoms as shown in a retrospective analysis of 64 women from the Framingham cohort. Physical therapists provide instruction on range of motion and strengthening exercises, as well as the use of canes and other assistive devices; these lead to decreased pain and improved mobility. Good data are lacking regarding the use of thermal modalities (e.g., the application of hot or cold packs), wedged insoles to correct for varus and valgus knee deformities, and taping the medial knee to realign the patella; however, these are relatively innocuous and may be beneficial in some patients. Use of transcutaneous electrical nerve stimulation and tidal irrigation of the knee is controversial.

Pharmacologic

U.S. Food and Drug Administration (FDA)-approved medications include acetaminophen, capsaicin cream, nonsteroidal antiinflammatory drugs (NSAIDs), cyclooxygenase-2 (COX-2) inhibitors, intraarticular steroids, opiates, and intraarticular hyaluronic acid. Popular alternative treatments include glucosamine and chondroitin. Acetaminophen, in doses up to 4 g per day, is considered the drug of first choice (use with caution in patients with liver disease). Capsaicin cream can be used to supplement this or other medications the patient may be taking for OA; there are no data supporting its use as monotherapy. NSAIDs are considered the next step in patients not responding to a combination of acetaminophen and capsaicin cream. They may be combined with a cytoprotective agent (e.g., misoprostol 200 μg twice a day) in patients who are at high risk for NSAID-induced ulcers (age >65 years, prior history of ulcer disease, and concomitant steroids or anticoagulants); alternatively, a COX-2 inhibitor may be used.

Intraarticular steroids are usually reserved for patients whose joints have effusions or demonstrate other signs of inflammation, such as warmth and erythema. It is recommended that they not be administered in a single joint more than once every 3 months, because repeated injections may damage intraarticular structures. Prior to joint injection, the joint fluid should be aspirated and sent for crystal examination, cell count, Gram stain, and culture.

Opiates are typically used for patients with acute pain flare-ups refractory to other modalities. Due to their addictive potential, it is suggested that they not be used more than 14 days at a time.

Relatively new to the armamentarium of medications used for OA is intraarticular hyaluronic acid. It is a component of proteoglycan molecules that acts to replace the rheologic properties of synovial fluid, so-called viscosupplementation. Data from experimental models suggests that it also increases endogenous hyaluronan synthesis, decreases degradation of proteoglycans, and insulates pain fibers. The two available preparations, hylan G-F 20 and sodium hyaluronate, have been found to be beneficial in the treatment of OA of the knee when injected once weekly for 3 or 5 consecutive weeks, respectively. At present, use of this therapy is limited due to its cost (average $500–$600) and the lack of data clearly indicating the optimal candidates for therapy; specifically, there are no guidelines indicating at what intervals and how often these injections can be repeated.

In the past few years, the use of glucosamine and chondroitin for the treatment of OA has gained popularity in the United States. They are naturally occurring constituents of cartilage proteoglycan and have been used individually or in combination for the treatment of OA in Europe for decades. This practice is supported by several European trials that yielded favorable results. *In vitro* data suggest that they increase endogenous proteoglycan synthesis and prevent further cartilage breakdown, a so-called chondroprotective effect. Based on the earlier European studies, these compounds appear to offer some benefit to patients with OA; however, as pointed out in a recent meta-analysis by McAlindon et al., methodologic flaws inherent in these earlier trials led to overestimates of true benefit. An ongoing National Institutes of Health trial may help clarify their role in the treatment of OA. Presently, they have not received FDA approval for this indication.

Surgical

Patients with OA who have pain and significant limitation of activities of daily living despite adequate pharmacologic and nonpharmacologic therapy should be referred to an orthopedic surgeon for evaluation. There is good evidence to date that in the hands of an experienced surgeon, total joint arthroplasty provides significant pain relief and functional improvements.

Review the Difference Between Conventional Nonsteroidal Antiinflammatory Drugs and Cyclooxygenase-2 Inhibitors.

In the past few years, our understanding of the biology of the COX enzyme has increased dramatically. We now know that there are at least two isoforms of the enzyme, COX-1 and COX-2. COX-1 is constitutively expressed and plays a key role in homeostatic functions such as protection of the gastric mucosa. COX-2, on the other hand, appears to be an inducible isoform involved in the inflammatory response and other pathologic processes. Conventional NSAIDs inhibit both isoforms, whereas, as their name implies, COX-2 inhibitors are much more selective inhibitors of COX-2. This property is responsible for their lower incidence of gastrointestinal ulceration, as shown in endoscopic studies. Whether they are a more cost-effective approach to preventing gastrointestinal ulceration than an NSAID combined with a cytoprotective agent is unknown.

Case

Mr. Smith is a 59-year-old carpenter, with a past medical history significant for hypertension and peptic ulcer disease, who comes to your office with pain in his left knee of several months' duration. He denies any trauma to his left knee. He describes the pain as soreness, which is 4 out of 10 in severity and worsened with walking and squatting. It is slightly improved with over-the-counter (OTC) analgesics and non–weight bearing. He has occasional swelling in his knee, and he sometimes feels that his knee is going to give way. A friend of his claimed to have had great success with glucosamine and chondroitin and suggested that he give them a try. The patient requests your opinion on this matter.

Physical examination reveals a weight of 250 pounds, height of 6 feet 1 inch (body mass index = 33), and blood pressure of 140/90 mm Hg. In general, he appears overweight and in no apparent distress. Cardiopulmonary examination is unremarkable. Examination of the left knee reveals a mild varus deformity and crepitation. There is no effusion or warmth. Anteroposterior and lateral views of the left knee reveal narrowing of the medial tibiofemoral joint space and osteophytes.

1. What are some nonpharmacologic approaches to treating this patient?
2. What medications would you use to treat this patient? Is he a candidate for arthroplasty at this time? Why or why not?
3. Would you recommend that he try glucosamine and chondroitin?

Case Discussion

What Are Some Nonpharmacologic Approaches to Treating This Patient?

A suitable nonpharmacologic approach to this patient may begin with instruction on joint protection. Examples include using well-cushioned jogging shoes as primary footwear; using wedged insoles to compensate for his varus deformity; and seeking alternatives to prolonged standing, kneeling, and squatting that may be required while on the job. Because our patient is overweight, an individualized exercise program aimed at muscle strengthening and weight loss also would be useful.

What Medications Would You Use to Treat This Patient? Is He a Candidate for Arthroplasty at This Time? Why or Why Not?

Based on the patient's history, he may already be using acetaminophen, but it is important to quantify how much and how often he is taking this remedy. If he were not responding to acetaminophen alone, capsaicin cream could be added. If he failed to respond to this combination, a COX-2 inhibitor could be tried; his history of peptic ulcer disease makes use of NSAIDs less favorable. He should also be counseled to avoid OTC medications that contain salicylates.

It would be premature to refer the patient for surgery, because he does not appear to have severe, debilitating disease and has not yet had an adequate trial of nonsurgical modalities.

Would You Recommend that He Try Glucosamine and Chondroitin?

Because the production of glucosamine and chondroitin is not currently regulated by the FDA, there is speculation regarding their safety. Therefore, unless he uses a brand from a company that is well known and trusted by him, it is probably best that he avoid these preparations.

Suggested Reading

Abramowicz M, ed. Hyaluronan injections for osteoarthritis of the knee. *Med Lett* 1998;40:69–70.

Creamer P, Hochberg M C. Osteoarthritis. *Lancet* 1997;350:503–509.

Deal C L, Moskowitz R W. Nutraceuticals as therapeutic agents in osteoarthritis: the role of glucosamine, chondroitin sulfate, and collagen hydrolysate. *Rheum Dis Clin North Am* 1999;25:379–395.

Hochberg M C, Altman R D, Brandt K, et al. Guidelines for the medical management of osteoarthritis: part II osteoarthritis of the knee. *Arthritis Rheum* 1995;38:1541–1546.

Lane N E, Thompson J M. Management of osteoarthritis in the primary-care setting: an evidence-based approach to treatment. *Am J Med* 1997;103(suppl):25–30.

McAlindon T E, LaValley M P, Gulin J P, et al. Glucosamine and chondroitin for treatment of osteoarthritis: a systematic quality assessment and meta-analysis. *JAMA* 2000;283:1469–1475.

85

Gout

Rebecca Babcock Bair

- Discussion *536*
- Case *537*
- Case Discussion *538*

1. What is the clinical presentation of an acute gouty attack?
2. What is the pathogenesis of acute gouty arthritis?
3. What are the four clinical stages of gout?
4. What is the gold standard for diagnosing gout?

Discussion

What Is the Clinical Presentation of an Acute Gouty Attack?

The clinical presentation consists of sudden onset of exquisitely painful arthritis. In early gout these attacks usually involve only one joint, but later in the course of disease attacks may be polyarticular. In the majority of first gouty attacks, the first metatarsophalangeal joint (the great toe) is the site of the acute arthritis. Ninety percent of gout patients experience first metatarsophalangeal pain at some point in the course of their disease. Many patients report acute onset of joint pain at night. In addition to pain, there is often erythema, swelling, and warmth of the involved joints. There may be systemic signs of infection such as leukocytosis and fever. The arthritis then remits completely and then recurs with increasing frequency.

What Is the Pathogenesis of Acute Gouty Arthritis?

Gout is characterized by deposition of monosodium urate crystals in the joints. The biochemical hallmark of gout is increased serum urate concentration. Urate, the end product of purine oxidation, is a waste product that has no physiologic role. Increased serum urate concentration is a result of either overproduction or underexcretion of serum urate. In 90% of patients, gout is caused by an underexcretion of serum urate. After an average of 30 years of increased serum urate concentration, urate begins to crystallize in the synovial fluid. The inflammatory response to the crystals is produced by a variety of mechanisms, including (a) phagocytosis of the crystals by leukocytes, (b) activation of the kallikrein system, (c) activation of complement, and (d) urate-mediated destruction of white blood cells and release of lysosomal products into the synovial fluid.

What Are the Four Clinical Stages of Gout?

Gout progresses through four clinical phases: asymptomatic hyperuricemia, acute gouty arthritis, intercritical gout (disease-free intervals), and chronic tophaceous gout. Although asymptomatic hyperuricemia may last a lifetime without arthritic symptoms, the risk of gout increases with the degree and duration of hyperuricemia. The phase of asymptomatic hyperuricemia ends with the first attack of gouty arthritis or nephrolithiasis. Asymptomatic hyperuricemia is common and should not ordinarily be treated.

The sudden onset of pain, erythema, limited range of motion, and swelling of the involved joint characterize acute gouty arthritis. It is predominantly a disease of the lower extremities. The attack usually begins at night and may be triggered by a specific event such as trauma, alcohol ingestion, ingestion of drugs, dietary excess, or surgery.

Following recovery from acute gouty arthritis, the patient reenters an asymptomatic phase called intercritical gout. This phase provides the physician with an opportunity to modify underlying acquired causes of hyperuricemia, including ethanol ingestion, medications (thiazides, furosemide), and obesity.

The arthritis then recurs with increasing frequency over time in untreated patients. Approximately 60% of patients have a second attack within the first year. Polyarticular involvement also becomes more common. After years of recurrent gouty arthritis, tophi (urate crystal deposits) develop in cartilage, tendons, and the bursae of some patients. This phase is known as chronic tophaceous gout.

What Is the Gold Standard for Diagnosing Gout?

The gold standard for diagnosing gout is identifying monosodium urate crystals in synovial fluid, within leukocytes, or in extracellular fluid using a polarized microscope. Monosodium urate crystals are needle shaped and strongly negatively birefringent under polarized light. Reliance on clinical presentation, serum urate concentration, or response to nonsteroidal agents does not replace direct evaluation of synovial fluid and may lead to an inaccurate diagnosis. The synovial fluid leukocyte counts are elevated from 2,000 to 100,000 cells/mm^3 in acute gouty arthritis. Because infection can coexist with urate crystals, joint fluid Gram stain and cultures should be obtained.

Case

A 73-year-old man with a history of hypertension and alcohol abuse presents with sudden onset of left knee pain, which awoke him from sleep. The patient denies any trauma to the area or any history of knee surgery. He currently denies any other joint complaints but he recalls experiencing severe "big toe" pain approximately 2 months ago, which seemed to resolve without any treatment.

Examination reveals a blood pressure of 170/90 mm Hg, pulse of 80 beats/min, and temperature of 36.0°C. The left knee is diffusely erythematous, swollen, and warm. It is exquisitely tender to palpation, and there is limited range of motion. No areas of skin breakdown are apparent.

1. What are the possible etiologies of his knee pain and what further tests are indicated?
2. How is acute gouty arthritis treated?
3. What medications are used to prevent recurrent attacks?

Case Discussion

What Are the Possible Etiologies of His Knee Pain and What Further Tests Are Indicated?

Acute monoarthritis is a potential medical emergency. Acute gouty attacks must be differentiated from acute infectious arthritis (septic joint), other crystal deposition diseases, osteoarthritis, fractures, ligamentous injury, and meniscal injury.

Investigation should include joint aspiration of synovial fluid for leukocyte count, Gram stain, culture, and an examination for crystals. In the patient described here, aspiration of synovial fluid confirmed the presence of monosodium urate crystals.

How Is Acute Gouty Arthritis Treated?

Acute gout can be treated with NSAIDs, corticosteroids, or colchicine. The sooner the drug therapy is initiated, the quicker the patient will respond. NSAIDs are first-line agents, and they are given at high doses tapered over several days. NSAIDs should be avoided or used cautiously in patients with renal dysfunction, peptic ulcer disease, and poorly compensated congestive heart failure. In the patient described here, an NSAID was initiated which resulted in quick resolution of his symptoms. In addition he was counseled about weight loss and limiting his alcohol intake.

If NSAIDs are contraindicated, corticosteroids are a safe alternative. A short course of oral prednisone (40–60 mg/day) can be given. Intraarticular injections of a corticosteroid are usually very effective, and aspiration of the joint alone can sometimes greatly reduce the pain of gout.

Colchicine exerts its effect by inhibiting the phagocytosis of urate crystals and by blocking the release of chemotactic factor. Colchicine is less favored now than in the past because its onset of action is slow and it causes gastrointestinal side effects. The drug is usually administered orally with a dose of 1 mg initially followed by 0.5 mg every 2 hours until abdominal comfort or diarrhea develops. Colchicine is safe except in patients who have renal or hepatic dysfunction or in the elderly who may be prone to dehydration. Colchicine may be given intravenously if oral administration is not possible. However, the risk of systemic toxic effects is much greater with intravenous therapy than with oral therapy.

What Medications Are Used to Prevent Recurrent Attacks of Gout?

Acute attacks of gout may be prevented by daily small doses of either colchicine or nonsteroidal antiinflammatory drugs. Identifying and correcting the cause of increased serum urate concentration or administering drugs that inhibit urate synthesis or increase its excretion can prevent gout. A single gouty attack does not usually justify life-long treatment with urate-lowering drugs. Hyperuricemic therapy should be initiated in patients with frequent gouty attacks, tophi, or urate nephropathy. Hyperuricemic drug therapy should not be started until an acute attack of gouty arthritis has ended because of the risk of increased mobilization of uric acid stores.

Two classes of drugs are available: uricosuric drugs and xanthine oxidase inhibitors. Uricosuric drugs increase the urinary excretion of urate. In contrast, xanthine oxidase inhibitors block the final step in urate synthesis, reducing the production of urate. A potential complication of these drugs is the precipitation of acute attacks of gout due to the sudden change in the serum urate concentration. The risk can be minimized by concurrently administering prophylactic drugs, delaying urate-lowering therapy until several weeks after the last attack of gout, and beginning therapy with a low dose of the urate-lowering drug.

Determination of 24-hour urine urate excretion can help to identify the most appropriate urate-lowering drug. Uricosuric agents should be used in most patients with gout who are found to be "underexcretors" (24-hour urinary urate excretion of <330 mg/day). Probenecid is the most frequently used uricosuric medication. The main risk associated with this drug involves the increase in the urinary excretion of urate that occurs soon after initiation of therapy. This can lead to urate crystals in the urine and deposition of uric acid in the renal tubules, pelvis, or ureter, causing renal colic or the deterioration of renal function. Initiating therapy at a low dose can reduce these risks. Colchicine or nonsteroidal agents should be continued for the first 6 to 12 months of therapy because gouty attacks may increase after beginning uricosuric drugs. The starting dose of probenecid is 250 mg orally twice daily. A reasonable goal is to reduce the serum uric acid concentration to less than 6 mg/dL. The uricosuric effect of probenecid is reduced in patients with renal insufficiency, and the drug has little effect in patients with a creatinine clearance of less than 60 mL/min. Uricosuric agents are contraindicated in patients with a history of nephrolithiasis.

Allopurinol, an inhibitor of xanthine oxidase, is indicated in patients with increased urate production. However, it is effective in lowering serum urate concentrations in patients with overproduction or underexcretion of urate (or both). The risk of precipitating acute gout is reduced if therapy is begun with a low dose (50–100 mg/day), which is slowly increased over a period of 3 to 4 weeks. The goal of therapy is to reduce the serum urate concentration to less than 6 mg/dL. Once again, colchicine or nonsteroidal agents should be continued for the first 6 to 12 months of therapy. The dosage of allopurinol must be adjusted in patients with renal failure. Allopurinol is the drug of choice in patients with severe tophaceous gout and in patients with a history of impaired renal function (creatinine clearance of <50 mL/min), urate nephropathy, or nephrolithiasis.

The patient described here began to experience frequent attacks of gout despite prophylaxis with daily colchicine. A 24-hour urine urate excretion revealed that he was an underexcretor. Probenecid was initiated at a dosage of 250 mg twice daily, which was gradually increased to achieve a serum urate level of less than 6 mg/dL.

Suggested Reading

Becker M A, et al. Gout. In: *Primer on the rheumatic diseases.* Atlanta Georgia. Arthritis Foundation, 1988:195–207.

Emmerson B. The management of gout. *N Engl J Med* 1996;334:445–451.

Springfield D, et al. Molecular and cellular biology of inflammation and neoplasia. In: Simon SR, eds. *Orthopaedic basic science.* Rosemont, Illinois: American Academy of Orthopaedic Surgeons, 1994:257.

86
Rheumatoid Arthritis

S. Sam Lim
Doyt Conn

1. What is rheumatoid arthritis?
2. What are the extraarticular manifestations of rheumatoid arthritis?
3. How is it diagnosed?
4. Why is early detection important and how does this affect treatment?
5. Does rheumatoid arthritis affect the spine?

Discussion
What Is Rheumatoid Arthritis?

Rheumatoid arthritis (RA) is a chronic, symmetric polyarthritis that can lead to deformity and destruction of joints due to erosion of cartilage and bone. The presumed etiologic agents inciting the inflammatory response that results in disease are unknown (although there are many hypotheses, including bacterial or viral pathogens). Multiple genes are likely associated with susceptibility and severity of RA. Pathologically, this unknown antigen (or antigens) activates susceptible T-lymphocytes with certain major histocompatibility complex (MHC) molecules, causing both T- and B-cell proliferation. Within a rheumatoid joint space, the inflammatory cascade leads to synovial hyperplasia, congestion, edema, and fibrin exudation. In later stages, this uncontrolled inflammation ultimately may lead to pannus formation, granulation tissue resulting from proliferation of synovial blood vessels and fibroblasts. The pannus grows much like a benign tumor, actively invading cartilage, releasing digestive enzymes, leading to periarticular bone and cartilage destruction characteristic of RA. One must not forget, however, that the scope of inflammation in RA may go beyond the joint space. Clinically evident extraarticular manifestations of RA occur in 20% of patients, with subclinical involvement occurring even more frequently.

What Are the Extraarticular Manifestations of Rheumatoid Arthritis?

- General
  - Fatigue, malaise

- Skin
  - Rheumatoid nodules
  - Vasculitis
- Eyes
  - Keratoconjunctivitis sicca
  - Episcleritis, scleritis
- Lungs
  - Pleural effusion
  - Interstitial fibrosis
  - Bronchiolitis obliterans organizing pneumonia (BOOP)
- Heart
  - Pericarditis, myocarditis
- Kidneys
  - Amyloidosis
- Hematologic
  - Anemia
- Neurologic
  - Compression neuropathies
  - Mononeuritis multiplex

Rheumatoid arthritis is truly a systemic disease. In general, fatigue and malaise are common complaints. The presence of rheumatoid nodules may be helpful diagnostically and generally indicate more severe disease. The dry eyes and dry mouth (keratoconjunctivitis sicca) associated with Sjögren syndrome and RA often are overlooked unless specific questions are asked about these symptoms. Episcleritis and scleritis involve inflammation of the eyes, with the latter having the capability to erode through the sclera and into the choroid, causing scleromalacia perforans. Pulmonary involvement in an autopsy series was found to be extremely common. Inflammation of the pleura can produce pleural fluid findings characterized by a markedly low glucose when compared with serum and a white blood cell count usually less than 5,000/mm³. Interstitial fibrosis can be a result of the disease itself or secondary to medications (i.e., methotrexate). Rheumatoid nodules can present anywhere in the lung parenchyma, as well as near the pleura. BOOP may be a complication of RA or drug therapy. Symptomatic pericarditis is rare and is usually associated with an overall disease flare. Rheumatoid nodule–like lesions can appear almost anywhere in the heart, possibly disrupting the valves or causing conduction delay. Kidney involvement is rare, in contrast to systemic lupus erythematosus (SLE). Most kidney problems are secondary to the use of nonsteroidal antiinflammatory drugs (NSAIDs), gold, or penicillamine. In advanced RA, amyloidosis may occur in the kidney. An anemia of chronic disease can be a result of chronic inflammation. Neurologically, wherever a peripheral nerve enters an inflamed synovium or tendon sheath, there is the possibility of a compression neuropathy, such as carpal tunnel syndrome. Vasculitis may complicate RA and can result in palpable purpura, leg ulcers, distal sensory neuropathy, and mononeuritis multiplex.

How Is It Diagnosed?

The diagnosis of RA is based on careful history taking and physical examination, as well as review of any pertinent laboratory data. Essential to diagnosis is evidence of joint inflammation, or synovitis, of multiple joints. RA synovitis involves peripheral joints (hands, wrists, elbows, knees, ankles, and toes), sparing the distal interphalangeal joints of the hands, and is symmetric. However, the initial presentation can often vary, lacking characteristic symmetry. The onset is usually insidious over a period of several weeks. Although rare, acute, explosive polyarthritis may occur. Recognizing the RA pattern of joint involvement allows one to suspect and then diagnose RA.

The American College of Rheumatology has established criteria for the diagnosis of RA. Although not initially intended for individual diagnostic purposes, they have become useful as a guide in establishing the diagnosis (Table 86.1). The first four criteria involve articular manifestations and must be involved for at least 6 weeks. Upon initial presentation, other causes of synovitis must be excluded. If an effusion is detected, the joint fluid should be aspirated as part of the initial workup to document inflammation and to rule out any crystals. Morning stiffness is almost always a feature of synovitis and is prolonged, lasting more than 1 hour as opposed to the brief 5 to 10 minutes of "gelling" seen in osteoarthritis.

Rheumatoid nodules occur at some point in up to 50% of RA patients and are strongly associated with rheumatoid factor positivity. Rheumatoid nodules tend to occur along areas of increased trauma such as the extensor surface of the forearm, flexor surface of the fingers, ischial area and Achilles tendon. It is sometimes difficult to distinguish a gouty tophus from a rheumatoid nodule, in which case an aspiration or biopsy of the nodule is indicated. Methotrexate can promote rheumatoid nodule formation.

It is important to remember that there are no laboratory tests, histologic findings, or radiographic features that confirm the diagnosis of RA. Laboratory tests must always be viewed in the context of the clinical picture. The presence of rheumatoid factor (RF), an immunoglobulin that binds to the Fc portion of immunoglobulin G, may be helpful in the diagnosis of RA. In a patient with multiple joints involved in the RA pattern of involvement, the presence of RF helps establish the diagnosis. It must be remembered that RF has been found in at least 1% of the normal population. In addition, positive results are found in other disease states, such as subacute

Table 86.1. Criteria for the Classification of Rheumatoid Arthritis (RA)

Criterion[a]	Definition
1. Morning stiffness	Morning stiffness in and around the joints, lasting at least 1 hour before maximal improvement
2. Arthritis of three or more joint areas	At least three joint areas (out of 14) simultaneously having soft tissue swelling or fluid; the 14 possible areas are right or left PIP, MCP, wrist, elbow, knee, ankle, and MTP joints
3. Arthritis of hand joints	At least one area swollen in a wrist, MCP, or PIP joint
4. Symmetric arthritis	Simultaneous involvement of the same joint areas (as defined in criterion 2) on both sides of the body
5. Rheumatoid arthritis	Subcutaneous bony nodules over bony prominences, extensor surfaces, or in juxtaarticular regions
6. Serum rheumatoid factor	Demonstration of abnormal amounts of serum rheumatoid factor
7. Radiographic changes	Radiographic changes typical of RA on posteroanterior hand and wrist radiographs, including erosions or unequivocal bony decalcification

A patient is said to have RA if he or she has satisfied at least four of these seven criteria.
[a]Criteria 1 through 4 must have been present for at least 6 weeks.
PIP, proximal interphalangeal; MCP, metacarpophalangeal; MTP, metatarsophalangeal.

bacterial endocarditis, SLE, liver disease, tuberculosis, sarcoidosis, and syphilis, among others. It is found in about 85% of RA patients. Once RF positivity has been established, there is no need to repeat the test. Nor is there utility in following titers. RF positivity may correlate with a more severe disease course, rheumatoid nodule formation, and extraarticular manifestations.

Rheumatoid arthritis virtually always affects the hands and wrists. Radiographs are not only used to assist in diagnosis, they are useful in assessing disease progression as well. Radiographic evidence of RA includes periarticular soft tissue swelling, uniform loss of joint space (nonuniform loss points more toward osteoarthritis), marginal erosions progressing to severe erosions of subchondral bone, and subluxations (partial dislocation of a joint). It is important to realize that radiographic evidence of erosions can become apparent only after several months of active disease. These erosions are the end point of the destructive process radiographically. Because they are irreversible, they mark a point of no return.

Why Is Early Detection Important and How Does This Affect Treatment?

The way we approach the treatment of RA has undergone a change over recent decades. Initially, in what was called the pyramid concept, therapy entailed a plan of sequential drug administration starting at the bottom of the pyramid from what was thought to be the least toxic drugs moving up to the more toxic ones. Salicylates or other NSAIDs occupied the bottom, first-line therapies. The first-line NSAIDs were thought to provide relatively rapid analgesia. There was even some thought that they might effectively slow the progression of the disease. What we know now is that NSAIDs do not stop disease progression. Inevitably, after considerable progression of the disease, physicians would turn to the second-line agents known as disease-modifying antirheumatic drugs (DMARDs).

What studies have suggested now is that much of joint damage, which ultimately results in disability, occurs early in the course of the disease. This has shifted thinking into the current concept of treating RA earlier and more aggressively with DMARDs, hoping to change the course of the disease in its early state before much joint damage has occurred. One study followed 681 patients from Northern Saskatchewan meeting criteria for RA. They were followed for an average of 11.9 years to identify the frequency and severity of disability as well as factors predictive of subsequent disability. Follow-up included assessment of functional ability and routine laboratory and radiographic data. The results showed that functional class, disability index, and radiologic deterioration all progressed as a function of disease duration. Moreover, the rate of progression of disease was most marked early in the course of RA. Another study out of The Netherlands showed that more than 80% of patients with RA of less than 2 years duration had joint space narrowing on plain radiographs of the hands and wrists, whereas two thirds had erosions.

Does Rheumatoid Arthritis Affect the Spine?

We cannot forget to mention that cervical spine instability may occur at C1–C2. Here, the transverse ligament of C1 or the odontoid process itself becomes lax or destroyed by inflammation. This instability can result in cord compression. Symptoms range from neck pain, which can radiate over the occiput or down the thoracolumbar spine when the neck is flexed. Most commonly, patients complain of gradual paresthesias and weakness in the hands. Lateral flexion and extension radiographs should be taken to document the degree of subluxation in a symptomatic patient. Stabilization of the cervical spine is of utmost importance whenever RA patients are either emergently or electively intubated.

Case

A 34-year-old female postal worker comes to your office with a chief complaint of bilateral hand and knee pain for 6 months. She reports that her pain gradually started in both her wrists and knuckles, then recently began involving her knees. Her complaints are worst in the morning when she feels very fatigued and her joints are "stiff and swollen." They start feeling better after "a hot shower" and tolerable 3 hours later as she is part way into her delivery route. She has taken a variety of over-the-counter NSAIDs but has required higher and more frequent doses to ease her pain and swelling. She comes to you because she can no longer climb all the stairs on her delivery route secondary to pain and swelling, especially in her knees.

She has no significant past medical history except for some childhood asthma. Her medications include various over-the-counter NSAIDs. She tolerated them well, taking them at the "maximum labeled dose." She is married and monogamous. She has not traveled away from home in a couple of years. She denies any recent trauma, illness, fever, chills, sore throat, diarrhea, or dysuria. She does not report dry eyes, dry mouth, rash, oral ulcers, or chest pain.

She is afebrile and normotensive. Her examination reveals a fit-appearing woman in moderate discomfort. Significant findings include bilateral wrist, MCP, and proximal interphalangeal (PIP) joint warmth, redness, and swelling. She has limited movement of these joints secondary to swelling and pain. She is unable to make a closed fist. Her elbows are warm and extend just short of full extension. There are no palpable nodules or rash. Her knees are obviously swollen, red, and warm. You easily demonstrate ballottement of the patella.

Her leukocyte count is 8,000 cells/mm^3 with a hemoglobin of 12 g/dL, a hematocrit of 36%, and platelets of 300,000. The erythrocyte sedimentation rate is 75 mm/h. Her chemistries are normal, and she is rheumatoid factor positive. Her synovial fluid is yellow with a leukocyte count of 30,000 and no crystals. Urinalysis yields no useful findings. Her hand films reveal soft tissue swelling around the joints and juxtaarticular osteoporosis.

1. What is the differential diagnosis for acute polyarthritis in this patient?
2. How do you treat rheumatoid arthritis?
3. What are some new developments in the treatment of rheumatoid arthritis?

Case Discussion

What Is the Differential Diagnosis for Acute Polyarthritis in This Patient?

This patient clearly has polyarthritis (inflammation of more than four joints). The symmetrical involvement of the PIPs, MCPs, wrists, elbows, and knees for more than 6 weeks is practically diagnostic of RA. The morning stiffness, anemia, and thrombocytosis all go along with the significant amount of inflammation present. Less likely causes of inflammatory polyarthritis include SLE and seronegative spondyloarthropathies. SLE can present with an RA-like polyarthritis. However, our patient exhibits no other clinical features such as fever, rash, oral ulcers, serositis, or evidence of renal disease. Seronegative spondyloarthropathies (ankylosing spondylitis, Reiter's syndrome, psoriatic arthritis, and arthritis associated with inflammatory bowel disease) are characterized by spondylitis, sacroiliitis, and inflammation of the eyes and ligamentous insertions (enthesopathy). The joint pattern is usually oligoarthritic (involvement of two to four joints), asymmetric, and involves large, lower extremity joints. Polyarticular gout can present like RA but is highly unlikely in a premenopausal woman in this clinical setting. Infectious etiologies are equally unlikely in this woman. Disseminated neisserial infection presents with migratory polyarthritis, tenosynovitis, and cutaneous pustular lesions. Sarcoidosis also can present with polyarthritis but with fewer joints. In the acute form, it always involves the ankles.

How Do You Treat Rheumatoid Arthritis?

Initial treatment of every patient with RA should consist of education. It is important that patients feel a sense of control over their disease. They must be educated to the chronic, waxing and waning nature of their disease in order to anticipate and prepare for it. In some patients, the type, extent, and manner in which educational material is presented may be more important than drug therapy. Occupational and physical therapy are underused, underappreciated, and have an important impact. They can teach joint protection, instruct in exercises leading to maintenance or improvement in joint function, and help in splinting of inflamed or painful joints.

The goals of treatment are to alleviate pain, control inflammation, and prevent joint destruction. The initial pain and inflammation can be partially alleviated by NSAIDs. Newer agents that selectively block cyclooxygenase-2 do not differ substantially in terms of efficacy to that of the traditional NSAIDs. Their advantage arises from decreased gastrointestinal bleeding. Glucocorticoids are the most potent suppressors of inflammation and are very effective. Although not traditionally grouped with the other DMARDs, low-dose glucocorticoids have been shown in some studies to significantly impact progression of disease. In a 2-year blinded study of 128 patients with RA of less than 2 years duration, the group receiving 7.5 mg/day of prednisolone showed little radiographic progression of disease compared with those that received placebo. Doses should range from 5 to 10 mg of prednisone once or twice daily for symptomatic relief. Doses ranging from 40 to 60 mg/day of prednisone are unnecessary and should be avoided unless treating systemic extraarticular manifestations such as rheumatoid vasculitis. Calcium and multivitamin supplementation should always accompany glucocorticoid usage. A baseline bone densitometry study should be considered in those anticipating long-term use.

Prevention of joint destruction for the reasons stated earlier should be approached using the appropriate DMARD as early as possible in the disease course. DMARDs are agents capable of modifying disease course in a more fundamental and prolonged manner than NSAIDs. They must by definition change the course of RA for at least 1 year as evidenced by sustained improvement in physical function, decreased inflammatory synovitis, and slowing or prevention of structural joint damage. For patients with mild disease, hydroxychloroquine is often the first drug of choice because of ease of use and its favorable toxicity profile. Retinopathy is an extremely rare side effect, but patients should be screened for it biannually. Other possibilities are sulfasalazine or gold. For patients with moderately active or severe disease, methotrexate is regarded as the DMARD of first choice. The initial dosage is usually 7.5 to 10 mg/wk, titrated up to an average dosage of 15 to 20 mg/wk given orally. If gastrointestinal upset develops or there is a question about the absorption of the drug, it can be given intramuscularly or intravenously. In the hands of an experienced clinician or rheumatologist, methotrexate is well tolerated and can be effectively taken for many years. Complete blood count with platelets and differential along with liver function tests are mandatory and should be monitored frequently early in the treatment coarse with the ultimate goal of monitoring every 2 months. Concomitant alcohol use increases the risk of methotrexate-induced hepatotoxicity and should be avoided. Methotrexate in patients with hepatic or renal insufficiency or with severe lung disease can be associated with a syndrome of pulmonary hypersensitivity with dyspnea, cough, or fever. The incidence of stomatitis, GI upset, hair thinning, and bone marrow suppression may be reduced with supplemental folate (usually 1 mg/day).

Sometimes combinations of DMARDs are used with enhanced effectiveness without increased toxicity. Cyclosporine has been used with benefit in combination with methotrexate.

What Are Some New Developments in the Treatment of Rheumatoid Arthritis?

This is an exciting time to be studying and treating RA. Scientific investigation into the pathogenesis of RA is now at the immunologic and molecular levels. Because of this, for the first time in over 10 years, we have new treatments available for RA. Working at the immunologic level, an inhibitor of pyrimidine synthesis called luflunomide was recently approved for the treatment of active RA. We are also learning more about the cytokines involved in the inflammatory cascade, of which tumor necrosis factor-α (TNF-α) is a potent inflammatory cytokine. Etanercept is a soluble receptor for TNF-α approved for use in severe RA. Infliximab, approved for use in Crohn's disease and now for RA, is a monoclonal antibody against TNF-α that also shows promise. In addition, there are more than 80 drugs currently being developed for the treatment of RA. The challenge for the future is to determine how these new drugs will fit into our therapeutic approach to RA.

Suggested Reading

Kirwan J R. The effect of glucocorticoids on joint destruction in rheumatoid arthritis. *N Engl J Med* 1995;142–146.

Primer on the rheumatic diseases, 11th ed. Atlanta: Arthritis Foundation, 1997.

Sherrer Y S, et al. The development of disability in rheumatoid arthritis. *Arthritis Rheumatism* 1986;April:494–500.

van der Heijde, et al. Biannual radiographic assessments of hands and feet in a three-year prospective followup of patients with early rheumatoid arthritis. *Arthritis Rheumatism* 1992;January:26–34.

XVI
Urology

87

Benign Prostatic Hyperplasia

Erica Brownfield

1. What are the risk factors for benign prostatic hyperplasia?
2. What is the natural history of benign prostatic hyperplasia?
3. What is the differential diagnosis of obstructive voiding symptoms in men?
4. What is the diagnostic approach for benign prostatic hyperplasia?
5. What are the treatment options for benign prostatic hyperplasia?
6. What is the role, if any, of prostate-specific antigen testing in benign prostatic hyperplasia?

Discussion

What Are the Risk Factors for Benign Prostatic Hyperplasia?

The single most important risk factor for benign prostatic hyperplasia (BPH) is age. The prevalence of BPH in autopsy studies increases from 8% in men 31 to 40 years of age, to 40% to 50% in men 51 to 60, to over 80% in men over age 80. Many years ago, BPH was the leading cause of renal failure in men (now surpassed by diabetes and hypertension).

The second most important risk factor for the development of BPH is normal testicular function. Men with congenital deficiency of 5α-reductase activity (the enzyme that converts testosterone to dihydrotestosterone in the prostate and other androgen-sensitive tissues) have a rudimentary prostate throughout life, and reducing serum testosterone concentrations in men with BPH causes partial regression of the hyperplasia.

Race has some influence on the risk for severe BPH requiring surgery. It has been shown that younger African-American men (<65 years) may need surgical treatment more often than white men with BPH.

There is no consensus on the role of smoking and its association with BPH. However, chronic alcoholism is known to cause low serum testosterone concentrations, and autopsy findings suggest a weak inverse relationship between BPH and cirrhosis. There is no known association between sexual activity or vasectomy and BPH.

It is possible that a family history of early prostatectomy is a risk factor for BPH. Hereditary BPH could account for 9% of all cases requiring surgery and for more than 50% in men under 60 years of age.

What Is the Natural History of Benign Prostatic Hyperplasia?

The natural history of BPH depends somewhat on baseline symptoms. As a general rule, BPH is slowly progressive and requires some form of treatment. However, up to 30% of patients with mild BPH have spontaneous regression of symptoms without treatment. There is no convincing evidence that BPH is an independent risk factor for prostate cancer.

What Is the Differential Diagnosis of Obstructive Voiding Symptoms in Men?

In diagnosing BPH, one needs to exclude other causes of a man's symptoms by history, physical examination, and several simple tests. Disorders that can produce similar symptoms include:

- Urethral stricture
- Bladder neck contracture
- Bladder calculi
- Neurogenic bladder
- Urinary tract infection and prostatitis
- Bladder cancer
- Prostate cancer

What Is the Diagnostic Approach of Benign Prostatic Hyperplasia?

Obtaining a detailed medical history is important in diagnosing BPH. In addition to asking the patient about obstructive (hesitancy, straining, weak stream, terminal dribbling, prolonged voiding) and irritative (frequency, urgency, nocturia, urge incontinence) symptoms, it is important to ask about the following:

- Medication use (e.g., diuretics, anticholinergics, sympathomimetics)
- Presence of gross hematuria or pain in the bladder region
- History of urethral trauma, urethral instrumentation, or urethritis
- Symptoms of neurologic disease that would suggest a neurogenic bladder
- Comorbidities (e.g., diabetes, hypercalcemia, congestive heart failure)

American Urology Association Symptom Score

The American Urology Association (AUA) Symptom Score is recommended by the Agency for Health Care and Policy Research (AHCPR) for the initial assessment of patients presenting with symptoms of BPH. The symptom score is figured on a 5-point scale of 0 (not present) to 5 (almost always present). Symptoms are classified as mild (0–7 total score), moderate (8–19 total), and severe (20–35 total). The score is a useful way to assess symptoms over time. It is a reliable and valid instrument (Fig. 87.1).

Question	Not at All	Less Than 1 Time in 5	Less Than Half the Time	About Half the Time	More Than Half the Time	Almost Always
1. During the last month or so, how many times did you most typically get up to urinate from the time you went to bed at night until the time you got up this morning?	None ☐	1 Time ☐	2 Times ☐	3 Times ☐	4 Times ☐	5 or More ☐
2. During the last month or so, how often have you had to urinate again less than 2 hours after you finished urinating?	☐	☐	☐	☐	☐	☐
3. During the last month or so, how often have you found you stopped and started again several times when you urinated?	☐	☐	☐	☐	☐	☐
4. During the last month or so, how often have you found it difficult to postpone urination?	☐	☐	☐	☐	☐	☐
5. During the last month or so, how often have you had a weak urinary system?	☐	☐	☐	☐	☐	☐
6. During the last month or so, how often have you had to push or strain to begin urination?	☐	☐	☐	☐	☐	☐
7. During the last month or so, how often have you had a sensation of not emptying your bladder completely after you finished urinating?	☐	☐	☐	☐	☐	☐

Figure 87.1. American Urological Association Symptom Index

For each patient with symptoms suggesting BPH, a digital rectal examination should be performed to assess prostate size, consistency, symmetry, and the presence of nodules. A neurologic examination, including rectal sphincter tone, should be performed.

A urinalysis is indicated to look for evidence of white blood cells and red blood cells to suggest infection, stone, or tumor. Serum creatinine should be measured because an abnormal value could indicate underlying renal or prerenal disease or bladder outlet obstruction.

Postvoid Residual Urine Volume

Measurement of a postvoid residual volume (PVR) should be obtained in patients whose symptoms or signs suggest incomplete bladder emptying. These include significant obstructive voiding symptoms, urinary incontinence (which could mean overflow secondary to outflow obstruction), elevated serum creatinine, or evidence of urinary tract infection. Obtaining a PVR (which can be done in the office) involves passing a urinary catheter immediately after micturition to quantify the amount of urine remaining in the bladder. Although a variety of urinary catheters can be used, using a Foley catheter is often preferred because it can be left in the bladder pending further urologic evaluation if the patient has significant obstruction as indicated by a very high PVR (generally >250 mL). Although the PVR is poorly reproducible, an elevated PVR suggests significant obstruction (most often due to BPH) that, if uncorrected, may lead to renal damage and recurrent urinary tract infections. An estimated PVR can be obtained with a bladder scanner that does not require catheterization or radiologic assistance.

Urodynamic Studies

Urodynamic studies provide objective measurement of intravesicular pressure and peak urinary flow. In a subset of patients with poor bladder emptying and BPH, they can be useful for determining if bladder atony or neurogenic bladder are also present. When appropriate, these tests are generally ordered and performed by the consulting urologist.

Radiologic Studies

Renal ultrasonography is indicated in patients with an elevated creatinine to look for evidence of urinary obstruction (e.g., hydronephrosis). Patients with hematuria not due to glomerular disease are best evaluated further with an intravenous pyelogram.

Urethrocystoscopy

Urethrocystoscopy is not routinely recommended but may be indicated in some patients prior to consideration of surgery.

What Are the Treatment Options for Benign Prostatic Hyperplasia?

The main goals of treatment in BPH are to improve quality of life by decreasing symptoms and to prevent the complications of BPH (e.g., acute urinary retention and irreversible bladder decompensation, renal failure secondary to obstructive uropathy, and urinary tract infections). Due to the high level of effectiveness of currently available medical therapies (e.g., α-adrenergic blockers and 5α-reductase inhibitors), surgical intervention is needed in only a small subset of patients.

The AHCPR recommends using the AUA symptom score to make a treatment decision analysis. Men with mild symptoms (AUA ≤7) should be followed in a strategy of "watchful waiting." Each year, the AUA score should be recalculated and men should be reassured. Patients with moderate to severe symptoms (AUA ≥8) should be given information of benefits and harms of watchful waiting and full range of treatment options.

Any man with BPH and urinary retention, persistent symptoms despite medical therapy, or complications secondary to BPH should be evaluated by a urologist.

Drug Therapy

Alpha-adrenergic blockers are the mainstay of BPH treatment. They bind to and block α-adrenergic receptors present on smooth muscle cells in the prostatic urethra and bladder outlet, reducing smooth muscle tone. They reduce obstructive voiding symptoms in 60% to 80% of patients and produce a 50% overall improvement of urinary flow rates. The three drugs approved by the U.S. Food and Drug Administration for BPH are doxazosin, terazosin, and the newer agent, tamsulosin. The main side effects of α-adrenergic blockers have included orthostatic hypotension, dizziness, and weakness. For this reason, patients are initially started on the lowest dose at night for 3 days followed by a blood pressure check and gradually increased over a few weeks. Tamsulosin, believed to act selectively in the urinary tract, has the fewest systemic side effects and can be started at full dosages (0.4 mg daily) on day 1.

5α-reductase inhibitors (e.g., finasteride) decrease the size of the prostate gland; therefore, they may be better for men with marked prostatic enlargement. They increase peak urinary flow rates, decrease symptoms by approximately 20%, and may decrease the need for future surgery. They are often used in conjunction with α-adrenergic blockers. Because 5α-reductase inhibitors decrease prostate-specific antigen (PSA) levels by up to 50%, many clinicians will double the PSA values obtained in patients using these drugs and interpret accordingly. The main side effects of these drugs include decreased libido and erectile dysfunction. Finasteride is the only 5α-reductase inhibitor approved in the United States.

Herbal Therapies

Saw palmetto may be more efficacious than placebo and comparable with finasteride in terms of symptom improvement and urinary flow rates. Believed to work via 5α-reductase inhibition, like finasteride, it decreases PSA levels by up to 50%, such that PSA levels must be interpreted accordingly. There are limited data on saw palmetto and no standardization of preparations.

Other Drugs

There is a lack of efficacy and potential for side effects with other antiandrogens. Gonadotropin releasing hormone (GnRH) agonists are not recommended as a standard of care, possess significant side effects (e.g., hot flashes and decreased libido), and are prohibitively expensive.

Invasive Therapies

Transurethral resection of the prostate (TURP) has been the mainstay of BPH treatment, producing the best overall improvement of both symptoms and objective voiding parameters in men with severe symptoms. With available medical therapies, use of TURP has markedly declined. Complications include impotence, incontinence, and retrograde ejaculation.

Use of other invasive procedures (e.g., transurethral incision of the prostate, open prostatectomy) and newer technologies (e.g., urethral stents, laser prostatectomy, microwave therapy, and electrovaporization) should be individualized, taking into account the patient's urologic and medical condition, patient preference, and urologist's level of expertise.

Table 87.1. Normal Values of PSA

	Reference Ranges of PSA	African-American Men
Age 40–49	0–2.5 ng/mL	0–2 ng/mL
Age 50–59	0–3.5 ng/mL	0–4 ng/mL
Age 60–69	0–4.5 ng/mL	0–4.5 ng/mL
Age 70–79	0–6.5 ng/mL	0–5.5 ng/mL

PSA, prostate-specific antigen.

What Is the Role, if Any, of Prostate-Specific Antigen Testing in Benign Prostatic Hyperplasia?

Benign prostatic hyperplasia, prostatitis, and acute urinary retention can all elevate PSA levels and may make PSA interpretation difficult. Digital rectal examination does not change PSA to a clinically important degree. All men should be educated about causes of PSA elevation, the limited ability to distinguish elevated PSA secondary to BPH versus organ-confined prostate cancer, and the potential need for further invasive work-up if the PSA is elevated (Table 87.1).

Case

A 58-year-old African-American man with a history of hypertension and reflux gastritis presents with daily urinary straining, hesitancy, decreased urinary stream, and nocturia of a few months duration. He started to drink more fluids during the day to help with urination, but this did not work. In the past few days, he has felt bloated and his urine output has diminished. His current medications include atenolol and prilosec. He does not smoke, and he drinks one glass of scotch per night. On examination his blood pressure is 150/82 mm Hg, pulse is 64 beats/min, and respirations are 14 breaths/min. He has unremarkable cardiac and pulmonary examinations. His abdomen has suprapubic distension and mild tenderness. His prostate is firm, smooth, and enlarged; there are no palpable nodules. Laboratory studies show a blood urea nitrogen of 56 mg/dL, creatinine of 2.9 mg/dL (baseline 1.0), and potassium of 5.8 mmol/liter. A urinalysis reveals a specific gravity of 1.050, 1+ protein, and hyaline casts.

1. Given his presentation, what is your immediate concern and what should you do?
2. After the immediate treatment is initiated, what are the therapeutic options?
3. What is the likely disease progression in this patient?

Case Discussion

Given His Presentation, What Is Your Immediate Concern and What Should You Do?

The immediate concern for this patient is acute urinary retention secondary to bladder outlet obstruction. The first goal is to relieve the obstruction by placing a Foley catheter. The catheter should be left in the patient's bladder to allow continued urinary drainage. One should perform ultrasonography to rule out hydronephrosis and consult a urologist for further management.

After the Immediate Treatment Is Initiated, What Are the Therapeutic Options?

The initial treatment options in a patient with urinary retention due to BPH are surgery versus medical therapy. It is important to obtain a thorough history looking for factors that may have provoked urinary retention (e.g., over-the-counter cold preparations containing decongestants or antihistamines). In this patient with elevated creatinine, surgery should be recommended because persistent obstruction can lead to progressive renal damage. If the patient is not a surgical candidate or refuses surgery, the alternative is to leave the urinary catheter in place. In a patient with urinary retention and no evidence of renal damage (normal creatinine), it would be reasonable to initiate medical therapy with α-adrenergic blockers and finasteride (if the prostate is enlarged) to decrease prostate size and decrease the incidence of acute urinary retention. After about a week, the urologist can remove the urinary catheter and perform a voiding trial. If the patient cannot empty his bladder once the catheter is removed, the catheter should be replaced and definitive intervention planned accordingly. If the patient can urinate and the catheter is removed, the patient should be educated on the signs and symptoms of retention and should be followed closely. If urinary retention develops again, surgery should be considered.

What Is the Likely Disease Progression in This Patient?

Because the patient presented with severe symptoms, he will likely continue to have severe symptoms unless surgically treated. Approximately 50% of men who develop acute urinary retention will have a recurrence.

Suggested Reading

Barry M J, Fowler F J, Bin L, et al. The natural history of patients with BPH as diagnosed by North American urologists. *J Urol* 1997;157:10–15.

Barry M J, Roehrborn C. Management of benign prostatic hyperplasia. *Annu Rev Med* 1997;48:177–189.

Cunningham G, Kadmon D. Diagnosis of benign prostatic hyperplasia. *Up to Date* 2000;8.

Cunningham G, Kadmon D. Epidemiology and pathogenesis of benign prostatic hyperplasia. *Up to Date* 2000;8.

Garnick M. Screening for prostate cancer. *Up to Date* 2000;8.

McConnell J D, Barry M J, Bruskewitz R C, et al. BPH: diagnosis and treatment. Clinical practice guidelines. No. 8, 1994. AHCPR Publication No. 94-0582. Rockville, MD: Agency Health Care Policy and Research, U.S. Department of Health and Human Services.

Yalla S V, Sullivan M P, Lecamwasam H S, et al. Correlation of American Urological Association symptom index with obstructive and non obstructive prostatism. *J Urol* 1995;153:674–680.

88
Prostatitis
Daniel D. Dressler

1. What are the different types of prostatitis, and how are they defined and classified?
2. What is the epidemiology of prostatitis? What are its etiologies?
3. What are the common clinical features of acute and chronic prostatitis?
4. How is the diagnosis of prostatitis confirmed?
5. What are the management options for prostatitis, and what is the duration of therapy?

Discussion

What Are the Different Types of Prostatitis, and How Are They Defined and Classified?

Prostatitis can generally be classified into acute and chronic, bacterial and nonbacterial. In 1968, Meares and Stamey introduced techniques that led to formalized definitions and classification of prostatitis. However, in 1995 the National Institutes of Health developed a classification system to create a uniform standard with which to define the types of prostatitis, a standard by which all future research, clinical evaluation, and epidemiologic studies could be based. Comparison of these two classification systems is illustrated in Table 88.1.

What Is the Epidemiology of Prostatitis? What Are Its Etiologies?

Prostatitis accounts for approximately 1% of visits to primary care physicians and 8% of visits to urologists in the United States. It affects men of all ages, and has its greatest incidence in the 36 to 50 year age range. Bacterial causes are identified in a relatively small number of cases.

Acute bacterial prostatitis (type I) represents only 1% to 5% of all cases of prostatitis. It is characterized by a positive bacterial culture (on routine urinalysis). Predominant identifiable etiologies include *Escherichia coli* (80%) and *Proteus* species. Less commonly seen are *Klebsiella, Pseudomonas, Serratia,* and *Enterobacter.* Rare causes include *Enterococcus faecalis, Staphylococcus aureus,* and anaerobes.

Table 88.1. Classification of Prostatitis

Meares and Stamey Classification (1968)		NIH Classification (1995)[a]	
Category	Definition	Analogous Category	Definition
Acute bacterial prostatitis	Prostatic fluid Isolation of bacteria Purulence Systemic signs of infection	Type I: acute bacterial prostatitis	Acute infection of the prostate (culture positive)
Chronic bacterial prostatitis	Prostatic fluid WBCs on micro Isolation of bacteria No systemic signs of infection	Type II: chronic bacterial prostatitis	Recurrent infection of the prostate (culture positive)
Chronic nonbacterial prostatitis	Prostatic fluid WBCs on micro No isolation of significant bacteria	Type IIIA (*inflammatory*) Chronic nonbacterial prostatitis/chronic pelvic pain syndrome	WBCs in semen, expressed prostatic secretions, or postprostatic massage urine
Prostatodynia (chronic pelvic pain syndrome)	Prostatic fluid No WBCs on micro No isolation of bacteria Persistent symptoms	Type IIIB (*noninflammatory*) Chronic pelvic pain syndrome	No WBCs in semen, expressed prostatic secretions, or postprostatic massage urine
		Type IV Asymptomatic inflammatory prostatitis	No symptoms. Inflammation found incidentally by prostate biopsy or WBCs in semen/prostatic secretions in evaluation of other disorders

[a]Adapted from Executive Summary Chronic Prostatitis Workshop, National Institutes of Health/NIDDK (www.niddk.nig.gov/health/urolog, 12/95); with permission. WBCs, white blood cells.

Chronic bacterial prostatitis (type II) often presents as recurrent urinary tract infections. It represents approximately 5% to 10% of all cases of prostatitis, and organisms are cultured from prostatic fluid using methods described below.

Chronic nonbacterial prostatitis (type IIIA), or culture-negative inflammation (white blood cells, WBCs) in prostatic fluid, is diagnosed in 40% to 65% of all patients with prostatitis. The etiology of the inflammation is unknown. Many have proposed infectious etiologies, such as *Chlamydia, Mycoplasma, Ureoplasma, Trichomonas,* or viral agents; however, most studies do not support these claims. Other proposed etiologies include autoimmune or hypersensitivity reactions, but evidence for these mechanisms has been minimal.

Chronic pelvic pain syndrome (type IIIB) presents with symptoms of prostatitis, but neither organisms nor inflammatory cells are isolated from urinalysis or prostatic secretions. It comprises approximately 20% to 40% of all cases.

What Are the Common Clinical Features of Acute and Chronic Prostatitis?

Common signs and symptoms consistent with acute versus chronic prostatitis are presented in Table 88.2.

Table 88.2. Signs and Symptoms of Prostatitis

Symptoms and Signs	Acute Prostatitis	Chronic Prostatitis
Duration of symptoms	Days	>6 mo
Systemic symptoms and signs	Fever, rigors, tachycardia, myalgias, arthralgias	Fatigue, myalgias, arthralgias
Urinary symptoms	Dysuria, frequency, urgency, acute urinary retention	Dysuria, frequency
Pain: quality	Severe	Often dull, aching (variable)
Pain: location	Perineal, penile, rectal, and/or low back	Perineal, pelvic, penile (especially penis tip), low abdomen, low back, rectal, testicular, and/or ejaculatory
Prostate examination[a]	Exquisitely tender, warm, tense, enlarged, smooth textured	Normal to enlarged and boggy; usually nontender (variable examination)

[a]Avoiding prostate examination in patients with suspected acute prostatitis due to the risk of inducing bacteremia is recommended throughout the urologic literature; however, little if any evidence to support this risk has been documented.

How Is the Diagnosis of Prostatitis Confirmed?

A patient with suspected acute prostatitis should provide a mid-stream urine sample for dipstick testing and urine culture, and should have two sets of blood cultures drawn. Prostate massage prior to obtaining a urine specimen, thought to increase culture yield, is generally not recommended in acute prostatitis because it is typically very painful and there is a theoretical risk of precipitating bacteremia. In addition, pathogens are almost always isolated from urine.

Patients presenting with characteristic signs and symptoms of acute prostatitis, but with normal urinalyses, should undergo investigation for other etiologies. Serious illnesses with similar clinical presentations include testicular torsion and Fournier gangrene. Immediate urologic consultation should be obtained if these diagnoses are suspected.

Procedures to obtain prostatic secretions for analysis can be useful in the diagnosis of chronic prostatitis. Meares and Stamey introduced a four-cup examination of expressed prostatic secretions in 1968. Although this test has been considered the standard for evaluating chronic prostatitis, it has significant limitations. First, the procedure has never been properly evaluated for validity or diagnostic accuracy in a well-controlled setting. Second, leukocytes in prostatic fluid may be caused by common conditions other than prostatitis, such as urethritis, prostate stones, or recent ejaculation. Finally, routine use of the localization test has been adopted neither by primary care physicians nor urologists, likely because it is a time-consuming procedure. In 1997, Nickel published an inexpensive, more expedient localization procedure, the premassage and postmassage test, which was already in use by many urologists. The details of each of the localization procedures are enumerated below.

To assure an adequate specimen is obtained using the localization procedure, the clinician should ascertain and instruct as follows:

1. No recent antibiotics (within the previous month)
2. No recent ejaculation (within the previous 2 days)
3. Bladder should be full but not distended
4. No evidence of active urethritis or urinary tract infection
5. Retract the foreskin of uncircumcised men throughout the procedure

Table 88.3. Localization Procedures

Localization Procedure	Meares and Stamey (1968)	Nickel (PPMT) (1997)
Technique	1. **VB1:** Collect the first 10 mL voided urine 2. Discard the next 100 mL voided 3. **VB2:** Collect 10 mL mid-stream urine 4. **EPS:** Vigorously massage the prostate (1 min) and collect any expressed prostatic secretions 5. **VB3:** Collect the first 10 mL urine voided after the massage 6. Transport all specimens to laboratory immediately for microscopy and quantitative culture	1. **Pre-M:** Mid-stream urine specimen 2. Vigorously massage the prostate (1 min) from periphery toward midline 3. **Post-M:** Urine specimen produced immediately after prostate massage 4. Transport specimens to laboratory for microscopy and quantitative culture
Interpretation	1. All specimens yield less than 10^3 CFU/mL → **negative test for bacterial prostatitis** 2. VB3 specimen or EPS specimen yields a colony count of 10-fold or more greater than the VB1 specimen → **chronic bacterial prostatitis (type II)** 3. VB1 specimen yields a colony count greater than other specimens → **urethritis or specimen contamination** 4. All specimens yield at least 10^3 CFU/mL → **Unable to interpret, possible cystitis** (in this case treat the patient for 2–3 days with an antibiotic that does not penetrate the prostate but will sterilize bladder urine; then repeat the procedure)	1. Pre-M culture negative, post-M culture positive, and post-M WBC positive → **chronic bacterial prostatitis (type II)** 2. Pre-M culture negative, post-M culture negative, and post-M WBC positive → **chronic abacterial prostatitis (type IIIA)** 3. Pre-M culture negative, post-M culture negative, and post-M WBC negative → **noninflammatory pelvic pain syndrome (type IIIB)** 4. Pre-M culture positive, post-M culture positive, and post-M WBC positive → **cystitis ± type II**

VB, voided bladder specimen; pre-M, premassage; EPS, expressed prostatic secretions specimen; post-M, postmassage; CFU, colony-forming units.

6. Clean the glans penis well with providone-iodine or soap and water
7. One of the two localization procedures from Table 88.3 above should then be performed.

The sensitivity and specificity of the Nickel technique above has been reported as 91% for each. No role has been effectively established for the use of prostate ultrasonography in the diagnosis of prostatitis, although it may be useful in refractory or type II prostatitis to exclude abscess or prostatic stones. Psychological factors, including depression and somatization, can play an etiologic role in chronic prostatitis. However, definitive evidence including causality has yet to be established. Obtaining a serum prostate specific antigen level is not useful in the diagnosis of prostatitis, and should be discouraged in such a setting.

What Are the Management Options for Prostatitis, and What Is the Duration of Therapy?

The usefulness of antibiotics in the treatment of prostatitis has not been well studied in a randomized, controlled fashion. Most studies have small numbers of patients, have no placebo, and do not use consistent definitions of disease, doses of therapy, duration of therapy, or periods of follow-up. Thus, even review articles, consensus statements, and various guidelines differ somewhat in their recommendations. Although the levels of evidence for antibiotic use are low (level III and IV evidence), experts continue to recommend an antibiotic trial in the setting of a clinical diagnosis of prostatitis. Poor penetration of the prostate by penicillins and cephalosporins should limit their use in prostatitis.

The treatment strategy for acute prostatitis includes rest, adequate fluid repletion, and analgesia with nonsteroidal antiinflammatory drugs (NSAIDs). Acute urinary retention should be treated with a transurethral catheter or suprapubic catheterization if necessary. Empiric antibiotic therapy should be started immediately. The decision to admit to the hospital and choice of oral versus parenteral antibiotics should be guided by the clinical severity. Appropriate antibiotic regimens include ciprofloxacin (500 mg twice daily orally or 400 mg twice daily intravenously) and ofloxacin (400 mg twice daily). Newer quinolones, presumed to have similar efficacy, have not been adequately studied. Alternatives to quinolones include trimethoprim-sulfamethoxazole (160/800 mg twice daily) or ampicillin with gentamicin if enterococcal infections are suspected or confirmed. The standard duration of antibiotic therapy is 4 weeks. Failure to respond to therapy should arouse suspicion, and the clinician should search for prostatic abscess via transrectal ultrasonography or computed tomography of the prostate.

In chronic bacterial prostatitis (type II) the antibiotic regimen should be based on antimicrobial sensitivities. Quinolones are first-line therapy, and alternative agents include trimethoprim (200 mg twice daily), trimethoprim-sulfamethoxazole (160/800 mg twice daily), and doxycycline (100 mg twice daily). Although the recommended duration of antibiotic therapy is variable, most groups advocate at least a 4-week course, potentially extending therapy for up to 12 weeks. In culture-negative chronic prostatitis (type III), most sources favor an antibiotic trial similar to that for type II prostatitis. However, symptoms should be monitored frequently (every 2 weeks) and antibiotics continued only if symptomatic improvement is documented. Failure to respond to antibiotics or other therapies should prompt urology referral. Repeated or prolonged courses of antibiotics in this group should be avoided.

Other symptom-modifying therapies that may be effective in nonbacterial prostatitis include (ordered from highest to lowest levels of evidence):

1. Transurethral or transrectal microwave thermotherapy
2. Alpha receptor blocking agents with dose titration based on symptoms (studies used terazosin and alfuzosin)
3. NSAIDs
4. Stress management
5. Allopurinol (additional studies needed)

Case

A healthy 47-year-old man presents with a 5-day history of lower abdominal pain and dysuria. He has no fever, chills, or other systemic symptoms. He denies any prior urinary infections or other urinary complaints, including hesitancy, urgency, and frequency. He is sexually active only with his wife of 22 years, but admits to a vague discomfort with ejaculation for the past 3 or 4 weeks. He denies any penile discharge or testicular pain. He takes no medications, uses no illicit drugs, and does not smoke or drink alcohol. His family history is unremarkable.

A physical examination reveals a well-developed white man in no distress with a temperature of 37.2°C, pulse of 84 beats/min, blood pressure of 110/70 mm Hg, and respiratory rate of 16 breaths/min. His abdominal examination is remarkable only for mild suprapubic tenderness with deep palpation. Bowel sounds are active and there is no distention, rebound, or guarding. External genitalia are normal, and inguinal lymph nodes are nonpalpable. The rectal examination is remarkable for a mildly enlarged prostate that is smooth and nontender. A urinalysis performed in the office reveals 8 to 12 WBCs per high-power field.

A urine culture is sent, and the patient is sent home with a 7-day course of trimethoprim-sulfamethoxazole for treatment of a presumptive urinary tract infection. He returns to your office 3 weeks later with persistent symptoms. His culture from 3 weeks earlier revealed no growth, and repeat urinalysis in the office today is completely normal.

1. What is the diagnosis and classification?
2. What is your next step in this patient's diagnostic evaluation?
3. What are your therapeutic options in this patient?

Case Discussion

What Is the Diagnosis and Classification?

It is unlikely that this patient has a urinary tract infection with a negative urine culture. Other diagnostic possibilities include urethritis due to a sexually transmitted disease, but this is supported neither by his history nor by any discharge on examination. Prostatitis is common in a patient his age and with his symptom complex. If he does have prostatitis, the classification by the new National Institutes of Health system is likely a nonbacterial prostatitis or chronic pelvic pain syndrome (type III), the most common type.

What Is Your Next Step in This Patient's Diagnostic Evaluation?

The patient's initial visit, with postrectal examination urinalysis positive for WBCs, suggests an inflammatory prostatitis (type IIIA), but a true prostatic massage (1 minute, vigorous) was not performed. Such examination followed by repeat urinalysis and culture may help diagnose a chronic bacterial prostatitis (type II) if the culture grows an organism. Bacterial growth with antibiotic sensitivity would help guide antibiotic management. If his postmassage culture is negative, he would be classified as type III, and the presence or absence of WBCs in his postmassage urinalysis would further subclassify him into inflammatory (type IIIA) or noninflammatory (type IIIB) chronic pelvic pain syndrome. Urethral culture for *Chlamydia* and *Gonococcus* will help narrow the diagnosis.

What Are Your Therapeutic Options for This Patient?

It is important to remember that this patient is not acutely ill or toxic, and waiting for the results of the diagnostic evaluation is appropriate. Nevertheless, even a non-bacterial prostatitis may prompt an antibiotic trial. If empiric therapy is initiated after diagnostic evaluation, a quinolone is the first-line agent in prostatitis and would also treat a potential urethritis. Doxycycline is another choice that could play a similar dual role. Other choices include trimethoprim alone or trimethoprim-sulfamethoxazole. Alternatively, single therapy with an α-blocking agent or NSAID while waiting for culture results may provide interim symptomatic relief. A follow-up visit in 1 to 2 weeks to review the results of his cultures and evaluate symptomatic improvement is indicated. If all cultures are negative and his symptoms are improving on antibiotic therapy, continuing the antibiotic for a 4- to 6-week course may be done. If his symptoms are not improving on 2 weeks of antibiotic therapy (with negative cultures), urologic referral may be necessary.

Suggested Reading

Clinical Effectiveness Group. National guideline for the management of prostatitis. *Sex Transm Infect* 1999;75(suppl 1):46–50.

Collins M M. Diagnosis and treatment of chronic abacterial prostatitis: a systematic review. *Ann Intern Med* 2000;133:367–381.

Johansen T E. The role of antibiotics in the treatment of chronic prostatitis: a consensus statement. *Eur Urol* 1998;34:457–466.

Lipsky B A. Prostatitis and urinary tract infection in men: what's new; what's true? *Am J Med* 1999;106:327–334.

Nickel J C. Prostatitis: evolving management strategies. *Urol Clin North Am* 1999;26:737–751.

89

Microscopic Hematuria

Stacy M. Higgins

1. How is microscopic hematuria defined?
2. What are the common etiologies of microscopic hematuria? Do these change based on age or sex?
3. How can the history and physical examination assist in the differential diagnosis of hematuria?
4. What is the utility of laboratory and radiologic testing in the workup of hematuria?
5. In patients for whom no etiology can be found, what is the appropriate follow-up?

Discussion

How Is Microscopic Hematuria Defined?

Anywhere from three to eight red blood cells (RBCs) per high-power field (HPF) is accepted as the upper limit of normal for hematuria, although significant urologic disease may still be present even with so-called normal levels of RBC excretion. The range is probably age and sex related; the prevalence of all degrees of microscopic hematuria increases with age. The arbitrary nature of the definition of microscopic hematuria will lead to some patients with disease escaping assessment, while others with no pathologic cause will be investigated. There is no relation to the seriousness of the underlying cause and the degree of hematuria, so hematuria should be considered a symptom of serious disease until proven otherwise.

Hematuria is a relatively common finding. The prevalence of hematuria on dipstick testing ranges from 2% to 16%, and on urine microscopy lies between 1% and 5%. Physiologic excretion of RBCs can occur at low levels in young healthy people, resulting from trauma during sexual intercourse or urine contamination with menstruation. Vigorous exercise also can cause hematuria, although this is a diagnosis of exclusion. With increasing age, hematuria, whether persistent or transient, requires more detailed diagnostic testing to rule out malignancy because of the increased prevalence of uroepithelial, renal cell, and prostate cancers.

Microscopic hematuria is often detected on a urinalysis obtained as part of a general physical examination, hospital admission, or preoperative evaluation. It is a common problem that can affect up to 13% of the general population. Because of its intermittent occurrence and the low incidence of significant associated urologic disease, screening of all adults for microscopic hematuria with dipstick testing is not currently recommended. Many patients with microscopic hematuria are asymptomatic and have no evidence of genitourinary or systemic disease. As clinicians, we need to understand the occurrence and significance of microscopic hematuria when deciding on the most appropriate diagnostic evaluation, balancing the cost of a full evaluation with the possibility of an occult malignancy.

What Are the Common Etiologies of Microscopic Hematuria? Do These Change Based on Age or Sex?

The causes of microscopic hematuria (Table 89.1) range from conditions posing little risk to the patient to potentially life-threatening conditions such as malignancy. In adults the most common causes of hematuria include neoplasm, kidney stones, inflammation (including infection), and benign prostatic hyperplasia. Other less common causes include trauma, obstruction from non–tumor-related etiologies, hematologic abnormalities, vascular abnormalities, benign familial hematuria and exercise-induced hematuria. Immunoglobulin A (IgA) nephropathy (Berger disease) is the most common cause of glomerular hematuria.

Risk factors for urothelial carcinoma include tobacco use, exposure to aniline dyes, dietary nitrites and nitrates, analgesic abuse, urinary schistosomiasis, cyclophosphamide, pelvic irradiation, chronic cystitis, and bacterial infections associated with urinary calculi and obstruction of the upper urinary tract.

How Can the History and Physical Examination Assist in the Differential Diagnosis of Hematuria?

Because of the wide range of pathologies leading to hematuria, a careful history and examination help to direct the investigation pathway. For example, recent menstruation, urinary tract instrumentation, or sexual trauma suggest that the most appropriate approach may be repeating the urinalysis at a later date. Symptoms of fre-

Table 89.1. Most Frequent Causes of Hematuria by Age and Sex

Age 0–20 yr
Acute glomerulonephritis
Acute UTI
Congenital urinary tract anomalies with obstruction
Age 20–40 yr
Acute UTI
Bladder cancer
Urolithiasis
Age 40–60 yr
Acute UTI
Bladder cancer
Urolithiasis
Age >60, females
Acute UTI
Bladder cancer
Age >60, males
Acute UTI
Benign prostatic hyperplasia
Bladder cancer

UTI, urinary tract infection.

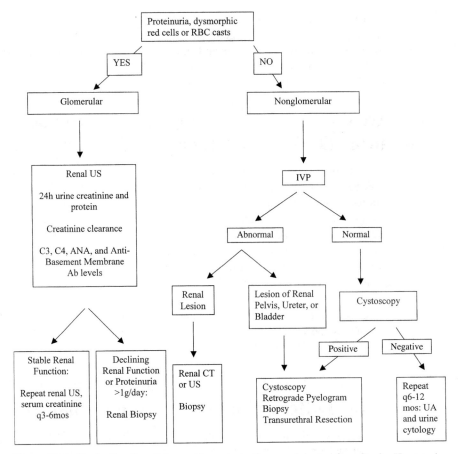

Figure 89.1. Evaluation for etiology of hematuria. Source: Adapted from Paola: Hematuria: Essentials of Diagnosis. *Hospital Practice,* Nov, 15, 1990.

quency and dysuria suggest the presence of a urinary tract infection or prostatitis. Pain can point to the presence of nephrolithiasis, ureteric blood clot, or renal infarction. A recent streptococcal pharyngitis, a rash, or peripheral edema may signal the onset of a nephritic condition. The use of alcohol and tobacco should be quantified to assess the probability of papillary necrosis or bladder cancer. Occupational carcinogen exposure in the rubber or dye industries predisposes to transitional cell carcinoma. Foreign travel raises the possibility of schistosomiasis (the most common cause of hematuria worldwide) or malaria. Nonsteroidal antiinflammatory drugs may cause papillary necrosis, and certain chemotherapy agents can cause a hemorrhagic cystitis. Anticoagulation may predispose to hematuria, but it is usually the unmasking of an underlying genitourinary lesion. Family history may point to sickle cell anemia, hemophilia, polycystic kidney disease, Alport syndrome, and some forms of glomerulonephritis.

Significant signs on physical examination include fever, hypertension, rash, edema, enlarged prostate, hearing loss (Alport syndrome), or new heart murmur. Palpation may reveal a mass or tenderness in the abdomen or flank and an enlarged or nodular prostate. There may be external lesions of the genitalia and urethral opening, pointing toward a sexually transmitted disease. Pelvic examination will identify vaginal prolapse or other pathology as the source of blood.

What Is the Utility of Laboratory and Radiologic Testing in the Workup of Hematuria?

Urinalysis

Urinary dipstick analysis has a sensitivity of 91% to 100% and a specificity of 65% to 99% for greater than three RBCs/HPF. Hemoglobin, either free in urine or from urinary RBCs, will catalyze an oxidation reaction between the substances on the strip, resulting in a color change on the strip. For diagnosis, a freshly voided specimen should be obtained and examined within 30 minutes. In hypotonic urine or in urine left unexamined for more than 30 minutes, dipstick testing may be positive for blood while the urinalysis is negative for RBCs because of lysis, and the release of free hemoglobin. The combination of a positive dipstick and a negative urinalysis is also seen in hemoglobinuria and myoglobinuria. Because of its low specificity, a positive dipstick mandates urine microscopy examination.

Urine Microscopy

Glomerular disease is suggested by marked proteinuria, RBC casts, or a characteristic RBC morphology. Specifically, nonglomerular erythrocytes are isomorphic in shape, uniform in size, and resemble circulating RBCs. Conversely, in glomerular hematuria, the urinary erythrocytes are dysmorphic, distorted with irregular outlines, and often have small blebs extruding from their cell membrane. They are also characteristically heterogeneous in size. Proteinuria has been described with gross bleeding into the urinary tract distal to the kidneys. RBC casts are seen with acute interstitial nephritis, diabetic nephropathy, renal embolism, renal vein thrombosis, and exercise. Pyuria or white blood cell (WBC) casts suggest inflammation or infection of the urinary tract. Urinary eosinophils are commonly seen in acute interstitial nephritis.

Urine Culture

Urine cultures are used to look for infection as a possible cause of the hematuria. Men with cystitis need to undergo further workup because this is frequently the result of obstruction. After treatment of the infection, repeat urinalysis is warranted to ensure that hematuria has resolved, because urinary tract infections can coexist with other causes of hematuria.

Urine Cytology

In the detection of uroepithelial cancer, primarily transitional cell cancer of the bladder, urine cytology has a relatively low sensitivity of 67%, but a high specificity of 96%. Sensitivity of voided urine cytology is dependent on the number of urine specimens examined, the stage and grade of the bladder tumor, and the expertise of the cytopathologist. Analysis should be performed on a fresh urine specimen, bladder washings, or brushings of cystoscopic lesions. Cytology is more sensitive in detecting poorly differentiated than well-differentiated bladder cancer, and lesions that are sessile or *in situ* rather than papillary.

Blood Tests

Serum creatinine levels should be assessed to look for evidence of renal insufficiency; in black patients, sickle cell screening is warranted. In patients with evidence of glomerular disease, a complete workup includes antinuclear antibody, antiglomerular basement membrane, serum complement levels, cryoglobulins, streptococcal serologies, hepatitis B surface antigen, venereal disease research laboratory, human immunodeficiency virus, and blood cultures (when indicated).

Imaging

The main value of abdominal radiographs is to exclude urinary tract calcification, which may be due to calculi or infection (e.g., tuberculosis or schistosomiasis).

Urinary tract ultrasonography can detect renal masses and determine whether they are cystic, solid, or complex. It also can detect calcification with a reasonably high degree of accuracy. If normal, an ultrasonography scan will exclude all but the smallest renal cell malignancies. Because it poses no risk to the kidney, ultrasonography is particularly useful for patients with renal impairment or an allergy to contrast dye precluding the use of intravenous pyelography (IVP).

In IVP, contrast excretion gives rise to the nephrogram, pyelogram, and cystogram. The principal positive finding, a filling defect within the collecting system, may be due to urothelial malignancy, a radiolucent stone, or papillary necrosis resulting in a sloughed papilla, blood clot, or metastases. A postmicturition film gives a broad indication of the completeness of bladder emptying. IVP should not be performed in patients at high risk for contrast nephropathy.

The role of computed tomography (CT) is in the further evaluation of renal tract masses detected by IVP or ultrasonography. CT can pick up small renal masses not visible on ultrasonography and may be used to evaluate the renal tract in cases where ultrasonography was unsatisfactory. Finally, it has a greater sensitivity to the presence of calcification than the plain film.

The main purpose of cystoscopy when used diagnostically is to inspect the bladder, looking for evidence of papillary transitional cell carcinomas or any raised, red plaques to suggest a diagnosis of carcinoma *in situ*. Cystoscopy has 87% sensitivity for uncovering uroepithelial malignancy. It has been recommended that cystoscopy be performed in patients under 40 only when at increased risk for bladder carcinoma (positive or suspicious urinary cytology, history of tobacco use, or history of occupational exposures).

Renal Biopsy

There is no consensus on the indications for a renal biopsy in patients with hematuria. Patients with marked proteinuria, RBC casts, or dysmorphic urinary RBCs are more likely to have glomerular (medical) disease and benefit from biopsy. The most common findings on renal biopsy are mesangial proliferative glomerulonephritis (especially IgA nephropathy), thin basement membrane disease, diffuse proliferative glomerulonephritis, and normal renal tissue.

In Patients for Whom No Etiology Can Be Found, What Is the Appropriate Follow-Up?

Despite a complete and exhaustive workup, no specific cause for microscopic hematuria is identified in approximately 20% of patients. In patients for whom no etiology can be found, follow-up examinations revealed cancer in 1% to 3% of those with microscopic hematuria. After the initial workup, a typical follow-up regimen is to perform urinalysis and cytology every 6 months and a cystoscopy and IVP or ultrasonography every year, for up to 3 years if the hematuria persists.

Case

A 67-year-old man with a history of hypertension and smoking presents with symptoms of urinary urgency and hesitancy. He reports that his symptoms have been progressively worsening over the past year, and he frequently feels as though his bladder is not completely emptied after voiding. He comes in today because for the past week he has also had some burning with voiding. He denies fever, chills, back pain, nausea, vomiting, or gross hematuria. His occupational history is notable for working at a factory producing chemical dyes while in his early twenties. On examination, his blood pressure is 140/82 mm Hg, pulse 84 beats/min, and temperature 99.5°F. He has mild suprapubic discomfort and fullness on abdominal examination; on rectal examination, an enlarged, boggy, tender prostate without nodules is encountered. Urinalysis is positive for leukocyte esterase, nitrites, and hemoglobin, but otherwise normal. Urine microscopy reveals 10 to 20 WBCs, 10 to 20 RBCs, and bacteria, with no casts.

1. What are the possible etiologies of his symptoms?
2. What workup would you recommend?
3. What, if any, follow-up should be recommended?

Case Discussion

What Are the Possible Etiologies of His Symptoms?

Based on his age and sex, the most likely etiology of his symptoms is a urinary tract infection. The patient's symptoms suggest incomplete emptying of the bladder, possibly due to prostatic enlargement. The physical examination finding of an enlarged, boggy, tender prostate also raises the possibility of prostatitis and prostatic hyperplasia. Given his occupational history, bladder carcinoma also must be considered in the differential diagnosis. Information on his travel history should be obtained to rule out schistosomiasis as a possible cause. Given that pain is not a major component of the presentation, nephrolithiasis is unlikely.

What Workup Would You Recommend?

Studies should be ordered to help rule in or out possible diagnoses. To begin with, a urine culture should be ordered to check for infection. Passing a urinary catheter to assess for a postvoid residual volume will help evaluate if there is prostatic hyperplasia with incomplete emptying, increasing the susceptibility for bladder and prostate infection. Based on the history and physical examination, this is the most likely diagnosis.

The patient was empirically placed on ciprofloxacin 500 mg twice daily pending urine cultures and doxazosin 2 mg at bedtime for treatment of his obstructive voiding symptoms and for an elevated post void residual of 100 mL. Urine cultures returned positive for *Escherichia coli*.

What, if Any, Follow-Up Should Be Recommended?

Following treatment of his infection, his urinalysis should be repeated to ensure that his infections and the accompanying hematuria have resolved. If the hematuria persists, the next step would be IVP to evaluate for filling defects or masses. Urine cytology can help evaluate for bladder carcinoma, but given its low sensitivity, it cannot definitively rule it out. In cases where there is a high suspicion secondary to risk factors, as in this case, or because of age, a cystoscopy should be performed for direct bladder visualization. If cystoscopy is negative, but urine microscopy remains positive for RBCs, it is recommended to repeat the workup every 6 to 12 months, keeping in mind that older patients and males are at higher risk for bladder and prostate carcinoma.

Suggested Reading

Corwin H., Silverstein M. Microscopic hematuria. *Clin Lab Med* 1988;8:601–610.

Grossfield G, Carroll P. Evaluation of asymptomatic microscopic hematuria. *Urol Clin North Am* 1998;25:661–676.

Paola A. Hematuria: essentials of diagnosis. *Hosp Practice* November 15, 1990.

Rockall A G, Newman-Sanders A P G, et al. Haematuria. *J Postgrad Med* 1997;73:129–136.

Sutton J. Evaluation of hematuria in adults. *JAMA* 1990;263:2475–2480.

Thaller T, Wang L. Evaluation of asymptomatic microscopic hematuria in adults. *Am Fam Physician* 1999;60:1143–1151.

90
Erectile Dysfunction
Clyde Watkins, Jr.

1. What is the definition of impotence or erectile dysfunction?
2. Review clinically relevant erectile physiology.
3. What are the risk factors for erectile dysfunction?
4. How do you work up erectile dysfunction?
5. Who should see a urologist?
6. What treatment options are available for primary care providers?

Discussion
What Is the Definition of Impotence or Erectile Dysfunction?

Many clinicians use the terms impotence and erectile dysfunction (ED) interchangeably. However, impotence is a broad term that includes problems of libido, ejaculation, and orgasm, and erectile dysfunction is a distinct sexual problem. The National Institutes of Health Consensus Guidelines Development Panel defines ED as "the consistent inability to achieve or maintain an erection sufficient for satisfactory sexual performance."

Review Clinically Relevant Erectile Physiology.

The penis is innervated by both autonomic (parasympathetic and sympathetic) and somatic nervous systems. Sacral parasympathetic nerves govern erection and tumescence, whereas sympathetic nerves govern detumescence and ejaculation. Because of this dual innervation, either psychogenic (autonomic) or somatic (peripheral) stimuli, or a combination of the two, may initiate erection.

In the nonerect state, cavernosal smooth muscle tissue, as well as the arterial vessels of the penis, exist in a state of constriction. Current evidence indicates that the vasodilation and relaxation of cavernosal smooth muscle required for erection involves a nonadrenergic–noncholinergic mechanism mediated by nitric oxide.

Nitric oxide is released by neurons, endothelial cells, and corporal smooth muscle cells of the penis in response to sexual stimulation. After diffusing to corpus cavernosal smooth muscle cells, nitric oxide stimulates guanylate cyclase to produce cyclic guanosine monophosphate (cGMP), which serves as a second messenger to promote smooth muscle relaxation and vasodilation. Nitric oxide is then hydrolyzed by cGMP-specific phosphodiesterase (PDE) type 5.

What Are the Risk Factors for Erectile Dysfunction?

Age

The predominant risk factor for ED is age. In the Massachusetts Male Aging Study, a community-based survey of men 40 to 70 years of age, 52% of men reported having some degree of ED: complete ED in 10%, moderate ED in 25%, and minimal ED in 17% overall. Furthermore, the survey found that the severity of ED increased with advancing age.

Diabetes can affect both the vascular and neurologic systems. It is a common cause of ED, with half of diabetic men being affected. Additionally, ED occurs 10 to 15 years earlier in diabetic men than in the general population.

Atherosclerosis is a risk factor in 70% of cases of ED in men 60 years and over. ED may serve as an early marker for peripheral or cardiovascular disease.

Hypertension

The major risk of hypertension is its contribution to the overall risk of atherosclerosis. ED is a noted side effect of many of the medications taken to control hypertension.

Cigarette Smoking

Smoking is an independent risk factor for ED and potentiates the effects of other risk factors for atherosclerosis.

Renal Disease

Renal disease is frequently associated with ED with nearly half of male patients with uremia experiencing ED and 75% of dialysis-dependent men affected. Patients who have undergone renal transplantation tend to have persistence of their ED.

Pelvic Injury

Pelvic injury in general is associated with ED. One third of men in the United States with pelvic fracture and associated arterial injury are affected. In some cases, ED is due to nerve damage or impairment of penile blood flow following pelvic surgery. Up to 40% of men undergoing radical prostatectomy for adenocarcinoma have ED.

Spinal Cord Injury

Some degree of ED is present in 50% of men with lumbar injury. Some men may be able to achieve erection through central mechanism (thoughts), but the ability to achieve erection through direct stimulation tends to be lost or severely impaired.

Drug Abuse

Marijuana and alcohol, contrary to popular belief, depresses sexual function. Additionally, the hypogonadism, chronic liver damage, and neuropathy associated with chronic alcoholism strongly influence the incidence of ED.

Medications

The importance of a whole range of medications as risk factors should not be underestimated. Twenty-five percent of all ED cases may be attributed to medications taken for other conditions (Table 90.1).

Endocrine Abnormalities

Hypogonadotropic hypogonadism, hyperthyroidism, hypothyroidism, and hyperprolactinemia are responsible for ED in less than 5% of cases. However, all of these conditions are risk factors for ED and may exacerbate symptoms caused by other factors. ED is often the presenting complaint in men with pituitary adenomas.

Psychogenic Abnormalities

Erectile dysfunction is primarily an organic disease. However, psychological factors, including loss of self-confidence, performance anxiety, poor partner communication, and marital conflict, are often important contributing factors. Patients who are already anxious or depressed are prone to ED, which in turn can exacerbate their anxiety and depression. Performance anxiety causes detumescence through increasing adrenaline levels and the resultant increased adrenergic tone. The prevalence of purely psychogenic ED is open to debate. Depending on the age and source of patients studied, estimates of pure psychogenic ED vary from 10% to 30%. Other psychogenic factors such as depression, marital discord, dysfunctional attitudes, sexual phobias, religious inhibition, or traumatic past experience are capable of causing ED and are treatable by psychotherapy.

Table 90.1. Medications Associated with Erectile Dysfunction

Angiotensin-converting enzyme inhibitors
β-blockers
Calcium channel blockers
Centrally acting antiadrenergic agents
Flutamide
H$_2$ receptor blockers
Leuprolide
Thiazide diuretics
Phenothiazines
Selective serotonin reuptake inhibitors
Spironolactone
Tricyclic antidepressants

How Do You Work Up a Case of Erectile Dysfunction?

History

The majority of ED is a result of an organic disorder, but both organic and psychological factors are at play in the true cause of ED.

Get a Description of the Problem

Is the patient's complaint really ED, an age-related change in sexual functioning, or other sexual dysfunction (i.e., loss of libido, retrograde ejaculation) (Table 90.2). Was the onset sudden or gradual and over what time period did it develop?

Determine Whether the Libido Is Intact

In cases of decreased libido, the workup should focus on endocrine causes of sexual dysfunction libido.

1. Assess risk factors and/or symptoms that may suggest a secondary cause.
2. Assess the contribution of organic and psychogenic factors.

Answering yes to any of the following questions is suggestive of a predominantly psychogenic cause of ED.

- Do you ever wake up with an erection?
- When you masturbate, can you get an erection?
- Can you get an erection at any time, during any sexual activity, with any partner?

Physical Examination

The physical examination should be directed toward areas pertinent to the possible etiology.

- Search for signs of vascular disease
  - Diminished or absent peripheral pulses
- Genitourinary examination
  - Genital examination
  - Testicular size and consistency
  - Penile plaques
- Digital rectal examination
  - Rectal tone
  - Prostate examination
- Neurologic examination
  - Perineal sensation

Table 90.2. Age-Related Changes in Male Sexual Function

More time or more physical stimulation to achieve erection
More control over their ejaculations, but the flow is reduced
Tend not to be as hard, and the refractory period is prolonged
More likely to take medication that contributes to erectile dysfunction

- Rectal tone
- Cremasteric reflex

Laboratory Evaluation

Basic laboratory tests to order when evaluating ED include serum chemistries, lipids, and glucose. All other tests are warranted only when indicated by the history and physical. Testosterone and prolactin levels are generally not indicated in the primary evaluation of ED, unless the initial history and physical suggest an endocrinologic cause.

Specialized Diagnostic Testing

Definitive diagnostic testing is time consuming, tedious, and expensive. A specialist should generally use diagnostic testing after a primary care evaluation has failed to resolve the problem or if surgical intervention is planned.

Who Should See a Urologist?

Most patients with ED can be managed within a primary care setting. Special circumstances may indicate the need for a specialist referral for further diagnostic testing or management. Table 90.3 outlines the criteria for appropriate specialist referral.

What Treatment Options Are Available for Primary Care Providers?

Modify Reversible Causes

- Prescription and nonprescription drug use
- Specific endocrinologic conditions (hypogonadism, thyroid disease)
- Pelvic trauma or anatomic conditions
- Life-style and psychosocial factors

First-Line Therapy

Sildenafil

Sildenafil is a type 5 phosphodiesterase inhibitor with a high specificity for corporal smooth muscle. It works by prolonging the action of nitric oxide and cGMP, thus

Table 90.3. Erectile Dysfunction: Criteria for Specialist Referral

Significant Peyronie disease or penile curvature
Patient with history of pelvic or perineal trauma
Vascular or neurosurgical intervention needed
Complicated endocrinopathy
Complicated psychiatric or psychosocial disorder
Patient or physician request for further evaluation

prolonging smooth muscle relaxation. Sildenafil is taken 1 hour before sexual activity and does not take effect until sexual stimulation occurs. Duration of activity is around 4 to 6 hours, and it is effective in 50% to 90% of patients. Side effects including flushing, headaches, gastrointestinal disturbances, and transient color blindness. There is a risk of priapism when erections last over 6 hours. Sildenafil is contraindicated in those using nitrate preparations and those with retinitis pigmentosa. Nitric oxide donors, such as nitroglycerin, in combination with sildenafil can cause severe and prolonged vasodilation that may cause hypotension and vascular collapse.

Alternative Oral Therapies

Yohimbine is an alpha-adrenergic receptor antagonist that acts as the adrenergic receptors in brain centers associated with libido and penile erection. Yohimbine's overall effect on erectile function is marginal. Its greatest effect has been noted to be in men with nonorganic erectile dysfunction.

Trazodone is thought to exert an effect on erectile function through its serotonergic and adrenergic activity. However, there are no clinical trials to support its effect on erectile dysfunction.

An oral form of phentolamine (peripheral vasodilator) and sublingual form of apomorphine (dopaminergic agonist that stimulates centers in the central nervous system to produce an erection) are currently being tested for commercial use.

Vacuum Constriction Devices

Vacuum constriction therapy consists of a vacuum device that is placed over the penis and the activation of a vacuum pump. Blood is drawn into the penis due to the subatmospheric pressure around the penis. A constriction device is then placed around the penis to hold the blood in place. Complications include painful ejaculation (10%–15%) and petechiae (if ring left on for >30 minutes). Contraindication to use of vacuum therapy includes those with severe coagulopathy and decreased manual dexterity.

Couples/Sexual Therapy

Sexual therapy can be beneficial in addressing more psychogenic causes of ED. It also can be beneficial to couples in managing their relationship in cases of organic ED.

Second- and Third-Line Therapies

Second- and third-line therapies should be selected based on failure, insufficient response, or adverse side effects associated with one or more of the first-line therapies, or patient and/or partner preferences. Candidates for second- and third-line therapies should be referred to a specialist for advanced diagnostic testing and treatment. These options consist of intercavernosal injection therapy, transurethral therapy, and the use of prostheses.

Case

Mr. K is a 65-year-old widower that you followed in your clinic for many years. He has a past history of hypertension, type 2 diabetes mellitus, and gastroesophageal reflux disease. He currently does not smoke (quit 5 years ago) and admits to heavy alcohol use in the past (quit 10 years ago). He presents complaining that "I have lost my nature." He states that at most times he cannot get an erection. On the times that he does have an erection they are very soft. This problem began approximately 14 months ago and has slowly worsened. It is a source of embarrassment for him. He still has a strong sexual desire and this problem has caused strain in his current relationship. He is very active, walking 2 miles per day, and is an avid golfer. Medications include glipizide XL 10 mg daily, omeprazole 20 mg daily, and hydrochlorothiazide/triamterene 25 mg/37.5 mg daily.

On physical examination, his blood pressure is 160/92 mm Hg, pulse 86 beats/min, and respiratory rate 20 breaths/min. He has no thyromegaly and has clear lungs and a 2/6 systolic murmur along the left sternal border radiating to the axilla. He has a normal abdominal examination. Rectal examination demonstrates good sphincter tone and a normal prostate. He has normal male genitalia; testicles are descended with normal size and consistency. Peripheral pulses are normal bilaterally, and no edema is present. A neurologic examination shows normal monofilament testing and a normal cremasteric reflex.

A laboratory assessment shows normal chemistries, except for an elevated random glucose at 246 mg/dL. His baseline electrocardiogram shows normal sinus rhythm with left ventricular hypertrophy and no evidence of prior myocardial infarction.

1. What are Mr. K's risk factors for erectile dysfunction?
2. What are Mr. K's treatment options?
3. Should testosterone levels be obtained routinely in the initial evaluation of erectile dysfunction?

Case Discussion

What Are Mr. K's Risk Factors for Erectile Dysfunction?

- Hypertension
- Type 2 diabetes
- Antihypertensive medications (hydrochlorothiazide/triamterene)
- Atherosclerosis

What Are Mr. K's Treatment Options?

The first steps in treatment of ED are to modify any reversible causes of ED. Mr. K had previously discontinued smoking and alcohol consumption. These are important reversible causes of ED, and a strong effort to convince patients to abstain from both tobacco and alcohol should be made. Mr. K can be switched from hydrochlorothiazide to another antihypertensive that is less closely associated with erectile dyfunction (e.g., an angiotensin-converting enzyme inhibitor or calcium channel blocker). Importantly, Mr. K's hypertension and diabetes should be aggressively controlled. Mr. K's treatment options include sildenafil therapy and a vacuum constriction device. Mr. K is a good candidate for both forms of therapy. He should be given his choice of therapy after discussing the risks and benefits for both. Even though he is not currently taking nitrates, if you prescribe sildenafil, he needs to be counseled on the dangers of using nitroglycerin in combination with sildenafil.

Should Testosterone Levels Be Obtained Routinely in the Initial Evaluation of Erectile Dysfunction?

Endocrine abnormalities account for less than 5% of all causes of ED. Androgen deficiency typically manifests as ED accompanied by a diminished libido and hypogonadism. Mr. K admits to a normal libido and has normal genitalia and secondary sex characteristics on physical examination. Given the low prevalence of androgen deficiency and the lack of supporting findings on initial evaluation, measurement of testosterone levels is of limited value.

Suggested Reading

Lue T F. Erectile dysfunction. *N Engl J Med* 2000;342:1802–1813.
Kuritzky L, et al. Management of impotence in primary care. *Comp Ther* 1998;24:137–146.
Position paper. The process of care model for evaluation and treatment of erectile dysfunction. *Int J Impot Res* 1999;11:59–74.

91
Scrotal Mass

Michael Benjamin

- Discussion *577*
- Case *579*
- Case Discussion *580*

1. What is the differential diagnosis of a scrotal mass?
2. What workup is indicated for outpatients with a scrotal mass?
3. What is the role of serum tumor markers in the diagnosis of testicular cancer?

Discussion
What Is the Differential Diagnosis of a Scrotal Mass?

Scrotal masses can present at any age, and may first come to the attention of either the clinician or the patient. The presence or absence of associated scrotal or testicular pain is an important clue in formulating a differential diagnosis. Common causes of a painful and painless scrotal mass are presented in Table 91.1.

Testicular torsion, a surgical emergency, is associated with the acute onset of severe scrotal pain. It is most common in children and young adults. On examination, the affected testis rides higher in the scrotal sac than the unaffected side, and can demonstrate a "bell-clapper" finding: the testicle is elevated, and its long axis rotated 90 degrees with respect to the unaffected testis. The cremasteric reflex (normally present in children to age 12) is typically absent. The overlying scrotum can be inflamed, and a reactive hydrocele may be found if sufficient time has passed since the onset of torsion. Color Doppler ultrasonography can help evaluate testicular artery blood flow if the diagnosis is in doubt: absent testicular artery blood flow can secure the diagnosis. Because irreversible testicular damage can occur within 12 hours of onset, prompt surgical exploration can save the affected gonad and prevent future episodes by fixation to the scrotal wall.

Torsion of the appendix testis can mimic true testicular torsion, but the pain is usually more subacute in onset. This diagnosis is not an emergency, because the torsion does not compromise testicular blood flow. The appendix testis is a remnant of the Müllerian duct system, present on the superior aspect of the testis. The diagnosis should be considered in the setting of normal testicular artery Doppler circulation and a small reactive hydrocele. Treatment is symptomatic, with rest, ice, and nonsteroidal antiinflammatory drugs (NSAIDs); surgical decompression may be necessary.

Epididymitis can present both acutely or subacutely, and is associated with scrotal pain. The epididymis is a linear structure on the posterior aspect of the testis connecting the testes to the vas deferens. It can become inflamed. Acute epididymitis can be accompanied by symptoms of systemic sepsis (fever, chills), and urinary

Table 91.1. Causes of Scrotal Mass

Painful scrotal mass
   Testicular torsion
   Torsion of the appendix testis
   Epididymitis
   Traumatic hematomas and rupture
   Henoch-Schönlein purpura
   Varicocele
   Cysts: epididymal, hydrocele, spermatocele
Painless scrotal mass
   Testicular carcinoma
   Postvasectomy epididymal swelling
   Idiopathic edema
   Varicocele
   Cysts: epididymal, hydrocele, spermatocele

---

tract symptoms such as frequency or dysuria. Physical findings include severe tenderness and swelling of the affected epididymis. A reactive hydrocele may be present, along with inflammation of the overlying scrotum, similar to torsion. For this reason, a sonogram of the testis may help distinguish torsion from epididymitis in the setting of acute pain and scrotal erythema. Acute epididymitis usually has a bacterial etiology, and can be accompanied by cystitis or prostatitis. The acuity of the illness frequently warrants intravenous antibiotics and hospital observation. Cases in younger men tend to be associated with sexually acquired pathogens such as *Chlamydia trachomatis* or *Neisseria gonorrhoeae,* whereas older men tend to have enteric pathogens as the cause. Antibiotics of choice include intravenous fluoroquinolones or ampicillin with gentamicin.

Epididymitis can have a subacute presentation, and can be associated with trauma or sexual activity, without a bacterial etiology. Physical findings are often less pronounced than with acute cases. Treatment is with NSAIDs and intramuscular ceftriaxone with oral doxycycline or ofloxacin to cover chlamydia, gonorrhea, and gram-negative organisms.

Testicular trauma is a significant cause of acute scrotal pain or mass from a reactive hydrocele. Rupture of the testis is diagnosed with ultrasonography, and should be referred for immediate surgical repair.

Vasculitis can affect the testis and present with pain. For example, Henoch-Schönlein purpura is the constellation of purpura, arthralgia, immunoglobulin A nephropathy, gastrointestinal bleeding, and occasionally scrotal pain. Treatment is with ice and NSAIDs.

A varicocele is a common cause of a scrotal mass. Symptoms may or may not include pain, and the mass may be large or small. A varicocele is a dilatation of the pampiniform plexus of veins. It is more common on the left, due to the higher pressures in the left spermatic vein. Right-sided lone varicoceles are less common, and usually prompt a search for underlying causes of compression of the right spermatic vein (i.e., cancer or other mass lesions). Typically, the mass enlarges during a Valsalva maneuver. There is evidence that varicoceles contribute to infertility; therefore referral to a urologist for surgical ligation may be indicated for men with infertility. Otherwise, treatment is supportive.

Cysts are common causes of painless scrotal masses. Spermatoceles are cysts arising from the epididymis, whereas hydroceles are cysts lined by the tunica vaginalis surrounding the testes. Reactive hydroceles can be associated with trauma, epididymitis, or testicular cancer. Treatment involves watching over time, or surgical excision.

Testicular cancer, another important cause of scrotal mass, is usually painless and most commonly presents in men 18 to 30 years of age. Testicular germ cell tumors are most common, and are classified into seminomas and nonseminomatous cancers.

What Workup Is Indicated for Outpatients with a Scrotal Mass?

Frequently, patients will present with some component of pain with their testicular mass. If the pain is acute and there is a reasonable suspicion of testicular torsion, immediate urologic consultation is indicated. If the disease presentation is more subacute, a trial of antibiotics is indicated to empirically treat for epididymitis.

If symptoms have not resolved within 2 weeks, testicular ultrasonography is indicated to help diagnose testicular cancer. Germ cell tumors typically show microcalcifications, hypoechoic masses, and intratesticular incorporation. Definitive treatment of testicular cancer involves orchiectomy, radiotherapy, or retroperitoneal lymph node dissection. Some patients will go on to require chemotherapy, either for high-risk or recurrent disease.

Painless testicular masses should be considered carcinoma until proven otherwise, and should be handled accordingly with immediate referral to a urologist.

What Is the Role of Serum Tumor Markers in the Diagnosis of Testicular Cancer?

Serum tumor markers are useful in limited situations. Alpha-fetoprotein is elevated in nonseminomatous tumors only, whereas β-human chorionic gonadotropin (β-HCG) and lactate dehydrogenase can be elevated in both types of germ cell tumors. These markers are followed throughout the course of diagnosis and treatment, and increasing levels can help secure the diagnosis of carcinoma. Unfortunately, the tests are not sensitive enough to meaningfully screen for disease, for example β-HCG is elevated in less than 20% of seminomas.

Case

A 19-year-old man is seen in the urgent care center complaining of an acutely tender and swollen left scrotal mass. He reports waking up with a sensation of fullness and heaviness of the left scrotum. On examining himself, he noted a tender nodular mass of the posterior part of the left testicle. Subsequently, the tenderness has worsened, and he left early from his job at a restaurant to be evaluated. He reports no history of trauma or previous mass. He reports a recent breakup with his girlfriend of 6 months, with whom he had been sexually active. He is convinced he has cancer, because a friend died of testicular cancer. The examination reveals an apprehensive young man in mild distress. Temperature is 100.5°F, blood pressure 105/65 mm Hg, pulse 95 beats/min. On genitourinary examination, the scrotum is erythematous and tender on the left side, and the epididymis is swollen and tender on that side as well. The testes are freely mobile and not tender to palpation. No discharge is present at the urethra, and rectal examination reveals a nontender prostate and brown stool. No inguinal lymphadenopathy is present, and the cremasteric reflex is absent.

1. What might be the cause of this patient's scrotal mass?
2. What is the next step in diagnosing the cause of the illness?
3. What treatment should be undertaken?

Case Discussion

What Might Be the Cause of This Patient's Scrotal Mass?

Several components of the history and physical examination are suspicious for epididymitis. The presentation is fairly acute, but there is no history of trauma to suggest testicular torsion. The history includes sexual activity, and young women commonly carry chlamydia asymptomatically. The physical examination findings of scrotal erythema and tenderness are worrisome, because these can occur in both torsion and epididymitis. The epididymal tenderness and mobility of the testes point to a diagnosis of epididymitis.

What Is the Next Step in Diagnosing the Cause of the Illness?

A urinalysis would be helpful in the evaluation of this patient because it may show white blood cells consistent with an infection. The epididymal tenderness is suggestive of acute epididymitis, but the lack of sexual activity for 6 months makes a sexually transmitted disease somewhat less likely. Testicular ultrasonography is advised for this patient, because the acuity of the presentation and the scrotal erythema make the diagnosis of testicular torsion possible. Ultrasonography is a low-risk procedure with a potential benefit of saving a testis from infarction, given the timing of this patient's presentation. If testicular torsion is in the differential diagnosis, an immediate consultation with a urologist is warranted in the event that the patient needs emergent surgical intervention.

What Treatment Should Be Undertaken?

If ultrasonography suggests a diagnosis of testicular torsion, the treatment is immediate surgical decompression. Otherwise, the Centers for Disease Control and Prevention recommends an intramuscular dose of ceftriaxone and 10 days of oral doxycycline, or 10 days of oral ofloxacin for treatment of chlamydial or gonococcal epididymitis. Referral for urologic evaluation for possible reactive hydrocele or carcinoma would then be reserved for patients failing to improve on antibiotics.

Suggested Reading

Al Mufti R A, Ogedegbe A K, Lafferty K. The use of Doppler ultrasound in the clinical management of acute testicular pain. *Br J Urol* 1995;76:625.

Bosl G J, Motzer R J. Medical progress: testicular germ-cell cancer. *N Engl J Med* 1997;337:242.

Doherty A P, Bower M, Christmas T J. The role of tumour markers in the diagnosis and treatment of testicular germ cell cancers. *Br J Urol* 1997;79:247.

Eyre R C. Evaluation of scrotal pathology. *Up to Date Online* 1999. http://www.uptodate.com/

92
Nephrolithiasis
Byard F. Edwards

- Discussion   *582*
- Case   *585*
- Case Discussion   *586*

1. Why do renal calculi form?
2. How does the medical practitioner diagnosis nephrolithiasis?
3. How does the medical practitioner evaluate nephrolithiasis?
4. How does the medical practitioner treat nephrolithiasis?
5. When should the urologist be consulted?

Discussion
Why Do Renal Calculi Form?
High Ion Concentrations

Urinary ions of calcium (Ca), oxalate, phosphate (PO_4), uric acid (UA), cystine, magnesium, and ammonium develop urinary stones from soluble complexes that enlarge preformed crystals or create new crystals. Ion concentrations may be undersaturated (not prone to crystal formation), metastable (likely to increase current crystal size, but not create new crystals), or unstable (likely to form new crystals). Since the urine ion concentration from non–stone-forming patients frequently is metastable with regard to calcium oxalate, additional factors determine stone formation.

Nucleation

Spatial orientation of a surface's charged sites determine whether crystal lattices will form and grow on that surface. This is known as epitaxial matching. Monosodium urate, uric acid, and hydroxyapatite are good epitaxial fits for calcium oxalate crystal formation. Calcium phosphate plaques in the renal papillum (i.e., Randall plaques) provide a nucleus for calcium oxalate crystals and provide fixed platforms favoring the crystals' development into stones. Collecting duct epithelial cells also can act as a nucleus for calcium oxalate and provide an additional anchor for stone growth.

Electrostatic Attraction

Charged surfaces on crystals rapidly create aggregate masses.

Insufficient Crystal Inhibition

Pyrophosphate adsorbs to and inhibits the growth of hydroxyapatite and calcium oxalate crystals. Stone formers frequently have reduced urinary concentrations of pyrophosphate. Citrate inhibits calcium oxalate crystal nucleation, aggregation, and growth into stones by complexing with calcium and increasing the calcium oxalate concentration needed for metastability. Urinary citrate concentrations are reduced with metabolic acidosis (presumably by increased proximal tubule resorption), hypokalemia, distal renal tubular acidosis, diarrhea, and renal impairment. Magnesium inhibits stones by complexing with oxalate, thereby reducing the formation of calcium oxalate crystals. Glycopeptides and nephrocalcin, a glycoprotein, bind to the crystal's face, thereby inhibiting crystal growth, aggregation, and adherence to the epithelium. Abnormal peptides with impaired binding to the crystals may be present in stone formers.

Urine pH

Uric acid and cystine are less soluble, but calcium phosphate is more soluble in acidic solutions. A urine pH of less than 6 predisposes a patient to uric acid stones. Urea splitting organisms (*Proteus, Providencia, Klebsiella, Pseudomonas,* and enterococci) generate ammonium ion, raise the urine pH over 7, and induce a metastable state for struvite stones that consist of magnesium, ammonium, and phosphate.

How Does the Medical Practitioner Diagnose Nephrolithiasis?

Presentation

Renal stones are not symptomatic until they cause obstruction or infection. Acute urinary obstruction induces extreme, colicky pain in the affected flank or costovertebral angle that radiates to the scrotum in males or labium majorus and round ligament in females. The patient is restless and constantly seeks new positions for pain relief. The embryonic proximity of the gonads and kidneys facilitates the referred pain through shared autonomic nerve fibers. Additional symptoms arising from the autonomic nerves include visceral pain, nausea, vomiting, and ileus. Renal colic can be misdiagnosed as appendicitis, colitis, gastroenteritis, ectopic pregnancy, pancreatitis, posterior gastric or duodenal ulcer, abdominal aortic dissection, or salpingitis. As the stone migrates through the ureter and approaches the ureterovesicular junction, urinary frequency and urgency occur. Gross hematuria may not be present. Fever is absent unless an infection is present.

Examination

Fist percussion over the affected kidney evokes pain. Abdominal findings are benign except for tenderness over the calculus on deep palpation and reduced bowel sounds if ileus is present.

Imaging

An abdominal film (kidneys/ureter/bladder) is diagnostic in 80% to 90% of patients with radiopaque (calcium oxalate, calcium phosphate, cystine, and struvite) stones that are not obscured by phleboliths, gas, or feces. Intravenous pyelography (IVP), if not contraindicated by renal failure, will outline a filling defect for an incomplete stone obstruction, or show a hazy outline of the affected renal pelvis and ureter if a complete obstruction is present. The urinary filtration of the dense radiopaque solution can accelerate the stone's passage. Spiral computed tomography (CT) can be used to localize multiple stones; ultrasonography may miss stones less than 5 mm in diameter, but can be used to adequately assess for hydronephrosis and polycystic kidney disease.

How Does the Medical Practitioner Evaluate Nephrolithiasis?

Urinalysis shows hematuria in 90% of renal colic cases, and the spun sediment may show crystals. Calcium oxalate crystals are bipyramidal or dumbbell shaped; urate crystals are amorphous or cuboidal; cystine crystals are hexagonal; struvite crystals are "coffin lid" rhomboid in shape. Calcium oxalate and uric acid crystals are birefringent under polarized light. A low urine pH favors the existence of uric acid and cystine stones, while a high pH favors calcium phosphate, and struvite stones. The presence of bacteria is always clinically significant and necessitates differentiating between a staghorn calculus and stones colonized with bacteria.

Blood chemistries should include potassium, bicarbonate, creatinine, calcium, phosphorus, uric acid, and intact parathyroid hormone (PTH) level. Hypokalemia and hypobicarbinemia suggest the presence of type I or II renal tubular acidosis (RTA). Only type I has increased incidence of nephrolithiasis resulting from hypercalciuria, hypocitraturia, and alkaline pH. Elevated serum calcium and lowered phosphorus levels hint at hyperparathyroidism. Although PTH promotes renal tubular calcium resorption, the filtered calcium load is greatly increased from bone demineralization and increased gut calcium absorption. The net result is increased calciuria. Hypercalciuria also may result from increased levels of vitamin D, granulomatous diseases, malignancies, hyperdynamic bone syndromes, Cushing disease, furosemide use, and familial disorders. Up to 40% of calcium stone formers have hypercalciuria (>4 mg/kg body weight/24 h) and 25% have hyperuricosuria (>800 mg/24 h).

Urine chemistries should be assayed several weeks after the obstruction has resolved and consist of 24-hour urine collections for sodium, potassium, calcium, phosphorus, oxalate, uric acid, citrate, cystine, creatinine, magnesium, and urine volume. High concentrations of sodium, calcium, phosphorus, oxalate, cystine, and uric acid or low concentrations of potassium, citrate, magnesium, and reduced urine volume promote stone formation. Adequacy of the collection can be assessed by the measured creatinine as discussed in Chapter 62.

Patients should strain their urine through nylon, coffee filter, or other finely meshed material when experiencing renal colic and submit the collected stones for analysis. In the United States, calcium oxalate accounts for about 75%, uric acid and struvite for 10%, and cystine for 1% of the stones. However, this distribution differs in different cultures. In Israel, uric acid accounts for 75% of the stones.

How Does the Medical Practitioner Treat Nephrolithiasis?

Most stones pass spontaneously without medical intervention. Fifty percent of stones 4 to 6 mm pass spontaneously; only 10% of stones greater than 6 mm pass spontaneously.

Hospitalization is required for inadequate fluid maintenance, uncontrolled pain, acute renal failure, or pyelonephritis. Intravenous fluids are required to maintain a high urine output if nausea and vomiting prevent the patient from ingesting 2 to 3 L of fluids per day.

Analgesia can usually be achieved with intravenous or oral nonsteroidal antiinflammatory medicines. However, narcotics should be used as needed. Antibiotics are not indicated unless an infection is present.

When Should the Urologist Be Consulted?

Stones less than 5 mm that do not pass in 48 hours, or stones larger than 5 mm will likely require further intervention. The options of therapy include extracorporeal shock wave lithotripsy (ESWL), ureteroscopy, percutaneous nephrolithotomy, and open surgery. Open surgery is the least desirable option and is required in less than 1% of cases for unusually large stones. ESWL can reduce 85% of obstructing stones to passable gravel, but multiple sessions may be required for larger stones and stones lodged in the distal ureter. ESWL is the therapy of choice for stones less than 1 cm lodged in the upper ureter. Staghorn calculi require percutaneous endoscopic lithotomy with ultrasonic or electrohydraulic probes used to fragment the stone. Ureteroscopy can remove all stones lodged in the ureter, but is more invasive than ESWL.

Case

Mr. Y, a 47-year-old man with a previous medical history of pancreatitis and gout, was cycling on some country roads during a particularly hot summer day. That evening, after noticing his urine was rather dark, he drank an extra glass of water before going to bed. He awoke in the early hours of the morning to an excruciating pain in his left side that could not be quieted regardless of his position. As he paced the floor, the pain began to radiate to his scrotum. Now sweating and nauseous, he reattempted to urinate in the bathroom and begged his wife to call the doctor.

1. What predisposing conditions could have contributed to his renal colic?
2. What preventive therapy can be offered?
3. What is the risk for stone recurrence?

Case Discussion

What Predisposing Conditions Could Have Contributed to His Renal Colic?

The maintenance of dilute urine is essential to keep the urinary ions from forming crystals. Mr. Y exercised in hot weather without maintaining adequate water intake. Urine osmolarity and ion concentration increased as the kidney maximized water resorption. Once the ion concentration reached the metastable or unstable state, the crystals could aggregate through electrostatic attraction. The reduced urine volume prolonged the transit time and increased the probability that the aggregating mass could reach an obstructing size.

Mr. Y's history of pancreatitis may have resulted in chronic malabsorption and steatorrhea. Calcium normally binds oxalate in the gut, preventing its absorption. In malabsorption states, the calcium is complexed with the dietary fats and the oxalate is absorbed into the body, increasing the probability for oxalate stone formation.

Mr. Y's history of gout predisposes him to hyperuricemia and hyperuricosuria. Urinary uric acid crystals can form uric acid stones or act as a nidus for calcium oxalate and calcium phosphate stone formation. Postprandial alkaline tide may be reduced in gouty patients, causing a low urine pH in the morning and an increased risk for uric acid stone formation.

What Preventive Therapy Can Be Offered?

- Maintenance of a dilute urine. Mr. Y should be advised to drink at least 2 to 3 L of water per day or more if he has increased losses through sweat, vomiting, or diarrhea. The urine should always be pale if not clear in color.
- Potassium citrate, 20 mEq orally three times daily, increases urinary citrate levels, inhibits calcium oxalate formation, alkalinizes the urine to inhibit uric acid and cystine stone formation, inhibits calciuria, and supplements potassium for those patients on thiazide diuretics.
- Allopurinol, 300 mg orally daily, reduces uric acid synthesis and new stone formation in patients with hyperuricemia and hyperuricosuria.
- Thiazide diuretics, hydrochlorothiazide 50 mg orally twice daily, decrease calcium stone formation by increasing calcium resorption in the proximal and distal tubules.
- Acetazolamide, 250 mg orally each day at bedtime, prevents nocturnally acidic urine in gouty patients.
- Cholestyramine, 4 g orally twice daily, binds oxalate in the bowel lumen to prevent enteric hyperoxaluria.
- Dietary changes:
  - Dietary purines contribute 50% to the excreted uric acid load. A reduction in beef, poultry, and fish consumption is prudent.
  - Sodium should be limited to 2 g per day to prevent increased calciuria.
  - Ascorbic acid should be limited to less than 1,000 mg per day to prevent hyperoxaluria.
  - Calcium should not be restricted in the diet. Increased oxalate absorption in the gut occurs with calcium restriction.
  - Restriction of oxalate rich foods is of limited benefit.

What Is the Risk for Stone Recurrence?

Recurrence peaks at 2 to 3 years, with 50% having additional stones by 5 years and 60% by 10 years. For those who have recurrent stones, the interval between the stones usually shortens with each successive stone passage.

Suggested Reading

Asplin J R, Favus M J, Coe F L. Nephrolithiasis. In: *Brenner and Rector's the kidney*, 6th ed. Philadelphia: WB Saunders, 2000:1774–1810. Available at: http://home.mdconsult.com/das/book/body/0/877/957.html

Craig S. Renal calculi. In: Emedicine: EmergencyMedicine/Genitourinary. Available at: http://www.emedicine.com/emerg/topic499.htm

Kidney stones. In: Urologychannel. Available at: http://www.urologychannel.com/kidneystones/index.shtml

National Institute of Diabetes and Digestive and Kidney Diseases (NIDDK). Available at: www.niddk.nih.gov/

Subject Index

A page number followed by a "t" indicates a table and a page number followed by an "f" indicates a figure.